VIVIAN LEE

vivian.lee@medtronic.com
763-526-2005

AF779521

Pacemakers and Implantable Cardioverter Defibrillators: An Expert's Manual

PACEMAKERS AND IMPLANTABLE CARDIOVERTER DEFIBRILLATORS

AN EXPERT'S MANUAL

EDITED BY

AMIN AL-AHMAD MD, FACC, FHRS
Assistant Professor, Department of Medicine, Stanford University School of Medicine,
Associate Director of the Cardiac Arrhythmia Service, and Director of the Cardiac Electrophysiology Laboratory,
Stanford University, Stanford, California

KENNETH A. ELLENBOGEN MD, FACC, FAHA, FHRS
Kontos Professor of Medicine, Chair of the Division of Cardiology, and Director of Cardiac Electrophysiology
in the Department of Internal Medicine, Virginia Commonwealth University, Richmond, Virginia

ANDREA NATALE MD, FACC, FHRS
Executive Medical Director, Texas Cardiac Arrhythmia Institute, St. David's Medical Center, Austin, Texas;
Consulting Professor, Division of Cardiology, Stanford University, Stanford, California; Clinical Associate Professor of Medicine,
Case Western Reserve University, Cleveland, Ohio; Senior Clinical Director, EP Services, California Pacific
Medical Center, San Francisco, California; and Director of Interventional EP, Scripps Green, San Diego, California

PAUL J. WANG MD, FACC, FHRS
Professor, Department of Medicine, Stanford University School of Medicine,
and Director of the Cardiac Arrhythmia Service, Stanford University, Stanford, California

cardiotext PUBLISHING
Minneapolis, Minnesota

Cardiotext Publishing, LLC
3405 W. 44th Street
Minneapolis, MN 55410
USA

www.cardiotextpublishing.com

Any updates to this book may be found at: www.cardiotextpublishing.com/titles/detail/9780979016462

Comments, inquiries, and requests for bulk sales can be directed to the publisher at:
info@cardiotextpublishing.com.

♾ Printed on acid-free paper.

FSC Mixed Sources
Cert no. SW-COC-001271
© 1996 FSC

This book is printed on 100% FSC-certified paper from well-managed forests, where people, wildlife, and the environment benefit from the forestry practices. Forest Stewardship Council certification is globally recognized for ensuring well-managed forests.

Cover and book design by Zan Ceeley, Trio Bookworks

Library of Congress Control Number: 2010924259
ISBN-13: 978-0-9790164-6-2

Printed in Canada

15 14 13 12 11 10 1 2 3 4 5 6 7 8 9 10

To my wife, Rola, for her love and patience. To my three wonderful kids, Maya, Dana, and Mohammad, for being the sunshine of my life; and to my mother and father, for the constant support and inspiration.
Amin Al-Ahmad

To my wife, Phyllis, and my three wonderful kids, Bethany, Amy, and Michael.
Kenneth A. Ellenbogen

To my wife, Marina, my daughters, Veronica and Eleonora, and the memory of my father, Domenico.
Andrea Natale

To my loving wife, Gloria, my wonderful daughters, Margaret and Catherine, and the memory of my parents, Samuel and Lillian.
Paul J. Wang

CONTENTS

About the Contributors *xi*

Preface *xv*

PART I PACEMAKER SYSTEMS

1 Pacemaker Systems: The Basics of Pulse Generator Design and Engineering 3
HUGH THOMAS MCELDERRY AND JOHN C. EVANS

2 Pacemaker and Implantable Cardioverter Defibrillator Lead Design 19
ANDREA M. RUSSO

3 Pacemaker Timing Cycles: Ventricular Based and Atrial Based 65
FRED KUSUMOTO

4 Algorithms for Minimizing Right Ventricular Pacing 79
MICHAEL O. SWEENEY

5 Normal Pacemaker Sensing, Abnormal Sensing, and Automatic Sensing 117
CARSTEN W. ISRAEL

6 Pacemakers and Atrial Arrhythmias: Detection and Treatment 147
DAVID S. KWON AND BYRON K. LEE

7 Miscellaneous Pacing Algorithms 157
George H. Crossley and Robert Andrew Pickett

8 Automatic Threshold Measuring Algorithms 165
Marco V. Perez, Henry H. Hsia, Paul C. Zei, Mintu P. Turakhia, Paul J. Wang, and Amin Al-Ahmad

9 Sensor-Driven Pacing 179
Chu-Pak Lau, Chung-Wah Siu, and Hung Fat Tse

10 Interpretation of Device Diagnostics 203
Jordan M. Prutkin and Robert W. Rho

PART 2 IMPLANTABLE CARDIOVERTER DEFIBRILLATORS

11 Basic ICD Systems 229
Jane Chen

12 ICD Lead Design 239
Gautham Kalahasty and Kenneth A. Ellenbogen

13 Sensing in ICDs 265
Sergio L. Pinski

14 ICD Therapy—ATP 295
Karin K. M. Chia, Luigi Di Biase, Paolo Pieragnoli, Giuseppe Ricciardi, Laura Perrotta, Robert Canby, Amin Al-Ahmad, Mark S. Wathen, Andrea Natale, and Luigi Padeletti

15 ICD Therapy—Shock 309
T. Jared Bunch, Jeffrey S. Osborn, and John D. Day

16 Discrimination Algorithms and Arrhythmia Detection 317
Irina Suman Horduna and Paul Khairy

17 Pacing with an ICD System: What Are the Issues? 361
Robert F. Rea

18 Assessing Defibrillation Efficacy at ICD Implant 369
Charles D. Swerdlow and Paul J. DeGroot

PART 3 BIVENTRICULAR PACING SYSTEMS

19 Basics of Biventricular Pacing Systems: Principles and Timing Cycles 399
Ravi Ranjan and Joseph E. Marine

20 Programming to Avoid Phrenic Nerve Stimulation during Left Ventricular Pacing 415
Paul J. Wang, Amin Al-Ahmad, Henry H. Hsia, Paul C. Zei, and Mintu P. Turakhia

21 AV and VV Optimization 419
Jeffrey H. Chung, Robert J. Kim, and Kenneth M. Stein

22 Electromagnetic Interactions from Magnetic Resonance Imaging in Patients with Implantable Arrhythmia Devices 433
Saman Nazarian and Henry R. Halperin

Index *443*

ABOUT THE CONTRIBUTORS

Editors

Amin Al-Ahmad, MD, FACC, FHRS, Assistant Professor, Department of Medicine, Stanford University School of Medicine, Associate Director of the Cardiac Arrhythmia Service, and Director of the Cardiac Electrophysiology Laboratory, Stanford University, Stanford, California

Kenneth A. Ellenbogen, MD, FACC, FAHA, FHRS, Kontos Professor of Medicine, Chair of the Division of Cardiology, and Director of Cardiac Electrophysiology in the Department of Internal Medicine, Virginia Commonwealth University, Richmond, Virginia

Andrea Natale, MD, FACC, FHRS, Executive Medical Director, Texas Cardiac Arrhythmia Institute, St. David's Medical Center, Austin, Texas; Consulting Professor, Division of Cardiology, Stanford University, Stanford, California; Clinical Associate Professor of Medicine, Case Western Reserve University, Cleveland, Ohio; Senior Clinical Director, EP Services, California Pacific Medical Center, San Francisco, California; and Director of Interventional EP, Scripps Green, San Diego, California

Paul J. Wang, MD, FACC, FHRS, Professor, Department of Medicine, Stanford University School of Medicine, and Director of the Cardiac Arrhythmia Service, Stanford University, Stanford, California

Contributors

T. Jared Bunch, MD, Intermountain Heart Rhythm Specialists, Cardiovascular Department, Intermountain Medical Center, Murray, Utah

Robert Canby, md, Department of Biomedical Engineering, University of Texas, Austin, Texas

Jane Chen, md, fhrs, facc, Associate Professor of Medicine, Director, Electrophysiology Fellowship Program, Washington University School of Medicine, St. Louis, Missouri

Karin K. M. Chia, mbbs, fracp, Cardiac Arrythmia Service, Department of Medicine, Cardiovascular Medicine, Stanford University, California

Jeffrey H. Chung, md, Fellow, Maurice R. & Corinne P. Greenberg Division of Cardiology, Department of Medicine, Weill Medical College of Cornell University, New York, New York

George H. Crossley, md, fhrs, facc, Clinical Professor of Medicine, St. Thomas Research Institute and the University of Tennessee College of Medicine, Nashville, Tennessee

John D. Day, md, Intermountain Heart Rhythm Specialists, Cardiovascular Department, Intermountain Medical Center, Murray, Utah

Paul J. DeGroot, ms, Medtronic, Inc., Minneapolis, Minnesota

Luigi Di Biase, md, Texas Cardiac Arrhythmia Institute, St. David's Medical Center, Austin, Texas; Department of Cardiology, University of Foggia, Foggia, Italy; Department of Biomedical Engineering, University of Texas, Austin, Texas

John C. Evans, md, Fellow, Clinical Cardiac Electrophysiology, Stanford University School of Medicine, Stanford, California

Henry R. Halperin, md, ma, Division of Cardiology/Cardiac Arrhythmia, Johns Hopkins University, Baltimore, Maryland

Irina Suman Horduna, md, ccds, Electrophysiology Fellow, Electrophysiology Service, Montreal Heart Institute, University of Montreal, Canada

Henry H. Hsia, md, facc, Associate Professor of Medicine, Cardiac Electrophysiology and Arrhythmia Service, Stanford University Medical Center, Stanford, California

Carsten W. Israel, md, Assistant Professor of Medicine and Cardiology, J. W. Goethe University, Frankfurt, Germany; Head of the Department of Cardiology, Evangelical Hospital, Bielefeld, Germany

Gautham Kalahasty, md, Assistant Professor of Medicine, Division of Cardiology, Department of Internal Medicine, Virginia Commonwealth University, Richmond, Virginia

Paul Khairy, md, PhD, Associate Professor of Medicine, Canada Research Chair in Electrophysiology and Adult Congenital Heart Disease, and Director of the Adult Congenital Heart Center, Montreal Heart Institute, University of Montreal, Canada

Robert J. Kim, MD, FACC, Assistant Professor of Medicine, Maurice R. & Corinne P. Greenberg Division of Cardiology, Department of Medicine, Weill Medical College of Cornell University, New York, New York

Fred Kusumoto, MD, Associate Professor of Medicine, Mayo School of Medicine, Director of Electrophysiology and Pacing, Division of Cardiovascular Diseases, Department of Medicine, Mayo Clinic Florida, Jacksonville, Florida

David S. Kwon, MD, PhD, Electrophysiology Fellow, Cardiac Electrophysiology and Arrhythmia Service, Division of Cardiology, University of California, San Francisco, California

Chu-Pak Lau, MD, FRCP, FRACP, Honorary Clinical Professor, Division of Cardiology, Department of Medicine, University of Hong Kong, Queen Mary Hospital, Hong Kong, China

Byron K. Lee, MD, Assistant Professor of Medicine, Cardiac Electrophysiology and Arrhythmia Service, Division of Cardiology, University of California, San Francisco, California

Joseph E. Marine, MD, Associate Professor of Medicine, Johns Hopkins University School of Medicine; Director of Electrophysiology, Johns Hopkins Bayview Medical Center; Staff Electrophysiologist, Johns Hopkins Hospital, Baltimore, Maryland

Hugh Thomas McElderry, MD, Division of Cardiovascular Diseases, University of Alabama, Birmingham, Alabama

Saman Nazarian, MD, Division of Cardiology/Cardiac Arrhythmia, Johns Hopkins University, Baltimore, Maryland

Jeffrey S. Osborn MD, Intermountain Heart Rhythm Specialists, Cardiovascular Department, Intermountain Medical Center, Murray, Utah

Luigi Padeletti, MD, Department of Heart and Vessels, University of Florence, Florence, Italy

Marco V. Perez, MD, Fellow, Cardiac Electrophysiology, Division of Cardiovascular Medicine, Stanford University, Stanford, California

Laura Perrotta, MD, Department of Heart and Vessels, University of Florence, Florence, Italy

Robert Andrew Pickett, MD, St. Thomas Research Institute, Nashville, Tennessee

Paolo Pieragnoli, MD, Department of Heart and Vessels, University of Florence, Florence, Italy

Sergio L. Pinski, MD, Head, Section of Cardiac Pacing and Electrophysiology, Cleveland Clinic Florida, Weston, Florida

Jordan M. Prutkin, MD, MHS, Acting Assistant Professor, Division of Cardiology, University of Washington, Seattle, Washington

Ravi Ranjan, MD, PhD, Fellow, Clinical Electrophysiology, Division of Cardiology, Johns Hopkins University School of Medicine, Baltimore, Maryland

Robert F. Rea, MD, Associate Professor of Medicine; Consultant, Cardiovascular Diseases; Director, Implantable Cardiac Electrical Device Service; Mayo Clinic, Rochester, Minnesota

Robert W. Rho, MD, Associate Professor of Medicine, Division of Cardiology, University of Washington, Seattle, Washington

Giuseppe Ricciardi, MD, Department of Heart and Vessels, University of Florence, Florence, Italy

Andrea M. Russo, MD, FACC, FHRS, Professor of Medicine, UMDNJ/Robert Wood Johnson Medical School; Director, Cardiac Electrophysiology; Director, Cardiac Ablation and Arrhythmia Services; Cooper University Hospital, Camden, New Jersey

Chung-Wah Siu, MBBS, Cardiology Division, University Department of Medicine, University of Hong Kong, Queen Mary Hospital, Hong Kong, China

Kenneth M. Stein, MD, FACC, Senior Vice President and Associate Chief Medical Officer, Cardiac Rhythm Management Group, Boston Scientific Corporation, Natick, Massachusetts

Michael O. Sweeney, MD, Director, Cardiac Pacing and Implantable Device Therapies, Brigham and Women's Hospital; Associate Professor of Medicine, Harvard Medical School, Boston, Massachusetts

Charles D. Swerdlow, MD, Division of Cardiology, Department of Medicine, Cedars-Sinai Medical Center, and the David Geffen School of Medicine, UCLA, Los Angeles, California

Hung Fat Tse, MD, PhD, FRCP, FHKCP, Specialist in Cardiology, William M. W. Mong Professor in Cardiology, Academic Chief, Cardiology Division, University Department of Medicine, University of Hong Kong, Queen Mary Hospital, Hong Kong, China

Mintu P. Turakhia, MD, MAS, Instructor of Medicine, Stanford University, Stanford, California; Director, Cardiac Electrophysiology, Palo Alto Veterans Affairs Health Care System, Palo Alto, California

Mark S. Wathen, MD, Heart and Vascular Center, Cookeville Regional Medical Center, Cookville, Tennessee

Paul C. Zei, MD, Clinical Assistant Professor, Stanford University School of Medicine, Stanford, California

PREFACE

THE FIELD OF CARDIAC ARRHYTHMIAS has evolved greatly over the past twenty years as implantable devices have become increasingly utilized to help manage patients with cardiac arrhythmias. As devices have become more complex—with multiple programmable features and many different algorithms—the potential for interactions and confusing behavior is more common than ever. Whether troubleshooting a pacemaker tracing or assessing the cause of an inappropriate shock, a clear understanding of device function is crucial. Knowledge of device function and device algorithms is a must for clinicians implanting and managing these devices.

The goal of *Pacemakers and Implantable Cardioverter Defibrillators: An Expert's Manual* is to provide a reference text written by experts in the field that provides a detailed understanding of the different algorithms and the interactions that can occur across different device manufacturers.

This book is intended to serve as an aid to practicing electrophysiologists, fellows in training, as well as allied professionals, such as nurses and cardiovascular technicians, for both day-to-day use and to use as a study guide for certification examinations.

Pacemakers and Implantable Cardioverter Defibrillators is divided into three sections: The first section covers pacing and includes a range of topics from the basic understanding of the pulse generator to timing cycles and sensor driven pacing. The reader will gain insight that will not only be an in-depth look at pacing, but will also serve as a foundation for the other sections of the book. The second section on the implantable cardioverter defibrillator offers chapters that not only discuss arrhythmia detection and device classification, but also device testing and therapy. The third section builds on the prior sections to cover the topics of biventricular pacing and interactions with implantable devices, as with MRI.

We believe that *Pacemakers and Implantable Cardioverter Defibrillators* is a comprehensive and detailed examination of device algorithms and programming options, and a valuable companion to any clinician interacting with patients with implantable devices. We are sincerely hopeful that the reader finds this book to be helpful for everyday clinical practice.

—The Editors

PART I
PACEMAKER SYSTEMS

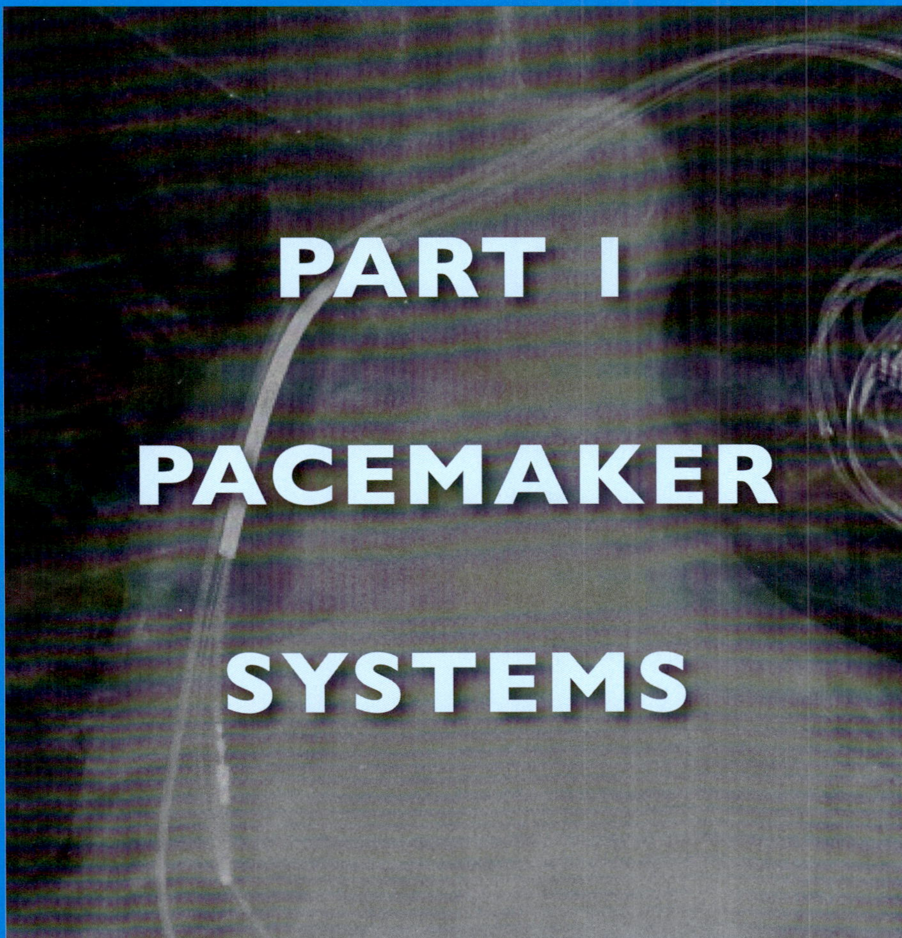

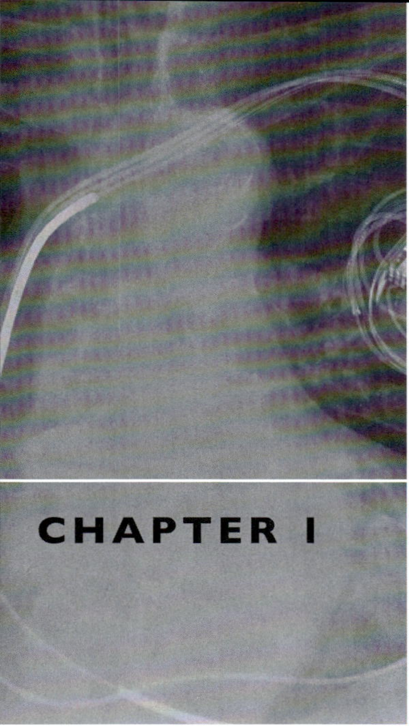

Pacemaker Systems

The Basics of Pulse Generator Design and Engineering

CHAPTER 1

Hugh Thomas McElderry and John C. Evans

Pacemaker Pulse Generator

In its most simplified representation, the artificial pacemaker consists of the two major components: a pulse generator and the leads connecting the generator to the heart. The major functions of the pacemaker pulse generator are to power the device and to generate the impulses that go from the leads to the heart in accordance with specified programming. The major components of the pulse generator, responsible for these functions, are the battery and the small computer controlling the output of the device, a hybrid circuit consisting of a microprocessor, resistors, and many other components. The battery and hybrid circuit are packaged together in a casing made of titanium with a translucent epoxy header to allow for connection to leads (see Fig 1.1). Because leads are discussed elsewhere, this chapter focuses on the pulse generator, specifically its components and implications for the clinical care of patients with implanted cardiac pacemakers.

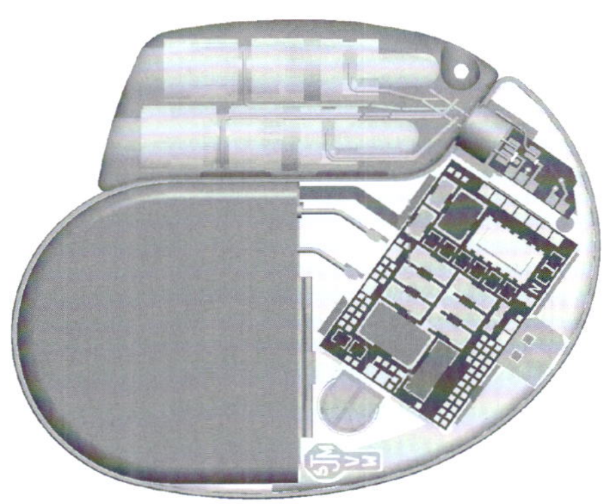

Fig 1.1 Structure of a pacemaker pulse generator. Notice the major components include the battery, the hybrid circuit, and the epoxy header for attaching leads. The battery, 25% of the total volume of the device, is in a hermetically sealed titanium can with the hybrid circuit. (Courtesy of St. Jude Medical. Used with permission.)

Pacemakers and Implantable Cardioverter Defibrillators: An Expert's Manual. © 2010 Amin Al-Ahmad, Kenneth A. Ellenbogen, Andrea Natale, and Paul J. Wang, eds. Cardiotext Publishing, ISBN: 978-0-9790164-6-2.

Pacemaker Hardware

The first pacemakers consisted of approximately 10 discrete components in addition to the battery.[1] These pulse generators were asynchronous, nonprogrammable single chamber devices. Although, the pacemakers of today serve the same primary role, the components to accomplish this goal have gone through several evolutionary changes. The hybrid circuit houses the integrated circuits and components needed for pacemaker functions. The integrated circuits contain data storage and memory elements, telemetry components, sensors, analog amplifiers, analog filters, analog-to-digital converters, and the hardware responsible for delivering the pacing pulse. Every manufacturer and model pulse generator is slightly different, but they all have some basic components in addition to the microprocessor that is responsible for the programming of the pacemaker.

Sensing intrinsic activity

The analog signal of the intrinsic cardiac electrical activity needs to be converted into a digital signal for processing. Before this is accomplished the intrinsic signal is amplified and filtered. It is then converted to a digital signal and processed. Intrinsic signals can have very small amplitudes and thus require amplification. Some pacemakers have the option of setting a sensitivity as low as 0.1 mV. This requires clean amplification as well as significant filtering in order to reliably sense signals at 0.1 mV without oversensing noise. The ideal filter would allow P and R waves to be sensed unobstructed, but would filter out all other signals such as myopotentials, EMI, other noncardiac signals, as well as undesirable cardiac signals such as T waves and far-field R waves. Band pass filters are implemented, which allow only the frequencies within a certain range to be seen. Lower frequency signals such as respiration artifact and higher frequency signals such as myopotentials are filtered out. The signal is then passed through an analog-to-digital converter, which measures the intrinsic signal as a series of discrete values. The microprocessor then analyzes these signals and acts on them based on the defined programming. Feedthrough filters also play an important role in decreasing the effect of electromagnetic interference in pacing systems.

Random-Access Memory (RAM) and Read-Only Memory (ROM)

The code or series of instructions the microprocessor runs is called firmware. This code can either be stored in random-access memory (RAM), read-only memory (ROM), or a combination of both. RAM is simply an array of transistors in a device. It is both readable as well as writeable by the microprocessor and thus has the advantage that it can be changed and used for short-term storage. Despite the technology used in personal computers that implement a quantity of RAM in the order of magnitude of gigabytes, billions of bytes of data, current pacemakers have a quantity of RAM in the order of magnitude of kilobytes, just thousands of bytes of data. As RAM is simply an array of transistors, each transistor requires a steady amount of current to reliably store data. It is desirable to minimize this current drain.

The quantity of RAM in a pacemaker is limited by a number of factors. The RAM used in pacemakers has an extremely low leakage current, which allows for extended device longevity. There are also physical size constraints within the pulse generator that limit the amount of RAM that can be used. Newer pacemakers are trending to collect an increasing amount of diagnostics such as rate histograms, lifetime trends, and stored electrograms. This data is stored in RAM. The relatively slow telemetry speeds of inductive pacemakers can also limit the amount of RAM, as clinicians may not be willing to wait long periods of time to download all of the data in a large quantity of RAM.

Not only is the RAM used for storing diagnostic data, the code itself is often stored on RAM. The execution of the code also occurs from the RAM space, and is used for housing variables, function call trees, and general processor operation. Even if the code is stored in the read-only memory, ROM, the device will still contain some RAM for code execution and data storage.

ROM has been in used in some pacemakers and it provides the advantage as well as the disadvantage of being able to permanently store the code into ROM. The advantage of ROM code is that it is permanent, cannot be changed, and is more robust. This provides a higher level of stability and reliability than code stored in RAM.

Sometimes the architecture of the system is designed for the use of ROM code as well as allowing the code to be upgraded if needed. Through architectural design some ROM code links to data on a RAM-based system, thus allowing for the stability of the permanent storage of the code while still allowing some sections of the code to be upgraded. If a software glitch that compromises the patient's safety is discovered, it is desirable to correct the software glitch by upgrading the code rather than explanting and replacing the system.

Another advantage of ROM is that it is not susceptible to the rate of data errors that are common in RAM failures. All current pacemakers implement RAM, and thus they all are susceptible to RAM failures. A RAM failure is also sometimes known as a bit flip whereby the data stored in a transistor, either a 0 or 1, is actually represented by the incorrect value. Technology is now available to self-correct the majority of these errors. This level of error correction does not protect against something known as a hard error. This is when a value of a bit in RAM, either 0 or 1, cannot be changed. A hard error is rare in comparison to the frequency of bit flips.

Telemetry control

Implantable medical devices such as pacemakers and defibrillators require periodic follow-up to ensure the system is working properly. Both at routine follow-up and when an issue is suspected, telemetry allows for communication between the device and a programmer. The system is checked to ensure adequate battery voltage, lead integrity, pacing threshold, and other parameters.

Inductive telemetry

Until recently, all available pacemakers in the United States communicated with programmers by way of inductive or near-field telemetry. This technology is based on inductive coupling between two closely placed coils using the mutual inductance between these coils. The first coil and circuitry is sealed in the pacemaker "can" while the second coil is located in the "wand" which connects to the programmer.

The wand allows communication in real time to and from the pacemaker and the programmer. Intracardiac electrograms, measured battery voltage, lead impedance, and current consumption in the selected pacing programs are some of the parameters that can be displayed and documented via the programmer. The wand is also used to program features such as pacing mode and parameters.

Wireless communication

In addition to inductive telemetry, many pacemakers also have radiofrequency (RF) telemetry technology, which makes telemetry from a base station possible. Although we are unaware of malicious attacks to implantable defibrillators that use RF, it has been shown that security and privacy vulnerabilities exist.

Home monitoring

Transtelephonic monitoring (TTM) of pacemakers, which has been performed for decades,[2] allows the early identification of pacing system failure or battery depletion. This modality was developed to monitor the function of pacing systems at a time when pulse generator and lead longevities were much less predictable.

The typical TTM system includes wristband electrodes, a magnet, and a device to transmit the recorded strip over a regular telephone line. Each transmission is initiated with a rhythm strip (electrocardiographic lead I), after which the patient is instructed to place the magnet in the skin overlying the pacemaker in order to record the "magnet rate." The rhythm strips transmitted allow the analysis of the atrial and ventricular rhythm and rate, appropriateness of sensing and capture, and the magnet rate which can indicate the proximity to elective replacement time. Some devices can perform automatic threshold tests with magnet placement.

Future hardware

Advances in technology have increased the desired requirements of pacemakers. As the quantity of diagnostic data stored in the pacemaker increases, the time it takes to telemeter this data to a programmer increases as well. Faster telemetry speeds to decrease this telemetry time and improve efficiency in the clinical setting are desired. Faster telemetry speeds are possible at a cost of increased energy demands on the device. RF telemetry offers increased speed as well as freedom to perform daily remote monitoring checks without requiring the patient to place a wand over the pacemaker utilizing inductive telemetry. RF is possible again, but at the cost of increased energy. Patient notifiers, either vibratory or audible, may also be desirable features but they increase current consumption. All current and future capabilities must function within these energy limitations imposed by the next major part of the pulse generator, the battery.

Battery

The battery in a pacemaker accounts for the majority of the size and weight of the device. Battery characteristics determine the functional life of a pacemaker, as well as the capability of certain pacemaker functions. Therefore, significant effort is put into improving and optimizing battery technology.

The ideal pacemaker battery would be small and lightweight, yet contain a large amount of energy. It would have a low self-discharge rate to promote longevity. The ideal battery would not generate any gaseous byproducts in the reaction, converting chemical to electrical energy, allowing it to be hermetically sealed within the pulse generator to ensure moisture does not invade the pacemaker and damage the device. The ideal battery would also have predictable and reliable performance to ensure that the clinician could accurately determine the elective replacement time.

The volume and the mass of the battery represent a significant portion of the total pulse generator. In the case of the pacemaker seen in Fig 1.1, the battery is 2.8 cc and is 25% of the total volume of the pulse generator. Advances in technology have allowed for more efficient digital circuitry, which has enabled a smaller battery to be utilized. A smaller battery in turn translates into a smaller pulse generator with similar longevity to previous generations.

Battery chemistry

The battery produces energy that is generated by its chemical components. Lithium has the highest specific energy and thus is often used in batteries where size is important. In 1972 the first lithium-based pacemaker battery was implanted.[3] Since the late 1970s pacemakers have almost exclusively used lithium-based batteries.[1] Over the years a number of different lithium-based chemistries have been used, but today virtually all pacemakers use lithium iodine chemistry. The lithium iodine battery has many of the characteristics of the ideal pacemaker battery, which have lead to its adoption over the last three decades.

A number of different battery chemistries were used prior to lithium batteries. The most popular battery in first-generation pacemakers was the zinc mercuric oxide battery. Over three million mercury cells were implanted between 1960 and 1976.[4] Each cell has a voltage of 1.35 and thus five or six batteries were often placed in series to provide the required voltage for pacing. These cells also produced hydrogen gas, which prevented the pacemaker from being hermetically sealed.[5] Because they could not be hermetically sealed, body fluids could leak into the device resulting in sudden failure.[6] Another characteristic rendering the zinc mercuric oxide battery less than optimal is the limited longevity caused by a high rate of self-discharge at body temperature.

Nickel cadmium battery cells were also used in the first generations of devices. These batteries needed to be recharged every few weeks.[6] To recharge the battery a wand containing a large coil was placed over the device. As an electric current passes through a coil of wire it creates an electromagnetic field. This electromagnetic field induces a current in a similar coil of wire located in the pacemaker. This induced current was used to charge the nickel cadmium batteries.

Nuclear-powered pacemakers have been used as well. The first nuclear-powered pacemaker was implanted in 1970.[7] Plutonium-238 was the isotope utilized, with a half-life of 89 years. The radioactive decay created heat that was then converted into electricity. In the era of the zinc mercury batteries that seldom lasted more than 2 years,[8] the nuclear-powered pacemaker had a longevity that was limited only by the amount of radioactive plutonium contained in the pacemaker. These pacemakers were not as common as the mercury-powered batteries, and in the 1970s fewer than 3000 nuclear-powered pacemakers had been implanted worldwide.[7]

The common lithium iodine battery has a high internal resistance that increases as the cell is discharged.[9] This can limit the speed at which the battery can supply electrons to the circuit and thus limit the instantaneous current. Pacemakers have traditionally operated in the microampere range, and thus this characteristic of the lithium iodine battery has not been a significant limitation. Although features such as RF telemetry and patient notifiers are used infrequently, they do require a significantly higher amount of current while they are being operated and would require different battery chemistry than the common lithium iodine systems. ICDs batteries commonly have a lithium silver vanadium oxide (SVO) chemistry and have the ability to deliver current on the ampere range.

Wilson Greatbatch has designed a QMR battery, which is a mid-rate battery offering a current supply in the mA range between that of current pacemaker and ICD battery chemistries.[9] Lithium carbon monofluoride (CFx) is a battery chemistry that offers similar characteristics of the lithium iodine cells such as the relatively flat voltage discharge curve, and high energy density. It also has a low internal resistance and has been used in some drug-infusion pumps, neurostimulators, and pacemakers. An additional benefit of the CFx technology is that the case of the battery can be made of titanium, which not only provides a weight savings over stainless steel, but it is more MRI compatible.

Battery longevity

Given that the calculation of the elective replacement time is primarily based on pacemaker battery, it is important for the battery voltage to slowly decay as the battery nears depletion. However, for energy supply to the electronics, it is desired for the battery voltage to remain constant. The lithium iodine battery provides the combination of both a steady voltage during the life of the battery as well as predictable voltage decay near the end of the life of battery. Figure 1.2 displays the voltage decay curve of a typical lithium iodine battery. The battery voltage is approximately 2.78 V at beginning of life. The voltage remains relatively constant over the life of the battery until its precipitous decline. Approximately 90% of the stored energy in the lithium iodide battery has been depleted once the battery voltage reaches 2.65 V. A battery voltage of 2.55 V relates to approximately 95% energy consumption. The predictable decay allows the physician to reliably anticipate end of battery life early enough for elective device

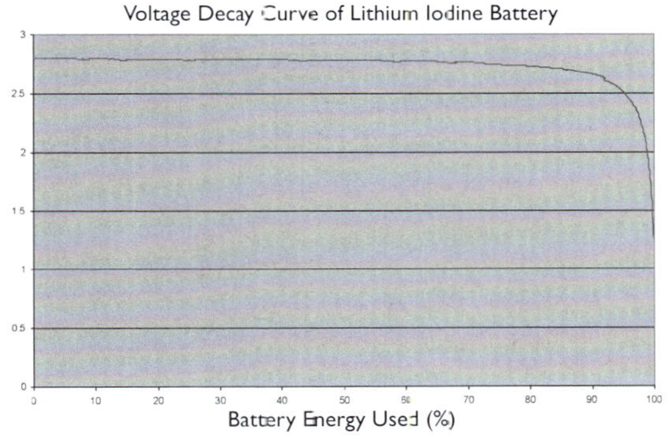

Fig 1.2 Voltage decay curve of lithium iodine battery. Notice the relatively constant voltage until nearly 90% of the battery energy is expired.

replacement. In some low-voltage pulse generators the microprocessor is able to measure the amount of energy consumed over time. It may then use these values to more accurately predict the time of elective replacement based on the energy capacity in the battery and the measured energy consumption. Each specific battery, as well as pacemaker, may have different voltage indicators for the elective replacement indicator (ERI) as well as end of life (EOL). See Fig 1.2.

The longevity of the pacemaker battery is dictated by the combination of the battery size and the current drain from the energy used by the pacemaker. It is commonly known that the more energy delivered to the heart in the form of pacing pulses, the higher the current drain on the battery and accordingly the pacemaker will have a decreased longevity. The delivery of the pacing pulses to the myocardium is not 100% efficient and thus some energy is used internally to the pacemaker in the delivery of the pacing pulses. Therefore, the current drain from the battery is made up of both the amount of energy consumed to deliver the pacing pulses to the myocardium and the quiescent current, also called the housekeeping current. The quiescent current is the amount of energy required to keep the pacemaker functioning, sensing, and storing diagnostics even if all the pacing pulses are inhibited.

First-generation pacemakers did not have telemetry, programmability, diagnostics, or other advanced features that increase the quiescent current. As noted previously, today's pacemakers have inductive and radiofrequency (RF) telemetry, rate responsive sensors, patient notifiers, high levels of automaticity and extensive amounts of memory for the collection of diagnostics and stored electrograms, and advanced algorithms such as automatic capture verification. Despite all of these additional features, today's pacemakers use smaller batteries and last longer than the first generation of pacemakers.

Battery drain

The current drain from a battery is not constant and varies throughout the cardiac cycle. A higher demand is placed on the battery during the pacing pulse delivery. For simplicity the current drain is calculated as the average current drain. This includes the quiescent current as well as the current needed to deliver the pacing pulses. The quiescent current is the sum of all the current drain from powering the electronics within the pacemaker not including the energy delivered to the myocardium. For nominal settings in most pacemakers this value is on the order of 10 to 20 microamps (μA). Similarly, the energy stored in a battery is measured in amp hours (Ah). Today's pacemaker batteries have a capacity of approximately 0.5 to 2 Ah.[10]

New developments in pacemaker and lead technology have decreased pacing capture thresholds and have made the pacemaker internal circuitry more efficient. As a result, the amount of energy required to safely maintain consistent capture of the myocardium has decreased significantly. For example, pacing in the ventricle only (VVI), at a rate of 60 bpm at 2.5 V and 0.4 ms into 500-Ω lead with 100% pacing consumes < 2 μA of current. With a nominal current drain of about 10 μA, only 2 μA is due to the pacing and the other 8 μA are from the quiescent current. Therefore, in this example, the current from the pacing pulse is responsible for 20% of the current drain on the battery. As such, if no pacing stimuli were delivered the battery would last approximately 25% longer. Although the exact numbers change for each pacemaker manufacturer, model, lead interface, and patient, the concepts remain the same. The energy output in terms of voltage and number of pacing pulses delivered is inversely related to the longevity of the pacemaker.

Many factors affect the number of pacing pulses delivered. Given a specific set of programmed parameters, the percent pacing will differ based on different patient conditions. Patients with complete heart block can be expected to pace 100% in the ventricle, whereas those patients with other indications may only pace a small percentage of the time. However, given a specific condition there is a number of programming parameters that can affect the number of delivered pacing pulses which directly affect longevity.

The programmed base rate can affect the number of pacing pulses. For example, while considering only VVI devices for simplicity, increasing the base rate from 50 bpm by 20% to 60 bpm will increase the number of pacing pulses delivered by 10% and increase the current drain from pacing pulses by 10%. At nominal values this is approximately 2 μA. Therefore, this increase in rate will only increase the current drain by 0.2 μA. This will have a very minimal impact on longevity due to the significantly higher quiescent current. Figure 1.3 shows the relationship between total current changes and the programmed base rate for two separate voltage outputs. The energy required by each pacing pulse will impact the total energy consumption. For example, by doubling the stimulation rate, the number of pacing pulses will be doubled, which in turn will double the pacing current drain caused by pacing. The total pacing current is composed of both pacing current drain and quiescent current drain. Therefore, the proportion of quiescent current drain to pacing current drain can vary differently with different parameters. The effect can be more significant when higher-energy pacing pulses are required. As shown in Fig 1.3, these factors negatively affect longevity and can compound to increase their effects. If the percent pacing is < 100%, then this mild increase in total current consumption will be even less significant. Changes in base rate will not affect battery longevity as long as the patient's intrinsic rate is above the programmed base rate because there will be no change in the number of pacing pulses.

Current Drain at Various Rates, VVI, 500Ω, .4ms

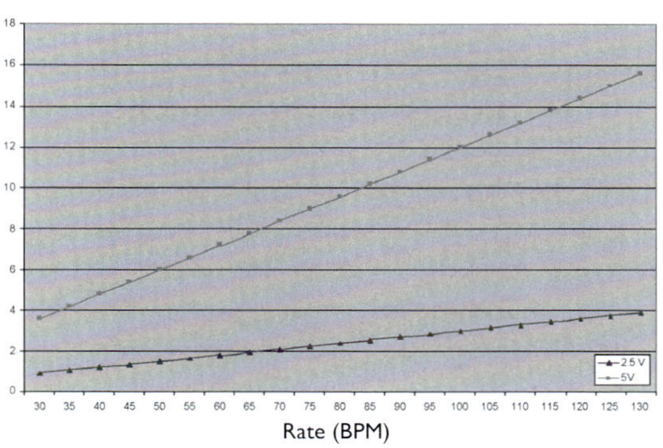

Fig 1.3 Current consumption vs. pacing rate. Current drain due to pacing increases linearly with increased pacing rates in the setting of 100% pacing, and that the energy demands are greater with higher output. Notice that a doubling of the pulse amplitude from 2.5 to 5 V causes approximately four times the current drain.

Another common programmed parameter that significantly affects the percent pacing in dual chamber devices is the AV delay. The shorter the programmed AV delay the more likely the device is to pace. With the emergence of data that demonstrates unnecessary right ventricular pacing leads to left ventricular dysfunction, devices should be programmed to avoid unnecessary right ventricular pacing.[11] A high percentage of ventricular pacing is still desirable for cardiac resynchronization therapy (CRT) devices in which the AV delay is programmed to ensure ventricular pacing.

The pacing rate and AV delay are the two main factors that influence the number of paced beats. However, there is a number of advanced algorithms that either directly or indirectly modify the rate and AV delay and therefore can have a significant impact on the percent pacing and quantity of paced beats.

Several manufacturers have an atrial overdrive algorithm with the intent of decreasing atrial arrhythmias in some patients.[12,13] These algorithms use the same fundamental principle of pacing faster than the intrinsic atrial rate although there are slight differences among them. These algorithms will typically have atrial pacing percentages > 90%.[14] For patients with paced AV delays programmed shorter than the intrinsic conduction interval, ventricular pacing will also be increased. Although there is some debate about the clinical benefit of these algorithms and the potential negative impact of increasing right ventricular pacing, there is no debate that these algorithms increase the amount of pacing and thus decrease the longevity of the pulse generator.[15]

In a normal heart, the intrinsic rate will increase with exercise or stress. Many patients who meet criteria for pacemaker implantation are chronotropically incompetent such that their heart rate does not increase appropriately with exercise. For these patients, pacemakers have features that attempt to mimic the normal heart rate acceleration. These sensors measure a variety of parameters in an attempt to accurately gauge exercise or stress and then increase the heart rate appropriately. A number of different sensors are available, but the most common is the activity sensor which usually contains an accelerometer to measure movement. Other sensors measure body temperature, QT intervals, minute ventilation, and/or myocardial contractility. All of these sensors use some energy to operate which can cause either a negligible or substantial current drain based on the technology used. However, when pacemakers are programmed to actively increase the patient's rate during activity, the sensor will determine how significantly to accelerate the patient's rate as well as the duration of this temporary change in pacing rate. The amount of current drain can be more pronounced with these algorithms if they result in an increase in pacing of more than one chamber.

During atrial fibrillation (AF), it may be desired to increase the ventricular pacing rate compared to sinus rhythm. Due to the lack of atrial contraction during AF, raising the ventricular pacing rate can help increase cardiac output. For patients with a CRT device, several algorithms have been designed to ensure biventricular pacing during atrial fibrillation. The automatic mode switching feature may temporarily increase the base rate in the ventricle while the patient is mode switched due to AF or other rapid atrial arrhythmias. Other ventricular rate-smoothing algorithms work by increasing and decreasing the ventricular programmed rate based on the running average of the intrinsic heart rate. Thus, as the intrinsic rate increases the programmed rate will follow it. This offers the benefit of increased CRT in heart failure devices as well as a benefit of less heart rate variability.[16] These algorithms can help clinically by increasing the rate when needed especially in nontracking modes.

A number of common algorithms can temporarily decrease the rate. The two most common are rest rate and hysteresis. To mimic the heart's natural slowing during sleep or rest, most pacemakers have a sleep or rest rate. When these algorithms are enabled, they will temporarily decrease the rate based on either the time of day or automatically based on data from the sensor showing the patient is sedentary. Hysteresis may be used to permit the atrial or ventricular escape interval to be longer than the pacing interval. As a result, the intrinsic heart rate must decrease to a lower value than the pacing rate in order for pacing to commence.

Amplitude of pacing pulses

The amount of energy required to depolarize the myocardium varies from patient to patient as well as over time. The threshold in a patient can change due to maturation of the lead/tissue interface, disease conditions, pharmacological influences, the time of day, as well as other factors.[17–19] The standard of care has been to provide a 2:1 or 3:1 safety margin in terms of energy, which may be achieved with 2:1 safety margin with respect to voltage or a 3:1 safety margin with respect to pulse width. For example, a capture threshold of 1V at 0.4 ms may be programmed to 2 V at 0.4 ms. It is expected that the higher the programmed voltage the more energy is being delivered to the myocardium and the faster the battery will drain. However, there is no direct correlation between the energy consumed from the battery and the energy delivered to the myocardium. Due to inefficiencies in the pacemaker circuitry, these values differ.

The energy delivered to the patient can be determined from the programmed voltage (V), the programmed pulse width, and the lead impedance (R). The formula used to calculate this value is:

$$E = \frac{V_{programmed} V_{programmed} \text{ Pulse Width}}{R}$$

To calculate the amount of energy consumed from the battery a similar formula can be used:

$$E = \frac{V_{supply} V_{programmed} \text{ Pulse Width}}{R}$$

Both of these formulas make some assumptions that lead to a slight difference between the true and calculated values. For example, the internal capacitance in the pacing system is not being taken into account, which causes the amount of energy delivered to the patient to be slightly less than the calculated values. Most pacemakers operate with a working battery voltage of 2.5 to 2.8 V. Thus, the circuits normally rely on a 2.5-V power supply, and thus, the pacing voltage supplies are typically multiples of 2.5 V. Commonly, pacemakers have power supplies of 2.5 V, 5 V, and 7.5 V.[19] The power supply used is dependent on the programmed pacing voltage. For pacing voltages of 2.5 V and below, the 2.5-V power supply is used. For programmed voltages of 2.75 to 5 V, the 5-V supply is used, and for pacing voltages of 5.5 to 7.5 V the 7.5-V, power supply is used.

The efficiency of the pacing circuitry is dependent on the programmed pacing voltage as well as voltage of the needed power supply within the pacemaker. Figure 1.4 shows the energy delivered to the patient's heart as well as the energy consumed from the pacemaker battery for a lead impedance of 500 Ω and a pulse duration of 0.4 ms. When the programmed voltage is increased from 2.5 to 2.75 V, the energy delivered to the patient increases from 5 to 6.1 μJ. However, the energy consumed from the battery increases from 5 to 11 μJ. This is due to the relatively low efficiency of pacing at a voltage that requires the use of the voltage doubler, the 5-V power supply. The same phenomenon can be seen when pacing more than 5 V when the voltage tripler is needed to create the 7.5-V power supply. Increasing the pacing voltage will increase the energy consumed from the battery. However, there is no direct correlation between pacing voltage and battery consumption. Both energy delivered and programmed voltage are important in determining pacemaker longevity.

The effect of the voltage doubler can vary at different pulse widths. In Fig 1.4, the pacemaker current consumption is compared to the programmed pulse amplitude. As seen in Fig 1.5, the effects of the voltage doubler and tripler significantly impact the current drain of the pacemaker. The pulse amplitude can either be manually or automatically programmed. Automatic algorithms include Capture Management by Medtronic, AutoCapture by St. Jude Medical, and Automatic Capture by Boston Scientific. Some of these algorithms have beat-by-beat capture verification, and others perform a capture threshold test periodically. The algorithms can

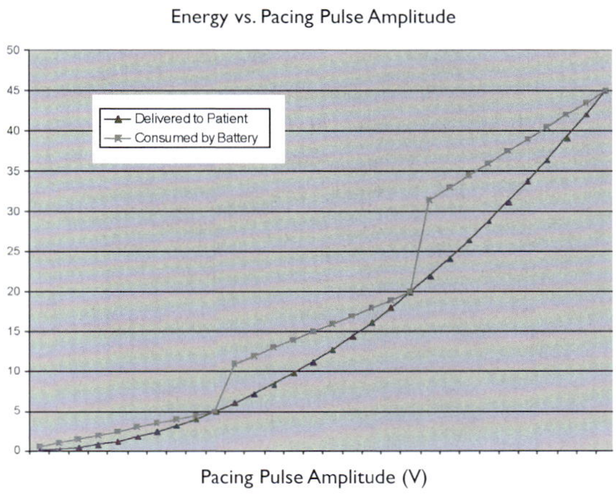

Fig 1.4 Energy consumption vs. pacing pulse amplitude. Due to the using a 2.78-V battery, a voltage doubler or tripler must be used to deliver higher pulse amplitudes. The steps in the energy consumption curve demonstrate that despite incremental increases in energy delivery to patient with higher pulse amplitudes, there is inefficiency when utilizing the voltage doubler and tripler.

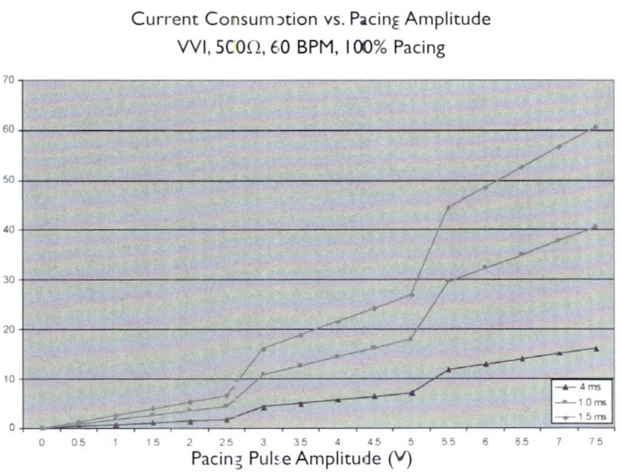

Fig 1.5 Current consumption vs. pacing amplitude for several pulse durations. Note the significant increase in current drain by increasing pulse amplitudes > 2.5 V and > 5 V across pulse durations. The graph demonstrates that despite jumps in energy consumption that at these voltages, the incremental increase in energy consumption by increasing pulse duration remains proportional.

then adjust the programmed pacing amplitude in an attempt to reduce the current drain while still maintaining an adequate safety margin. In some devices these algorithms have been shown to increase longevity by 55% compared to standard programming and by 6% when compared to low output programming.[21]

Pulse width of pacing pulses

Although the pulse amplitude is the most common parameter used to adjust the energy delivered to capture the myocardium, the programmed pulse width is another alternative. By adjusting these two values the clinician is able to optimize the longevity while still ensuring an appropriate safety margin.

From the previous formula of

$$E = \frac{V_{supply} V_{programmed} \text{ Pulse Width}}{R}$$

it can be observed that the energy consumed as well as the energy delivered to the patient is directly proportional to the pulse width. If the pulse width is doubled, the energy is also doubled. This is not true for the voltage. As the voltage is squared in the formula, if the programmed voltage is doubled, then the energy is quadrupled.

As shown in Fig 1.6, the difference in energy delivered compared to the energy consumed is related to the programmed pulse amplitude. The farther apart these plots are the greater the loss in efficiency. By altering the pulse width, the desired amount of energy can be delivered at a more-optimal pacing pulse amplitude. This concept can be seen in Fig 1.7 where the longevity of a St. Jude Medical model 5826 Zephyr XL is shown at various delivered pacing energies. The pacing energy is shown for both 0.4 ms as well as 1.0 ms. The highlighted section shows the drop in longevity when programming the pulse amplitude from 2.5 to 5 V. As 2.5 and 5 V are the most efficient pacing voltages in this device, the longest longevity at a specific required pacing energy can be obtained by programming the pulse width to a value that causes the pulse amplitude to be 2.5 or 5 V.

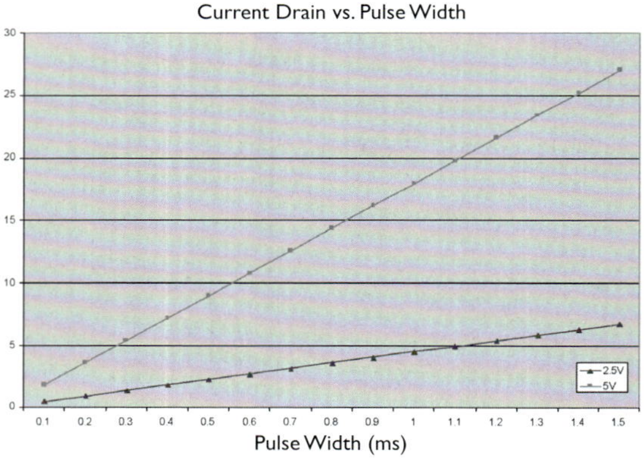

Fig 1.6 Current drain vs. pulse width. Notice the linear relationship of current drain with increasing pulse width. Also of note, doubling the pulse amplitude from 2.5 to 5 V increases current drain four-fold.

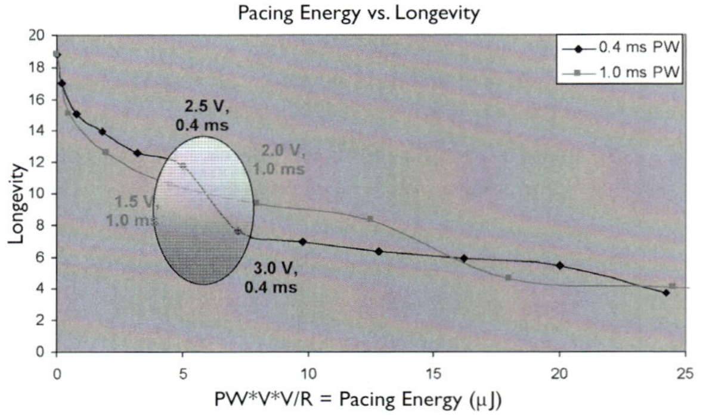

Fig 1.7 Pacing energy vs. battery longevity. Notice that increasing the pacing energy by increasing the pulse amplitude above the battery voltage, necessitating the use of a voltage doubler, has a much greater impact on battery longevity than a similar increase in energy of increasing the voltage at a greater pulse duration that remains below the battery voltage.

Lead impedance

Although the lead impedance is not a programmed parameter, it can significantly alter the longevity of the pulse generator. The lead impedance is inversely proportional to the energy delivered in a pacing pulse. As shown in Fig 1.8, as the impedance doubles the energy in a pacing pulse is halved, assuming the voltage and current remain constant.

There has been some debate over the efficacy of using high-impedance leads to extend device longevity. High-impedance pacing leads have a high-current density due to the small diameter of the lead tip. An example of a high-impedance lead is the CapSure Z (Medtronic, Inc.), which has surface area of 1.2 mm^2.[22] This surface area is significantly less when compared to the standard impedance lead such as the CapSure SP (Medtronic, Inc.), which has a surface area of 5.8 mm^2.[20]

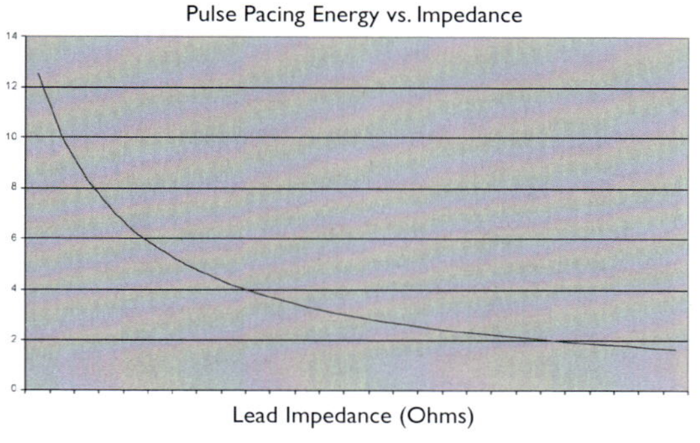

Fig 1.8 Pacing pulse energy vs. lead impedance. Notice the inverse exponential relationship between higher pacing impedance and pacing pulse energy.

Some studies have shown that patients who require ventricular pacing > 50% of the time can benefit from an increase in longevity of 18 months if a high-impedance lead is used compared to a standard impedance lead.[22] Other studies evaluating the long-term comparison between standard and high-impedance leads report only a small effect on pulse generator longevity.[10,23]

Again using the formula

$$E = \frac{V_{programmed} V_{programmed} \text{ Pulse Width}}{R}$$

we can determine that increasing the impedance will decrease the energy consumed assuming all other variables are held constant. The approximate nominal battery voltage of a lithium iodine battery is 2.78 V, so this can be used to aid in determining the average current drain from pacing from one lead. Using the common values for longevity calculations, a pulse amplitude of 2.5 V and a pulse width of 0.4 ms at a rate of 60 bpm, and the formula

$$E = \frac{V_{programmed} V_{programmed} \text{ Pulse Width}}{R*Rate*V_{battery}}$$

the current drain due to pacing pulses is calculated to be 1.8 μA with an impedance of 500 Ω and 0.9 μA with a lead impedance of 1000 Ω. With devices that have a relatively high quiescent current of 17.6 μA, this savings of 0.9 μA is only a savings in longevity of < 5%.[10] With faster pacing rates, larger required pacing amplitudes, and pulse generators with a lower quiescent current, the savings from high-impedance leads will be more significant.

Pacemaker failure

Despite advances in design and construction that place pacemakers among the most reliable electronic devices ever created, they remain susceptible to unpredictable behavior and failure. The understanding of pacemaker construction presented thus far aids in recognition of how these failures and unusual behaviors can manifest themselves. It only requires failure at one critical location to result in potentially catastrophic consequences leading to inappropriate sensing or pacing.

Issues with devices can be recognized at several different time points including in-house quality assurance testing preformed by all manufacturers, during preimplant testing, and after implant. It is, of course, ideal to recognize a potential problem prior to implant. If a device is explanted due to an issue recognized after implantation, the device should be returned to the manufacturer for evaluation. Detection of new failure mechanisms is facilitated by careful evaluation of explanted devices. In fact, it is the recommendation of the HRS Task Force on Device Performance Policies and Guidelines that all extracted devices be returned to the manufacturer for evaluation regardless of the indication for removal. This is the best way to ensure that each device is appropriately evaluated.

Common versus nonrepetitive component failure

As stated previously, pacemakers have an inherent failure rate attributable to random component failure. This rate is estimated at 0.8 per 1000 devices implanted.[24] When a device is returned to the manufacturer, every effort is made to identify the potential failure mechanism and/or component. If after evaluating these devices the manufacturer determines that multiple devices have a common failure mechanism, then the manufacturer is required to report this information to the Food and Drug Administration (FDA), even if the failure rate is lower than the expected random component failure rate.

Despite all efforts to uncover potential issues during quality assurance testing, many issues do still occur after device implant. Often these failures are not recognized until years after the device is manufactured and thousands of devices have been implanted. These issues have been a problem ever since pacemakers were first manufactured, but as the absolute number of devices implanted has increased, so have the number of patients affected by these issues.

Once a problem is recognized the FDA may elect to place the device on recall based on the potential impact to the patient. The FDA has established a hierarchy for device recalls based on the potential impact to the patient. A level I recall is associated with a reasonable chance that the issue could cause serious injury or death. A level II recall is less serious and presents either a possibility that the device will cause temporary or reversible health problems, or that there is a remote chance that the device will cause serious health problems. A level III recall is a situation that results in little chance the device could cause health-related issue. Due to the nature of pacemakers and the patients receiving them, recalls typically fall into the Level I or II category. The HRS Task Force on Device Performance Policies and Guidelines has recommended a change in language to more clearly communicate the significance of these failure mechanisms to physicians and patients. The Task Force suggested changing Level I Recall to Class I advisory notice or safety alert. They also recommend changing Level II and III Recall to simply advisory notice or safety alert.

Often the manufacturer, in their communication letter to physicians, will make recommendations for management of patients with affected devices, but ultimately, the management of such recalls rests on a decision from the physician and patient. In all patients the risks of device replacement must be weighed against the patient outcome if a device fails. Although pulse generator change is a relatively simple procedure, the risks may not be so trivial. The risks most importantly include infection and damage to leads. In a retrospective review, the risk of reoperation at 60 days was 1.24%,[25] but other analyses have estimated the risk of complication to be as high as 8%.[26]

When evaluating the risk to the patient, several issues need to be considered. Devices may fail in either a predictable or unpredictable fashion. If an issue arises such as premature battery depletion, but does so in a predictable fashion, then accelerated follow-up rather than immediate generator change is generally advisable. In devices in which an issue may occur without warning, the results of sudden loss of pacemaker function must be considered when evaluating the patient for pacemaker generator change. In general, pulse generator replacement is reserved for the pacemaker-dependent patient who would be at greatest risk should a device fail. Elective generator change should only be considered if the anticipated nonrandom failure rate is greater than the expected random component failure rate.

Notable recalls and advisories

Sudden unpredictable failure of the device places the patient at the greatest risk. Table 1.1 includes a number of pacemaker recalls. The more recent advisories will be discussed as they are most likely to remain clinically relevant. Those failures that exceed the nonrandom component failure rate are the most significant as the physician may determine the risk-to-benefit ratio favors early pulse generator replacement.

FDA Level	Date Issued	Manufacturer	Models	At risk	Event Rate	Mechanism
II	2/5/07	Vitatron	T60, C60			Problem with retrograde conduction test can inhibit pacing if patient's intrinsic rate falls below the lower programmed rate
II	10/6/06	St. Jude Medical	Identity			Programmer incorrectly reports battery voltage, expected battery longevity and Elective Replacement Indicator (ERI) status
II	6/24/06	Guidant	Insignia, Nexus	31000	0.1–0.22	Low-voltage capacitor malfunction leading to unpredictable premature battery depletion or loss of pacing output
II	11/29/05	Medtronic	Sigma			Interconnect wire separation due to weakened bond from cleaning process during manufacturing
II	10/25/05	ELA Medical	Symphony, Rhapsody			Metal migration in the manufacturing process
I	7/18/05	Guidant	Discovery, Pulsar, Meridian	77500	0.31–0.88	Gradual loss of hermetic seal leading to device failure
II	7/20/04	Medtronic	Kappa 701, 901			Problem with programmer interface
II	6/23/03	Guidant	Multiple			Inadequate soldered electrical connection at an integrated circuit
II	5/6/03	Guidant	Multiple			Battery longevity overestimated when in fallback mode for high-rate atrial activity
II	11/4/02	St. Jude Medical	Tempo, Meta			Potential loss of output
II	9/22/05	Guidant	Insignia	41000	0.017–0.037	Foreign material in a crystal timing component
I	3/15/02	Medtronic	Kappa		0.02	Fractured power supply wires

Table 1.1 FDA Issued Pacemaker Generator Recalls

Loss of hermetic seal. As stated earlier in the chapter, pacemaker pulse generators are hermetically sealed to prevent fluid intrusion into the pulse generator. This fluid could potentially damage the internal components of the device. In July of 2005, the FDA issued a Level I recall on a large subset of Guidant Discovery, Pulsar, and Meridian pacemakers totaling approximately 75,000 devices. As a result of returned product analysis, the manufacturer determined that the hermetic seal encasing the pulse generator had failed, allowing moisture to damage various internal components. In some of these devices, in which rate responsive pacing was enabled, patients experienced inappropriate pacing at the upper sensor rate prior to more serious failures including loss of output. The expected failure rate for these devices due to breach of the hermetic seal has been estimated between 0.31% and 0.88%.

For patients who are not pacemaker dependent, Guidant has made several recommendations including accelerated follow-up. They have also suggested the rate sensor be programmed Off for patients who do not have chronotropic incompetence. Additionally, they recommend evaluating the device's response to turning the rate sensor On at rest at the time of pacemaker follow-up. If the device paces at the maximum sensor rate at rest, then it is likely that moisture has entered the device. This is a potential mechanism for early detection of a problem before more severe issues occur. Unfortunately not all devices have exhibited this; thus, it cannot be relied upon for early detection of impending device failure. Based on this, Guidant has recommended consideration of pulse generator change for pacemaker-dependent patients.

Interconnect wires. Based on return product analysis, Medtronic discovered an issue in a subset of their Kappa 600/700/900 and Sigma 100/200/300 pacemakers manufactured between 2000 and 2002. The issue was first reported in 2005, and a second cohort of devices was later included in May 2009. This total device population is approximately 36,000, which represents about 2% of the total Medtronic Kappa and Sigma series devices implanted. The specific component failure involved separation of redundant interconnect wires. Devices which fail in this mechanism may present clinically as loss of rate response, premature battery depletion, loss of telemetry, or no output. The predicted lifetime failure rate for devices still implanted is 4% in the Sigma group and 1.1% in the Kappa group.

In their letter to physicians, Medtronic noted an additional subset of 96,000 pacemakers in which the occurrence of this issue was much lower. The observed rate in this device population was 0.04% and modeled to be as high as 0.12%. Both of these figures are less than the nonrepetative failure rate and therefore no intervention is recommended in this device population.

Patient-device interaction. On some occasions the interaction of the device with the patient characteristics can be meaningful. In March 2002, Medtronic issued an advisory on a subset of their Kappa 600 and 700 series of pacemakers. The advisory was issued based on fractures encountered in the power supply wires. While the overall fracture rate was determined to be relatively low at 0.016%, the failure rate in devices implanted in a submuscular pocket was 5%. This increase in failure rate is likely due to increased stress placed on the device caused by flexing of the pulse generator can due to the overlying pectoralis muscle. This failure mode often presents as an intermittent problem and can be recognized as an electrical reset with the device serial number registering as "000000". There is a potential that the fracture will present as loss of all pacemaker function, rather than an intermittent problem. Thus it was recommended that patients with a subpectoral implant who are pacemaker dependent consider elective generator change.

References

1. Ohm OJ, Danilovic D. Improvements in pacemaker energy consumption and functional ca-

pability: four decades of progress. *Pacing Clin Electrophysiol.* 1997;20(1 Pt 1):2–9.

2. Dreifus LS, Pennock R. Newer techniques in cardiac monitoring. *Heart Lung.* 1975;4(4):568–572.
3. Greatbatch W, Holmes CF. The lithium/iodine battery: a historical perspective. *Pacing Clin Electrophysiol.* 1992;15(11 Pt 2):2034–2036.
4. Parker B. A vindication of the zinc-mercury pacemaker battery. *Pacing Clin Electrophysiol.* 1978;1(1):148–149.
5. Wnek GE, Bowlin GL. *Encyclopedia of Biomaterials and Biomedical Engineering.* New York: Informa Healthcare USA; 2008:1484.
6. Moses H, Miller B, Moulton K, Schneider J. *Pacemaker Technology. A Practical Guide to Cardiac Pacing.* Philadelphia, PA: Lippincott Williams & Wilkins; 2000:31.
7. Furman, S. Nuclear pacemakers. *Pacing Clin Electrophysiol.* 1979;2(2):135–136.
8. Bernstein A. Classification of cardiac pacemakers. In: El-Sherif N, Samet P, eds. *Cardiac Pacing and Electrophysiology.* Philadelphia, PA: WB Saunders. 1991:494–503.
9. Greatbatch W, Holmes CF, Takeuchi ES, Ebel SJ. Lithium/carbon monofluoride (Li/CFx): a new pacemaker battery. *Pacing Clin Electrophysiol.* 1996;19(11 Pt 2):1836–1840.
10. Shepard RK, Ellenbogen KA. Leads and longevity: how long will your pacemaker last? *Europace.* 2009;11(2):142–143.
11. Wilkoff BL, Cook JR, Epstein AE, et al. Dual-chamber pacing or ventricular backup pacing in patients with an implantable defibrillator: the Dual Chamber and VVI Implantable Defibrillator (DAVID) Trial. *JAMA.* 2002;288(24):3115–3123.
12. Carlson MD, Ip J, Messenger J, et al. A new pacemaker algorithm for the treatment of atrial fibrillation: results of the Atrial Dynamic Overdrive Pacing Trial (ADOPT). *J Am Coll Cardiol.* 2003;42(4):627–633.
13. De Voogt W, De Vusser P, Lau C, et al. Overdrive atrial septum stimulation in patients with paroxysmal atrial fibrillation (AF) and class 1 and 2 pacemaker indication (OASES). Paper presented at: Annual Scientific Sessions of the Heart Rhythm Society; May 17, 2003; Washington, DC. 2003.
14. Gold M, Fain E, Ip J, Al E. Frequent ventricular pacing attenuates the benefit of dynamic atrial overdrive for the prevention atrial fibrillation. *Heart Rhythm.* 2004;1:S65. Abstract 201.
15. Gillis AM. Selective pacing algorithms for prevention of atrial fibrillation: the final chapter? *Heart Rhythm.* 2009;6(3):302–304.
16. Sulke N, Silberbauer J, Boodhoo L, et al. The use of atrial overdrive and ventricular rate stabilization pacing algorithms for the prevention and treatment of paroxysmal atrial fibrillation: the Pacemaker Atrial Fibrillation Suppression (PAFS) study. *Europace.* 2007;9(9):790–797.
17. Biffi M, Sperzel J, Martignani C, Branzi A, Boriani G. Evolution of pacing for bradycardia: AutoCapture. *Eur Heart J Suppl.* 2007;9 (suppl I):I23–32.
18. Barold SS, Winner JA. Techniques and significance of threshold measurement for cardiac pacing. Relationship to output circuit of cardiac pacemakers. *Chest.* 1976;70(6):760–766.
19. Danilovic D, Ole-Jørgen O. Pacing threshold trends and variability in modern tined leads assessed using high resolution automatic measurements: Conversion of pulse width into voltage thresholds. *Pacing Clin Electrophysiol.* 1999;22(4):567–587.
20. Roos M, Kobza R, Erne P. Early pacemaker battery depletion caused by a current leak in the output circuitry: rectification not exchange. *Pacing Clin Electrophysiol.* 2007;30(5):705–708.
21. Boriani G, Rusconi L, Biffi M, et al. Role of ventricular AutoCapture function in increasing longevity of DDDR pacemakers: a prospective study. *Europace.* 2006;8(3):216–220.
22. Scherer M, Ezziddin K, Klesius A, et al. Extension of generator longevity by use of high impedance ventricular leads. *Pacing Clin Electrophysiol.* 2001;24(2):206–211.
23. Etsadashvili K, Hintringer F, Stuhlinger M, et al. Long-term results of high vs. normal impedance ventricular leads on actual (Real-Life) pacemaker generator longevity. *Europace.* 2009;11(2):200–205.
24. Maisel WH Pacemaker and ICD generator reliability: meta-analysis of device registries. *JAMA.* 2006;295:1929–1934.

25. Kapa S, Hyberger L, Rea RF, Hayes DL. Complication risk with pulse generator change: Implications when reacting to a device advisory or recall. *Pacing Clin Electrophysiol.* 2007;30(6):730–733.

26. Gould PA, Krahn AD. Complications associated with implantable cardioverter-defibrillator replacement in response to device advisories. *JAMA* 2006;295:1907–1911.

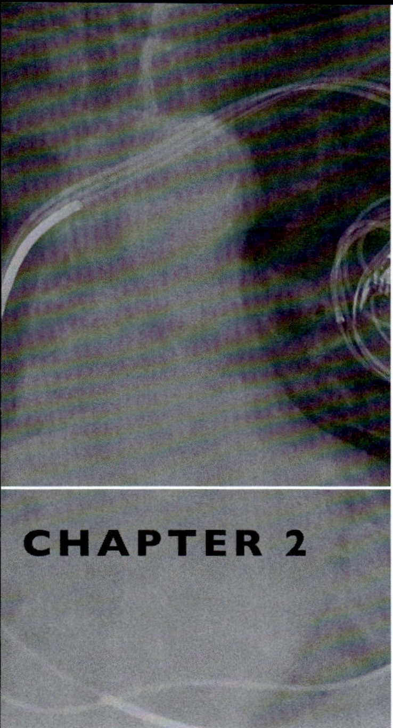

CHAPTER 2

Pacemaker and Implantable Cardioverter Defibrillator Lead Design

Andrea M. Russo

Introduction

The clinical benefits of permanent pacemakers and implantable cardioverter defibrillators (ICDs) have been well-established, and there has been a recent expansion of indications for device therapy.[1,2] These devices have improved the survival and quality of life for millions of patients throughout the world. At present, endocardial (or transvenous) leads are the mainstay of therapy. However, these intravascular leads may often be considered the "weakest link" of the device system. As cardiac implantable electronic device (CIED) implantation continues to rise, and younger patients who receive devices may require multiple generator replacements throughout their lifetime, lead technology becomes increasingly important. Challenges regarding evaluation of lead performance have been well recognized, and recommendations regarding policies and guidelines regarding performance have been published.[3] An expert consensus statement regarding the suggested monitoring of CIEDs, which may be helpful in detecting early lead failure, has also been published.[4]

Pacemaker lead development preceded ICD lead development by many years. In addition to providing bradycardia pacing, ICD leads are more complex due to requisite defibrillation circuits. However, both pacemaker and ICD lead systems must provide reliable sensing and pacing.

This chapter reviews lead design and the evolution in technology of transvenous atrial and ventricular pacing leads, ICD leads, and left ventricular (LV) leads used for cardiac resynchronization therapy (CRT). Modes of lead failure are also discussed.

Pacemakers and Implantable Cardioverter Defibrillators: An Expert's Manual. © 2010 Amin Al-Ahmad, Kenneth A. Ellenbogen, Andrea Natale, and Paul J. Wang, eds. Cardiotext Publishing, ISBN: 978-0-9790164-6-2.

Pacemaker Leads

Most pacemaker system problems are due to failure of some component of the lead. Lead components include the electrode, the conductor, the insulation, and the connector pin[5] (Fig 2.1). Leads must function in a very harsh environment within the heart, and must be constructed of materials that provide mechanical stability while allowing flexibility. They must also provide adequate electrical conductive and resistive properties, provide durable insulation, and maintain good contact with the myocardium.

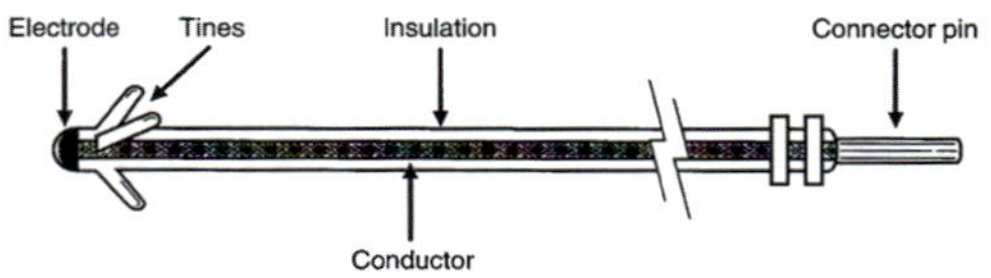

Fig 2.1 Basic components of a pacing lead include the electrode, conductor, insulation, and connector pin. In this example, a passive fixation mechanism is present with tines.[5] (Courtesy of Wiley-Blackwell. Used by permission.)

Intrinsic lead and electrode factors influence lead performance and impact on sensing or pacing. In addition to these lead and electrode factors, other extrinsic factors may also influence sensing and pacing function, including myocardial factors (such as fibrosis or infarction), metabolic factors (such as electrolyte abnormalities), drugs (such as amiodarone), and timing from implantation. Intrinsic lead and electrode factors, including lead polarity (unipolar vs. bipolar), electrode size and shape, electrode material, lead insulation, fixation mechanism, and steroid elution are discussed in the following sections.

Lead Polarity

According to strict definition, all pacemaker circuits may be considered "bipolar," as electrons flow from the cathode to the anode. However, the terms "unipolar" and "bipolar" refer to the number of electrodes on the pacemaker lead that have contact within the heart.[6] A unipolar lead has one electrode at the tip of the lead, the "cathode" or negatively charged end, which is in contact with the heart muscle (Fig 2.2). With a unipolar system, the pulse generator serves as the "anode," or positively charged end. Current flows from the negatively charged tip of the lead to the heart muscle and then to the positively charged pulse generator, completing the circuit. In contrast, a bipolar pacemaker lead has both electrodes within the heart (Fig 2.2). The tip electrode is the negatively charged "cathode," and a proximal electrode ring, located a short distance from the tip electrode, serves as the positively charged "anode."

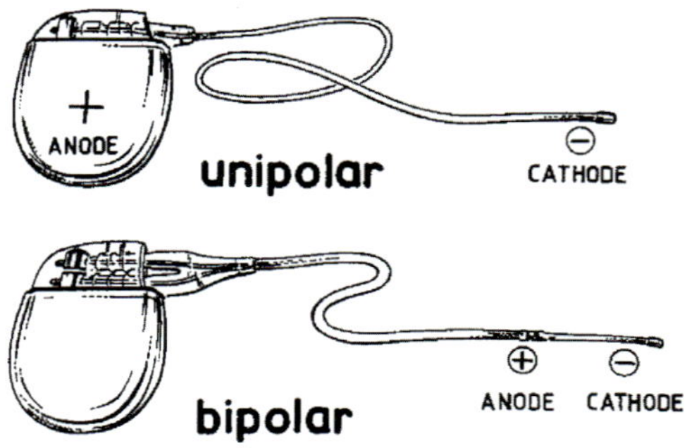

Fig 2.2 Unipolar and bipolar pacemaker leads. A unipolar lead has only one electrode at the tip of the lead, referred to as the *cathode,* which lies within the heart. The *anode* lies on the surface of the pulse generator. A bipolar lead has both the cathode and the anode located in close proximity to each other on the end of the lead, both of which lie within the heart.[6] (Courtesy of Wiley-Blackwell. Used by permission.)

At present, bipolar leads are much more commonly implanted than unipolar pacing leads. Early in development, bipolar leads were large, stiff, and difficult to implant. However, bipolar leads are now also small and easy to implant, similar to unipolar leads. Both types of leads are reliable and have low pacing thresholds. In addition, sensing amplitudes are similar with unipolar and bipolar leads using modern pacemaker systems.[7]

The biggest problem related to unipolar leads is the potential for oversensing and inhibition of pacing, which could be especially problematic in pacemaker-dependent patients. As the unipolar system has a larger interelectrode distance, extending from the distal tip electrode to the pulse generator, the unipolar sensing system will "see" more of the heart as it detects the intracardiac signal, and therefore unipolar systems are more susceptible to crosstalk. This includes the inappropriate sensing of the atrial stimulus artifact by the ventricular channel in a dual chamber pacing system, which can result in inhibition of ventricular output, and could be life threatening in pacemaker-dependent patients. Due to the smaller amplitude of the pacing stimulus, crosstalk is less common with bipolar systems.[6] Unipolar pacing systems are also more likely than bipolar systems to cause oversensing of skeletal muscle myopotentials, which may occur during muscle activity such as lifting or reaching, resulting in inhibition of pacing. A bipolar lead with more closely spaced electrodes, both of which are located within the heart, is less likely to record these far-field electrical signals. A bipolar lead is less likely to oversense ventricular electrograms in the atrial channel. This latter type of sensing of far-field electrical signals may result in inappropriate mode switching. Skeletal muscle stimulation may also occur during unipolar pacing, especially at high outputs, due to the proximity of skeletal muscle to the pulse generator, which is not typically seen with bipolar pacing systems.[6,7] It is particularly important for ICD systems to be bipolar, as this minimizes inappropriate oversensing of far-field intracardiac or extracardiac signals and thereby minimizes inappropriate ICD therapy.

It should be noted that a bipolar lead can be programmed in a unipolar mode, if desired. This may be advantageous when a lead is failing due to a fracture or insulation break. Programming the lead to unipolar pacing or sensing may improve function.

Unipolar pacing can be distinguished from bipolar pacing based on the size of the pacer stimulus on electrocardiography, as a unipolar pacing spike is much larger than a bipolar pacing spike. In fact, the bipolar pacing stimulus may be difficult to see on the surface 12-lead ECG or on pacemaker transtelephonic or other remote monitoring systems. When only one surface lead is recorded on remote monitoring, the paced beats may be difficult to distinguish from underlying conducted beats with a wide QRS, as these pacer spikes may not be visible.

Electrode Size

Earlier pacemaker lead electrodes had a larger surface area in contact with the endocardium, which resulted in a low pacing lead impedance and high current drain. As the cathodal surface area was reduced in size, higher current densities were obtained. This resulted in a lower pacing threshold and higher impedance at the electrode-tissue interface (400 to 800 Ω). Subsequently, leads with smaller distal electrodes (4 to 6 mm^2) and even higher impedance values were developed. Eventually, distal electrodes with very small surface areas (1.2 mm^2) and even higher impedance values of > 1000 Ω were developed.[8–10]

According to Ohm's law, $I = V/R$, the increased pacing impedance (associated with the smaller electrode size) results in a decrease in current. The high-impedance leads also have very low pacing thresholds, resulting in less current drain, which should increase pacemaker generator longevity.[8,9,11,12] Sensing characteristics of these high-impedance leads are similar to previous standard leads.[8,11,12] Although dislodgment rates were initially questioned, a very low rate of dislodgment was seen with the small surface area (1.2 mm^2) high-impedance lead when careful lead positioning and securing techniques were utilized.[10]

Polarization

Polarization refers to the electrochemical impedance generated at the electrode-tissue interface. As the stimulus is delivered, layers of oppositely charged ions surround the electrode. These layers of charge reach peak at the termination of the pulse stimulus, and then gradually dissipate. This polarization impedes the movement of charge from the electrode to the myocardium, leading to the need for increased voltage. Polarization develops with increased pulse duration, and one way to reduce polarization is to shorten pulse duration. Certain electrode materials may also reduce polarization. In addition, the polarization effect increases as the electrode surface area is reduced. The ideal lead would have a low polarization, as well as a high electrode impedance and low resistance of the conductor. Modern electrode design incorporates a small radius (to increase electrode impedance) with a porous and irregular surface (to maximize surface area and reduce polarization).[5,13]

Polarization occurs at the electrode-myocardium interface due to the electrical current from the tip of the electrode to the tissue, and the accumulation of ions in the myocardium gives rise to an afterpotential, which is recorded after a pacing stimulus.[13] Certain pacemaker pulse generators have a function that allows automatic assessment of pacing thresholds (such as "AutoCapture"). Low-output stimulation, just above the pacing threshold, is delivered while the device assesses whether the stimulus has captured the myocardium. By maintaining a stimulus amplitude of only 0.5 to 0.7 V above threshold, the longevity of the pacemaker generator can be increased. To allow a reliable determination of capture, the device must be able to distinguish between the myocardial depolarization-evoked response and the electrode polarization signal. If the polarization signal is detected by the pacemaker, it could be confused with myocardial depolarization, leading to pacing at an output below the true threshold. This type of automatic assessment of pacing threshold is most reliably performed by using low polarization leads. Use of non–low polarization leads can lead to incorrect threshold determination and non-capture,[14] which could be a serious problem in pacemaker-dependent patients.

Electrode Design

An electrode with a small radius and large surface area will result in optimal stimulation and sensing thresholds. Earlier electrode models had a smoother surface. Porous electrodes were designed to help reduce lead dislodgment and to reduce excessive threshold rises compared to previous smooth tip electrodes. Electrodes with a textured surface result in an increased surface area without an increase in electrode radius. This can be achieved by a variety of designs, including microscopic pores, coatings of microspheres, or wire filament mesh.[5] Porous electrodes, which have this complex surface structure, have low polarization properties.

Two types of porous electrodes are illustrated in Fig 2.3.[15] Histological examination comparing porous and smooth electrodes has demonstrated tissue in-growth throughout the porous electrode interior and a fibrotic capsule that was about half the thickness of the capsule seen with solid electrodes. R-wave stability and improved anchoring were also seen with the porous electrode.[16] The porous design allows the geometric area to be small, with a large total electrode surface area that includes the internal spaces within the electrode pores.[15] Electrodes with porous designs have been shown to have better stimulation thresholds in humans.[17] Active fixation leads may also include a porous electrode utilized as a surface cathode. The screw is used as the fixation mechanism, but is electrically inert, not utilized for sensing or pacing.

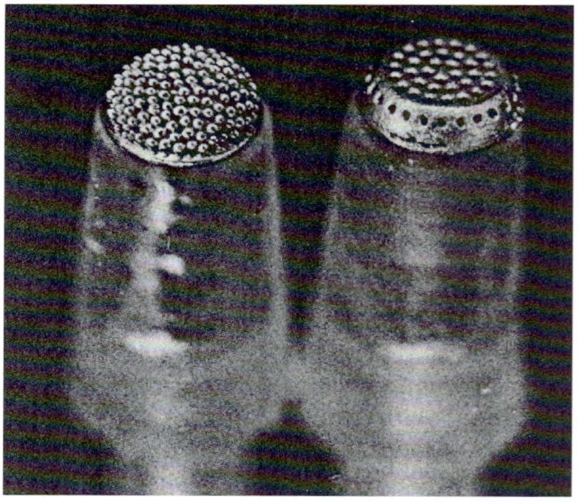

Fig 2.3 Two porous electrodes. The sintered porous electrode is shown on the left and the laser porous electrode is shown on the right.[15] (Courtesy of Wiley-Blackwell. Used by permission.)

Electrode Material

The choice of metals used for electrodes is important with regard to long-term function. The ideal electrode should minimize degradation over time and avoid any excessive foreign body reaction with excessive fibrosis. Metals such as zinc, copper, mercury, nickel, lead, and silver are associated with toxic reactions with the myocardium, while stainless steel alloys are susceptible to corrosion.

Materials that have been utilized for electrodes include platinum, platinum-iridium, Elgiloy (which is an alloy of cobalt, iron, chromium, molybdenum, nickel, and manganese), carbon coating a titanium or graphite core, and iridium oxide.[5,18–20] Microscopic corrosion has been noted with platinum-iridium and Elgiloy electrodes, without consistent clinical adverse effects. Corrosion appears to be directly related to the duration of electrode implantation.[18] Carbon electrodes may be the least susceptible to corrosion. Vitreous carbon has excellent mechanical strength, biocompatibility, and is inert in body tissues.[5,19] Carbon tip electrodes also have lower chronic stimulation thresholds, when compared with platinum and Elgiloy.[19,20]

Lead Conductors

The conductor of the lead is a wire that conducts electrical current from the pacemaker generator to the tip electrode to allow pacing. Unipolar leads have one conductor while bipolar leads have two. Alloys for conductors typically used in pacing leads include MP35N (cobalt, nickel, chromium, and molybdenum), Elgiloy, and nickel-silver.[5] Conductor coils may be of unifilar, multifilar, or cable design, as illustrated in Fig 2.4. The multifilar and cable designs allow the conductor to be more flexible and more resistant to fracture.[5]

Bipolar leads require two conductors. The original design used a parallel arrangement, with subsequent technology using a coaxial design, which is now commonly used (Fig 2.5). Bipolar leads that have a coaxial design include an inner coil extending to the distal electrode and an outer coil terminating at the proximal electrode (Fig 2.5, upper right). With this design, the conductor coils are separated by a layer of inner insulation. The coaxial design allows introduction of a stylet, which is passed through the inner lumen.

Advancements in technology have allowed the development of thin bipolar leads, which have an outside diameter similar to unipolar leads. The single strands of conductor wire are coated with a thin layer of ethylene tetrafluoroethylene (ETFE) insulation. Therefore, two or more conductors can be placed into a single coil to form the lead body[21,22] (Fig 2.5, lower right). These leads have demonstrated good acute and chronic stimulation thresholds, with a relatively low, short-term failure rate.[22]

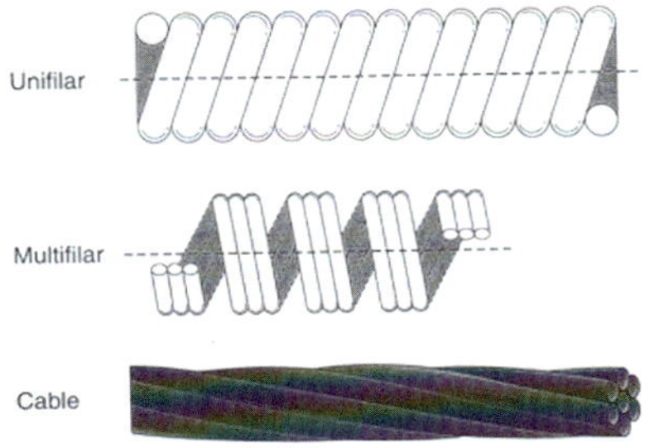

Fig 2.4 Conductor coils may have unifilar, multifilar, or cable design.[5] (Courtesy of Wiley-Blackwell. Used by permission.)

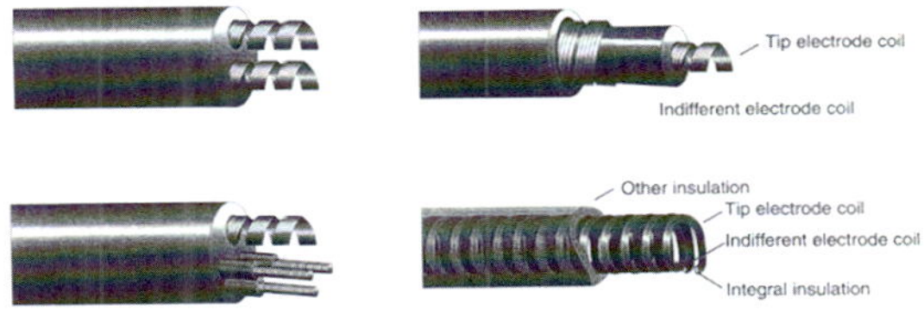

Fig 2.5 Options for conductor construction. **Upper left**: Parallel multifilar coils; **Lower left**: Parallel multifilar coil and three single cables; **Upper right**: Bipolar coaxial design with an inner multifilar coil surrounded by insulation, an outer multifilar coil, and outer insulation; **Lower right**: Individually coated wires wound together in a single multifilar coil for bipolar pacing.[5] (Courtesy of Wiley-Blackwell. Used by permission.)

Insulation

Insulation material extends from the tip of the lead to the lead connector. Insulation material used for pacemaker leads includes polyurethane or silicone. Silicone has been used for pacemaker leads since the 1960s, and polyurethane was introduced in 1979.[23] Each has its potential advantages and disadvantages.

Silicone has a high biocompatibility and biostability, but a relatively low tear strength.[13] Because it could be easily damaged during implantation, a thick layer of silicone was necessary, and this resulted in a lead diameter much larger than leads composed of polyethylene.[23] Silicone also has a high coefficient of friction, which made it difficult to pass one lead next to the other during implantation from a single subclavian stick with the original version of the silicone lead.[23] To overcome this, leads could be coated with a more lubricious material to allow easier handling. A stronger silicone was subsequently manufactured in later years, allowing silicone leads to be thinner than originally constructed.

Polyurethanes have an excellent biocompatibility and were initially thought to have good biostability.[23] Polyurethane has high tensile and tear strengths, as well as high cut resistance and superior compressive properties, making it possible to construct leads of smaller diameter than silicone leads.[5,23] Polyurethane also has a high flexibility and a low coefficient of friction.[13,24] Therefore, unlike silicone, two leads can be passed more easily side-by-side during implantation.

However, a poor long-term performance has been noted with polyurethane.[24,25–29] The two polyurethane polymers that have had the widest use are Pellethane 80A and Pellethane 55D, and the high failure rate occurred primarily in leads insulated with the P80A polymer. The probability of failure of one Medtronic bipolar polyurethane ventricular lead (Model 4012) was 21% at 6 years postimplantation.[27] Insulation failure may present clinically as muscle stimulation, oversensing, undersensing, loss of capture, reduced lead impedance, or premature battery depletion. An early sign of impending lead failure is diminishing electrogram amplitude, which may occur several months prior to clinical manifestations of lead failure.

Leads composed of Pellethane 80A were shown to have insulation degradation or "environmental stress cracking (ESC)" when explanted.[25] It is thought that microscopic cracks initially developed in the P80A polymer during manufacturing, with propagation of the cracks deeper into the insulation following environmental stress.[5] These cracks subsequently resulted in failure of the lead insulation. Environmental stress cracking is caused by the tendency of soft and hard segments of the lead to separate, causing damage to the surface.[23] More severe damage may occur in areas of the lead exposed to stress or strain, such as the region near the lead connector or the site of the ligature or between the clavicle and the first rib, when a subclavian puncture is used for access. Leads with Pellethane 80A insulation are more prone to insulation failure when the subclavian venous approach is used, compared to the cephalic vein approach.[30] It was suggested that pacemaker-dependent patients implanted with earlier polyurethane leads should be considered for prophylactic replacement due to the high failure rate.[27,28]

Metal-induced oxidation (MIO) is another mechanism of failure for polyurethane leads. An adverse chemical reaction may occur when the conductor produces corrosion products, which can lead to oxidative degradation of the polyurethane insulation from the inside.[13] These adverse reactions appear to be design- and model-specific, and not relevant to all polyurethane leads. This can be minimized by coating the conductor.[13]

The current polyurethane leads now typically utilize Pellethane 55D for insulation, which is stiffer and harder than Pellethane 80A. Long-term studies of leads using Pellethane 55D have shown better performance compared to Pellethane 80A.[13,31] The leads using Pellethane 55D appear less susceptible to environmental stress cracking.[23] However, due to the stiffness of Pellethane 55D leads, they are thought to be more prone to right ventricular perforation.[31] Leads may now also have a combination of silicone and polyurethane insulation materials. To avoid excessive stiffness at the tip of the lead, the distal end of the lead may include silicone for insulation. In addition, silicone may be placed between the conductor and the polyurethane, in an attempt to minimize metal-induced oxidation.[13]

Subsequent studies suggested improved reliability of other leads made from polyurethane insulation.[32] It was suggested that the early failure rate might have been related to the design of particular leads, as opposed to the insulation material itself. However, most data suggest that Pellethane 80A is not an acceptable insulation material for pacemaker leads.

Fixation Mechanisms

Endocardial leads have either active or passive fixation mechanisms that provide stability. The current passive fixation leads typically utilize tines, which are extensions of the insulation material that protrude backward just proximal to the electrode tip (Fig 2.1). This allows attachment of the lead to the right atrium or right ventricle by becoming entrapped within trabeculation in the heart. In addition to tines, other passive fixation mechanisms tried in the past included wedge tip or flanges, wings, or fins.[13,23] Compared to older style passive fixation leads, tined ventricular leads had a lower dislodgment rate.

Active fixation leads have a screw at the distal end, and this screw may or may not be an electrically active component of the lead. The original screws were fixed and unprotected, potentially placing endovascular and valvular structures at risk of damage. Subsequently, a mannitol covering over the screw was utilized, which was designed to dissolve within several minutes. After the capsule dissolved, the screw on the tip of the lead could be fixed in the cardiac chamber by rotating the lead over the stylet. The more common active fixation mechanism is now a retractable screw (Fig 2.6). A clothespin-type instrument is used to extend and retract the screw during implantation by turning the connector pin. All active fixation leads result in some trauma to the endocardium and myocardium, and steroid elution at the base of the screw has resulted in significantly improved stimulation thresholds, which is discussed in a future section.

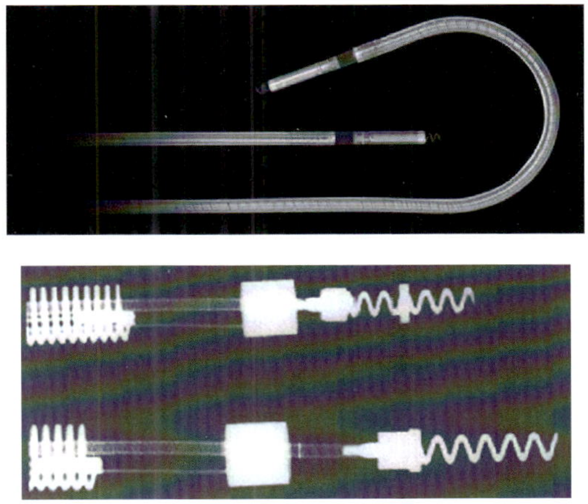

Fig 2.6 Active fixation lead. **Top**: St. Jude Medical Tendril lead with a retractable screw (courtesy of St. Jude Medical). **Bottom**: Radiographic appearance of a retractable screw mechanism where the screw is extended in the lower image, and retracted in the upper image.[5]

Advantages of active fixation leads include the ability to place the lead at various sites in the ventricle or atrium, as well as a low dislodgment rate. Active fixation leads may be preferable when positioning the RV lead on the septum rather than at the apex. In addition, active fixation atrial leads may be preferable for patients with surgically removed RA appendages, distorted chamber anatomy, or severe tricuspid regurgitation. On occasion, the retraction mechanism of the screw may fail during implantation when multiple attempts are required for repositioning, necessitating insertion of a new lead, but this is not common with current technology.

Extensive myocardial fibrosis typically develops with passive fixation leads. Although fibrosis may also occur at the attachment of active fixation leads to the myocardium, active fixation leads may be easier to extract than passive leads. With current technology, both active and passive leads perform well, with low rates of dislodgment. The selection of active or passive mechanism is now largely based on physician experience and preference.

Connectors

Current leads and connectors conform to standards that require leads to have a 3.2-mm diameter bipolar connector pin. This is referred to as an industry standard known as IS-1 (international standard 1). Historically, the older unipolar leads were 5 mm or 6 mm in diameter and bipolar leads had a bifurcated connector.[5] The presence of this current industry standard prevents incompatibility between leads and connectors blocks, which would otherwise require use of lead adaptors. Therefore, leads from one manufacturer can be matched with pulse generators from another manufacturer without the need for any additional hardware.

Steroid-Eluting Leads

A normal rise in stimulation threshold occurs following lead implantation, which is due to an inflammatory response at the electrode-tissue interface. Prior to use of steroid-eluting leads, the stimulation threshold would rapidly rise within the first 24 hours and then peak at 1 week. Over the next 6 to 8 weeks, the threshold would eventually fall, but typically remained at a level higher than the implantation value but lower than the peak threshold. In addition, prior to steroid elution, active fixation leads would typically have higher pacing thresholds than passive leads at implantation, and this threshold would decline rapidly within the first 15 to 30 minutes following implantation. This was felt to be related to acute injury as the screw was advanced into the myocardium. With the advent of steroid-eluting leads, these early and late rises in stimulation threshold are markedly reduced or essentially eliminated.

Dexamethasone sodium phosphate has been used in steroid-eluting electrode systems. Steroid elution is available in both active and passive leads, and multiple studies have demonstrated the effectiveness of steroid-elution in obtaining very low acute and chronic stimulation thresholds, with near elimination of the acute rise in stimulation threshold early post-implantation.[33–35] The beneficial effect of the steroid is thought to be due to a reduction in inflammatory response at the electrode tip. A "flat" response in pacing threshold was seen during 18-month follow-up using a passive fixation lead with steroid elution (Medtronic CapSure SP) when compared to another passive fixation nonsteroid-eluting lead (Telectronics Encor) and active fixation (Medtronic Bisping electrically active and Telectronics Accufix electrically inactive nonsteroid-eluting) leads[33] (Fig 2.7). This beneficial effect of steroid elution is important in reducing current drain, thus increasing pulse generator longevity.

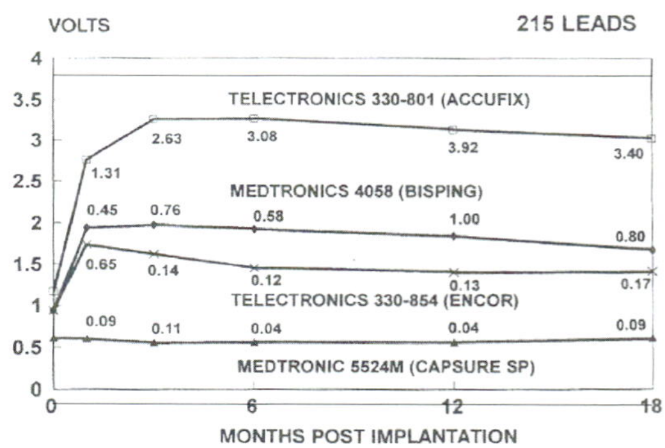

Fig 2.7 Bipolar stimulation thresholds for active and passive fixation leads, with and without steroid-elution. The Medtronic CapSure SP lead (passive fixation, steroid-eluting) had better pacing thresholds postimplantation at all periods of follow-up, compared to another passive nonsteroid-eluting lead (Telectronics Encor) and active fixation (Medtronic Bisping and Telectronics Accufix) leads ($p < 0.05$).[33] (Courtesy of Wiley-Blackwell. Used by permission.)

Lead Advisories and Recalls

One of the most serious and potentially life-threatening pacemaker lead advisories involved an atrial lead. In November of 1994, a Telectronics atrial lead was recalled due to reported fractures noted in the J-shaped retention wire utilized in Accufix leads (models 330-801 and 329-701). The electrically inactive J-retention wire lies beneath the outer insulation, and was welded at the distal end to the anode, free at its proximal end. Although the lead may function normally when fracture occurs, the retention wire may protrude outside of the lead insulation, causing potential damage to cardiac or other vascular structures, or this wire may embolize to the lung vasculature. Cardiac or other vascular tears have led to death. Periodic fluoroscopy was recommended to evaluate the lead and exclude protrusion of the retention wire.[36,37] There was initially some controversy as to whether these leads should be extracted. It has been suggested that leads with retention wire fracture should be extracted, with continued regular fluoroscopic screening for those leads that demonstrated a normal fluoroscopic appearance.[38] The shape of the Accufix lead after implantation was a strong predictor of fracture, and a lower threshold for lead extraction was indicated in patients with non–J-shaped leads.[37,39,40] The hazard of J-wire fracture decreased over time from implantation.

Telectronics Encor leads also had J-shaped retention wires. Compared to the wire of the Accufix leads, which lies just beneath the outer insulation, the Encor wires were located deeper within the cathode conductor.[13] Fracture and protrusion of the wire in these Encor leads appeared to be related to the way the lead was implanted, with trauma during implantation potentially leading to lead deformity. Fluoroscopy was recommended on at least one occasion for these leads.

Other pacing lead advisories have also been issued, involving leads made by various manufacturers. Most of these advisories were related to reduced lead survival, with a lead survival probability "below expectations." The cause of lead failure is most often associated with lead insulation, and less often associated with conductor failure. Each manufacturer is required to provide regular lead performance reports, and this information is available upon request or on the manufacturer's web site. Patient management recommendations are also included in the physician notification letters when advisories are issued, and this may include suggestions for enhanced follow-up.

Implantable Cardioverter Defibrillator Leads

ICD lead technology and implantation approach have changed substantially since approval of the first ICD system in 1985. The initial implantation approach was epicardial, with subsequent approval of the first endocardial ICD lead in 1993. Lead technology has had a significant impact on the ease of implantation and performance of ICD systems. This chapter describes the design and characteristics of ICD leads, focusing on the evolution of lead technology over the past 15 years.

Similar to a pacemaker lead, the ICD lead is responsible for sensing and pacing. It is composed of electrodes, conductors, insulation, connectors, and a fixation mechanism. However, ICD leads must be designed somewhat differently than pacemaker leads due to the need for high-voltage shock therapy for defibrillation. Leads may be located in epicardial, endocardial, or extrathoracic locations and systems may include a combination of these lead locations. Epicardial systems were the first systems studied clinically, and are briefly discussed. These epicardial systems have been essentially supplanted by endocardial (transvenous) systems, which are the main focus of this chapter.

Historical Perspective — Epicardial ICD Lead Systems

Since the pioneering work of Michel Mirowski in the 1960s and 1970s, there have been rapid advancements in ICD lead technology. With thoracotomy systems, epicardial defibrillation patches were implanted through median sternotomy, lateral thoracotomy, subxiphoid, or subcostal approach. Sensing options typically included use of epicardial sensing electrodes or an endocardial sensing lead inserted through a transvenous approach to the right ventricle (RV), which was tunneled to the abdomen for connection to the pulse generator. Transvenous access may also have been used for placement of an additional shocking lead or coil in the superior vena cava (SVC).

The first human implants utilized a titanium spring electrode positioned in the SVC and an epicardial patch for defibrillation.[41,42] Sensing was initially performed utilizing the high-voltage electrodes, but this was supplanted by the use of separate epicardial or endocardial rate sensing leads due to sensing problems. Complications of the initially implanted defibrillation lead systems included migration of the SVC coil. Due to potential adverse effects of SVC lead migration on defibrillator function, the SVC electrode/epicardial patch electrode configuration was supplanted by the epicardial patch/patch electrode configuration, which demonstrated better defibrillation efficacy and avoided the problem of SVC lead migration.[43] Figure 2.8 illustrates an epicardial patch lead system, including epicardial rate sensing leads.[44]

As epicardial lead implantation requires a thoracotomy, it was associated with significant morbidity and mortality, with a perioperative surgical mortality rate as high as 5%. However, many patients undergoing epicardial ICD implantation may have also undergone other concomitant cardiac surgery at the time of patch lead placement, likely increasing the operative risk. Other concerns with epicardial implantation include infection that can spread directly from the pocket to leads lying on the heart. Subsequent bypass graft surgery or valve replacement may also be difficult due to fibrosis if patches were placed directly on the heart, rather than outside the pericardium. Patients with epicardial patches in place may also be resistant to external defibrillation due to an increase in transthoracic impedance.

A high rate of lead malfunction was identified with epicardial patch leads. Many patients with fractured leads were asymptomatic and were identified during routine surveillance X-ray and formal lead testing. Pericardial constriction may also be seen as a complication of epicardial patch placement.

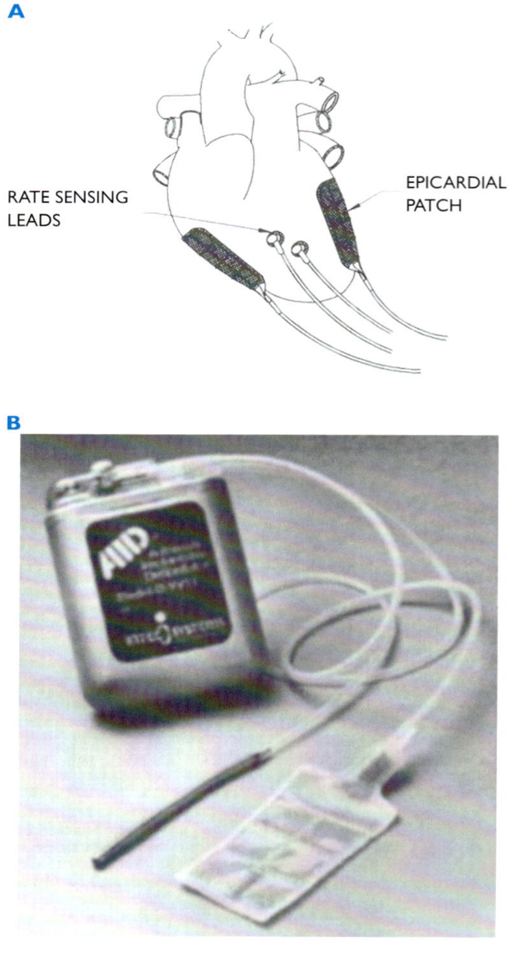

Fig 2.8 Epicardial patch lead system. **A**: Schematic of epicardial defibrillation patches and epicardial sensing rate leads.[44] **B**: Initial model of a rectangular epicardial patch, with an SVC electrode.[44]

Malfunctions of epicardial pace/sense leads are also common, occurring in 3% to 15% of patients.[45–49] This often presented with inappropriate ICD discharges due to oversensing and was typically related to lead fracture. The presence of an adaptor also increased the risk of sensing lead problems with epicardial systems. With epicardial pacing leads, there was also a high incidence of elevated pacing thresholds or complete loss of capture.

Endocardial ICD Lead Systems

Although the concept of transvenous defibrillation was first developed by the early work of Michel Mirowski, widespread application was limited due to high defibrillation energy requirements. This was subsequently solved by advancements in device technology. The development of a transvenous lead with both shock and sensing functions with ease of implantation permitted more widespread use of ICDs. Initially, subcutaneous patches were routinely utilized as part of the defibrillation system. After lead design improved and biphasic waveform and active can technology became available, which reduced defibrillation energy requirements, the addition of subcutaneous leads was rarely needed.

There are several advantages to an endocardial system. A transvenous lead system obviates the need for a thoracotomy procedure and reduces morbidity and mortality associated with the procedure. Transvenous systems result in less patient discomfort and more rapid surgical recovery. Hospital stay and costs are also reduced.

Integrated Bipolar versus Dedicated Bipolar Leads

Functions of a transvenous ICD lead include sensing, pacing, and shock delivery. Leads types include true bipolar and integrated bipolar leads (Fig 2.9). ICD leads, which have true bipolar sensing and pacing capabilities, have separate tip and ring electrodes designed for sensing and pacing, similar to permanent pacemaker leads. Leads with true bipolar sensing are less likely to manifest sensing errors. However, true bipolar leads have a longer distance from the tip to the distal defibrillation coil in the RV, compared with integrated leads. ICD leads with integrated sensing and pacing capabilities have only a single tip electrode, and the distal defibrillation coil is used as the anode for sensing and pacing functions. The electrograms obtained from an integrated bipolar lead will have a more "unipolar" appearance due to the larger surface area for sensing compared with the electrograms from a dedicated bipolar lead. One advantage of ICD leads having integrated bipolar sensing and pacing functions is that there is a shorter tip to defibrillation distance. Because the defibrillation coil is closer to the myocardium of the right ventricle, there may be an advantage with respect to defibrillation success.[50]

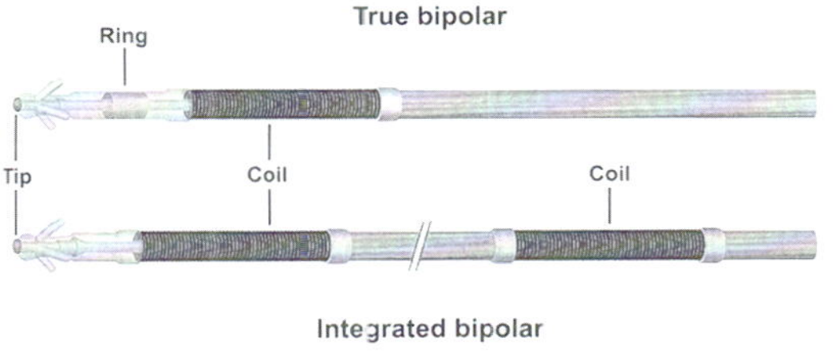

Fig 2.9 True bipolar and integrated bipolar ICD leads. **Top**: True bipolar leads sense between the distal tip and proximal ring, which are dedicated for pacing and sensing. **Bottom**: Integrated bipolar leads pace and sense between the tip and the distal coil. The distal coil is used for sensing, pacing, and defibrillation.[5] (Courtesy of Wiley-Blackwell. Used by permission.)

Integrated bipolar leads may be more susceptible to sensing problems. In earlier integrated bipolar lead designs, there was a short (6 mm) distance from the lead tip to the distal coil in an attempt to minimize far-field oversensing. However, problems with sensing may occur postshock as the amplitude of the electrogram may diminish significantly after shock delivery. This could potentially result in failure to redetect VF. Redesign of integrated bipolar leads subsequently included a greater distance between the lead tip and distal coil (12 mm), which minimizes reduction of the postshock electrogram amplitude and essentially eliminates this problem. Delay with capture has also been noted following shock delivery, resulting from a temporary increase in pacing threshold. To compensate for this, devices can now be programmed to higher pacing outputs following shock delivery.

Single and Dual Coil Defibrillation Leads

ICD leads may have one or two coils utilized for defibrillation. Single coil defibrillation leads have one coil that lies in the RV, which may be designated as the cathode. When used in conjunction with an active or "hot" can defibrillator, the shell of the device may be the defibrillation anode. However, polarity can be easily reversed non-invasively using modern ICDs. Dual coil defibrillation leads have an additional proximal coil that typically lies within the HRA/SVC junction. The proximal coil can be used alone as the defibrillation anode, or it can be combined with an active can as a combined defibrillation anode. Dual coil systems may have a slightly better defibrillation threshold compared to single coil systems.

Insulation

Insulation influences lead reliability. The most frequently used insulation materials are silicone, polyurethane, and fluoropolymers. Insulation materials were previously discussed in more detail in the pacemaker lead section. Advantages and disadvantages of silicone and polyurethane were already reviewed.

Concerns have been raised about polyurethane in some pacemaker leads, with reports of a high rate of failure due to insulation problems.[27] An increased long-term failure rate was noted with leads utilizing Pellethane 80A, related to metal ion oxidation and environmental stress cracking. In contrast, another polyurethane (55D) is stiffer and has a good reliability.[51] Coating of the conductor with a fluoropolymer layer can prevent metal oxidation, but fluoropolymer use may be limited by the stiffness of the material.[50]

Based on prior experience with pacemaker leads, contemporary ICD leads utilize several insulating materials. The insulating body is usually made of silicone. An outside polyurethane layer is used to reduce the coefficient of friction and reduce scar formation, while protecting against abrasion. Because the polyurethane is not in direct contact with the conductors, metal ion oxidation is avoided. The conductors are also often insulated with an extra layer of a fluoropolymer.[50]

Figure 2.10 (A) depicts a schematic cross-section of defibrillation leads, as well as cross-sectional photographs (B–D) of leads from three different manufacturers.[51] This demonstrates incorporation of both silicone and polyurethane insulation materials with various thicknesses of insulation.

A

B

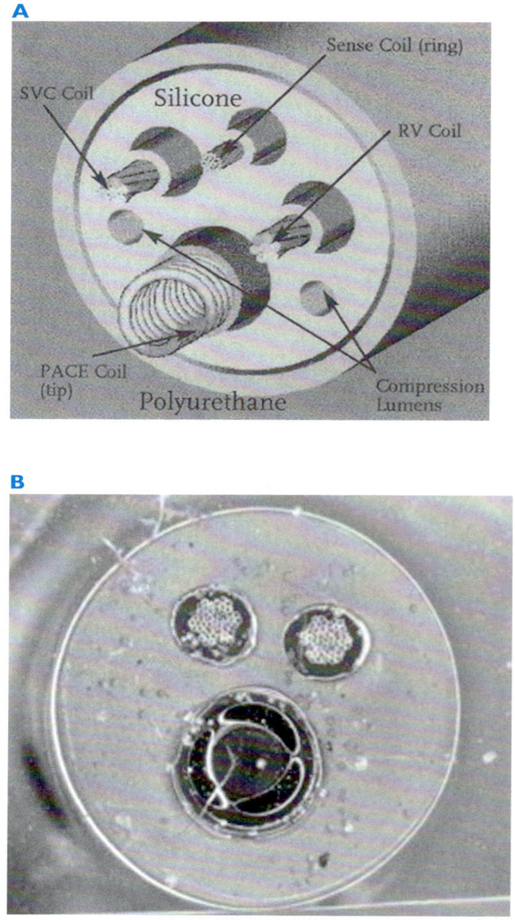

Fig 2.10 A–D Defibrillation lead insulation. **A** demonstrates a schematic view of a Medtronic lead that utilizes both silicone as an inner insulation and polyurethane as an outer insulation. (Courtesy of Medtronic, Inc. Used with permission.) The cross-section of the insulation in a Guidant ENDOTAK Reliance lead is shown in **B**, Medtronic Sprint Quattro Secure lead in **C**, and St. Jude Riata lead in **D**. (Cross-sectional views courtesy of Guidant, Inc.[51])

Fig 2.10 (cont.)

C

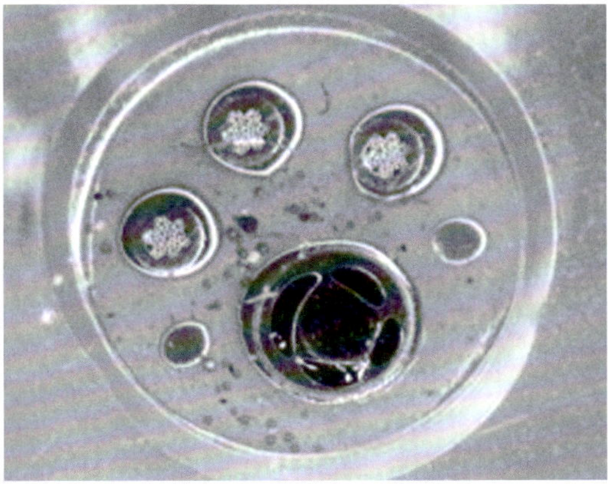

D

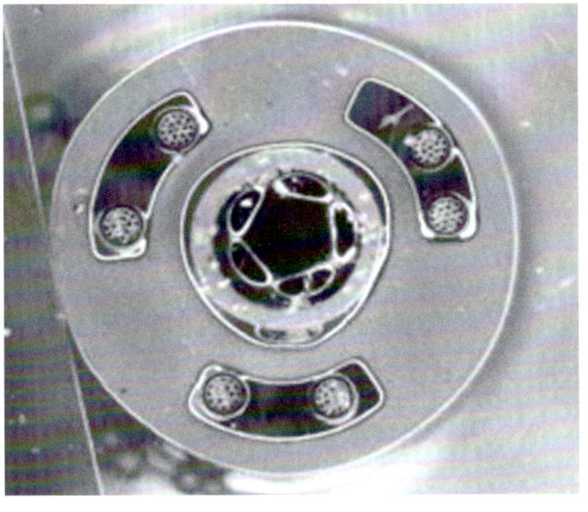

Conductors and Electrodes

To deliver current efficiently, conductors with a low resistance will minimize voltage losses. This can be achieved by using a composite wire of Drawn Brazed Strand or Drawn Filled Tube construction (Fig 2.11). These wires combine low-resistance metals such as silver, stainless steel, MP35N (an alloy of nickel, cobalt, chromium, and molybdenum), titanium, or other high strength metal to obtain a strong and low resistance wire.[52] The wires can then be formed into coils (for Drawn Filled Tube) or twisted into cables (for Drawn Brazed Strand wire). Coils provide a lumen for passage of a stylet. The coils can be arranged concentrically or in parallel, combining the wires needed for defibrillation, sensing, and pacing (Fig 2.12). Parallel pathways are now more frequently utilized, as this prevents the lead body from becoming too large or stiff.[52]

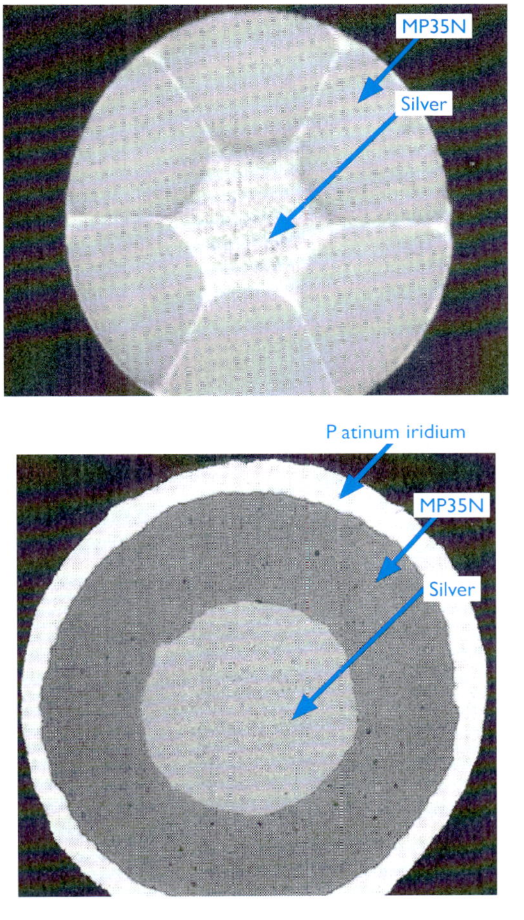

Fig 2.11 Defibrillator conductors. **Top**: Cross-sectional photograph of Drawn Brazed Strand composite wire showing six stainless steel strands and silver in the center between the strands and on the outer surface. The low-resistance silver is drawn between and around the high-strength MP35N an alloy of nickel, cobalt, chromium, and molybdenum. **Bottom**: Cross-sectional photograph of Drawn Filled Tube composite wire showing the low-resistance inner conductor (silver), a high-strength shell (MP35N), and metal outer layer (platinum iridium) for use as an electrode.[52]

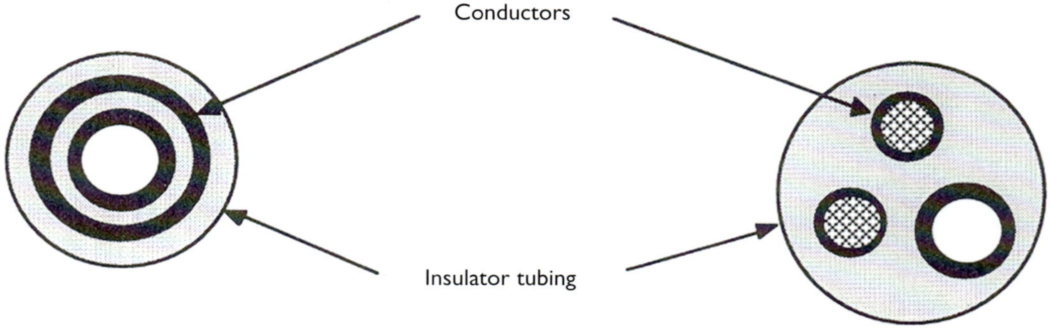

Fig 2.12 Potential lead construction configurations. The left figure demonstrates a concentric two-conductor configuration and the right figure demonstrates the parallel construction of two Drawn Brazed Strand cables and a Drawn Filled Tube coil. The Drawn Filled Tube coil contains a center lumen for a stylet.[52]

Although the electrode design for defibrillation leads varies among manufacturers, the choice for materials is somewhat standard. The material utilized for the electrodes is limited to high-conducting, low-corrosion, biocompatible, and biostable materials.[44] Most electrodes are composed of platinum, platinum alloy (such as platinum-iridium), or titanium.[44,52] Platinum is very resistant to corrosion in the body, and is very conductive, with proven long-term reliability demonstrated in pacemaker leads.[44] Use of other metals in defibrillation systems, such as carbon electrodes, has been promising.[53,54]

Electrode designs vary among manufacturers, including single wire coil, multi-wire braid, or ribbon designs. Lead design and material limitations include issues regarding impedance, fatigue life, stiffness and corrosion.[44] One of the most important concerns is fatigue performance, and the lead should be built to outlive the pulse generator, as patients may require multiple generator replacements throughout the years.

In addition to fatigue, sources of physical stress on the conductor of the defibrillation lead include potential compression or fracture at the junction of the clavicle and first rib, or kinking of the lead within the defibrillator pocket.[55,56] Leads may pass through the subclavius muscle or costoclavicular ligament before entering the subclavian vein, leading to soft tissue entrapment and potential lead damage. The cephalic vein approach is often preferable for lead longevity and minimizes lead fracture from subclavian crush injury.

High-voltage defibrillation systems typically have impedance measures ranging from 20 to 80 Ω (remaining < 100 Ω). Epicardial patches demonstrate impedance values at the lower end of this range, whereas transvenous systems are typically in the 40 to 80 Ω range. Impedance values outside this range suggest a problem with the lead system. High-voltage values > 100 Ω suggest conductor fracture and values < 20 Ω suggest insulation failure. In addition, following shock delivery, a large disparity between the programmed energy and the delivered energy suggests lead conductor failure.

ICD Lead Design

Similar to pacemaker leads, ICD leads may have a coaxial construction or multi-lumen lead construction (Fig 2.13). The coaxial construction is characterized by a coiled conductor with an outside insulation layer, surrounded by another conductor, in a layered design, with an insulating layer between each of the conductors (Fig 2.13a). A stylet can be inserted through a channel inside the innermost conductor during implantation. Examples of leads with this type of construction include the earlier Transvene Medtronic leads (Minneapolis, MN) and the TVL Ventritex leads (St. Jude Medical/Ventritex, Sunnyvale, CA).[50]

The multi-lumen design has coiled and straight conductors running in parallel through a single insulating body, with additional insulating layers covering each conductor (Fig 2.13b). There are also extra lumens inside the multi-lumen body, which increase the lead's resistance to compression. A stylet can be inserted through a coiled conductor to the lead tip during implantation. Examples of this type of design include the ENDOTAK 60, ENDOTAK 70, ENDOTAK-DSP, Endurance, and Reliance leads from Guidant, Medtronic's Sprint lead family, and the St. Jude Medical/Ventritex SPL and Riata lead family. The multi-lumen construction is now favored, and has the advantage of a smaller size with more conductors fitting into a smaller lead.[50]

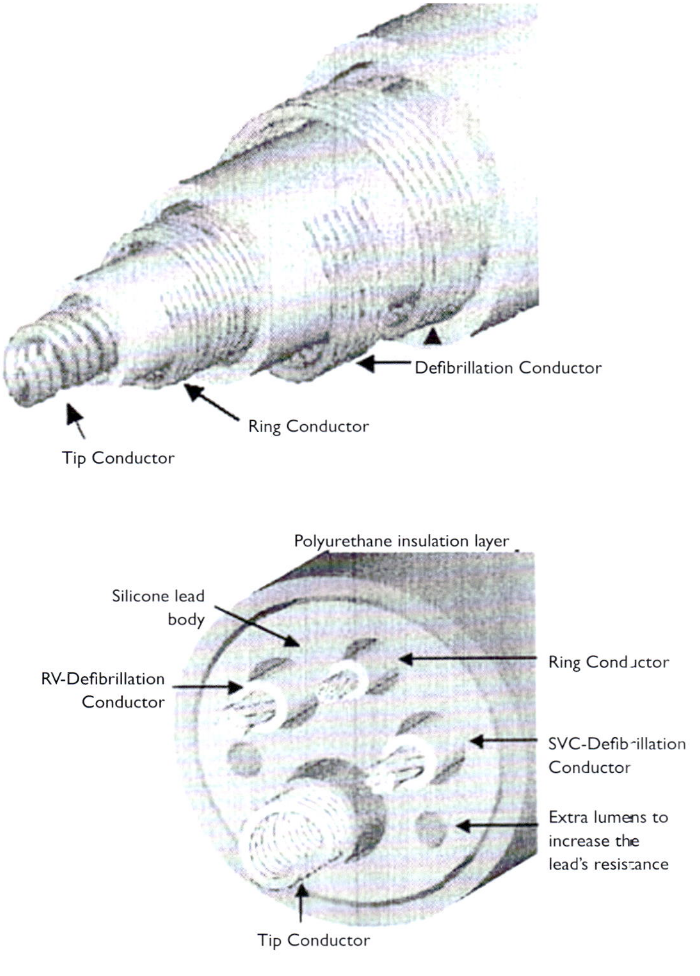

Fig 2.13 ICD lead design. **A**: Coaxial lead construction demonstrating a single coil defibrillation lead with true bipolar sensing and pacing. The tip and ring conductors are responsible for sensing and pacing, while the defibrillation conductor is responsible for defibrillation. **B**: Multilumen lead construction of a dual coil defibrillation lead with true bipolar sensing and pacing. The tip and ring conductor are responsible for sensing and pacing, while the distal defibrillation conductor in the RV and the proximal defibrillation conductor in the SVC are responsible for defibrillation.[50] (Courtesy of Wiley-Blackwell. Used by permission.)

The details regarding the design and specifications of individual leads from different manufacturers are summarized in Table 2.1.

Size and Surface Area

The initial endocardial leads were large in caliber with a lead body diameter measuring 12 Fr and were subsequently downsized to between 6.6 Fr to 8.2 Fr. One of the earliest endocardial leads was manufactured by Intec/CPI (Pittsburgh, PA), which had a 16-mm^2 distal platinum-iridium tip, utilized for pacing and sensing, and distal 4.3 cm^2 and proximal 8.5 cm^2 platinum electrodes with helically wound coils utilized for defibrillation.[57] This lead was the predecessor of CPI/Guidant's ENDOTAK endocardial lead (CPI/Guidant, St. Paul, MN), first implanted in 1988, which received approval as the first endocardial defibrillation system in 1993. This lead has undergone several modifications, and multiple other endocardial leads from other manufacturers are now available. Various lead specifications, including lead size and surface area, are outlined in Table 2.1. Figure 2.14 illustrates two currently available endocardial leads from different manufacturers.

Implantation Site

Rapid advancements in ICD technology have occurred since approval of the first device in 1985. Initially, devices were implanted in the abdominal region using epicardial patch systems. This was followed by long endocardial leads inserted through the subclavian, cephalic, or axillary vein and tunneled to the abdominal region. Since the early 1990s, ICDs have been implanted like pacemakers in the infraclavicular position. This was the result of development of the transvenous lead system, as well as improvements in ICD technology (such as biphasic waveforms and active can systems) that allowed a reduction in pulse generator size.

Connectors

The connector is the part of the lead secured to the pulse generator. One of the connectors has a lumen through which a stylet can be passed during insertion of the lead into the heart. The lead connector must fit into the pulse genera-

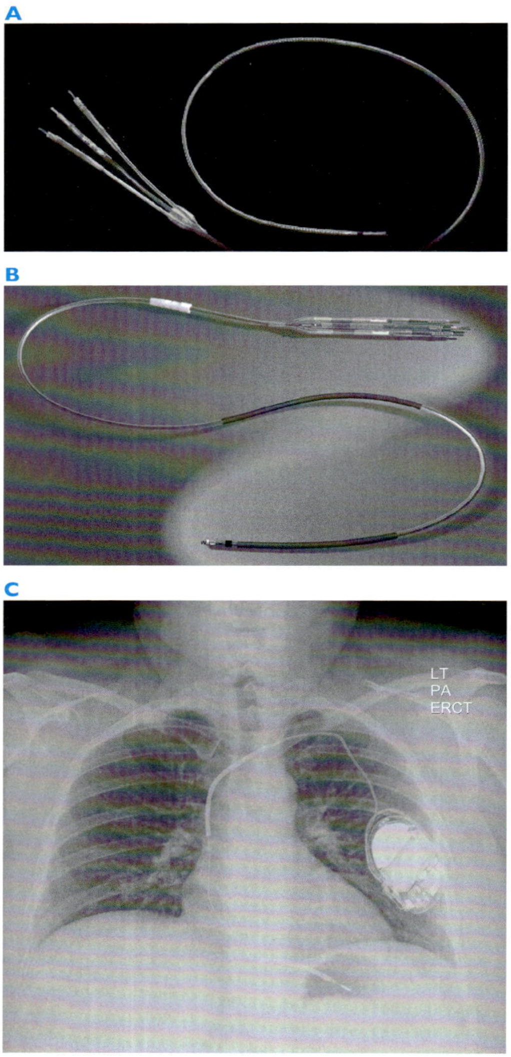

Fig 2.14 Endocardial lead systems. Examples of currently available transvenous ICD lead systems are shown. **A**: St. Jude Riata dual coil transvenous active fixation ICD lead (courtesy of St. Jude Medical). **B**: Medtronic Sprint Secure Model 6947 dual coil active fixation lead, with screw in the extended position (courtesy of Medtronic). **C**: Radiograph demonstrating positioning of a transvenous dual coil lead, with the distal coil at the RVA and proximal coil at the SVC/HRA junction.

tor header. During the implantation procedure, the pin of the lead connector should be clearly visualized by the implanting physician as it extends past the inner connector block before the set-screw is tightened.

The current standard for connectors includes a "DF-1" connection for the high-voltage portion, and an "IS-1" connection (6-mm termination) for the pace/sense portion of the lead (Fig 2.15). Due to the current standardization of the connections between the lead and pulse generator, different leads can be exchanged with pulse generators made by different manufacturers. Incompatibility of the lead connector with the pulse generator would require use of adaptors, which could reduce reliability of the system.

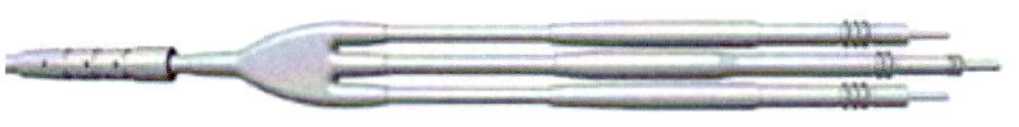

Fig 2.15 Connectors. This is an example of current connectors from the Sprint family of leads. The proximal end of the lead is composed of three connections, which are inserted separately into the header of pulse generator (courtesy of Medtronic).

At the present time, the proximal end of the lead is composed of three connections, which are inserted separately into the header of pulse generator. A new connector, "IS-4" (IS-4 terminal) may soon replace the current standard in defibrillation systems. This single connector includes both defibrillation and pacing elements, and would be connected to the pulse generator as a single unit. One potential disadvantage of this new system may be the inability to easily "cap" the proximal defibrillation coil, if a high defibrillation threshold (DFT) is noted and alternative configurations for DFT testing are necessary. However, the noninvasive capability of "eliminating" the proximal coil from the defibrillation system is now available in some ICD systems and obviates this problem.

Adaptors and Extenders

Lead adaptors may sometimes be needed to connect new replacement pulse generators to old pre-existing leads or to tie electrode combinations, such as connecting an SVC coil to a subcutaneous patch to allow them to work together as a common electrode. Extenders may be utilized if additional length is needed to match the two components. These adaptors and extenders must be reliable with similar performance characteristics present in the lead, as adaptor failure can result in failure of the defibrillator system. Older adaptors utilized medical adhesive to seal the set-screw, whereas newer adaptors use a set-screw seal.[52]

Lead Fixation

Similar to pacemaker leads, the distal tip of the defibrillation lead is fixed within the heart using either passive fixation tines or active fixation screws to assure lead stability (Fig 2.16, see following page). For active fixation leads, a retractable screw mechanism is typically present. The main advantage of active fixation is that the lead may be positioned in multiple locations, and is not limited to an RV apical location. In addition, active fixation leads may offer some advantage with respect to subsequent easier removal with extraction systems compared to passive leads.

Leads should also be anchored at the venous puncture site to help reduce lead dislodgment. Sutures should be tied around suture sleeves and not directly on the lead itself, to reduce insulation problems at the site of the ligature. Care should be taken to avoid excessive kinking or undue pressure on the leads in the pocket, to reduce insulation problems or connector fracture.

Steroid Elution

The benefits of steroid-eluting leads have been demonstrated for permanent pacemaker leads, and were previously discussed in the pacemaker lead section. Dexamethasone sodium phos-

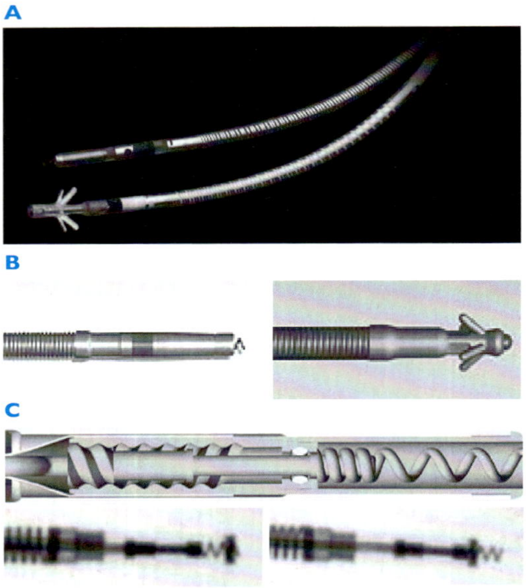

Fig 2.16. ICD lead fixation. Similar to pacemaker leads, ICD RV lead fixation may be either passive (tines) or active (retractable screw). **A**: Passive and active fixation systems in a St. Jude Medical Riata leads (courtesy of St. Jude Medical). **B**: Close-up views of the lead tips of Medtronic Sprint 6942 and 6943 leads, with active and passive fixation mechanisms (courtesy of Medtronic). **C**: Schematic of the retractable screw mechanism on a Boston Scientific lead (top) with the fluoroscopic appearance of the screw in the fully retracted (left) and fully extended (right) positions. (© Boston Scientific Corporation or its affiliates. All rights reserved. Used with permission of Boston Scientific Corporation.)

phate at the electrode-tissue interface helps to maintain chronically low stimulation thresholds. Steroid elution reduces the inflammatory response and attenuates the connective tissue reaction at the tip of the lead, resulting in a decrease in the peaking of pacing threshold, without adversely influencing chronic ventricular electrogram amplitude. This allows devices to be programmed at low pacing outputs to help increase device longevity. Defibrillator leads now also incorporate steroid elution.

Role of Lead Performance in Sensing Function

In addition to the defibrillation function of ICD leads, leads must provide reliable sensing of intracardiac signals to detect ventricular tachyarrhythmias and differentiate them from supraventricular rhythms. The system's ability to sense depends on the quality of the electrogram, the input amplifier, as well as the detection algorithm of the pulse generator. During the initial implantation procedure, R-wave amplitudes ≥ 5 mV tend to correlate with adequate ventricular electrogram amplitudes during VF, allowing appropriate detection of tachyarrhythmias. Although it is crucial to sense small amplitude signals during VF, it is also important for the defibrillator system to avoid oversensing of other intracardiac signals, such as T waves, or extracardiac signals, such as noise or myopotentials during sinus rhythm. Device amplifiers and detection algorithms are crucial for appropriate sensing; however, the need for high-quality lead performance with stability of electrograms is also essential. Endocardial leads may be associated with fibrotic reactions within the endocardium, and this could result in deterioration of intracardiac electrograms, thus impacting sensing function.

A registry of pacemaker and ICD pulse generators and leads identified that disrupted insulation accounted for 29% of ICD lead failures.[58] Failure of the conductor, electrode, fixation mechanism, or pin were identified as other causes of lead failure. Oversensing with delivery of inappropriate shocks was the most frequent consequence of ICD lead failure. Lead failure may also manifest as high or low impedance, noncapture, undersensing, or failure to defibrillate. Routine in-office or remote ICD follow-up to evaluate impedance and sensing/pacing functions may help detect unexpected lead failures before they become clinically manifested.

It is also important that rapid redetection of VF occurs after delivery of an unsuccessful first shock. As mentioned in a previous section, integrated bipolar leads were initially found to have longer redetection times than sensing with dedicated bipolar leads due to reductions in postshock R-wave amplitudes. This is likely due to the high-voltage field resulting in local myocardial stunning that is most apparent immediately postshock.[59] This may be due to lead design, specifically distance of the distal defibrillating coil from the rate-sensing cathode, when the distal defibrillating coil is utilized as the rate-sensing anode.[60] The problem improved when the spacing between the rate-sensing tip of the electrode and the distal coil was increased.[59,61] The redetection malfunction was never seen in patients with integrated bipolar systems when the distal coil to ring electrode distance was > 6 mm.[61] It should be noted that the distal end of the coil was separated from the tip electrode by only 6 mm in the early Guidant ENDOTAK-C 60 series, with a wider spacing (12 mm) in the subsequent ENDOTAK 70 series leads and in endocardial leads made by other manufacturers (Tables 2.1 and 2.2, see pages 52–61).

Subcutaneous Electrodes

Subcutaneous (SQ) patches, most often implanted in the left axillary region, have been utilized with endocardial defibrillation lead systems to lower the DFT. In addition to the axillary location, the SQ patch may be implanted in a more apical position. Prior to active can technology, the patch was also occasionally implanted in a high chest position beneath the left clavicle.

Array electrodes may also be implanted subcutaneously to lower the DFT. Both Boston Scientific and Medtronic have approved subcutaneous array electrodes for this purpose. The Boston Scientific lead is composed of three electrically common multifilar lead elements joined to a silicone yoke that attaches to a lead body and ends in a single, 6.1-mm titanium terminal pin. Each lead element is 25mm long and has a 6-Fr diameter, and is tunneled subcutaneously in the left lateral chest using a peel-away sheath. The pin is connected to the proximal coil of the endocardial lead using a Y adaptor. Use of the SQ array lead may lower the DFT by 10 J or more. Medtronic's system has a single element electrode for this purpose.

Other Defibrillator Electrodes

Although less of a problem with modern device technology, with availability of biphasic waveforms and active can devices, other additional electrodes may be added to achieve an adequate safety margin for defibrillation. When a single coil RV defibrillation lead results in an inadequate DFT, a separate SVC coil can be implanted. The addition of a coronary sinus (CS) defibrillation lead may also result in a reduction in the DFT. For example, a 7-Fr monopolar defibrillation lead (Medtronic model 6881) with a 50-mm coil electrode having a 90-mm^2 surface area can be inserted in the CS or SVC. Implantation of a transvenous lead system incorporating leads in the RVA, SVC, and CS or the combination of leads in the RVA, CS and subcutaneous patch have been shown to result in adequate DFTs at implantation. Implantation of a nonthoracotomy system that incorporates a CS lead has been found to be safe and effective. Due to the absence of any mechanism for active or passive fixation on the CS lead, the rate of dislodgment of CS leads used for defibrillation may be higher than RV leads. CS perforation does not appear to be a problem. Although there may be some evidence for thrombus formation in the CS, this does not appear to be a clinically significant issue.

Lead Determinants of Defibrillation Threshold (DFT)

Improvements in device technology, such as use of biphasic waveforms and active cans, have resulted in improved defibrillation efficacy, virtually eliminating the need for thoracotomy systems. Although advancements in device technology have clearly made a major impact on reduction of defibrillation requirements, the performance of the ICD system still depends in part on lead performance. Lead design characteristics, including conductor materials, wire thickness, lead body diameter, and lead construction technique will determine efficacy of the lead. The goal is to produce a lead that has low DFTs through a more uniform current distribution to the heart or a higher efficiency in delivering current. As shock distribution becomes nonuniform, DFTs will increase. If a lead is less efficient, DFTs will also be higher because a portion of the energy intended for delivery to the heart is lost near the surface of the defibrillation electrodes or inside the lead itself.[62]

Four basic design rules should be followed to enhance energy delivery through the lead, and include (1) minimizing electrode pullback, (2) delivering current to the apex, (3) minimizing energy loss within the lead, and (4) using efficient electrodes.[62]

(1) Electrode pullback: The term *pullback* is used to describe the distance between the lower active edge of the RV defibrillation electrode and the RV apex. In dedicated bipolar leads, sensing and pacing are performed through a pair of electrodes, separate from the defibrillation electrode (Fig 2.17). Sensing is accomplished utilizing an electrode at the tip of the lead and a ring electrode 1 to 2 cm proximal from the tip. The shocking electrode is proximal to these dedicated sensing/pacing electrodes. Medtronic and Biotronik ICD leads, and some St. Jude Medical leads, have utilized dedicated bipolar sensing. In contrast, in an integrated bipolar lead, rate sensing is accomplished between the catheter tip electrode and the RV defibrillation electrode. Therefore, the RV defibrillation electrode is typically closer to the tip of the lead because the separate rate sensing ring is not required (Fig 2.17). Many of the leads manufactured by St. Jude Medical, Boston Scientific, Telectronics, and Intermedics have incorporated this integrated bipolar strategy (Table 2.1).

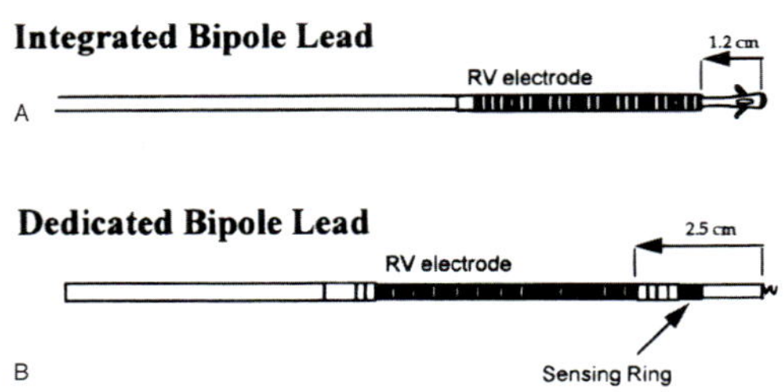

Fig 2.17 Design pullback. The impact of integrated bipolar and dedicated bipolar sensing methods on catheter design and the magnitude of the RV electrode pullback are illustrated. **A**, Leads using integrated bipolar sensing/pacing methods (from the tip to the RV defibrillation electrode) typically have a shorter pullback distance (eg, 1.2 cm in this figure). **B**, Leads using dedicated bipolar sensing/pacing methods have larger distances from the catheter tip to the active RV defibrillation electrode due to the presence of the sensing ring (e.g., 2.5 cm in this figure).[62] (Courtesy of Wiley-Blackwell. Used by permission.)

Endocardial leads with dedicated bipolar sensing must use a larger pullback (such as 2.5 cm in the Medtronic Transvene series) to provide space for the sensing ring between the tip of the lead and the RV defibrillation coil (Table 2.2). Even small differences in pullback may impact DFT.

(2) Location of current delivery: The goal in lead design is to deliver current as deep into the apex of the heart as possible. In addition to electrode pullback, the current distribution as it leaves the RV electrode is also important.[62] In addition to the resistance of the RV electrode material, the termination method in which the internal lead conductor is connected to the RV electrode can affect current distribution from the RV defibrillation electrode. Almost all endocardial defibrillation leads are constructed with the proximal termination technique, which connects the high-voltage conductor inside the lead body to the proximal end of the RV defibrillation electrode (Fig 2.18).[62] To optimize current distribution from the RV defibrillation electrode, defibrillation leads may also incorporate an internal shunting wire to connect the proximal and distal ends of the RV electrode, making the delivery of current balanced from both ends (Fig 2.18a). If the conductor terminates in the distal end, the defibrillation current is strongest at the terminal point (Fig 2.18c).

(3) Energy loss within the lead: During shock delivery, some energy is dissipated as heat inside the conductors of the lead and never reaches the heart. A lead with high performance would be one with a low-resistance lead body. This reduces energy loss inside the lead by minimizing the resistance of the conductors in the lead, enhancing efficiency and lowering DFT.[62]

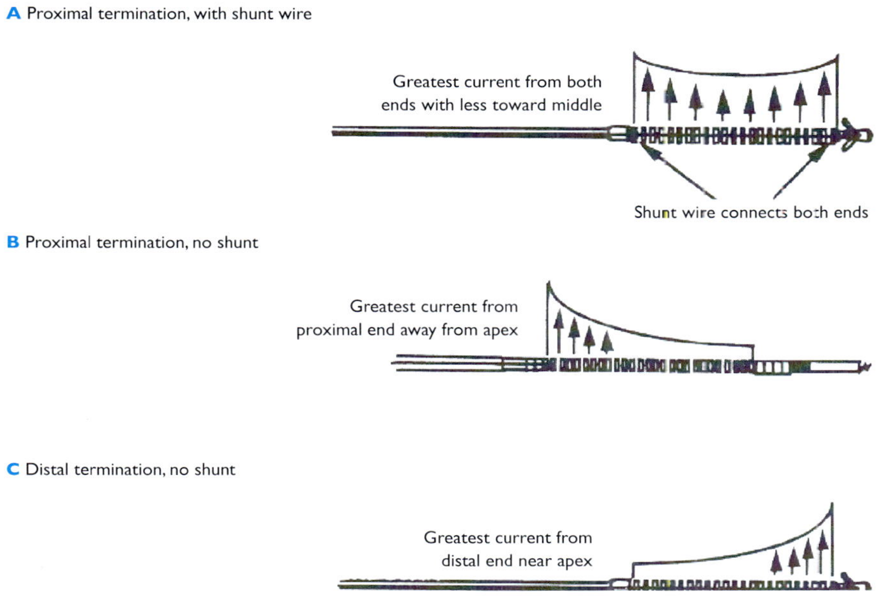

Fig 2.18 Distribution of defibrillation current along the defibrillation electrode: three methods of terminating the lead conductor to the RV electrode. **A**: The lead with the conductor terminated at the proximal end of the defibrillation electrode and a shunt wire connecting the proximal and distal electrode ends result in current delivery that is balanced from both ends of the electrode. **B**: A lead with the conductor terminated at the proximal end of the electrode and no shunt wire results in current delivery which is highest near the termination point at the proximal end and is weakest at the distal end near the apex of the heart. **C**: A lead with the conductor terminated at the distal end only, with no shunt wire, results in a defibrillation current that is strongest at the termination point at the distal end near the cardiac apex.[62] (Courtesy of Wiley-Blackwell. Used by permission.)

(4) Efficiency of electrodes: An additional goal for designing a high-performance lead is to use large, efficient electrodes. If the surface area of the defibrillation electrodes is too small, the ability to deliver current to the patient is limited.[62] An inefficient lead would have a high resistance and energy may be lost within a few centimeters of the electrode-heart interface. Design factors that influence electrode efficiency include the electrode material, the electrode's dimensions (length and diameter), and construction technique.[62] Increasing the length of the electrode may improve efficiency, but there are limitations on length of the RV defibrillation electrode due to the presence of the tricuspid valve. There appears to be a minimum SVC surface area needed to maintain defibrillation performance.[62]

Lead Coating

Coating of ICD leads with iridium oxide (IROX) results in a reduction of shock-induced polarization compared to an otherwise identical, uncoated lead.[63,64] Coating of transvenous leads with IROX (Model 497-20 Sulzer Intermedics, Inc, Angleton, TX, USA) exhibited lower DFTs than uncoated leads (Model 497-06, Sulzer Intermedics, Inc) in animal tests.[63,64] IROX coating applied to the surface of electrodes increases the microscopic surface area and reduces "crowding" of ions at the electrode-tissue interface by spreading out the charge, reducing the biphasic DFT.[63] However, these results could not be reproduced in humans (Biotronik, SPS 75 UP/BP, Berlin, Germany).[65] The reason for the discrepancy between human and animal data is unclear.

The increasing number of ICD implants is likely to result in an increased need for lead extraction. However, ICD lead extraction may be more complex than pacemaker lead extraction, as ICD leads are bulkier and shocking electrodes may uncoil with extraction techniques.[66] In addition, there is also a greater fibrotic reaction around the shocking coils due to the irregularity of the coils, leaving more space for inflammation and fibrous tissue in-growth. The ease of extraction may be improved with new Gore coated leads (Boston Scientific). This lead has a coating containing ePTFE, an expanded polytetrafluoroethylene polymer, which results in a reduction in the degree of fibrous tissue ingrowth at the shocking electrode surfaces. This Gore coating is electrically inert, without any effect on defibrillation thresholds.

Complications of ICD Leads

Complications of transvenous ICD leads include fracture, insulation breaks, dislodgment, perforation, and lead-header connection problems. The frequency of mechanical lead problems, such as lead dislodgment, perforation, subclavian crush, insulation breaks, or loose set-screws, has been reported to be 2% to 16% in large series.[45,48,67–81] An exceptionally high complication rate of 56% was seen in a single study in which ENDOTAK-C leads were utilized in conjunction with subcutaneous patch electrodes.[82] Using a Medicare database, the overall incidence of mechanical complications associated with ICD implantation has been reported to be 8.3% at 90 days.[83] The NCDR ICD registry has reported a lead dislodgment rate of 1% and perforation rate of 0.07%, but this is clearly an underestimation of complications due to inclusion of only in-hospital data.[84]

The true incidence of lead complications directly related to failure of the endocardial defibrillation lead itself will require continued long-term follow-up, as more lead problems will be detected with continued lead "wear and tear" over time. Due to expanding ICD indications and the number of patients receiving initial implants and replacements, the number of patients with longer follow-up will continue to increase. Fifteen percent of all ICD leads (Medtronic, St. Jude Medical, Biotronik, CPI, ELA) failed during a median follow-up of 934 days. The annual rate of ICD lead defects that require surgical intervention increased over time and reached 20% in 10-year-old leads, affecting all models in one study.[85] Women seemed to be more prone to lead failure.[85]

The reported incidence of lead-related complications varies widely, and may be due to patient selection, lead design, venous approach, implanter experience, pulse generator location, size of the pulse generator, and duration of follow-up. For example, a cephalic vein cutdown approach appears to be associated with a reduced incidence of lead failure compared to a subclavian venous stick. The risk of failure tends to increase over time, and appears to be particularly high during the first year following reoperation for battery depletion.[74] Problems also appear to be more frequent when adaptors between the pulse generator and the lead or extenders are used.[48]

In addition to mechanical complications, other complications related to endocardial lead systems include subclavian venous thrombosis or obstruction, particularly in patients who have multiple leads in place, and endovascular infection. Mechanical complications may also be seen with subcutaneous patches, including fractures, dislodgment, crinkling, and erosion. Fractures of patch leads may be initially asymptomatic and may be detectable by chest X-ray.

Acute Lead Failure

Acute lead failure is often caused by early lead dislodgment resulting in high stimulation thresholds, often requiring surgical intervention to correct the problem. A higher dislodgment rate may be seen with transvenous systems that use a separate SVC coil, as these defibrillation coils do not incorporate a fixation mechanism.[46] Dislodgment of the SVC lead may lead to an increase in the defibrillation threshold, or may be asymptomatic and detected on routine X-ray. A high incidence of lead dislodgment may be seen with defibrillation leads placed in the CS.[86] Earlier studies reported lead migration or dislodgment occurring in 10% of cases, with a reduction in the incidence of lead dislodgment (3%) later in the study, reflecting more experience and improved anchoring techniques.[86] Lead dislodgment may be asymptomatic or may result in oversensing or undersensing, when a sensing lead is involved, or ineffective defibrillation, when a defibrillation lead is involved.

Acute lead failure may also be due to cardiac perforation. This may result in pain, which is often pleuritic, high pacing thresholds, noncapture, undersensing, diaphragmatic pacing, or tamponade. A loose set-screw or loose connector may result in oversensing of noise, and may also occur early following implantation. These problems can be easily corrected with surgical intervention.

Chronic Lead Failure

Chronic lead failure is most often a result of insulation defects or fractured conductors. Signs of sensing lead failure may include oversensing or undersensing. Oversensing during the intrinsic rhythm may lead to inappropriate shocks, aborted shocks, or inhibition of pacing. Undersensing during VF may lead to failure of detection or prolonged arrhythmia detection leading to no therapy or a delay in therapy. Undersensing during the intrinsic rhythm may lead to inappropriate asynchronous pacing. Defects with the defibrillation portion of the lead may result in failure to effectively defibrillate ventricular arrhythmias.

Conductor fractures can lead to an increase in pacing impedance, intermittent loss of sensing or pacing, complete failure to sense or pace, or oversensing. Insulation defects may result in a decrease in pacing impedance and can also lead to oversensing or undersensing problems. If the insulation defect involves the outer insulation and the stress point is located at an extracardiac site, stimulation of the pectoral muscle or diaphragm may also be seen. If the inner insulation is also involved, intermittent or complete loss of pacing may also occur.[50] It should also be noted that insulation failure may be associated with normal values of impedance, sensing, and pacing thresholds at the time when lead failure is diagnosed.[74] Due to similar clinical manifestations of conductor and insulation problems, the exact cause of lead failure may not always be apparent, particularly before surgical intervention.

As previously discussed, polyurethane leads with a coaxial design are susceptible to inner insulation failure and shorts between the conductors, often caused by metal ion oxidation. Silicone-coated leads with multi-lumen design are prone to erosions of the insulation, particularly in abdominal locations, likely related to abrasion of the insulation resulting from direct contact of the lead with the large pulse generator.[50] Continuous or forceful traction of the lead during implantation may also result in tearing of the insulation. This emphasizes the importance of correct lead handling and the potential contribution of daily strenuous activities on lead reliability. Lead compression under the clavicle is a well-known cause of conductor failure or damage to the insulation. A lateral or cephalic vein cut-down approach may help reduce subclavian crush injuries.

Polyurethane coaxial leads, particularly with subpectoral ICDs, have been reported to have high failure rates.[74,87] The Medtronic Transvene single coil, coaxial polyurethane leads (model numbers 6936/6966) comprised 54% of ICD lead failures detected by a multicenter registry.[87] The mean time to failure for these leads was 4.8 ± 2.1 years, with an increased failure rate over time.[74,87,88] Lead survival analysis of the Medtronic polyurethane coaxial 6963 lead revealed a cumulative failure probability of 37% at a mean follow-up of 69 months in another study.[88] Insulation defects, pace/sense conductor fractures, or high-voltage coil fracture may be involved in the structural failure of these particular leads.[87] (It should be noted that the middle insulation layer of the 6936 lead is 80A polyurethane, the same polyurethane used to manufacture Medtronic 4004 and 4012 pacing leads, which also had a high failure rate.) A unique mode of failure of this lead included oversensing of electrical noise following shocks, and early detection of lead failure could be identified by short RR intervals on the counters.[88]

One study comparing the incidence of structural failure in a dedicated bipolar sensing lead (CPI BT-10) with that of an integrated lead (CPI ENDOTAK) in patients undergoing abdominal ICD implant found a failure rate of 17.8% with the BT-10 lead compared to 4.3% with the ENDOTAK lead after a mean follow-up of 29 months ($p < 0.01$).[69] Lead failure was thought to be related to insulation defects in all cases, typically with the problem occurring in the proximal portion of the lead within the generator pocket. One possible reason for the high failure rate may be related to trauma to the lead during tunneling, although tunneling technique was the same for both leads. Another potential reason for lead failure is the mechanical force of the heavy pulse generator against a non-reinforced lead, leading to insulation wear, with a lower rate of problems seen with the more reinforced ENDOTAK lead. Abdominal ICD implantation does appear to be associated with a higher lead failure rate, and this failure rate increases over time.[50] Mechanical stresses on the lead from tunneling to the abdomen and wear on the lead from a heavy pulse generator may contribute to insulation problems.

The first-generation endocardial defibrillation lead system (CPI ENDOTAK-C), often used in conjunction with a SQ patch, was associated with an extremely high rate of lead-related complications occurring in 56% of patients after a mean follow-up of only 51 weeks.[82] These complications included conductor fractures which could be fatal. Patch electrode conductor fractures were also observed. Due to an unacceptably high incidence of lead fracture, the high-energy conductor was changed from a coiled wire to Teflon-coated braided flexible cable, which appeared to solve this problem.[89]

The management of sensing lead failure in patients with integrated bipolar endocardial defibrillator leads (such as the ENDOTAK lead) is controversial. Although practice at some centers may be to replace the sensing lead alone, assuming the "independent" function of the sensing component in the circuit based on lead design, late failure of defibrillation has also been reported to occur years later. [90] This raises a concern about the long-term reliability of defibrillation once a sensing lead problem is diagnosed in patients with integrated bipolar leads. Therefore, revision using a new defibrillator lead may be considered.

Lead failure from conductor and/or insulation damage just beyond the stiff terminal ring of the IS-1 rate sensing terminal connector has been reported with one Guidant ENDOTAK lead (DSP model 0125). This lead was placed on advisory in 1999 with a technical memo reporting the potential problems with the long IS-1 terminal pin connector. Lead failure occurred in 3.5% of patients who underwent pectoral ICD implantation using a submuscular approach after a mean follow-up of only 16 months.[91] This was related to extension of the metal terminal ring beyond the header, when a smaller pulse generator was utilized, resulting in excessive stress and disruption of insulation or conductors in this area. Lead problems presented with asymptomatic oversensing or inappropriate shocks.

The Medtronic Sprint Fidelis ICD lead (6.6 Fr, models 6948 and 6949) was removed from the market in 2007 after 665 failures and five reported deaths. There was a greater-than-expected failure rate which was initially estimated to be 2.3% at 30 months. This lead is prone to early fracture of the pace/sense conductor and coil and the high-voltage conductor.[92,93] Pace-sense conductor and coil fractures can be detected by lead impedance measurements, assessment of short RR interval counters, threshold evaluation, and review of intracardiac electrograms. High-voltage conductor fracture may be clinically silent, but manifest by high impedance. Subsequent study has revealed that the failure rate was 3.75% per year, and the 3-year estimated lead longevity was only 88%, significantly lower than other contemporary ICD leads.[92] Most Sprint Fidelis failures were due to pace/sense conductor fracture, which often led to inappropriate shocks. The hazard of Sprint Fidelis fracture also appears to be increasing, whereas the failure rates of other ICD leads are low and stable over time. Although routine prophylactic replacement of this lead in all patients is not recommended, the decision about potentially replacing the lead at generator replacement should be individualized and based on patient history, clinical characteristics, and ICD/pacing indication.

Despite improvements in ICD lead technology, the lead itself does appear to be the "weakest link" in the ICD system. It is anticipated that the number of failing leads will continue to increase over time as more patients, particularly younger patients, have leads in place for many years with multiple generator replacements. The need for lead removal will likely also increase over time.

Reporting of Lead Failure

There have been inadequate reporting mechanisms to identify lead failure in the ICD industry. Device manufacturers provide product performance reports supplying information to physicians regarding device survivability, including information regarding particular devices that have a higher-than-expected failure rate. Some systems "on advisory" may warrant closer follow-up. Recommendations regarding policies and guidelines related to product performance have been published.[3]

Returned product analysis (RPA) provides a means for manufacturers to examine products that have been explanted and returned to the manufacturer, and this may help determine the mechanism of failure. However, most leads that have failed are not explanted; therefore reports of failure will be grossly underestimated by this type of reporting mechanism. In a prospective lead follow-up study, the Tachyarrhythmia Chronic System Study (TCSS), participating centers provided clinical observations related to leads, as well as information regarding whether the lead was explanted, abandoned, replaced, or if reprogramming was performed to rectify problems. This study did not require return of the lead for analysis to be counted as a "failing lead." The proportion of nonperforming leads detected by the TCSS was 2.2% compared to 0.5% using the RPA ($p < 0.001$).[94] Therefore, prospective follow-up of chronic leads by the TCSS provided a more accurate basis for determination of ICD lead failure than the RPA. In addition, a revision to the current NCDR ICD registry is also planned. This will now include information on specific leads at the time of initial ICD implantation and generator replacement, which will contribute to a better understanding of the frequency and time course of chronic lead failure.

Leads Used for Cardiac Resynchronization Therapy

Multiple clinical trials have demonstrated the benefit of CRT in the treatment of patients with congestive heart failure, LV dysfunction and a wide QRS, with and without ICD backup. The ACC/AHA/HRS Guidelines reflect these clinical trial results, and CRT therapy is indicated in patients with NYHA class III-IV congestive heart failure, LVEF ≤ 35%, and a wide QRS complex.[1]

Following visualization of the branches of the coronary sinus, which is typically performed using CS angiography, LV leads are placed into venous branches to pace the LV and thus resynchronize myocardial contraction. The site of LV pacing may play an important role in efficacy of resynchronization therapy. Therefore, it is important to be able to direct these leads into specific branches. This can be accomplished with leads that have a variety of shapes, and these shapes can be altered by use of a stylet-driven lead system. In addition, over-the-wire capability is also available to aid insertion of the lead into specific CS venous branches (Fig 2.19). More recent advancements in technology now also include a variety of inner and outer sheaths with different shapes, steerable sheaths, and even a steerable lead.

Many of the LV leads have preshaped distal curves, which are designed to increase stability within the CS branch. When the stylet is inserted into the distal tip of the lead, the lead is straightened. As the stylet is withdrawn, the

A

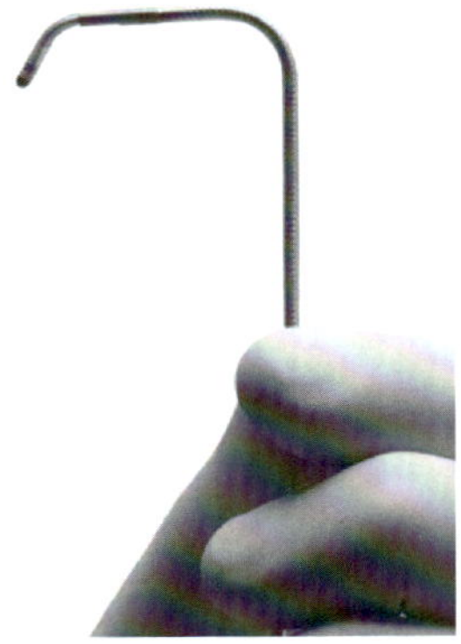

Fig 2.19 LV pacing leads. A variety of different LV pacing leads are now available with different sizes and shapes. **A**: Medtronic Attain bipolar LV lead. (Courtesy of Medtronic, Inc. Used with permission.) **B**: St. Jude QuickSite LV bipolar and unipolar leads with a variety of different S shapes. (Courtesy of Medtronic, Inc. Used with permission.) **C**: Biotronik Corox OTW BP Left Ventricular Lead (helical shape). (Courtesy of Biotronik. Used with permission.) **D**: Boston Scientific Acuity steerable steroid-eluting LV bipolar pace/sense lead with a pre-formed J shape. (© Boston Scientific Corporation or its affiliates. All rights reserved. Used with permission of Boston Scientific Corporation.) **E**: Boston Scientific Easytrak family of leads, including LV leads with tines. (© Boston Scientific Corporation or its affiliates. All rights reserved. Used with permission of Boston Scientific Corporation.) **F**: Attain StarFix active fixation LV lead with deployable lobes. (Courtesy of Medtronic, Inc. Used with permission.)

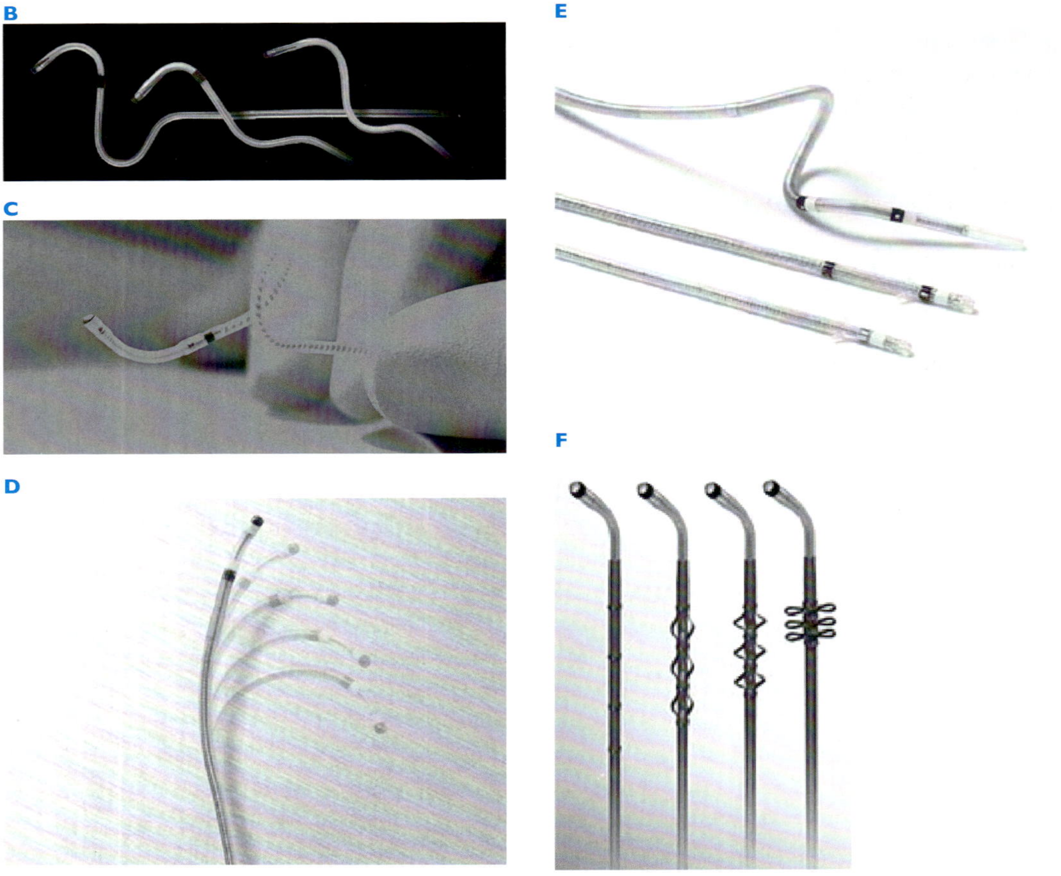

lead assumes its shape with a curve on the end. Many leads have a combination of stylet-driven and over-the-wire capabilities.

LV lead choices include unipolar and bipolar leads. Due to advancements in pulse generator technology, bipolar leads offer multiple pacing configuration choices, allowing selection of the configuration with the "best" threshold, while avoiding phrenic nerve stimulation. One advantage of unipolar leads is the small French size, with the smallest unipolar LV lead now at 4.1 Fr (Boston Scientific Acuity Spiral LV lead).

Advancements in lead technology also provide bipolar leads with much smaller caliber (5 Fr) than earlier leads (7 Fr and 6 Fr), and these bipolar leads may now also be maneuvered into small venous branches. Table 2.3 outlines specifications regarding LV leads (See pages 62–64).

It should be noted that LV leads have a higher rate of lead dislodgment than RV and RA leads. This is likely related to the absence of any "active" fixation mechanism. As noted previously, many of these leads have preshaped distal curves, which become apparent when the stylet is removed, designed to increase stability. Some LV leads have tines (Fig 2.19E), but the absence of trabeculation within the venous branches may still limit stability of these leads compared to RV leads. The size of the venous branch may also impact lead stability, and LV leads are available in a variety of sizes. In addition, one LV active fixation lead (Medtronic Attain StarFix) has deployable lobes to allow greater stability (Fig 2.19F). A 0% dislodgment rate has been reported with this active fixation lead.[95]

In addition to lead dislodgment, another complication of LV lead placement is diaphragmatic pacing. This is related to phrenic nerve stimulation, as this nerve may be in close proximity to lateral venous branches. The newer, smaller caliber leads tend to have lower pacing thresholds, and therefore pacing output may be minimized, often reducing or eliminating diaphragmatic pacing. LV lead technology now includes bipolar LV pacing capabilities, which allows multiple pacing configurations through CRT devices with enhanced programmability. The options available for pacing configurations will depend on the specific pulse generator model. Additional pacing configurations can be tested to reduce diaphragmatic pacing and improve LV pacing thresholds (Fig 2.20).

Some of the earliest CRT-ICDs did not have the availability of separate RV sensing, and the sensing circuit included both the RV and LV electrograms. In addition, prior to approval of the first CRT-ICD, an external adaptor was sometimes utilized to connect RV and LV leads for pacing, again resulting in a single sensing circuit that included both RV and LV electrograms. This often led to "double-counting" of the RV and LV signals, with inappropriate shock delivery for sinus tachycardia or atrial arrhythmias. With the current generation of CRT devices, separate RV sensing is routinely available, eliminating this problem.

Steroid-elution is frequently utilized with permanent pacing leads and ICD leads, and is also available with LV leads. Satisfactory pacing and sensing parameters have been demonstrated acutely and during follow-up of these

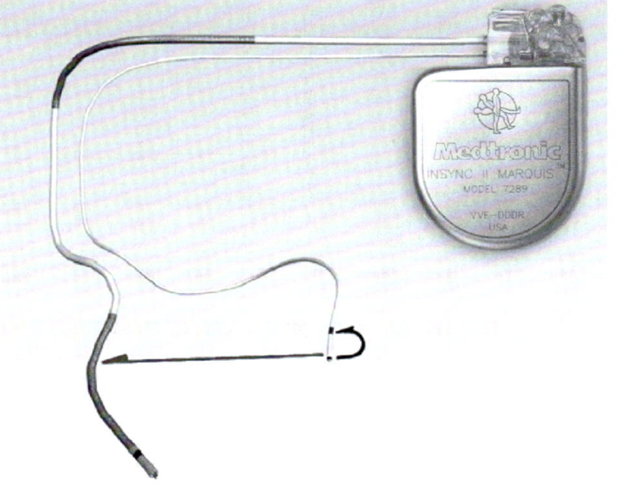

Fig 2.20 Bipolar LV lead and pacing options. In addition to LV bipolar pacing (LV tip to LV ring), the availability of a bipolar LV lead allows several different options for pacing, depending on enhanced programming options present in the selected pulse generator. For example, pacing may be performed between the LV tip and the RV coil, as shown here. (Courtesy of Medtronic, Inc. Used with permission.)

leads. Pacing threshold has been shown to stabilize 2 weeks after implantation and sensing threshold has remained stable from implant to 4-month follow-up.[96]

Summary and Future Outlook

ICDs have become the standard of care for secondary and now primary prevention of sudden cardiac death. Technological advances, including the development and refinement of ICD lead technology, have been largely responsible for the widespread expansion of ICD usage. However, lead failures remain an important complication of ICD therapy, despite technological advances. Insulation defects or fractured conductors may impact the quality of life of ICD patients, as well as impact device efficacy and costs. Additional advancements in lead technology are still clearly needed, especially given that more patients are receiving devices at a younger age and may require multiple generator replacements throughout their lifetime.

Lead development has so far focused on new materials and designs, size reductions, improved steering and handling, and maintenance of long-term reliability. The IS-1 pacing and DF-1 shocking standards for the lead/device interface may be updated to an IS-4 terminal, which will allow a reduction in the connector/header size. Newer lead designs may further aid in the ease of ICD lead extraction. Additional advances in LV lead technology may further increase the number of potential LV pacing configurations with availability of multiple LV electrodes. In addition, further investigation will hopefully determine ways to further increase the long-term reliability and reduce the failure rate of endocardial leads.

As the endocardial lead appears to be the weakest link in the ICD system, investigation is currently underway to evaluate the safety and efficacy of a totally subcutaneous ICD lead system. The initial prototypes (Cameron Health) include a subcutaneous coil implanted to the left of the sternum and an active can pulse generator implanted subcutaneously in the left chest.[97] However, these totally subcutaneous lead systems still involve leads, although implanted outside the venous system. Lead problems have been previously identified with subcutaneous patches, and subcutaneous coils are likely not immune to problems. Therefore, development of lead systems with better durability and greater resistance to damage is still needed. Finally, close follow-up of all ICD systems is still warranted to help detect early lead problems prior to clinical manifestations that may impact on morbidity, mortality, and quality of life of the ICD patient.

References

1. Epstein AE, DiMarco JP, Ellenbogen KA, et al. ACC/AHA/HRS 2008 guidelines for device-based therapy of cardiac rhythm abnormalities: a report of the American College of Cardiology/American Heart Association Task Force on Practice Guidelines. *J Am Coll Cardiol.* 2008;51:1–62.
2. Zipes DP, Camm AJ, Borggrefe M, et al. ACC/AHA/ESC 2006 guidelines for management of patients with ventricular arrhythmias and the prevention of sudden cardiac death: a report of the American College of Cardiology/American Heart Association Task Force and the European Society of Cardiology Committee for Practice Guidelines (Writing Committee to Develop Guidelines for Management of Patients With Ventricular Arrhythmias and the Prevention of Sudden Cardiac Death). *J Am Coll Cardiol.* 2006;48:247–346.
3. Maisel WH, Hauser RG, Hammill SC, et al. for the Heart Rhythm Society Task Force on Lead Performance Policies and Guidelines; American College of Cardiology (ACC); American Heart Association (AHA). Recommendations from the Heart Rhythm Society Task Force on Lead Performance Policies and Guidelines: developed in collaboration with the American College of Cardiology (ACC) and the American Heart Association (AHA). *Heart Rhythm.* 2009;6:869–885.
4. Wilkoff BL, Auricchio A, Brugada J, et al. for the

Heart Rhythm Society; European Heart Rhythm Association; American College of Cardiology; American Heart Association; European Society of Cardiology; Heart Failure Association of ESC; Heart Failure Society of America. HRS/EHRA expert consensus on the monitoring of cardiovascular implantable electronic devices (CIEDs): description of techniques, indications, personnel, frequency and ethical considerations. *Heart Rhythm.* 2008;5:907–925.

5. Hayes DL, Lloyd MA, Friedman PA. Clinically relevant basics of pacing and defibrillation. In: Hayes DL, ed. *Cardiac Pacing and Defibrillation: A Clinical Approach.* Malden, MA: Blackwell Publishing; 2000.
6. Mond HG. Unipolar versus bipolar pacing: poles apart. *Pacing Clin Electrophysiol.* 1991;14:1411.
7. Wiegand UK, Bode F, Bonnemeier H, et al. Incidence and predictors of pacemaker dysfunction with unipolar ventricular lead configuration. Can we identify patients who benefit from bipolar electrodes? *Pacing Clin Electrophysiol.* 2001;24:1383–1388.
8. Ellenbogen KA, Wood MA, Gilliagan DM, et al, and the CapSure Z Investigators. Steroid-eluting high-impedance pacing leads decrease short and long-term current drain: Results from a multicenter clinical trial. *Pacing Clin Electrophysiol.* 1999;22:39–48.
9. Moracchini PV, Cornacchia D, Bernasconi M, et al. High impedance low energy pacing leads: Long-term results with a very small surface area steroid-eluting lead compared to three conventional electrodes. *Pacing Clin Electrophysiol.* 1999;22:326–334.
10. Deshmukh P, Casavant D, Anderson K, Romanyshyn M. Stable electrical performance of high efficiency pacing leads having small surface, steroid-eluting pacing electrodes. *Pacing Clin Electrophysiol.* 1999;22:1599–1603.
11. Berger T, Roithinger FX, Antretter H, et al. The influence of high versus normal impedance ventricular leads on pacemaker generator longevity. *Pacing Clin Electrophysiol.* 2003;26:2116–2120.
12. Scherer M, Ezziddin K, Klesius A, et al. Extension of generator longevity by use of high impedance ventricular leads. *Pacing Clin Electrophysiol.* 2001;24:206–211.
13. Mond HG. Engineering and clinical aspects of pacing leads. In: Ellenbogen K, Wilkoff E., eds. *Clinical Cardiac Pacing and Defibrillation,* 2nd ed. Philadelphia: WB Saunders; 2000.
14. Luria D, Gurevitz O, Bar Lev D, et al. Use of automatic threshold tracking function with non-low polarization leads. *Pacing Clin Electrophysiol.* 2004;27:453–459.
15. Hirshorn MS, Holley LK, Skalsky M, et al. Characteristics of advanced porous and textured surface pacemaker electrodes. *Pacing Clin Electrophysiol.* 1983;6:525–536.
16. Amundson DC, McArthur W, Mosharrafa M. The porous endocardial electrode. *Pacing Clin Electrophysiol.* 1979;2:40–50.
17. Djordjevic M, Stojanov P, Velimirovic D. Target lead: Low threshold electrode. *Pacing Clin Electrophysiol.* 1986;9:1206.
18. Parsonnet V, Villaneuva A, Driller J, Bernstein AD. Corrosion of pacemaker electrodes. *Pacing Clin Electrophysiol.* 1981;4:289–296.
19. Elmqvist H, Schueller H, Richter G. The carbon tip electrode. *Pacing Clin Electrophysiol.* 1983;6:436–439.
20. Mugica J, Henry L, Attuel P, et al. Clinical experience with 910 carbon tip leads: Comparison with polished platinum leads. *Pacing Clin Electrophysiol.* 1986 9:1230–1238.
21. Mond HG, Grenz D. Implantable transvenous pacing leads: The shape of things to come. *Pacing Clin Electrophysiol.* 2004;27:887–893.
22. Breivik K, Danilovic D, Ohm OJ, et al. Clinical evaluation of thin bipolar pacing lead. *Pacing Clin Electrophysiol.* 1997;20:637–646.
23. Crossley GH. Cardiac pacing leads. In: *Cardiology Clinics,* Philadelphia: WB Saunders; February 2000.
24. Scheuer-Lesser M, Irnich W, Kreuzer J. Polyurethane leads: Facts and controversy. *Pacing Clin Electrophysiol.* 1983;5:454–458.
25. Byrd CL, McArthur W, Stokes K, et al. Implant experience with unipolar polyurethane pacing leads. *Pacing Clin Electrophysiol.* 1983;6:868–882.
26. Woscoboinik JR, Maloney JD, Helguera ME, et al. Pacing lead survival: Performance of different models. *Pacing Clin Electrophysiol.* 1992;15:1991–1995.

27. Hayes DL, Graham KJ, Irwin M, et al. A multicenter experiences with a bipolar tined polyurethane ventricular lead. *Pacing Clin Electrophysiol.* 1992;15:1033–1039.
28. Sweesy MW, Forney CC, Hayes DL, et al. Evaluation of an in-line bipolar polyurethane ventricular pacing lead. *Pacing Clin Electrophysiol.* 1992;15:1982–1985.
29. Hayes DL, Graham KJ, Irwin M, et al. Multicenter experience with a bipolar tined polyurethane ventricular lead. *Pacing Clin Electrophysiol.* 1995;18:999–1004.
30. Antonelli D, Rosenfeld T, Freedberg NA, et al. Insulation lead failure: Is it a matter of insulation coating, venous approach, or both? *Pacing Clin. Electrophysiol.* 1998;21:418–421.
31. Cameron J, Mond H, Ciddor G, Harper K, McKie J. Stiffness of the distal tip of bipolar pacemaker leads. *Pacing Clin Electrophysiol.* 1990;13:1915–1920.
32. Mugica J, Daubert JC, Lazarus B, et al. Is polyurethane lead insulation still controversial? *Pacing Clin Electrophysiol.* 1992;15:1967–1970.
33. Mond H, Hua W, Wang CC. Atrial pacing leads: The clinical contribution of steroid elution. *Pacing Clin Electrophysiol.* 1995;18:1601.
34. Crossley GH, Brinkler JA, Reynolds D, et al. Steroid elution improves the stimulation threshold in an active-fixation atrial permanent pacing lead. *Circulation.* 1995;92:2935–2939.
35. Mond H, Stokes KB. The steroid-eluting electrode: A 10-year experience. *Pacing Clin Electrophysiol.* 1997;19:1016–1020.
36. Kay GN, Brinker JA, Kawanishi DT, et al, Risks of Spontaneous Injury and Extraction of an Active Fixation Pacemaker Lead: Report of the Accufix Multicenter Clinical Study and Worldwide Registry. *Circulation.* 1999;100:2344–2352.
37. Parsonnet V, Roelke M, Bernstien AD, Stern M. Reduced frequency of retention wire fractures suggests that elective explantation of affected atrial leads is no longer indicated. *Pacing Clin Electrophysiol.* 2000;23:380–383.
38. Lloyd MA, Hayes D, Holmes DR Jr. Atrial J-pacing lead retention wire fracture: Radiographic assessment, incidence of fracture and clinical management. *Pacing Clin Electrophysiol.* 1995;18:95–964.
39. Saliba BC, Ardesia RJ, John RM, et al. Predictors of fracture in the Accufix atrial "J" lead. *Am J Cardiol.* 1997;80:229–231.
40. Kawanishi DT, Brinker JA, Reeves R, et al. Cumulative hazard analysis of J-wire fracture in the Accufix series of atrial permanent pacemaker leads. *Pacing Clin Electrophysiol.* 1998;21:2322–2326.
41. Mirowski M, Mower MM, Reid PR, Watkins L Jr. Implantable automatic defibrillators: Their potential in prevention of sudden coronary death. *Ann NY Acad Sci.* 1982;382:371–380.
42. Mirowski M, Reid PR, Mower MM, et al. Termination of malignant ventricular arrhythmias with an implanted automatic defibrillator in human beings. *N Engl J Med.* 1980;303:322–324.
43. Troup PJ, Chapman PD, Olinger GN, Kleinman LH. The implanted defibrillator: Relation of defibrillating lead configuration and clinical variables to defibrillation threshold. *J Am Coll Cardiol.* 1985;6:1315–1321.
44. Accorti PR. Leads technology. In: Singer I, ed. *Implantable Cardioverter Defibrillator.* Armonk, NY: Futura Publishing; 1994.
45. Almassi GH, Olinger GN, Wetherbee JN, Fehl G. Long-term complications of implantable cardioverter defibrillator lead systems. *Ann Thorac Surg.* 1993;55:888–892.
46. Korte T, Jung W, Spehl S, et al. Incidence of ICD lead related complications during long-term follow-up: Comparison of epicardial and endocardial electrode systems. *Pacing Clin Electrophysiol.* 1995;18:2053–2061.
47. Mattke S, Muller D, Markewitz A, et al. Failures of epicardial and transvenous leads for implantable cardioverter defibrillators. *Am Heart J.* 1995;130:1040–1044.
48. Stambler BS, Wood MA, Damiano RJ, et al. Sensing/pacing lead complications with a newer generation implantable cardioverter defibrillator: Worldwide experience from the Guardian ATP 4210 clinical trial. *J Am Coll Cardiol.* 1994;23:123–132.
49. Daoud EG, Kirsh MM, Bolling SF, et al. Incidence, presentation, diagnosis, and management of malfunctioning implantable cardioverter defibrillator rate sensing leads. *Am Heart J.* 1994; 128:892–895.

50. Gradaus R, Breithardt G, Bocker D. ICD leads: Design and chronic dysfunctions. *Pacing Clin Electrophysiol.* 2003;26:649–657.
51. Russo AM, Marchlinski FE. Engineering and construction of pacemaker and implantable cardioverter Defibrillator Leads. In: Ellenbogen KA, ed. *Clinical Cardiac Pacing, Defibrillation, and Resynchronization Therapy,* 3rd ed, Philadelphia: Saunders Elsevier; 2007.
52. Nelson RS, Gilman BL, Shapland JE, Lehmann MH. Leads for the ICD. In: Kroll MW, Lehmann MH, eds. *Implantable Cardioverter Defibrillator Therapy.* Massachusetts: Kluwer Academic Publishers; 1996.
53. Fotuhi P, Alt E, Callihan R, et al. Endocardial carbon braid electrodes: New approach to lowering defibrillation thresholds. *Pacing Clin Electrophysiol.* 1993;16:1919A.
54. Alt E, Theres H, Heinz M, et al. A new approach towards defibrillation electrodes: Highly conductive isotropic carbon fibers. *Pacing Clin Electrophysiol.* 1991;14:1923–1928.
55. Jacobs DM, Fink AS, Miller RP, et al. Anatomical and morphological evaluation of pacemaker lead compression. *Pacing Clin Electrophysiol.* 1993;16:434–444.
56. Magney JE, Flynn DM, Parsons JA, et al. Anatomical mechanisms explaining damage to pacemaker leads, defibrillator leads, and failure of central venous catheters adjacent to the sternoclavicular joint. *Pacing Clin Electrophysiol.* 1993;16:445–457.
57. Winkle RA, Bach SM, Mead RH, et al. Comparison of defibrillation efficacy in humans using a new catheter and superior vena cava spring left ventricular patch electrode. *J Am Coll Cardiol.* 1988;11;365–370.
58. Hauser R, Hayes D, Parsonnet V, et al. Feasibility and initial results of an internet-based pacemaker and ICD pulse generator and lead registry. *Pacing Clin Electrophysiol.* 2001;24:82–87.
59. Gold MR, Shorofsky SR. Transvenous defibrillation lead systems. *J Cardiovasc Electrophysiol.* 1996;7:570–580.
60. Gottlieb CD, Schwartzman DS, Callans DJ, Dillon SM, Marchlinski FE. Effects of high and low shock energies on sinus electrograms recorded via integrated and true bipolar nonthoracotomy lead systems. *J Cardiovasc Electrophysiol.* 1996;7:189–195.
61. Natale A, Sra J, Axtell K, et al. Undetected ventricular fibrillation in transvenous implantable cardioverter defibrillators: Prospective comparison of different lead system-device combinations. *Circulation.* 1996;93:91–98.
62. Lang DJ, Heil JE, Hahn SJ, Lindstrom CC, Derfus DL. Implantable cardioverter defibrillator lead technology: Improved performance and lower defibrillation thresholds. *Pacing Clin Electrophysiol.* 1995;18:548–559.
63. Niebauer MJ, Yamanouchi Y, Hills D, et al. Voltage dependence of ICD lead polarization and the effect of iridium oxide coating. *Pacing Clin Electrophysiol.* 2000;23:818–823.
64. Niebauer MJ, Wilkoff B, Yamanouchi Y, et al. Iridium oxide-coated defibrillation electrode: Reduced shock polarization and improved defibrillation efficacy. *Circulation.* 1997;96:3732–3736.
65. Gradaus R, Bocker D, Dorszewski A, et al. Fractally coated defibrillation electrodes: Is an improvement in defibrillation threshold possible? *Europace.* 2000;2:154–159.
66. Kantharia BK, Padder FA, Pennington JC, et al. Feasibility, safety, and determinants of extraction time of percutaneous extraction of endocardial implantable cardioverter defibrillator leads by intravascular countertraction method. *Am J Cardiol.* 2000;85:593–597.
67. Peters RW, Foster AH, Shorofsky SR, Nolan DA, Gold MR. Spurious discharges due to late insulation break in endocardial sensing leads for cardioverter defibrillators. *Pacing Clin Electrophysiol.* 1995;18:478–481.
68. Kron J, Herre J, Renfroe EG, et al., and the AVID Investigators. Lead and device-related complications in the Antiarrhythmics Versus Implantable Defibrillators Trial. *Am Heart J.* 2001;141:92–98.
69. Degeratu FT, Khalighi K, Peters RW, Shorofsky SR, Gold MR. Sensing lead failure in implantable defibrillators: A comparison of two commonly used leads. *J Cardiovasc Electrophysiol.* 2000;11:21–24.
70. Gold MR, Peters RW, Johnson JW, Shorofsky

SR for the World-Wide Jewel Investigators. *Pacing Clinical Electrophysiol.* 1997;20:208–211.

71. Grimm W, Menz J, Hoffmann J, et al. Complications of third-generation implantable cardioverter defibrillator therapy. *Pacing Clin Electrophysiol.* 1999;22:206–211.
72. Gupta A, Zegel HG, Dravid VS, Nierenberg SJ, Freiman DB. Value of radiography in diagnosing complications of cardioverter defibrillators implanted without thoracotomy in 437 patients. *Am J Radiol.* 1997;168:105–108.
73. Mehta D, Nayak HM, Signson M, et al. Late complications in patients with pectoral defibrillator implants with transvenous defibrillator lead systems: High incidence of insulation breakdown. *Pacing Clin Electrophysiol.* 1998;21:1893–1900.
74. Dorwarth U, Frey B, Dugas M, et al. Transvenous defibrillation leads: High incidence of failure during long-term follow-up. *J Cardiovasc Electrophysiol.* 2003;14:38–43.
75. Schwartzman D, Nallamouthu N, Callans DJ, et al. Postoperative lead-related complications in patients with nonthoracotomy defibrillator lead systems. *J Am Coll Cardiol.* 1995;26:776–786.
76. Brooks R, Garan H, Torchiana D, et al. Determinants of successful nonthoracotomy cardioverter defibrillator implantation: Experience in 101 patients using two different lead systems. *J Am Coll Cardiol.* 1993;22:1835–1842.
77. Zipes DP, Roberts D. Results of the international study of the implantable pacemaker cardioverter defibrillator. Intention-to-treat comparison of clinical outcomes. *Circulation.* 1995;92:59–65.
78. Raviele A, Gasparini G, for the Italian Endotak Investigator Group. Italian multicenter clinical experience with endocardial defibrillation: Acute and long-term results in 307 patients. *Pacing Clin Electrophysiol.* 1995;18:599–608.
79. Jones GK, Bardy GH, Kudenchuk PJ, et al. Mechanical complications after implantation of multiple lead nonthoracotomy defibrillator system: Implications for management and future system design. *Am Heart J.* 1995;130:327–333.
80. Lawton JS, Wood MA, Gilligan DM, et al. Implantable transvenous cardioverter defibrillator leads: The dark side. *Pacing Clin Electrophysiol.* 1996;19:1273–1278.
81. Eckstein J, Koller MT, Zabel M, et al. Necessity for surgical revision of defibrillator leads implanted long-term: causes and management. Circulation. 2008;117:2727–2733.
82. Tullo NG, Saksena S, Krol RB, Mauro AM, Kunecz D. Management of complications associated with a first-generation endocardial defibrillation lead system for implantable cardioverter defibrillators. *Am J Cardiol.* 1990;66:411–415.
83. Al-Khatib SM, Greiner MA, Peterson ED, et al. Patient and implanting physician factors associated with mortality and complications following implantable cardioverter-defibrillator implantation, 2002–2005. *Circ Arrhythm Electrophysiol.* 2008;1:240–249.
84. Hammill SC, Kremers MS, Stevenson LW, et al. Review of the registry's second year, data collected, and plans to add lead and pediatric ICD procedures. *Heart Rhythm.* 2008;5:1359–1363.
85. Kleemann T, Becker T, Doenges K, et al. Annual rate of transvenous defibrillation lead defects in implantable cardioverter defibrillators over a period of >10 years. *Circulation.* 2007;115:2474–2480.
86. Bardy GH, Hofer B, Johnson G, et al. Implantable transvenous cardioverter defibrillators. *Circulation.* 1993;87:1152–1168.
87. Hauser RG, Cannom D, Hayes DL, et al. Long-term structural failure of coaxial polyurethane implantable cardioverter defibrillator leads. *Pacing Clin Electrophysiol.* 2002;25:879–882.
88. Ellenbogen KA, Wood MA, Shepard RK, et al. Detection and management of an implantable cardioverter defibrillator lead failure: Incidence and clinical implications. *J Am Coll Cardiol.* 2003;41:73–80.
89. Moore SL, Maloney JD, Edel TB, et al. Implantable cardioverter defibrillator implanted by nonthoracotomy approach: Initial clinical experience with the redesigned transvenous lead system. *Pacing Clin Electrophysiol.* 1991;14:1865–1869.
90. Lawton JS, Ellenbogen KA, Wood MA, et al. Sensing lead-related complications in patients with transvenous implantable cardioverter defibrillators. *Am J Cardiol.* 1996;78:647–651.
91. Mera F, Delurgio DB, Langberg JJ, Moss EA,

Leon AR. Transvenous cardioverter defibrillator lead malfunction due to terminal connector damage in pectoral implants. *Pacing Clin Electrophysiol.* 1999;22:1797–1801.

92. Hauser RG, Hayes DL. Increasing hazard of Sprint Fidelis implantable cardioverter-defibrillator lead failure. *Heart Rhythm.* 2009;6:605–610.
93. Hauser RG, Kallinen LM, Almquist AK, Gornick CC, Katsiyiannis WT. Early failure of a small diameter high voltage implantable cardioverter defibrillator lead. *Heart Rhythm.* 2007;4:892–896.
94. Pratt TR, Pulling CC, Stanton MS. Prospective postmarket device studies versus returned product analysis as a predictor of system survival. *Pacing Clin Electrophysiol.* 2000;23:1150–1155.
95. Nagele H, Azizi M, Hashagen S, Castel MA, Behrens S. First experience with a new active fixation coronary sinus lead. *Europace.* 2007;9:437–441.
96. Achtelik M, Bocchiardo M, Trappe HJ, et al, on behalf of the Ventak CHF/Contak CD Clinical Investigation Study Group. Performance of a new steroid-eluting coronary sinus lead designed for left ventricular pacing. *Pacing Clin Electrophysiol.* 2000;23:1741–1743.
97. Bardy GH, Cappato R, Smith WM, et al. The totally subcutaneous ICD system (the S-ICD). (Abstract). *Pacing Clin Electrophysiol.* 2002; 24:578.

Table 2.1A Specifications of Boston Scientific Defibrillation Leads

Features	ENDOTAK	ENDOTAK	ENDOTAK	ENDOTAK	ENDOTAK	ENDOTAK	ENDOTAK	ENDOTAK
	60	70	0073/75	DSP 90	DSP 120	Endurance	Endur Rx	Endur EZ
	0060/62/64	0070/72/74	0113/15	0092/93/95	0123/25	0134/35/36	0144/45/46	0154/55/56
Defibrillation coils	RV/SVC	RV/SVC	RV/SVC	RV/SVC	RV/SVC	RV/SVC	RV/SVC	RV/SVC
Fixation mechanism	Tines	Tines	Tines	Tines	Tines	Tines	Tines	Screw
Sensing	Integ bipolar	Integ bipolar	Integ bipolar	Integ bipolar	Integ bipolar	Integ bipolar	Integ bipolar	Integ bipolar
Tip electrode	9 mm	9 mm	9 mm	8 mm	8 mm	2 mm	2 mm	6 mm
Steroid	No	No	No	No	No	No	Yes	Yes
Insulation	Silicone	Silicone	Silicone	Silicone	Silicone	Silicone	Silicone	Silicone
Coil electrode coating	NA	NA	NA	NA	NA	NA	NA	NA
Lead lengths (cm)	100	100	100,70	100	70	64,70,100	64,70,100	64,70,100
Lead body diameter	9.7/12 Fr	9.7/12 Fr	9.7/12 Fr	8.2/10 Fr	8.2/10 Fr	8.2/10 Fr	8.2/10 Fr	8.2/10 Fr
Tube design	coaxial	coaxial	coaxial	multilumen	multilumen	multilumen	multilumen	multilumen
Connector terminal								
Pace/sense	4.75 mm	4.75 mm	4.75 mm	IS-1	IS-1	IS-1	IS-1	IS-1
High voltage	6.1 mm	6.1 mm	6.1 mm	DF-1	DF-1	DF-1	DF-1	DF-1
Interelectrode spacing								
Tip-Ring	NA	NA	NA	NA	NA	NA	NA	NA
Tip-RV coil	6 mm	12 mm	12 mm	12 mm	12 mm	12 mm	12 mm	12 mm
Tip-SVC coil	10/13/16 cm	12/15/18 cm	15/18 cm	18 cm	18 cm	18 cm	18 cm	18 cm
Electrode surface area								
RV	295 mm^2	379 mm^2	379 mm^2	450 mm^2	450 mm^2	450 mm^2	450 mm^2	450 mm^2
SVC	617 mm^2	617 cm^2	617 mm^2	660 mm^2	660 mm^2	660 mm^2	660 mm^2	660 mm^2

Table 2.1A continues on following page

Chapter 2, Table 2.1A Specifications of Boston Scientific Defibrillation Leads.
(Modified from Ellenbogen KA, *Clinical Cardiac Pacing, Defibrillation, and Resynchronization Therapy*, 3rd Edition, Philadelphia: Saunders Elsevier, 2007)[51]

Table 2.1A (cont.) Specifications of Boston Scientific Defibrillation Leads

Features	ENDOTAK Reliance G 0174/75/76/77	ENDOTAK Reliance G 0164/65/66	ENDOTAK Reliance SG 0170/71/72	ENDOTAK Reliance G 0160/61	ENDOTAK Reliance 0157/58/59	ENDOTAK Reliance S 0137/38	ENDOTAK Reliance G 0184/85/86/87	ENDOTAK Reliance SG 0180/81/82
Defibrillation coils	RV/SVC	RV/SVC	RV	RV	RV/SVC	RV	RV/SVC	RV
Fixation mechanism	Tines	Screw	Tines	Screw	Screw	Screw	Screw	Screw
Sensing	Integ bipolar	Integ bipolar	Integ bipolar	Integ bipolar	Integ bipolar	Integ bipolar	Integ bipolar	Integ bipolar
Tip electrode	2 mm^2	5.7 mm^2	2 mm^2	5.7 mm^2	5.7 mm^2	5.7 mm^2	5.7 mm^2	5.7 mm^2
Steroid	Yes	Yes	Yes	Yes	Yes	Yes	Yes	Yes
Insulation	Silicone	Silicone	Silicone	Silicone	Silicone	Silicone	Silicone	Silicone
Coil electrode coating	ePTFE	ePTFE	ePTFE	ePTFE	ePTFE	ePTFE	ePTFE	ePTFE
Lead lengths (cm)	59,64,70,90	59,64,70	59,64,70	59,64	59,64,90	59,64	59,64,70,90	59,64,70
Lead body diameter	8.2 Fr	8.2 Fr	8.2 Fr	8.2 Fr	8.2 Fr	8.2 Fr	8.2 Fr	8.2 Fr
Tube design	multi-lumen	multi-lumen	multi-lumen	multi-lumen	multi-lumen	multi-lumen	multi-lumen	multi-lumen
Connector terminal								
Pace/sense	IS-1	IS-1	IS-1	IS-1	IS-1	IS-1	IS-1	IS-1
High voltage	DF-1	DF-1	DF-1	DF-1	DF-1	DF-1	DF-1	DF-1
Interelectrode spacing								
Tip-Ring	NA	NA	NA	NA	NA	NA	NA	NA
Tip-RV coil	12 mm	12 mm	12 mm	12 mm	12 mm	12 mm	12 mm	12 mm
Tip-SVC coil	18 cm	18 cm	NA	NA	18 cm	NA	18 cm	NA
Electrode surface area								
RV	450 mm^2	450 mm^2	450 mm^2	450 mm^2	450 mm^2	450 mm^2	450 mm^2	450 mm^2
SVC	660 mm^2	660 mm^2	NA	NA	660 mm^2	NA	660 mm^2	NA

Chapter 2, Table 2.1A (cont.) Specifications of Boston Scientific Defibrillation Leads.

Table 2.1B Specifications of Medtronic Defibrillation Leads

Features	Sprint	Sprint	Sprint	Sprint	Sprint	Sprint
	Fidelis	Fidelis	Fidelis	Fidelis	Quattro	Quattro Secure
	6930	6931	6948	6949	6944	6947
Defibrillation coils	RV	RV	RV/SVC	RV/SVC	RV/SVC	RV/SVC
Fixation mechanism	Tines	Screw	Tines	Screw	Tines	Screw
Sensing	True bipolar	True bipolar	True bipolar	True bipolar	True bipolar	True bipolar
Tip electrode	2.5 mm^2	4.2 mm^2	2.5 mm^2	4.2 mm^2	1.6 mm^2	5.7 mm^2
Steroid	Yes	Yes	Yes	Yes	Yes	Yes
Insulation	Polyurethane	Polyurethane	Polyurethane	Polyurethane	Polyurethane	Polyurethane
Coil electrode coating	Silicone	Silicone	Silicone	Silicone	Silicone	Silicone
Lead lengths (cm)	58,65,75,100	58,65,75,100	58,65,75,100	58,65,75,100	58,65,75,100	58,65,75,100
Lead body diameter	6.6 Fr	6.6 Fr	6.6 Fr	6.6 Fr	8.2 Fr	8.6 Fr
Tube design	multi-lumen	multi-lumen	multi-lumen	multi-lumen	multi-lumen	multi-lumen
Connector terminal						
Pace/sense	IS-1	IS-1	IS-1	IS-1	IS-1	IS-1
High voltage	DF-1	DF-1	DF-1	DF-1	DF-1	DF-1
Interelectrode spacing						
Tip-Ring	8 mm	8 mm	8 mm	8 mm	8 mm	8 mm
Tip-RV coil	12 mm	12 mm	12 mm	12 mm	12 mm	12 mm
Tip-SVC coil	NA	NA	18 cm	18 cm	18 cm	18 cm
Electrode surface area						
RV	513 mm^2	513 mm^2	513 mm^2	513 mm^2	585 mm^2	614 mm^2
SVC	NA	NA	663 mm^2	663 mm^2	819 mm^2	860 mm^2

Table 2.1B continues on following page

Chapter 2, Table 2.1B Specifications of Medtronic Defibrillation Leads.
(Modified from Ellenbogen KA, *Clinical Cardiac Pacing, Defibrillation, and Resynchronization Therapy*, 3rd Edition, Philadelphia: Saunders Elsevier, 2007)[51]

Table 2.1B (cont.) Specifications of Medtronic Defibrillation Leads

Features	Sprint Quattro Secure	Transvene	Transvene	Transvene
	6935	6936	6937a	6937
Defibrillation coils	RV	RV	SVC	SVC,CS
Fixation mechanism	Screw	Screw	—	—
Sensing	True bipolar	True bipolar	—	—
Tip electrode	5.7mm^2	10 mm^2	—	—
Steroid	Yes		—	—
Insulation	Polyurethane	Polyurethane	Silicone	Silicone
Coil electrode coating	Silicone	None	Silicone	Silicone
Lead lengths (cm)	58,65,75,100	65,75,110	35,58,65	35,52,58,110
Lead body diameter	8.6 Fr	10.5 Fr	7.5 Fr	6.9 Fr
Tube design	multi-lumen	coaxial		
Connector terminal				
Pace/sense	IS-1	IS-1	—	—
High voltage	DF-1	DF-1	DF-1	DF-1
Interelectrode spacing				
Tip-Ring	8 mm	12 mm	—	—
Tip-RV coil	12 mm	25 mm	—	—
Tip-SVC coil	NA	NA	—	—
Electrode surface area				
RV	614 mm^2	426 mm^2	—	—
SVC	NA	NA	125 mm^2	160 mm^2

Chapter 2, Table 2.1B (*cont.*) Specifications of Medtronic Defibrillation Leads.

Table 2.1C Specifications of St. Jude/Ventritex Defibrillation Leads

Features	TVL	TVL	SPL	Riata	Riata	Riata	Riata	Riata i
	RV02	RV01/1101	SP01/SP02	1570/71	1572	1580/81	1582	1560/61
Defibrillation coils	RV	RV	RV/SVC	RV/SVC	RV	RV/SVC	RV	RV/SVC
Fixation mechanism	Tines	Screw	Tines	Tines	Tines	Screw	Screw	Tines
Sensing	Integ bipolar	Integ bipolar	Integ bipolar	True bipolar	True bipolar	True bipolar	True bipolar	Integ bipolar
Tip electrode	6 mm^2	6 mm^2	6 mm^2	5 mm^2	5 mm^2	8 mm^2	8 mm^2	5 mm^2
Steroid	No	No	No	Yes	Yes	Yes	Yes	Yes
Insulation	Silicone	Silicone	Silicone	Silicone	Silicone	Silicone	Silicone	Silicone
Coil Electrode coating	None	None	None	None	None	None	None	None
Lead lengths (cm)	67	110	70	65	60, 65	60, 65, 75	60, 65, 75	60, 65, 75
Lead body diameter	10.5 Fr	10.5 Fr	6.7 Fr	6.7 Fr	6.7 Fr	7.6 Fr	7.6 Fr	6.7 Fr
Tube design	coaxial	coaxial	multi-lumen	multi-lumen	multi-lumen	multi-lumen	multi-lumen	multi-lumen
Connector terminal								
Pace/sense	IS-1	IS-1	IS-1	IS-1	IS-1	IS-1	IS-1	IS-1
High voltage	DF-1	DF-1	DF-1	DF-1	DF-1	DF-1	DF-1	DF-1
Interelectrode spacing								
Tip-Ring	NA	NA	NA	11 mm	11 mm	11 mm	11 mm	NA
Tip-RV coil	11 mm	11 mm	11 mm	17 mm	17 mm	17 mm	17 mm	11 mm
Tip-SVC coil	NA	NA	21 cm	17 cm (1570) 21 cm (1571)	NA	17 cm (1580) 21 cm (1581)	NA	17 cm (1560) 21 cm (1561)
Electrode surface area								
RV	470 mm^2	470 mm^2	480 mm^2	414 mm^2	414 mm^2	414 mm^2	414 mm^2	414 mm^2
SV	NA	NA	671 mm^2	663 mm^2	NA	663 mm^2	NA	663 mm^2

Table 2.1C continues on following page

Chapter 2, Table 2.1C Specifications of St. Jude/Ventritex Defibrillation Leads.
(Modified from Ellenbogen KA, *Clinical Cardiac Pacing, Defibrillation, and Resynchronization Therapy*, 3rd Edition, Philadelphia: Saunders Elsevier, 2007)[51]

Table 2.1C (cont.) Specifications of St. Jude/Ventritex Defibrillation Leads

Features	Riata i	Riata i	Riata i	Riata ST	Riata ST	Riata ST	Riata ST Optum
	1562	1590/91	1592	7000/1	7002	7010/11	7020/21
Defibrillation coils	RV	RV/SVC	RV	RV/SVC	RV	RV/SVC	RV/SVC
Fixation mechanism	Tines	Screw	Screw	Screw	Screw	Screw	Screw
Sensing	Int bipolar	Int bipolar	Int bipolar	True bipolar	True bipolar	Int bipolar	True bipolar
Tip electrode	5 mm^2	8 mm^2	8 mm^2	8 mm^2	8 mm^2	8 mm^2	8 mm^2
Steroid	Yes	Yes	Yes	Yes	Yes	Yes	Yes
Insulation	Silicone	Silicone	Silicone	Silicone	Silicone	Silicone	Poly/Silicone
Coil electrode coating	None	None	None	None	None	None	None
Lead lengths (cm)	60, 65, 75	60, 65, 75	60, 65, 75	60, 65, 75	60, 65, 75	60, 65, 75	60, 65, 75
Lead body diameter	6.7 Fr	6.7 Fr	6.7 Fr	6.3 Fr	6.3 Fr	6.3 Fr	6.3 Fr
Tube design	multi-lumen	multi-lumen	multi-lumen	multi-lumen	multi-lumen	multi-lumen	multi-lumen
Connector terminal							
Pace/sense	IS-1	IS-1	IS-1	IS-1	IS-1	IS-1	IS-1
High voltage	DF-1	DF-1	DF-1	DF-1	DF-1	DF-1	DF-1
Interelectrode spacing							
Tip-Ring	NA	NA	NA	11 mm	11 mm	NA	11 mm
Tip-RV coil	11 mm	11 mm	11 mm	17 mm	17 mm	11 mm	17 mm
Tip-SVC coil	NA	17 cm (1590) 21 cm (1591)	NA	17 cm (7000) 21 cm (7001)	NA	17 cm (7010) 21 cm (7011)	17 cm (7020) 21 cm (7021)
Electrode surface area							
RV	414 mm^2	414 mm^2	414 mm^2	367 mm^2	367 mm^2	367 mm^2	367 mm^2
SVC	NA	663 mm^2	NA	588 mm^2	NA	588 mm^2	588 mm^2

Table 2.1C continues on following page

Chapter 2, Table 2.1C (cont.) Specifications of St. Jude/Ventritex Defibrillation Leads.

Table 2.1C (cont.) Specifications of St. Jude/Ventritex Defibrillation Leads

Features	Riata ST Optim	Riata ST Optim	Riata ST	Riata ST Optim	Durata	Durata	Durata
	7022	7030/31	7040/41	7070/71	7120/21	7122	7130/31
Defibrillation coils	RV	RV/SVC	RV/SVC	RV/SVC	RVC/SVC	RV	RV/SVC
Fixation mechanism	Screw	Screw	Tines	Tines	Screw	Screw	Screw
Sensing	True bipolar	Integ bipolar	True bipolar	True bipolar	True bipolar	True bipolar	Integ bipolar
Tip electrode	8 mm^2	8 mm^2	3.5 mm^2	3.5 mm^2	6 mm^2	6 mm^2	6 mm^2
Steroid	Yes	Yes	Yes	Yes	Yes	Yes	Yes
Insulation	Poly/Silicone	Poly/Silicone	Silicone	Poly/Silicone	Poly/Silicone	Poly/Silicone	Poly/Silicone
Coil electrode coating	None	None	None	None	None	None	None
Lead lengths (cm)	60,65,75 cm	65 cm	60,65,75 cm	60,65,75 cm	60,65,(75) cm	60,65 cm	60,65 cm
Lead body diameter	6.3 Fr	6.3 Fr	6.3 Fr	6.3 Fr	6.3 Fr	6.3 Fr	6.3 Fr
Tube design	multi-lumen	multi-lumen	multi-lumen	multi-lumen	multi-lumen	multi-lumen	multi-lumen
Connector terminal							
Pace/sense	IS-1	IS-1	IS-1	IS-1	IS-1	IS-1	IS-1
High voltage	DF-1	DF-1	DF-1	DF-1	DF-1	DF-1	DF-1
Interelectrode spacing							
Tip-Ring	11 mm	11 mm	11 mm	11 mm	11 mm	11 mm	NA
Tip-RV coil	17 mm	17 mm	17 mm	17 mm	17 mm	17 mm	11 mm
Tip-SVC coil	NA	17 cm (7030) 21 cm (7031)	17 cm (7040) 21 cm (7041)	17 cm (7070) 21 cm (7071)	17 cm (7120) 21 cm (7121)	NA	17 cm (7130) 21 cm (7131)
Electrode surface area							
RV	367 mm^2	367 mm^2	367 mm^2	367 mm^2	367 mm^2	367 mm^2	367 mm^2
SVC	NA	588 mm^2	588 mm^2	588 mm^2	588 mm^2	NA	588 mm^2

Chapter 2, Table 2.1C (*cont.*) Specifications of St. Jude/Ventritex Defibrillation Leads.

Table 2.1D Specifications of Biotronik and Intermedics Defibrillation Leads

Features	Biotronik	Biotronik	Biotronik	Biotronik	Biotronik	Biotronik	Biotronik
	Kainox SL	Kainox RV	Kainox RV-S	Kentrox RV	Kentrox SL	Kentrox RV-S	Kentrox SL-S
	217,8,38,9,40	124-005	124-574	348090,91	7351-4,9,50	343080	345988,9
Defibrillation coils	RV/SVC	RV	RV	RV	RV/SVC	RV	RV/SVC
Fixation mechanism	Tines	Tines	Screw	Tines	Tines	Screw	Screw
Sensing	True bipolar	True bipolar	True bipolar	True bipolar	True bipolar	True bipolar	True bipolar
Tip electrode	6 mm^2	5 mm^2	5.3 mm^2	1.8 mm^2	1.8 mm^2	8.2 mm^2	8.2 mm^2
Steroid	No	No	No	Yes	Yes	Yes	Yes
Insulation	Silicone	Silicone	Silicone	Silicone	Silicone	Silicone	Silicone
Coil electrode coating	None	None	None	Yes	Yes	Yes	Yes
Lead lengths (cm)	75,100	75	74	65,75	65,75,100	65	65
Lead body diameter	10.5 Fr	8.7 Fr	10.5 Fr	9.3 Fr	9.3 Fr	9.3 Fr	9.3 Fr
Tube design	multi-lumen	multi-lumen	multi-lumen	multi-lumen	multi-lumen	multi-lumen	multi-lumen
Connector terminal							
Pace/sense	IS-1	IS-1	IS-1	IS-1	IS-1	IS-1	IS-1
High voltage	DF-1	DF-1	DF-1	DF-1	DF-1	DF-1	DF-1
Interelectrode spacing							
Tip-Ring	9 mm	9 mm	14 mm	9 mm	9 mm	11.5 mm	11.5 mm
Tip-RV coil	17 mm	15 mm	21 mm	16 mm	16 mm	18.5 mm	18.5 mm
Tip-SVC coil	13,16,18 cm	NA	NA	NA	16,18 cm	NA	16,18 cm
Electrode surface area							
RV	320 mm^2	300 mm^2	300 mm^2	310 mm^2	310 mm^2	310 mm^2	310 mm^2
SVC	600 mm^2	NA	NA	NA	480 mm^2	NA	480 mm^2

Table 2.1D continues on following page

Chapter 2, Table 2.1D Specifications of Biotronik and Intermedics Defibrillatior Leads. (Modified from Ellenbogen KA, *Clinical Cardiac Pacing, Defibrillation, and Resynchronization Therapy*, 3rd Edition, Philadelphia: Saunders Elsevier, 2007)[51]

Table 2.1D (cont.) Specifications of Biotronik and Intermedics Defibrillation Leads

Features	Biotronik	Biotronik	Biotronik	Biotronik	Intermedics	Intermedics	Intermedics
	Linox SD	Linox TD	Linox S	Linox T			
	350-053/4/5	351-337/8/9/ 340/335/336	351-333 351-334	351-353 351-354	497-05/06	497-19/20	497-23/24
Defibrillation coils	RV/SVC	RV/SVC	RV	RV	RV	RV	RV
Fixation mechanism	Screw	Tines	Screw	Tines	Screw	Screw	Screw
Sensing	True bipolar	True bipolar	True bipolar	True bipolar	—	—	—
Tip electrode	4.5 mm^2	1.8 mm^2	4.5 mm^2	1.8 mm^2	10 mm^2	8 mm^2	8 mm^2
Steroid	Yes	Yes	Yes	Yes	—	—	—
Insulation	Silicone	Silicone	Silicone	Silicone	Silicone	Silicone	Silicone
Coil electrode coating	—	—	—	—	None	IROX	IROX
Lead lengths (cm)	65,75	65,75,100	65,75	65,75	100	—	60,70,100
Lead body diameter	7.8 Fr	7.8 Fr	7.8 Fr	7.8 Fr	11 Fr	11 Fr	11 Fr
Tube design	multi-lumen	multi-lumen	multi-lumen	multi-lumen	—	—	—
Connector terminal							
Pace/sense	IS-1	IS-1	IS-1	IS-1	2 mm	IS-1	IS-1
High voltage	DF-1	DF-1	DF-1	DF-1	4.0 mm	DF-1	DF-1
Interelectrode spacing							
Tip-Ring	11 mm	9 mm	11 mm	9 mm	—	—	—
Tip-RV coil	17 mm	15 mm	17 mm	15 mm	6 mm	—	8 mm/6 mm
Tip-SVC coil	16 &18 cm	16 & 18 cm	NA	NA	—	—	—
Electrode surface area							
RV	290 mm^2	290 mm^2	290 mm^2	290 mm^2	440/880 mm^2	440 mm^2	440 mm^2
SVC	410 mm^2	410 mm^2	NA	NA	NA	NA	NA

Chapter 2, Table 2.1D (cont.) Specifications of Biotronik and Intermedics Defibrillation Leads.

Manufacturer	Model #s	Design pullback (cm)
CPI/Guidant	60 series	0.5
	70 series	1.2
	90 series	1.2
Medtronic	Transvene series	2.5
	Sprint series	1.2
Telectronics	040-068 & 069	1.8
Ventritex	TVL series	1.1
St. Jude Medical	Riata series	1.7
	Riata i series	1.1
Biotronik	Linox series	1.7/1.5

Chapter 2, Table 2.2 Design Pullback of RV Electrode
(Modified from Ellenbogen KA, *Clinical Cardiac Pacing, Defibrillation, and Resynchronization Therapy,* 3rd Edition, Philadelphia: Saunders Elsevier, 2007)[51]

Please note: Tables continue for this chapter on the following page.

Table 2.3 Specifications of LV Pacing Leads

Features	Guidant	Guidant	Guidant	Boston Sci	Boston Sci
	Easy Trak	Easy Trak 2	Easy Trak 3	Acuity Spiral	Acuity Steerable
	4510/11/12/ …13/37/38	4515/17/18/ …20/42/43/44	4522/24/25/ …27/48/49/50	4591/2/3	4554/5
Delivery	otw	otw	otw	otw	otw&stylet
Proximal lead body diameter	6 Fr	5.3 Fr	6.0 Fr	4.5 Fr	6.0 Fr
Distal lead body diameter	4.8 Fr	5.2 Fr	5.3 Fr	4.1 to 2.6 Fr	5.3 Fr
Distal shape	Straight	Straight	Spiral	Helical	J-shape
Fixation	Tines	Tines	3D spiral	Spiral	J-shape
Electrode config/ polarity	Unipolar	Bipolar	Bipolar	Unipolar	Bipolar
Connector terminal	LV-1 (10-13) IS-1 (37,38)	LV-1 (15-20) IS-1 (42-44)	LV-1 (22-27) IS-1 (48-50)	IS-1	IS-1
Insulation	Silicone w/ poly	Silicone w/ poly	Silicone w/ poly	Silicone w/ poly	Silicone w/ poly
Tip seal	No	No	No	No	No
Steroid	Yes	Yes	Yes	Yes	Yes
Lead lengths (cm)	65,72,80,90	80,90,100	80,90,100	80,90,100	80,90
Electrode surface area	3.5 mm^2	4.2 mm^2 (prox) 4 mm^2 (distal)	9 mm^2 (prox) 8.5 mm^2 (dist)	5.2 mm^2	9 mm^2 (prox) 7.8 mm^2 (dist)
Electrode spacing	NA	11 mm	11 mm	NA	8 mm
Tip electrode material	plat iridium	plat iridium	plat iridium	plat iridium	plat iridium

Table 2.3 continues on following page

Chapter 2, Table 2.3 Specifications of LV Pacing Leads.
(Modified from Ellenbogen KA, *Clinical Cardiac Pacing, Defibrillation, and Resynchronization Therapy,* 3rd Edition, Philadelphia: Saunders Elsevier, 2007)[51]

Table 2.3 (cont.) Specifications of LV Pacing Leads

Features	Medtronic	Medtronic	Medtronic	Medtronic	Medtronic
	Attain	Attain	Attain	Attain Ability	StarFix
	2187	4193	4194	4196	4195
Delivery	stylet	otw&stylet	otw&stylet	otw&stylet	otw&stylet
Proximal lead body diameter	6 Fr	4 Fr	6.2 Fr	4 Fr	5 Fr
Distal lead body diameter	5.4 Fr	5.4 Fr	4.5 Fr	5.1 Fr	5.3 Fr
Distal shape	Curved	Angled	Angled	Angled	Curved
Fixation	Curved	Angled	Angled	Angled	Deployable Lobes
Electrode config/ polarity	Unipolar	Unipolar	Bipolar	Bipolar	Unipolar
Connector terminal	IS-I	IS-I	IS-I	IS-I	IS-I
Insulation	Poly 55D	Poly 55D	Poly 55D	Poly, SI-PI	Poly
Tip seal	NA	Yes	Yes	Yes	Yes
Steroid	No	Yes	Yes	Yes	Yes
Lead lengths (cm)	58,65,75	78,88,103	78,88	78,88	78,88,103
Electrode surface area	5.8 mm^2	5.8 mm^2	5.8mm^2 (prox) 3.8mm^2 (dist)	5.8 mm^2 (ring) 5.8 mm^2 (tip)	5.8 mm^2
Electrode spacing	NA	NA	11 mm	21 mm	NA
Tip electrode material	Platinum	Platinum	Platinum	Platinum	Platinum

Table 2.3 continues on following page

Chapter 2, Table 2.3 (*cont.*) Specifications of LV Pacing Leads.

Table 2.3 Specifications of LV Pacing Leads

Features	St. Jude Aescula 1055K	St. Jude QuickSite 1056K	St. Jude QuickSite 1056/58T	St. Jude QuickFlex 1156/58T	Biotronik Corox OTW	Biotronik Corox OTW-S
Delivery	stylet	otw&stylet	otw&stylet	otw&stylet	otw&stylet	otw&stylet
Proximal lead body diameter	4.7 Fr	5.6 Fr	5.6 Fr	5.6 Fr	5.4 Fr	5.4 Fr
Distal lead body diameter	4.5 Fr	5 Fr	5 Fr	5 Fr	5.8 Fr	5.8 Fr
Distal shape	S curve	S curve	S curve	S curve height: 8 mm (1156) 16 mm (1158)	helix	straight
Fixation	curved	stepped circ	stepped circ	stepped circ	helix	straight
Electrode config/ polarity	Unipolar	Unipolar	Bipolar	Bipolar	Bipolar	Bipolar
Connector terminal	IS-1	IS-1	IS-1	IS-1	IS-1	IS-1
Insulation	Silicone	Silicone w/poly	Silicone w/poly	Silicone w/poly	Silicone w/poly	Silicone w/poly
Tip seal	NA	No	No	No		
Steroid	No	Yes	Yes	Yes	Yes	Yes
Lead lengths (cm)	75	75,86	75,86	75,86	77,87	77,87
Electrode surface area	6.8 mm^2	4.8 mm^2	4.8 mm^2	4.9 mm^2	5 mm^2	5 mm^2
(tip/ring, if bipolar)	NA	NA	14.7mm^2	7.4 mm^2	8 mm^2	8 mm^2
Electrode spacing	NA	NA	15 mm(1056) 20 mm(1058)	20 mm	18 mm	18 mm
Tip electrode material	TiN	Pt/Ir,TiN	Pt/Ir,TiN	Pt/Ir,TiN	Pt/Ir	Pt/Ir

Chapter 2, Table 2.3 (*cont.*) Specifications of LV Pacing Leads.

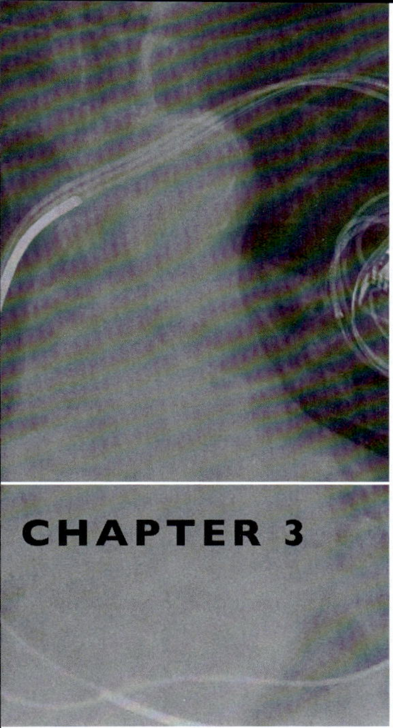

CHAPTER 3

Pacemaker Timing Cycles

Ventricular Based and Atrial Based

Fred Kusumoto

Introduction

Pacemakers were originally developed to provide rate support for patients with bradycardia. The earliest pacemakers were designed to "guarantee" ventricular rate support. However, as pacing therapy evolved basic pacemaker algorithms were altered to provide more consistent ventricular rates and to encourage intrinsic ventricular conduction. To achieve both of these goals, more complex timing cycles using a complex hierarchy were developed. Although useful, these algorithms can lead to apparent "abnormalities" and unexpected behaviors in pacemaker function that can erroneously be attributed to pacemaker malfunction.

Single Chamber Pacing

The timing cycles for single chamber pacing are fairly straightforward, but provide an introduction to our discussion of subtle differences in timing cycles used for dual chamber pacing. Although we think about the physiologic effects of cardiac activity, algorithms used by pacemakers are designed to respond to "cardiac events," whether it is a sensed signal or the delivery of a pacing output. In single chamber pacing, after a "cardiac event" is identified, the low rate timer is started. If the low rate timer expires without an intervening sensed event, a pacing output is delivered and the cycle repeats (Fig 3.1). Alternatively, if a sensed signal is observed before the low rate timer expires, most commonly a pacemaker will be programmed to not deliver a pacing stimulus (inhibited) and the low rate timer will be restarted.

The general functionality of the pacemaker is called the pacing mode and is commonly described using a three or four letter code that was

Pacemakers and Implantable Cardioverter Defibrillators: An Expert's Manual. © 2010 Amin Al-Ahmad, Kenneth A. Ellenbogen, Andrea Natale, and Paul J. Wang, eds. Cardiotext Publishing, ISBN: 978-0-9790164-6-2.

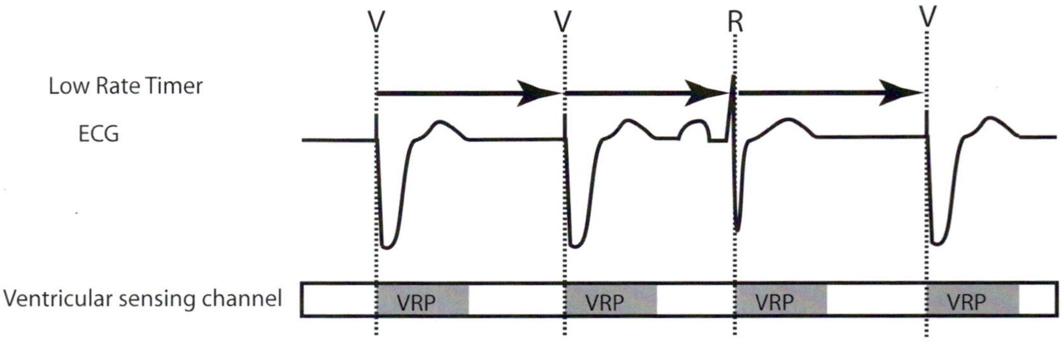

Fig 3.1 Timing cycles for a single chamber ventricular pacemaker programmed to the VVI pacing mode. With delivery of a ventricular stimulus (V), the low rate timer is initiated. If the low rate timer expires without an intervening sensed beat, a ventricular stimulus is delivered. If an R wave is sensed, the pacemaker inhibits (an inhibited or demand response) and the low rate timer is reset. After any ventricular activity (sensed or paced), a ventricular refractory period (VRP) is started to reduce the likelihood of spurious sensing of T waves.

originally developed in the 1970s and has remained largely unchanged for the past 30 years. In the pacing code, the first letter corresponds to the paced chamber(s), the second letter to the sensed chamber(s), and the third letter denotes the response to a sensed event. For single chamber devices, the first two letters will always be the same: either "A" or "V" depending on whether the lead is placed in the atrium or ventricle. For single chamber devices, the third letter is almost always an "I" to represent "inhibition" of the pacing output when an event is sensed as previously described. A fourth letter "R" is used to denote that sensor driven pacing or rate adaption algorithms have been turned "on." Although there have been several attempts to update the code to incorporate and provide a standardized classification of the complex multifunctional algorithms discussed in this textbook, none of these have become widely accepted.[1]

The basic function of timing cycles and algorithms for single chamber pacemakers vary little from manufacturer to manufacturer although there are some differences in the programmable values (Table 3.1). A low rate timer is employed along with a refractory period. For example, for a single chamber ventricular pacemaker programmed to the VVI pacing mode after a ventricular paced or sensed event, the low rate timer and the ventricular refractory period (VRP) will be started (Fig 3.1). The VRP is required to prevent inadvertent sensing of T waves in the ventricular channel. If the low rate timer expires without an intervening sensed event, a ventricular pacing stimulus is delivered. If a sensed ventricular event occurs after the VRP but before the low rate timer expires, the pacing stimulus will not be delivered (inhibited) and the timers will restart. Thus the device paces and senses in the ventricle and the response to a sensed event is inhibition (VVI pacing mode). Sorin single chamber ventricular pacemakers have a nonprogrammable refractory period set at 100 ms after a ventricular sensed event and 150 ms after a ventricular paced event with automatic extension of the refractory period by "retriggering" if deemed necessary by the device.

Single chamber atrial pacemakers work in the same way with a low rate timer and atrial refractory period (ARP). In this case the ARP is designed to prevent inadvertent sensing of intrinsic ventricular activity (R wave).

Dual Chamber Pacing

For dual chamber pacing, at a minimum two additional timing cycles are required: the AV interval and the upper rate limit. In addition, the low rate timer becomes more complex be-

Manufacturer	Popular Name (Model #)	LRL (bpm)	VRP/ARP (ms)
Medtronic	Adapta (ADSR01, ADSR03, ADSR06)	30–170	150–500/180–500
Boston Scientific	Altrua (S601)	30–150	200–500/150–500
St. Jude	Integrity (5160) Verity (5056, 5156, 5157) Victory (5610) Zephyr (5620, 5626)	30–170	125–500
Biotronik	Cyclos (349, 811) Philos (331, 446, 447, 599) Philos II (341, 826)	30–180	170–400
Sorin	Rhapsody (SR2210)	30–95	Automatic

Table 3.1 Ranges for Programmable Basic Values for Single Chamber Pacemakers from Different Manufacturers.

cause atrial signals, ventricular signals, or a combination of atrial and ventricular signals can be used to determine the "start" and "stop" of the timer.[2,3]

Atrioventricular Interval

The atrioventricular interval (AVI) is designed to mimic the PR interval and is initiated by an atrial event and stops with a ventricular event. If the AVI expires without a sensed ventricular event, a ventricular pacing output is delivered; conversely, if activity is sensed in the ventricular channel before the AVI expires, in most cases ventricular pacing is inhibited.

In actuality, the AVI is usually composed of several periods in the ventricular channel (Fig 3.2). In the ventricular channel, all manufacturers use a "blanking" period that is designed to prevent inadvertent "crosstalk" with the atrial pacing stimulus spuriously sensed on

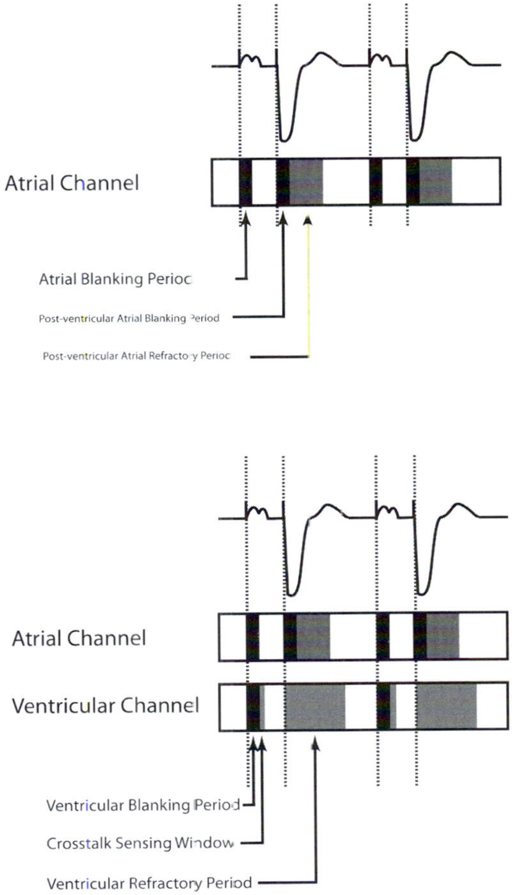

Fig 3.2 Refractory periods in dual chamber pacemakers. **Top**: Atrial channel only. Generally manufacturers will employ an atrial blanking period after an atrial paced event (and sometimes after an atrial sensed event) and a post-ventricular atrial blanking period (PVAB) and a subsequent postventricular atrial refractory period PVARP after a ventricular paced event (and sometimes after a ventricular sensed event). **Bottom**: Ventricular channel is added to the atrial sensing channel. In the ventricular channel, there is a ventricular blanking period, followed by a safety-pacing period to reduce the likelihood of inappropriate withholding of pacing therapy. After a ventricular paced event there is a ventricular refractory period (VRP).

the ventricular channel as ventricular activity. In addition, another window/period most commonly called the safety-pacing period (but also called the crosstalk detection window [St. Jude Medical], committed window [Sorin], or noise detection period) is often employed to prevent inappropriate withholding of ventricular stimuli in the presence of interference. Response to noise and safety pacing are fully discussed in Chapter 7, but for the purposes of this introductory discussion, if ventricular signals are sensed during this period the pacemaker assumes the possibility of "noise" and delivers a ventricular output at a short AVI. If the activity represented a premature ventricular contraction (PVC), the pacing output would have no effect (ventricular tissue is refractory), and conversely, if the signal represented noise, asystole is averted.

The AVI is programmable in all devices, but the available range may be limited based on the programmed lower and upper rate (Table 3.2). In addition to programming the AVI, most devices allow separate programming of different intervals depending on whether the interval was initiated with sensed atrial activity or atrial pacing. Because atrial depolarization is already proceeding when the pacemaker senses atrial activity, in most cases the sensed AVI is programmed to a slightly shorter value than the paced AVI. Table 3.2 provides a summary of some basic programmable parameters for different manufacturers. Instead of providing two separate parameters, both Boston Scientific and Biotronik allow the user to program a shorter sensed AV delay measured relative to the paced AV delay (Boston Scientific: "Sensed AV Offset," and Biotronik: "Sense Compensation").

Low Rate Timer

The low rate timer is referred to as the low rater, lower rate limit, basic rate, or base rate depend-

Manufacturer	Popular Name (model #)	AVI (ms)	Lower rate–Upper Rate (bpm)
Medtronic	Adapta (ADDR01, ADDR03, ADDR06, ADDRS1, ADDRL1) Versa (VEDR01) EnRhythm (P15o1DR)	SAV: 30–350 PAV: 30–350	30–210
Boston Scientific	Altrua (S602-6)	PAV: 10–400* Sensed AV offset from 0 –100.	30–150
St. Jude	Identity (5286, 5370, 5376, 5380, 5386, 5480) Integrity (5360, 5366) Verity (5256, 5356, 5357) Victory (5810, 5816) Zephyr (5820, 5826)	SAV: 30–325 PAV: 30–350	30–170
Biotronik	Cyclos 349, 799, 806) Philos (331, 443,598) Philos II (175, 341, 343, 826)	PAV: 30–300 Sense compensation: 0–120	30–185
Sorin	Reply Symphony (DR 2550) Rhapsody (DR 2510, 2530)	SAV: 30–250	30–185

Table 3.2 Ranges for Programmable Basic Values for Dual Chamber Pacemakers from Different Manufacturers.
*Depending on model; bpm, Beats per minute; AVI, AV interval; SAV, Sensed AV delay.

Manufacturer	Name used to describe the lower rate limit	Atrial/ventricular based
Medtronic	Lower Rate	MVP*: atrial based DDD: ventricular based with AVI compensation
Boston Scientific	Lower Rate Limit	Hybrid
St. Jude	Base Rate	Atrial based
Biotronik	Basic Rate	Atrial based
Sorin	Basic Rate	Atrial based

Table 3.3 Low Rate Timing Methods Used by Different Manufacturers *MVP: Managed Ventricular Pacing.

ing on manufacturer (Table 3.3). Regardless of the nomenclature, the low rate timer can be triggered by atrial events (atrial-based timing), ventricular events (ventricular-based timing), or a combination of both depending on the situation. It is important to remember that during everyday function, the pacing rate can be determined by a variety of timers. Although the low rate timer is often the usual timer "driving" the pacing rate, other timers such as a sleep or rest rate (usually programmed to a lower rate), a sensor-driven faster rate, or a rate-smoothing algorithm may be the basis for an observed pacing rate.

Ventricular-based timing

Originally all dual chamber pacemakers used ventricular-based timing. In this timing schema, ventricular events, whether sensed or paced, are used as the basis of the low rate timer. After a ventricular event, the atrial escape interval (AEI) determines the timing for the delivery of an atrial pacing stimulus. As shown in Fig 3.3, the AEI is determined as the low rate interval (timer) minus the programmed AVI.

In ventricular-based timing, the AEI is constant and this can lead to an apparent increase in heart rate in the presence of intrinsic ventricular conduction. In Fig 3, the low rate interval is programmed to 1000 ms (60 beats per minutes [bpm]) and the AVI is programmed to 250 ms giving an AEI of 750 ms. This is a reasonable programming setting for facilitating intrinsic

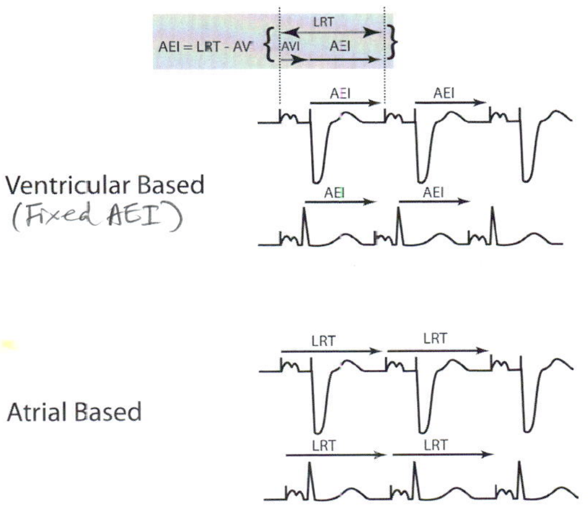

Fig 3.3 Different behavior of atrial-based (bottom) and ventricular-based (top) timing depending on whether intrinsic AV conduction is present. With ventricular pacing there is no difference between atrial- and ventricular-based timing. However, during ventricular-based timing, the atrial escape interval (AEI) is calculated as the difference between the low rate timer (LRT) and AVI (AEI = LRT – AVI). In traditional ventricular-based timing, the AEI remains fixed, so that in the presence of intrinsic ventricular conduction and a shorter AV delay, a faster rate than the programmed rate will be observed. In this example, if the low rate timer is programmed to a rate of 60 bpm (1000 ms) and the AVI is 250 ms, the AEI is 750 ms. If intrinsic AV conduction with an interval of 150 ms develops, with the fixed AEI the paced heart rate would be 67 bpm. With atrial-based timing, the heart rate will be determined by the low rate timer (LRT) and will be the same regardless of whether there is intrinsic conduction or ventricular pacing.

atrioventricular conduction. However, if normal intrinsic AV conduction is present (eg, the AP-VS interval is 150 ms), because the AEI is fixed, then the atrial-paced cycle lengths would shorten (900 ms or 67 bpm). This effect is magnified in the presence of a sensor-driven paced rate. Using the previously programmed values as an example, with a sensor-driven rate of 100 bpm, the AEI would be 350 ms (600 ms – 250 ms). In the presence of intrinsic AV conduction, atrial pacing stimuli would be delivered at 500 ms intervals (AEI + AV or 350 + 150 ms) and the pacing rate would actually be 120 bpm.

Atrial-based timing

Because of the possibility for faster heart rates in the setting of intrinsic conduction with pure ventricular-based pacing, all manufacturers have incorporated some form of atrial-based low rate timing in their current generation of pacemakers. In general terms, atrial-based pacing is present if the pacemaker uses atrial events for timing (or adjusting) the low rate timer. In pure atrial-based timing, an atrial event, whether paced or sensed, initiates the low rate timer. If the low rate timer expires without a sensed atrial event, an atrial pacing output is delivered. In this way regardless of whether ventricular pacing or intrinsic ventricular activity is present, behavior at the low rate timer will become more consistent. As a corollary to atrial-based timing, the AEI will vary and not necessarily be a fixed interval as it is in totally ventricular-based timing schemes. Timing systems used by different manufacturers are summarized in Table 3.3.

All pacing systems, whether atrial based or ventricular based, use a separate algorithm for timing in response to a PVC. A pacemaker generally defines a PVC as two consecutive ventricular sensed events without an intervening atrial signal. In some atrial-based systems (Biotronik), a PVC leads to reinitiation of the low rate timer that when it times out will result in an atrial stimulus. This leads to a compensatory pause and a single cardiac interval with a ventricular rate less than the programmed low rate timer (because it will represent the sum of the low rate timer and an AVI). Other atrial-based systems will use an abbreviated low rate timer (often the difference between the low rate timer and the programmed AVI) for delivery of the subsequent atrial stimulus. This would provide a response similar to a ventricular-based system. The different strategies to respond to PVCs that manufacturers have developed are summarized in Fig 3.4. It should be noted that

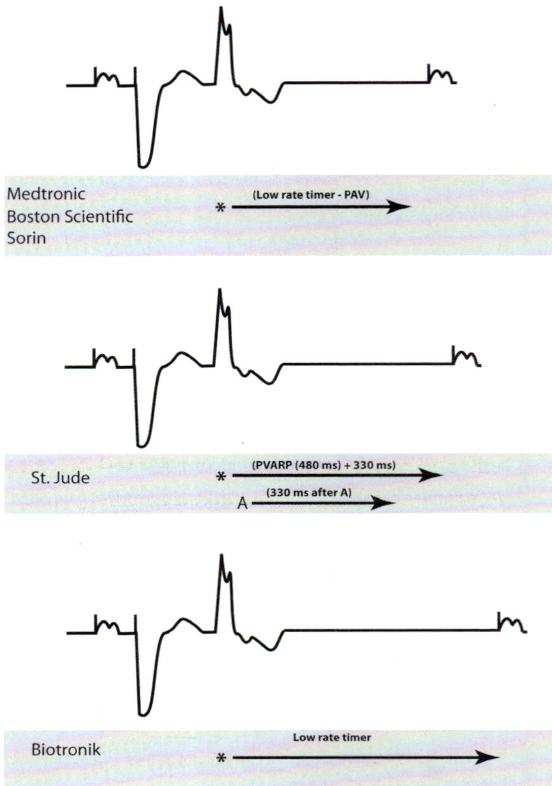

Fig 3.4 Different manufacturers response to a PVC. **Top**: Boston Scientific, Medtronic, and Sorin pacemakers will calculate the AEI as the difference between the low rate timer and the atrially paced AV interval (PAV). **Middle**: St. Jude Medical pacemakers use an algorithm based on the PVARP to calculate the timing of the next atrial pacing stimulus: PVARP + 330 ms. If atrial activity (A) is sensed within the PVARP, the 330 ms interval is started before the PVARP ends. **Bottom**: In Biotronik pacemakers that use a true atrial-based low rate timer, a pause that will result in an RR interval longer than what would be expected based on the programmed low rate (because of the additional time for AV conduction) will be observed.

because pacemakers generally define a premature ventricular response as two consecutive ventricular events without an intervening atrial signal, any situation that produces atrial sensing (true atrial activity due to a simultaneous premature atrial contraction or sinus beat with a PVC with a long coupling interval, far-field R wave, or noise) before the PVC will not trigger the expected PVC response.[4]

Medtronic

Currently available Medtronic pacemakers use atrial-based timing when programmed to the managed ventricular pacing (MVP) mode.[5] The MVP mode is discussed more fully in the chapter on minimizing ventricular pacing algorithms, but briefly the pacing system functions in the AAI mode with continuous monitoring of the ventricular channel. If two consecutive atrial signals are observed without an intervening ventricular signal, the pacing system "makes the diagnosis" of AV block and will deliver a ventricular stimulus 80 ms after the second atrial signal. The pacing stimulus is "committed" and any ventricular event sensed prior to ventricular pacing is considered invalid (a strategy similar to safety pacing). However, in the MVP mode, a PVC initiates a ventricular-based AEI that is calculated as the low rate timer (interval) minus the measured AVI (MAVI). When multiple missing ventricular signals in response to atrial events (presumably due to AV block) are identified, the device will switch to conventional dual chamber pacing that uses ventricular events for timing.

With conventional dual chamber pacing, Medtronic uses ventricular events for resetting the low rate timer (Fig 3.4). To mimic atrially based timing, the MAVI is compared to the programmed AVI with atrial pacing (paced AVI or PAV). The shorter interval is used to calculate the AEI (low rate interval – MAVI [PAV]). Under most conditions the MAVI will be shorter and will be used for calculating the AEI. In the presence of a PVC the AEI is calculated as the difference between the low rate interval and the PAV (low rate interval – PAV) as there is no MAVI to measure.

Boston Scientific

The most recent family of bradycardia devices offered by Boston Scientific uses a combination of atrial-based and ventricular-based timing depending on whether ventricular activity is paced or sensed. After a paced ventricular event, the device functions as a ventricular-based device with a fixed AEI before delivery of an atrial stimulus. However, if a sensed QRS complex is identified before the expiration of the AVI, the next atrial stimulus will be delivered after the AEI and the difference between the observed and programmed AVI have expired. The device switches to atrial-based timing until ventricular pacing resumes. In the presence of a PVC, Boston Scientific pacemakers utilize an algorithm similar to Medtronic pacemakers.

St. Jude Medical

St. Jude Medical uses atrial-based timing and calls the low rate timer the "base rate." Timing is based on atrial stimuli or sensed atrial activity. After a PVC, if atrial activity is sensed (presumably due to a retrograde P wave or sinus beat that blocked in the AV node) during the programmable postventricular atrial refractory period (PVARP), an atrial stimulus will be delivered after 330 ms if no intervening P wave is detected (Fig 3.4). If no atrial activity is sensed during the PVARP, the 330 ms interval starts once the PVARP ends.

Biotronik

Biotronik devices are atrially based and refer to the lower rate limit as the "basic rate." In response to a PVC, the low rate timer will start (ie, a single beat timing will be initiated by a ventricular event) and will deliver an atrial stimulus when the fully programmed interval is reached. This operation will lead to an apparent pause that is longer than would seem allowable by the programmed low rate timer (Fig 3.4).

Sorin (ELA)

Sorin pacemakers use atrial-based timing for their dual chamber pacing modes. Sorin has developed an interesting pacing mode called AAIsafeR.[6] In this pacing mode the device functions in the AAI mode (atrial-based timing by definition) and continuously monitors the PR and AR intervals. It defines a programmable PR interval > 350 ms and an AR interval > 450 ms as abnormal. The device will automatically switch to a dual chamber pacing mode using atrially based timing if > 2 consecutive blocked atrial events, > 3 blocked atrial events over the last 12 cycles, > 6 consecutive abnormal AR/PR intervals, or a >3-second pause. The device will change back to the AAI mode after 100 cycles or if 12 R waves are sensed in consecutive AA intervals. If the device must mode switch frequently (> 15 times/day for 3 days or > 45 times in a single day, the device will automatically limit the attempts to return to AAI to once a day.

In response to a PVC, Sorin uses a strategy similar to Medtronic and Boston Scientific pacemakers. The lower rate timer is reset with an AEI calculated as the difference between the basic rate and the AVI.

Upper Rate Limit

With the advent of dual chamber pacing systems that would sense atrial activity and deliver ventricular pacing in response to sensed atrial events, it was clear that a mechanism for eliminating the possibility of rapid repetitive ventricular pacing had to be developed. The upper rate limit is the maximal rate of allowable ventricular pacing and is also called the maximum tracking rate (St. Jude Medical, Boston Scientific, Sorin) or the upper tracking rate (Medtronic, Biotronik). The upper rate limit is timed from ventricular-paced events so it is always considered a ventricular-based timing cycle. The actual behavior of the pacemaker at or near the upper rate limit will depend on the relationship between the upper rate limit and the total atrial refractory period (TARP).[7]

Refractory Periods

Refractory periods are designed as an interval of time during which the pacemaker may sense physiologic activity that should not trigger a pacing response. From a physiologic standpoint, the refractory period can be thought of as an engineering means to mimic the normal refractory properties of the heart.

For example, after a sinus beat a very premature atrial beat is blocked if the AV node is refractory. Similarly, it is reasonable to design the device so that an early atrial beat will not lead to reinitiation of the AVI and an early ventricular pacing stimulus. All pacemakers use a timing period called the postventricular atrial refractory period or PVARP to mimic this response. Any sensed atrial activity in the PVARP is designated as an electrical signal generated by atrial tissue but the AVI is not initiated. Although a pacing response in not elicited, the activity is noted or "counted," thus facilitating identification of atrial arrhythmias.

The PVARP and the AVI are important for understanding the response of a pacemaker to higher atrial rates. The sum of the AVI and the PVARP is called the total atrial refractory period or TARP. During TARP, sensed atrial activity will not lead to triggering of the AVI and ventricular pacing. If the TARP is programmed to a value shorter than the upper rate timer, the patient will initially experience an AV Wenckebach response at high atrial rates. Conversely, if the TARP is programmed to a value longer than the upper rate timer, the patient will suddenly develop 2:1 AV block (Fig 3.5). All current pacemakers have a programmable option called dynamic PVARP that will adjust the PVARP based on prior rates. By shortening the PVARP at higher rates, 1:1 tracking of atrial activity at higher sinus rates is permitted. This feature is particularly important in younger patients with AV block. For example, if the AVI is programmed to 180 ms and the PVARP to 320 ms, the TARP would be 500 ms and 1:1 conduction will continue until a heart rate of 120 bpm. As the sinus rate increases beyond this value, atrioventricular block will develop. The programmed value of the upper rate limit dictates whether AV Wenckebach or 2:1 AV block is initially observed. Regardless of the relative values of the upper rate limit and TARP, once the sinus rate increases to a point that atrial activity

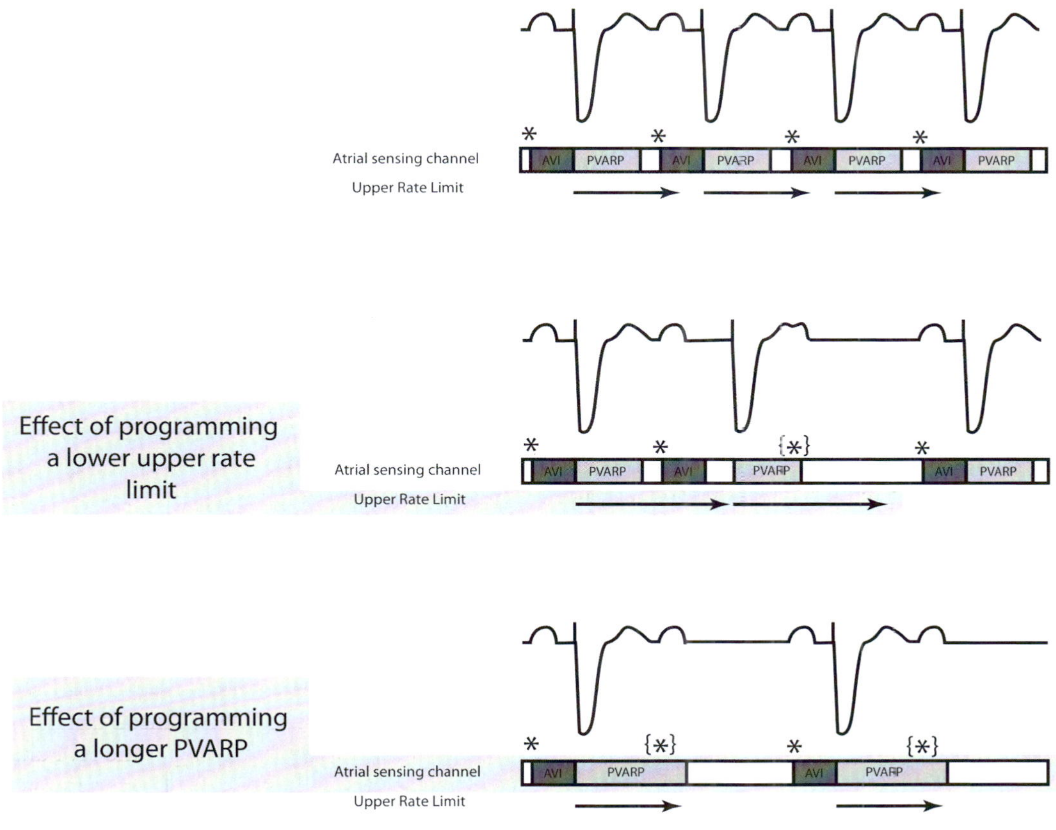

Fig 3.5 Upper rate behavior and relationships between the AVI, PVARP, and upper rate limit. **Top**: As long as the atrial rate (*) is slower than both the upper rate limit and the total atrial refractory period (TARP = AVI + PVARP) one-to-one tracking of atrial activity occurs. **Middle**: If the upper rate limit is programmed to a lower rate (longer interval), then a ventricular stimulus is not delivered until the upper rate limit "times out." This leads to an AV Wenckebach behavior with a "dropped QRS" when the atrial activity falls within the PVARP ({*}). **Bottom**: If the PVARP is increased (leading to a resulting increase in the TARP) to a value longer than the upper rate limit, sudden onset of 2:1 block will be observed.

is sensed at intervals shorter than the TARP, 2:1 block will occur.

Blanking Periods

Blanking periods are designed to prevent "cross-talk" between the atrial and ventricular leads. An atrial stimulus can produce enough voltage to be "seen" in the ventricular channel and a ventricular stimulus may be recorded in the atrial channel. The nomenclature can be confusing although can be thought of fairly simply in the following manner: In the ventricular channel, a blanking period is usually initiated after an atrial pacing stimulus is delivered, and in the atrial channel a blanking period is usually present after a ventricular stimulus (postventricular atrial blanking period or PVAB).

Conceptually the pacemaker defines any sensed activity in a blanking period as probable crosstalk from the other lead and it will not restart any timing cycles nor save it in the pacemaker memory. Refractory periods have been developed as a method to allow a specific response to physiologic activity within the chamber of interest. Examples would include a retrograde P wave produced by a PVC or rapid atrial activity due to atrial fibrillation, while blanking periods are designed to avoid spurious sensing from artificial sources (the pacemaker itself) or from inappropriate recording of a physiologic signal in the opposite channel (recording a far-field R wave in the atrial channel).

Manufacturers have developed different refractory periods and blanking periods with different strategies for managing crosstalk (Table 3.4). Some manufacturers have blanking periods after both paced and sensed events (Medtronic) whereas others use blanking periods only after paced events (Boston Scientific, St. Jude Medical). Programming of the PVAB period has become particularly relevant as clinicians have become more interested in using pacemakers and implanted cardiac devices as heart rhythm monitors. A long PVAB period could lead to undersensing of atrial tachyarrhythmias (Fig 3.6) whereas programming the interval too short could lead to spurious far-field R wave sensing that would inaccurately identify the "presence" of an atrial tachycardia. To provide programming options that reduce the likelihood of far-field ventricular sensing, some manufacturers provide a programmable blanking period after both sensed and paced ventricular events (Fig 3.7). As a general concept, because detection of atrial arrhythmias is emerging as one of the critical clinical functions for implanted devices, it is preferable to maximize the period that the pacemaker is scanning for abnormal atrial activity as much as possible.

Medtronic

Medtronic pacemakers have a nonprogrammable blanking period in a channel that occurs after a sensed or paced beat in that chamber. This period ranges from 50 to 100 ms and varies based on a proprietary algorithm. A programmable blanking period occurs in the sensing channel after an event in the other channel. After an atrial paced event, the ventricular channel has a programmable blanking period (postatrial ventricular blanking: 20 to 44 ms) and after a sensed or paced event in the ventricular channel, an atrial blanking period can be programmed from 130 to 350 ms.

Boston Scientific

In Boston Scientific pacemakers the ventricular blanking period after an atrial pacing event can be programmed from 30 to 200 ms and the postventricular atrial blanking period can be programmed from 30 to 200 ms after a ventricular paced event. Blanking periods are not provided after sensed events, either atrial or ventricular.

St. Jude Medical

Pacemakers from St. Jude Medical provide a blanking period in the ventricular channel after an atrial pacing event that can be programmed from 12 to 52 ms. St. Jude Medical pacemakers

Manufacturer	V Blanking (ms)	PVARP (ms)	PVAB (ms)
Medtronic	120–350*	150–500	120–350*
Boston Scientific	30–200	160–500	30–200
St. Jude Medical	12–52	125–500	60–200
Biotronik	32–72	200–775#	32–200
Sorin	250–Automatic	After PVAB–Automatic	45–155

Table 3.4 Ranges for Programmable Refractory Periods and Blanking Periods for Different Manufacturers.
* Depending on model #: Includes AVI; V, Ventricular; PVARP, postventricular atrial refractory period; PVAB, postventricular atrial blanking period.

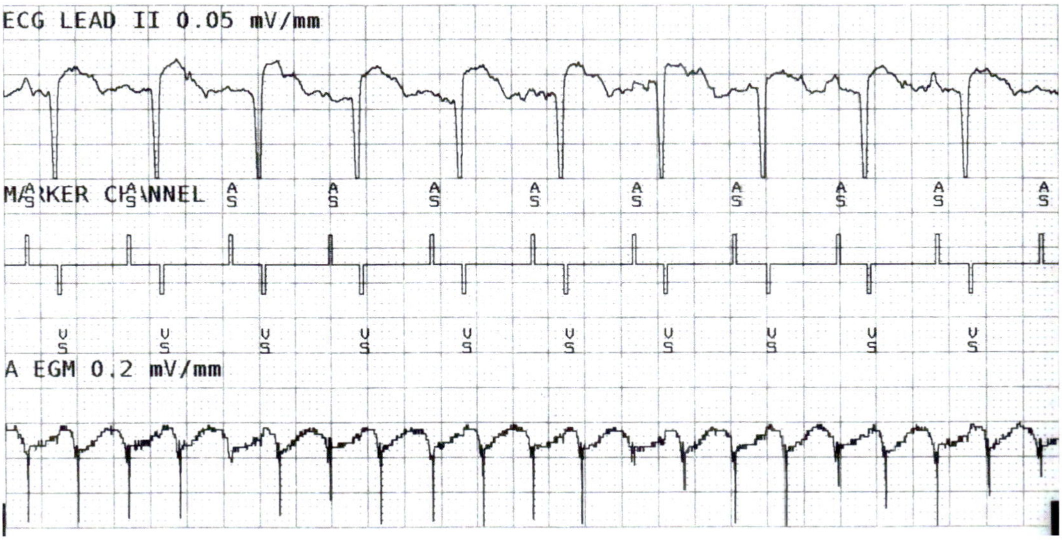

Fig 3.6 An example of underdetection of atrial tachycardia. Atrial electrograms reveal the patient is in a rapid atrial tachycardia not identified by the pacemaker because every other atrial signal is located within the blanking period. In this pacemaker, programming the PVARP to its minimal value still did not allow sensing of the abnormal atrial activity.

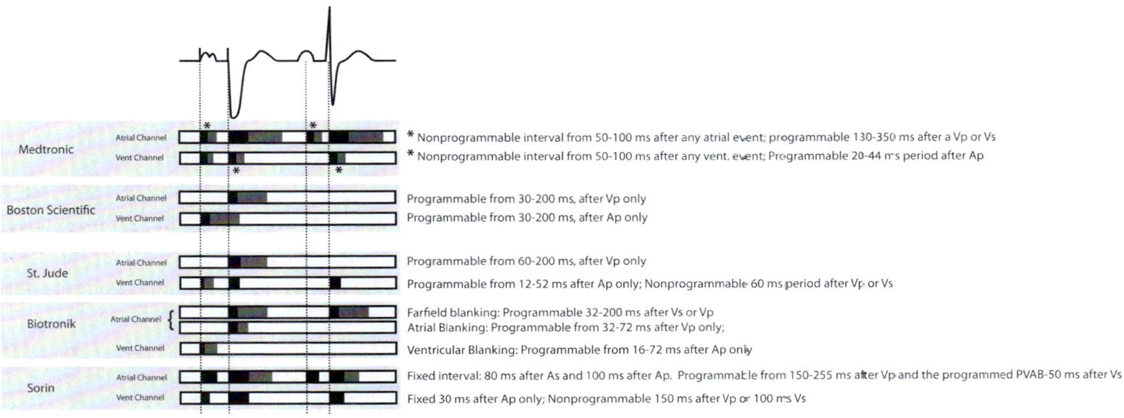

Fig 3.7 Manufacturers use different strategies for blanking periods and refractory periods. These periods are important for maximizing the likelihood that all clinically relevant atrial arrhythmias are identified while minimizing the likelihood of identifying artifacts due to noise or far-field activity. Black: Nonprogrammable portion; Dark gray: Programmable portion.

also have an "auto" feature that will repetitively add 12 ms intervals during the blanking period until a maximum of 52 ms.

In the atrial channel, a PVAB that can be programmed from 60 to 200 ms is available after a paced ventricular event.

Biotronik

Biotronik pacemakers provide a blanking period in each of the sensing channels. For the ventricular channel, a blanking period occurs after an atrial paced event ("Ventricular Blanking") and for the atrial channel, a blanking period occurs after a paced ventricular event ("Atrial Blanking"). In addition, in the atrial channel there is a programmable "Far-field Blanking" period that occurs after any ventricular event (sensed or paced).

Sorin

Sorin pacemakers use the term "Automatic (absolute) Refractory Period" rather than blanking period to describe a period that the pacemaker does not sense or pace and "Protection Period" to designate a period that the pacemaker will continue to sense but will not pace (analogous to a conventional refractory period). For the purpose of maintaining consistency in this discussion, the more widely used terms *blanking period* and *refractory period* will be used. The atrial channel has two separate "blanking" periods. First, a nonprogrammable 80-ms interval after an atrial sensed event and 100 ms after an atrial paced event. Second, the atrial channel has a PVAB that is programmable from 150 to 255 ms after a ventricular paced event and the programmed PVAB—50 ms after a ventricular sensed event. The ventricular channel also has two temporally separated blanking periods: a 30-ms blanking period after an atrial pacing output (none after an atrial sensed event), and a second blanking period after ventricular activity (100-ms blanking period after a ventricular sensed event and a 150-ms period after a ventricular paced event).

Magnet Response

Different manufacturers have similar yet subtly different responses to application of a magnet to the pacemaker (magnet mode) summarized in Table 3.5. For pacemakers, traditionally, the magnet turns the sensing circuitry "off" so that the pacemaker will function in the DOO pacing mode for any of the dual chamber modes (DDD, DDI, or DOO), VOO for any pacing mode that paces only the ventricle (VDD, VVI, or VOO), and AOO for any pacing mode that paced only the atrium (AAI, AOO). However, more recently manufacturers have provided programmable options for the magnet response. In some cases, manufacturers will use changes in magnet rates to help clinicians identify when a device is at or nearing battery depletion and should be followed more closely (intensified follow-up) or replaced (elective replacement interval).

Medtronic

The magnet mode for a Medtronic pacemaker will first do a Threshold Margin Test with three pulses at 100 ppm (pulses per minute) starting with the programmed amplitude and decreasing by 20% to the third pulse. After that the magnet rate will normally be 85 ppm but will decrease to 65 ppm at the elective replacement time.

Boston Scientific

Dual chamber pacemakers can be programmed to "Off" or "Asynch" In the "Asynch" response, the magnet rate is 100 ppm for beginning of life, 90 ppm for "Electric Replacement Near," and 85 ppm for elective replacement. If the pacemaker has been programmed to the "Off" response, no change in pacemaker function will be observed with magnet application. Turning the magnet response "Off" may be useful in selected situations when a patient is about to undergo magnetic resonance imaging (MRI).

St. Jude Medical

The pacemakers can be programmed to "Off" or "Battery Test." When the pacemaker is programmed to "Battery Test," the magnet rate gradually decreases with decreasing voltage from 98.6 ppm (Voltage > 2.75 V) to 66 ppm (voltage is ≥ 2.20 V). When the magnet rate reaches 86.3 ppm, the corresponding battery voltage is ≥ 2.5 V and the device has reached the elective replacement interval.

Biotronik

The magnet response to Biotronik devices can be programmed to "Asynchronous," "Automatic," and "Synchronous." When programmed to "Asynchronous," the pacemaker will pace at a fixed rate of 90 ppm. When programmed to "Automatic," the pacemaker will pace asynchronously at 90 beats for 10 cycles and then pace at the programmed low rate with appropriate sensing. When programmed to "Synchronous," the pacemaker will pace at the programmed low rate with sensing. The manufacturer set value is "Automatic." It is important for the clinician to remember that if a Biotronik pacemaker is

Manufacturer	Programmable Options (Nominal in bold)	Response
Medtronic	None	• Threshold Margin Test (Three pulses at 100 ppm with progressive 30% decrease in pacing amplitude) • Asynchronous pacing at 85 ppm • Asynchronous pacing at 65 ppm at ERI
Boston Scientific	**Async**	• Asynchronous pacing at 100 ppm • Asynchronous pacing at 90 ppm at ERN • Asynchronous pacing at 85 ppm at ERI
	Off	• No response to magnetic fields
St. Jude Medical	**Battery Test**	• Asynchronous pacing from 98.6 ppm (BOL) to 86.3 ppm (ERI) and 66 ppm (EOL) based on battery voltage
	Off	• No response to magnetic fields
Biotronik	**Automatic**	• 10 asynchronous pulses at 90 ppm followed by synchronous pacing at the programmed rate
	Synchronous	• Synchronous pacing at the programmed rate
	Asynchronous	• Asynchronous pacing at 90 ppm
Sorin	None	• Asynchronous pacing from 96 ppm (BOL) to 80 ppm (ERI) based on battery voltage

Table 3.5 Magnet Mode Options and Responses for Different Manufacturers.
BOL, beginning of life; ERI, elective replacement interval; EOL, end of life; ERN, elective replacement near; ppm, pulses per minute.

programmed to "Automatic" or "Synchronous," even with magnet application, the sensing circuit will be active.

The behavior of the device when it has reached elective replacement interval will also vary depending on the programmed magnet response. In the "Asynchronous" magnet mode the device will continue to pace at 80 ppm. With the "Synchronous" magnet mode the basic pacing rate will be decreased by 4.5% to 11%, and in the "Automatic" magnet mode the device will pace asynchronously at 80 ppm for 10 cycles and then decrease by 4.5% to 11%.

Sorin

The magnet rate for most Sorin pacemakers at beginning of life is 96 ppm and gradually decreases to 80 ppm when the elective replacement interval is reached (similar to St. Jude Medical pacemakers). With all Sorin pacemakers, while the magnet is applied, the pacemaker will pace with outputs of 5 mv/0.5 ms or the programmed value (if the programmed value is higher). Upon magnet removal, the pacemaker will continue to pace in the DOO pacing mode at the magnet rate for 8 beats. The first 6 beats are called the "capture test" with an AV delay of 94 ms (to increase the likelihood that ventricular pacing will be observed) followed by a 2-beat "rate test" in the DOO pacing mode at the programmed rate and AV delay.

Acknowledgments

I would like to thank Sarah Cornell, Janet Wright, Megan Cranston, Alex Chieu, Jim Gerrity, and Mike Brown for kindly providing manufacturer specific information for this chapter.

References

1. Bernstein AD, Daubert JC, Fletcher RD, et al. The revised NASPE/BPEG generic code for antibradycardia, adaptive-rate, and multisite pacing. North American Society of Pacing and Electrophysiology/British Pacing and Electrophysiology Group. *Pacing Clin Electrophysiol.* 2002 Feb; 25(2):260–264.
2. Hayes DL. Timing cycles of permanent pacemakers. *Cardiol Clin.* 1992 Nov;10(4):593–608.
3. Barold SS, Falkoff MD, Ong LS, et al. Timing cycles in DDD pacemakers. In: Barold SS, Mugica J, eds. *New Perspectives in Cardiac Pacing.* Mt. Kisco, NY: Futura Publishing; 1988:69–119.
4. Barold SS. Far-field R wave sensing causing prolongation of the atrial escape interval of DDD pacemakers with atrial-based lower rate timing. *Pacing Clin Electrophysiol.* 2003 Nov; 26(11):2188–2191.
5. Sweeney MO, Shea JB, Fox V, et al. Randomized pilot study of a new atrial-based minimal ventricular pacing mode in dual-chamber implantable cardioverter-defibrillators. *Heart Rhythm.* 2004 Jul;1(2):160–167.
6. Savouré A, Fröhlig G, Galley D, et al. A new dual-chamber pacing mode to minimize ventricular pacing. *Pacing Clin Electrophysiol.* 2005 Jan;28 Suppl 1:S43–S46.
7. Furman S. Dual chamber pacemakers: upper rate behavior. *Pacing Clin Electrophysiol.* 1985 Mar;8(2):197–214.

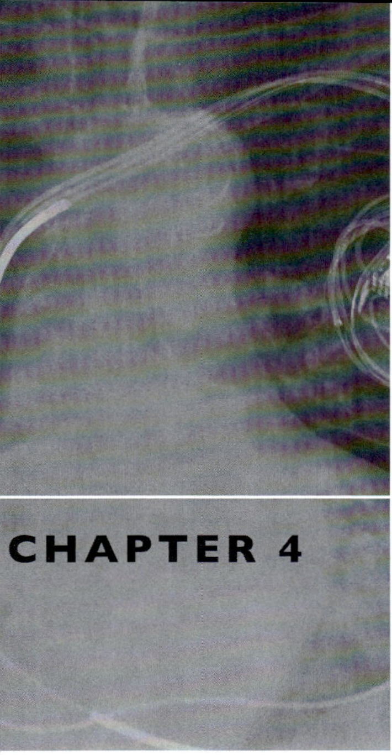

Algorithms for Minimizing Right Ventricular Pacing

CHAPTER 4

Michael O. Sweeney

Introduction

Exploration of the link between the sequence of cardiac electrical activation and mechanical function is one of the most exciting contemporary areas of research in cardiac pacing. Optimal left ventricular pumping function requires a normal electrical activation sequence derived from the synchronized participation of the distal components of the specialized conduction system (the main bundle branches and their ramifications). The left ventricle normally contracts rapidly and synchronously with little variation in the onset of electrical and mechanical activation throughout the wall. Synchrony of contraction is important because it results in a more effective and energetically efficient ejection. Ventricular asynchrony, most commonly due to conduction delay caused by left bundle branch block, results in paradoxical septal wall motion, delayed lateral wall contraction, reduced left ventricular pressure, mitral regurgitation, and reduced diastolic filling times. All of these effects contribute to reduced left ventricular pumping function.[1]

Clinical trials in patients with pacemakers for sinus node dysfunction (SND) or atrioventricular block (AVB) and implantable cardioverter defibrillators (ICDs) provide increasing evidence that desynchronization of ventricular electrical activation and contraction, induced by conventional right ventricular apex (RVA) pacing, is a serious threat for long-term cardiac morbidity and mortality.[2-6] The risk of heart failure is increased even in hearts with initially normal pump function and only having part-time ventricular pacing. This epidemiological data fits with knowledge from decades of pathophysiological research, indicating that RVA pacing creates abnormal contraction, reduced pump function, hypertrophy, and ultrastructural abnormalities.

Pacemakers and Implantable Cardioverter Defibrillators: An Expert's Manual. © 2010 Amin Al-Ahmad, Kenneth A. Ellenbogen, Andrea Natale, and Paul J. Wang, eds. Cardiotext Publishing, ISBN: 978-0-9790164-6-2.

Recognition of the chronic adverse effects of RVA pacing has stimulated interest in strategies to either eliminate or attenuate these effects using pacing modes that minimize ventricular pacing while providing bradycardia support at the atrial level. This approach is only suitable for patients in whom ventricular pacing is not obligatory and therefore applies almost exclusively to patients with SND unaccompanied by AVB. Because the vast majority of patients treated with pacemakers for SND have normal ventricular conduction (QRSd < 120 ms) and reliable AV conduction that remains stable over time,[7-10] preservation of normal ventricular activation by minimizing ventricular stimulation with atrial-dominant pacing support is feasible. Minimization of RVA pacing, as compared to conventional dual chamber pacing, has been shown to reduce the risk of persistent atrial fibrillation (AF) in SND.[10]

Efforts to optimize pacing mode or site should be greater in patients with longer expected duration of pacing, poorer cardiac function, and larger mechanical asynchrony. Awareness of the problem of desynchronization should also lead to more regular monitoring of cardiac pump function and mechanical asynchrony in any patient with ventricular pacing.

It is therefore suggested that the four goals of optimized pacemaker operation in patients with SND and normal ventricular conduction are (1) prevent symptomatic bradycardia, (2) provide physiologic chronotropic competence when necessary, (3) maintain AV synchrony when necessary, and (4) maintain normal ventricular activation sequence whenever possible.[11]

Pacing Strategies to Minimize Ventricular Pacing

As an atrial-dominant pacing strategy necessarily requires AV conduction, pacing platforms to minimize ventricular pacing can be conceptually grouped on the basis of paced AVI (PAVI) management: (1) no PAVI, (2) PAVI continuously operational, and (3) PAVI intermittently operational. Each of these approaches has advantages and limitations and a clinical superiority of any approach has not been demonstrated.

No AV Interval

The simplest approach to minimizing ventricular pacing in SND is single-chamber atrial pacing (AAIR). Atrial pacing is associated with reduced incidence of AF, thromboembolic events, congestive heart failure, and cardiovascular death compared to single-chamber ventricular pacing in SND.[8,12] Nonetheless, most patients with SND receive DDDR systems because of the small, but potentially serious risk of syncope due to progressive conduction system disease resulting in AVB[8,13-16] and because ventricular rate support is often required during AF. A ventricular lead is required for ICDs but many ICD patients receive dual chamber systems because of the need for physiologic pacing support[17-19] and the desire to exploit atrial activity for discrimination between supraventricular and ventricular tachycardias.

AV Interval Continuously Operational

The defining operational characteristic of the conventional dual chamber pacing platform is guaranteed ventricular pacing on every cardiac cycle. This is achieved by scheduling a ventricular pacing stimulus (VP) at the end of the PAVI. Conventional dual chamber pacing operation imposes restrictions on maximum allowable PAVIs, particularly during atrial sensing, in order to maintain sinus tracking at elevated rates and provide adequate detection windows for AF response algorithms. Dual chamber pacing operation in ICDs is even more complex and imposes further restrictions ("interlocks") on maximum allowable PAVIs to prevent competitive pacing during ventricular tachycardia (VT), which might result in detection failure due to inviolable cross-chamber blanking periods. Consequently, the maximum allowable PAVI during conventional dual chamber pacing operation has been in the range of 140 to 200 ms. PAVIs in this range have also been shown to optimize ventricular pump function during obligatory RVA pacing.[20]

Restricted PAVIs imposed by mode switching operation and other constraints of conventional dual chamber pacemaker and ICD timing cycles (see following) result in a high cumulative percent ventricular pacing (Cum%VP) in the majority of patients with SND, including those with intact AV conduction.[2,3] This high Cum%VP is due to the overlap of intrinsic AVIs (iAVI) with allowable PAVIs. Thus, conventional dual chamber pacing condemns the majority of patients with SND to a lifetime of "forced" ventricular desynchronization.[3]

Manipulation of PAVIs in conventional dual chamber modes among patients with intact AV conduction may permit "functional" AAIR operation and reduce unnecessary ventricular pacing. The goal of this approach is to maintain PAVIs longer than iAVIs so that the scheduled VP is continuously pre-empted by ventricular sensing. This can be achieved with either long static PAVIs or long dynamic PAVIs.

Long static PAVIs

Long static PAVIs (250–350 ms) are modestly effective in preventing unnecessary ventricular pacing in many pacemaker and ICD patients because of dynamic variation in AV conduction times.[16,21,22] Nonetheless, long static PAVIs attenuate the effect of ventricular pacing on left ventricular function seen at shorter PAVIs in some patients, though significantly increased left atrial diameters persist compared to AAIR pacing.[16]

Long dynamic PAVIs

Automatically adjusting PAVI extensions for promoting intrinsic AV conduction and reducing ventricular pacing are now featured in almost all contemporary dual chamber pacing systems. It is interesting to note that these features were initially developed more than 2 decades ago as a means for reducing current drain and extending pulse generator longevity rather than reducing morbidity associated with right ventricular stimulation.

These algorithms have a common architecture and consequently, overlapping performance characteristics. Regardless of specific implementation, the PAVI is periodically extended to permit emergence of intrinsic AV conduction. If a spontaneous ventricular event is sensed (VS) within the PAVI extension window, the scheduled VP is inhibited and the extended PAVI is maintained, resulting in functional AAIR pacing. Assuming that the PAVI extension exceeds the iAVI, ventricular pacing is suppressed. If a spontaneous ventricular event is not sensed during the PAVI extension, the scheduled VP is delivered when the PAVI times out. One or more cycles of ventricular pacing force the extended PAVI to collapse to the starting (usually nominal) value and conventional DDDR operation ensues.

Specific operational characteristics of automatic PAVI extensions

The pacemaker operates at two PAVIs, nominal (short) and long, in a three-stage process. Periodic PAVI extensions are scheduled according to elapsed time (ie, every 5 minutes) or number of cardiac cycles. The PAVI extension occurs incrementally (over several cycles) or instantly (between consecutive cycles). Single, multiple consecutive, or ratios of VPs eventually force PAVI collapse to the nominal (short) value. Future attempts may be permanently suspended if ventricular pacing commonly occurs during PAVI extensions. Differences between implementations exist for all three operating stages.

Medtronic Search AV and Search AV+ (Table 4.1 and Fig 4.1) Continuously updating blocks of the 16 most recent AV sequences are evaluated for relative timing relationships. Ventricular paced events or VS events that occur within 15 ms of the scheduled VP (at the extended PAVI) are classified as "late." VS events that occur more than 55 ms prior to the scheduled VP are classified as "early." VS events that occur between 15 to 55 ms before the scheduled VP are classified as "on time."

If ≥ 8/16 AV sequences are designated as "late," the PAVI is increased by 31 ms or to the

Search AV First Generation	SAV+ Second Generation
Maximum AVI=350 ms	Maximum AVI=600 ms
Continuously extends AVI in 31 ms increments until at least 8/16 VS events occur	Continuously extends AVI in 62 ms increments until at least 8/16 VS events occur
Reverts to programmed value if ≥ 8/16 VP events occur within extended AVI, or if ≥ 8/16 VS events are within 15 ms of extended AVI	Reverts to programmed value if ≥ 8/16 VP events occur within extended AVI
Max AVI Offset: 110 ms	Max Offset: 250 ms (in 10 ms increments)
Max SAV = 250 ms unless mode-switch off (interlock)	
Cycle Frequency: 1, 2, 4, 8, 16 hrs	Cycle Frequency: 15 min, 30 min, 1, 2, 4, 8, 16 hrs
No automatic deactivation; search repeats every 16 hours	Deactivated after 10 consecutive 16 hr search cycles (~1 week)
Dedicated diagnostic	Dedicated diagnostic

Table 4.1 Medtronic Search AV and Search AV + operation

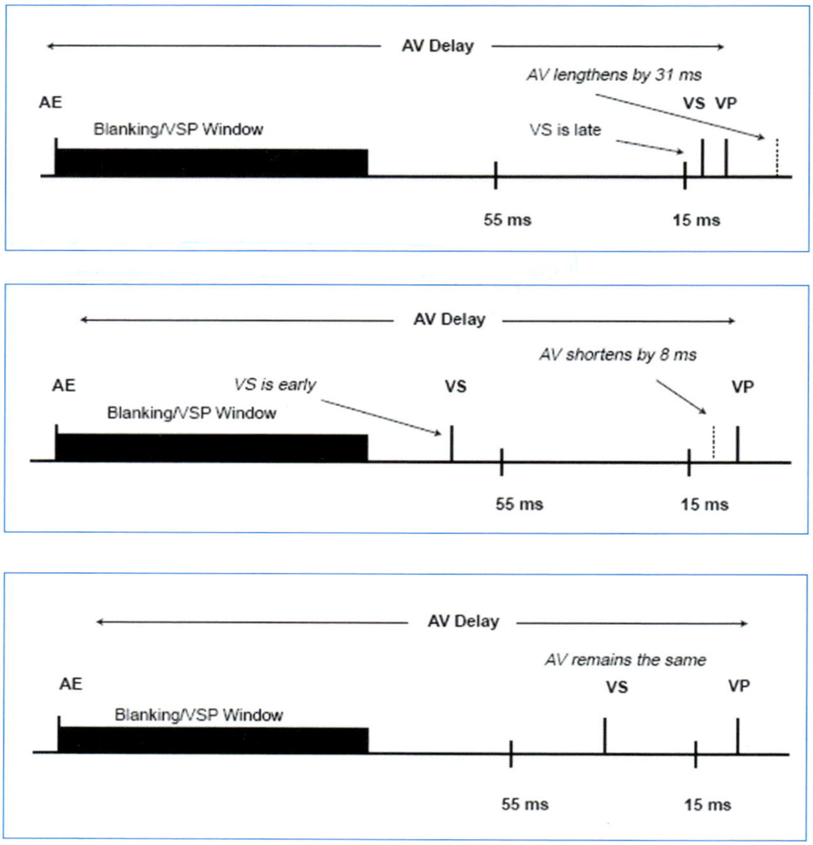

VS event classified as "late." AVI lengthens by 31 ms. This new value is used for the next 16 conduction sequences but will not exceed the maximum permitted AVI.

VS event classified as "early." AVI shortens by 8 ms and maintained for the next 16 conduction sequence.

VS event classified as "on time" (neither late nor early). No adjustments to the AVI are made for the next 16 conduction sequences.

Fig 4.1 Medtronic Search AV and Search AV+ operation.

maximum permitted PAVI. This value is maintained for the subsequent 16 AV sequences. If ≥ 8/16 AV sequences are designated as "early," the PAVI is decreased by 8 ms or the shortest permitted PAVI for the subsequent 16 AV sequences. If ≥ 8/16 AV sequences are neither "early" nor "late" the VS events are designated as "on time" and no adjustment to the PAVI is made over the subsequent 16 AV sequences. In this manner VS events are continuously maintained within a PAVI "window" that precedes the scheduled VP.

In the first iteration of Search AV the maximum permitted PAVI was 350 ms. Due to an interlock with mode switching operation, the maximum PAVI could only be achieved during atrial sensing by deactivating mode switch. This behavior introduced the possibility of sustained URL tracking during AF. Several adjustments were made to the second iteration of Search AV (SAV+). The maximum permitted PAVI was increased to 600 ms. The interlock with mode-switching operation during atrial sensing was eliminated. An adaptive paced AV blanking algorithm was added to reduce the probability of ventricular pacing in the vulnerable period following an undersensed ventricular premature beat (VPD). The PAVI search steps were increased from 31 to 62 ms and the geometric step frequency of search intervals was increased. The rule declaring VS events within 15 ms of the scheduled VP as "late" was eliminated. Finally, a stopping rule for PAVI searches was implemented after 10 consecutive failures at 16-hour intervals

Boston Scientific AV Search Hysteresis (Table 4.2) AV Search Hysteresis (AVSH) extends the PAVI for up to 8 consecutive cycles. As long as VS events are recorded, the extended PAVI is maintained. The PAVI will collapse to the programmed value upon the first VP within the 8-cycle search or after an unsuccessful 8-cycle search expires. The PAVI search frequency cycle frequency is programmable (32–1024 cycles in powers of 2) and a programmable PAVI increase (% 10–100 of programmed AVI) determines how much the PAVI will increase during a search cycle. This maximum PAVI was increased from 300 to 400 ms in the second iteration of AVSH; no other substantive changes were made.

AV Search Hysteresis First Generation	**AV Search Hysteresis Second Generation**
Maximum AVI = 300 ms Extends AVI to the programmed value (ms) AVI extension 10–100% of fixed or dynamic AVI Programmable in 10% increments (Nominal 30%) AVI Search Cycle 32–1024 cycles (powers of 2, ~0.5 to 176 min); Failed search resets time Algorithm activation ≥ 1 VS event outside extended AVI in first 8 cycles of each search Algorithm deactivation Single VP at extended AVI No VS within first 8 cycles of search AV Search Hysteresis Diagnostic Total number + number of successful AVI searches	Maximum AVI = 400 ms All other aspects of operation remain the same as first generation AVI extension

Table 4.2 Boston Scientific AV Search Hysteresis operation

St. Jude Medical AutoIntrinsic Conduction Search and Ventricular Intrinsic Preference (Table 4.3 and Fig 4.2) The St. Jude Medical AutoIntrinsic Conduction Search (AICS) employed a simple 3-stage PAVI hysteresis. The PAVI was extended up to a selectable maximum of 350 ms in 10-ms steps at fixed 5-minute duty cycles. A single VP or a failed search resets the duty cycle. The PAVI search could be linked to a rate hysteresis search interval, which was selectable in some models. AICS was inoperative at sinus or atrial pacing rates > 100 bpm, and the maximum PAVI extension was limited to 100 ms when ventricular AutoCapture was On.

AICS was modified and re-packaged as Ventricular Intrinsic Preference (VIP) in more recent St. Jude Medical pacing systems. The maximum PAVI remains fixed at 350 ms. The PAVI search duty cycle frequency and AVI increment are now programmable. Deactivation occurs when the number of consecutive VPs equals the programmed number of search cycles. The sinus or atrial pacing rate lockout was increased to 110 bpm. The purpose of these modifications is to provide leniency in the conditions forcing resumption of ventricular pacing at shorter PAVIs.

Other automatic AVI extension approaches: Biotronik, Vitatron, and ELA Biotronik offers an AV Hysteresis feature similar to that of Boston Scientific and St. Jude Medical. The PAVI is extended for up to 6 cycles (programmable) and is maintained as long as VS events are recorded. Similar to Boston Scientific, a single VP at any point or a failed search cycle forces collapse of the PAVI. The PAVI extension interval is programmable whereas the duty cycle frequency (every 180 cycles) is not. The maximum permissible PAVI is 300 ms.

Vitatron Refined Ventricular Pacing (RVP) utilizes a conventional 3-stage AV hysteresis approach with one unique difference relating to upper rate timing. The maximum permissible PAVI is 365 ms. In other AV hysteresis platforms, PAVI extensions necessarily extend total atrial refractory period (TARP). However, as atrial rate increases TARP and PAVI are shortened to maintain 1:1 tracking. This results in increased ventricular pacing fre-

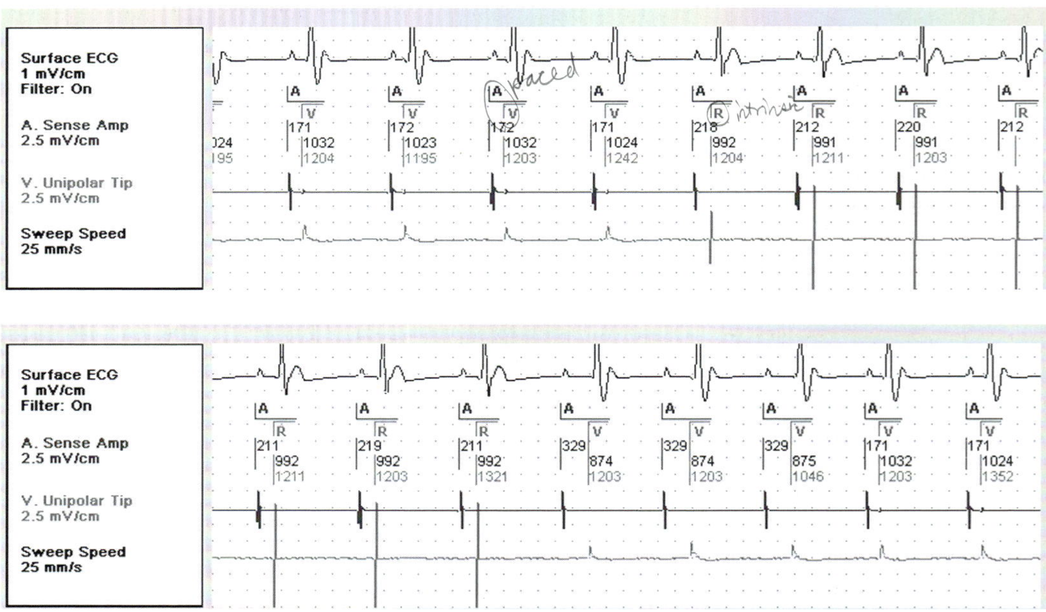

Fig 4.2 St. Jude Medical VIP operation. **Top**: Algorithm is activated by first sensed R wave during a search interval. **Bottom**: Algorithm is deactivated when number of consecutive VPs equals programmed number of search cycles (3, in this example).

Auto Intrinsic Conduction Search (AICS) First Generation	Ventricular Intrinsic Preference (VIP) Second Generation
Maximum AVI = 350 ms Extends AVI to the programmed value (ms) AVI extension +10 → 120 ms in steps of 10 ms AVI Search Cycle 5 minute intervals (non-programmable)\ Failed search resets timer Algorithm deactivation Single VP at extended AVI AICS is disabled when base rate ≥ 90 bpm, intrinsic atrial or atrial paced rate ≥ 90 bpm, Negative AV hysteresis is on No dedicated diagnostic to assess efficacy	Maximum AVI = 350 ms Extends AVI to the programmed value (ms) +50 → +150 in steps of 25 ms +150 → + 200 in steps of 10 ms AVI extension 30 sec, 1, 3, 5, 10, 30 min (nominal: 1 min) AVI Search Cycles (number of consecutive cycles AVI remains extended during search) 1, 2, 3 (nominal 1) Algorithm activation 1 intrinsic R wave s sensed during a search interval 3 consecutive R waves outside a search interval Algorithm deactivation Number of consecutive V Ps equals programmed number of search cycles VIP is disabled when base rate ≥ 110 bpm, intrinsic atrial or atrial paced rate ≥ 110 bpm, Negative AV hysteresis is on

Table 4.3 St. Jude Medical AICS and VIP operation

quency during atrial rate increases or lock out of PAVI extensions at high atrial rates. Vitatron pacemakers use a "physiologic band" to define normal vs. pathologic atrial rate. A physiologic atrial rate is calculated from the running average of the actual (sensed or paced) atrial rate. The physiologic band is defined by an upper boundary equal to the physiologic rate + 25 bpm (minimum value: 100 bpm) and the lower boundary by the physiologic rate – 15 bpm (or the sensor-indicated rate if higher). Atrial events above the upper boundary of the physiologic band are not tracked and trigger mode-switch. Because this approach does not rely on TARP to classify atrial events for AF recognition this should theoretically increase the success of PAVI extensions by eliminating upper rate timing cycle conflicts and reduce the risk of endless loop tachycardia (ELT).

ELA Automatic Mode Conversion (DDD/AMC) The ELA first-generation approach to automatic PAVI extensions (DDD/AMC) differed significantly from conventional AV hysteresis approaches. Though this approach was described as automatic mode switching between DDDR and AAIR, it was actually a form of PAVI hysteresis where every pacing cycle includes a scheduled VP. The PAVI is increased in 47-ms steps for 5 cycles (non-programmable) after 100 consecutive VP cycles or upon a transition from atrial pacing to atrial sensing. If 8 consecutive VS events occur during the PAVI extension, the PAVI is maintained at 31 ms longer than the average AVI of the previous 8 cycles (functional "AAI" mode). The maximum PAVI is 344 ms. A single VP during the PAVI extension forces collapse to the programmed value ("DDD" mode).

Performance of Automatic AVI Extensions for Minimizing Ventricular Pacing

There has been very little systematic comparison of the effectiveness of different algorithms for suppressing ventricular pacing. Most comparisons have been made between nominal settings, which yield virtually continuous ventricular pacing given that PAVI < iAVI in almost all situations, and a specific PAVI extension algorithm. Direct comparisons between different proprietary algorithms do not exist.

Some generalizations are possible. First-generation algorithms that force collapse of the extended PAVI after a single VP are heavily biased to ventricular pacing (Fig 4.3). Algorithms that permit a maximum PAVI of ≤ 300 to 350 ms are only modestly effective in suppressing ventricular pacing (Fig 4.4). The effectiveness of any algorithm is reduced by impaired baseline AV conduction and therefore reported results must be interpreted in the context of the study population.

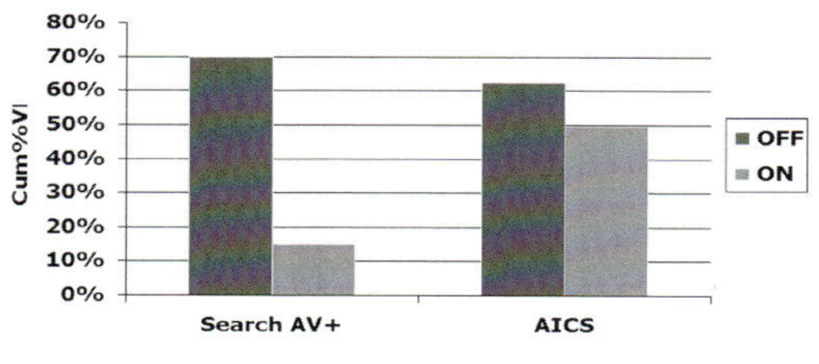

Fig 4.3 Comparison of ventricular pacing reduction using Medtronic Search AV+ and St. Jude Medical AICS. Among patients with 1:1 AV conduction, Search AV+ reduced Cum%VP from 70% to 15% (79% relative reduction) compared to nominal PAVI settings whereas AICS reduced Cum%VP from 62% to 50% (19% relative reduction).[61,62]

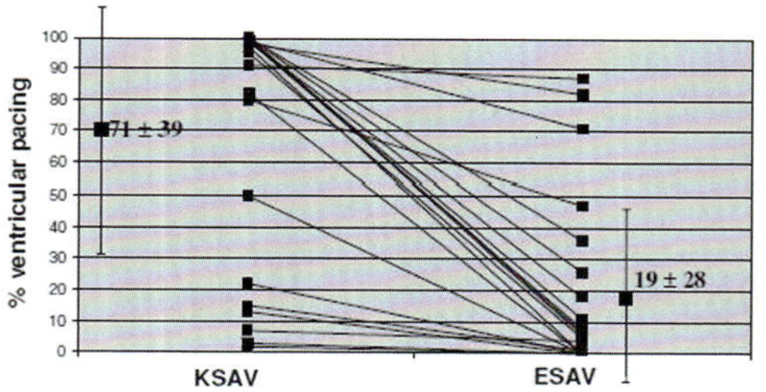

Fig 4.4 Comparison of Medtronic Search AV and Search AV+ for reducing ventricular pacing.[63] (Figure courtesy of Todd Sheldon, MS, modified by M. O. Sweeney, MD)

Examination of the performance of Boston Scientific AVSH in the INTRINSIC RV study highlights the general limitations and variable success of this algorithm approach to minimizing ventricular pacing. INTRINSIC RV tested the hypothesis that dual chamber ICDs programmed to minimize ventricular pacing would not be inferior to backup pacing at 40 bpm using single chamber ICD programming.[23] All patients received dual chamber ICDs programmed to DDDR with AVSH On at nominal settings (minimum pAVI = 90 ms, maximum pAVI = 200 ms, search interval 32 cycles, pAVI increase 50%) over rate range 60 to 130 bpm. Percent ventricular pacing was evaluated after a 1-week observation period and patients with > 20% ventricular pacing were excluded from the study. It was expected that > 80% of patients would pass this screening period and be enrolled. However, an interim analysis revealed that only one-third of patients would meet the enrollment criteria for reduced ventricular pacing at nominal AVSH settings.[24] After 1 week, atrial pacing was 24.6% ± 24.7%; RV pacing was 41.5% ± 29.7%, and 67.5% of patients had > 20% RV pacing. Based on these observations, the protocol was amended and AVSH programming was modified to include maximum pAVI = 300 ms with 100% increase. Additionally, recognizing the contribution of atrial pacing to PAVI extensions, a rate hysteresis offset of –20 bpm was added. Consequently, atrial pacing would not occur until the sinus rate reached 40 bpm. This was necessary due to an interlock between extended PAVIs at increasing rates and tachycardia detection programming requirements. After pacing protocol modification, atrial pacing was 9.4% ± 7.8%, ventricular pacing 14.6% ± 27.8%, and still 23% of patients had > 20% ventricular pacing and were excluded from the study. The consequence of the limitations imposed by AVSH is that among patients in whom < 20% ventricular pacing was achieved, atrial pacing was virtually eliminated and was still exceeded by ventricular pacing percentage. The unintended effect of these compromises was that AVS H mimicked ventricular-only single chamber operation in a dual chamber platform, whereas the stated goal was to provide functional AAIR pacing.[23]

The SAVEPACe trial used the Medtronic Search AV+ algorithm to test the hypothesis that minimization of ventricular pacing in sinus node disease would reduce the risk of AF.[10] After 1.7 years of follow-up in 1065 patients, median percent ventricular pacing was less in dual chamber minimal ventricular pacing vs. conventional dual chamber pacing (9.1% vs. 99%, $p < 0.001$), whereas atrial pacing was similar (71.4% vs. 70.4%, $p = 0.96$) (Fig 4.5). One hundred ten patients developed persistent AF (conventional dual chamber pacing, 68, or 12.7%, vs. dual chamber minimal ventricular pacing, 42, or 7.9%). The hazard ratio for development of persistent AF in dual chamber minimal ventricular pacing vs. conventional dual chamber pacing was 0.60 (95% confidence interval 0.41–0.88; $p = 0.009$), indicating a 40% relative risk reduction. This second-generation approach to minimizing ventricular pacing was highly effective and achieved the parallel goal of functional atrial pacing, unlike AVSH in the INTRINSIC RV study. However, it is important to recognize that the SAVEPACe population was enriched for reliable AV conduction by the requirements for a successful atrial pacing test at 100 bpm for 30 s.

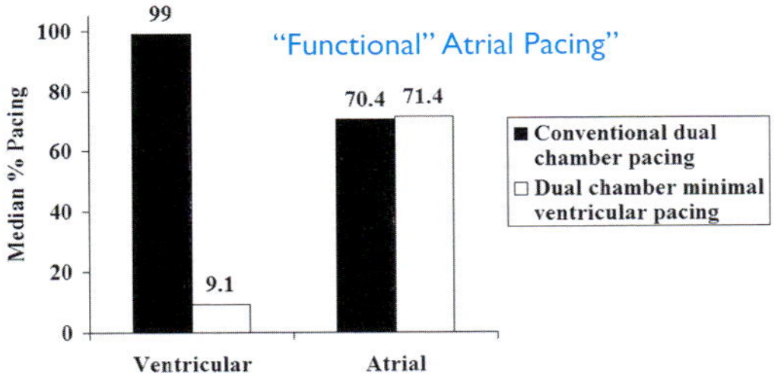

Fig 4.5 Reduction in ventricular pacing using Medtronic Search AV+ in the SAVEPACe trial.[10]

Limitations of Fixed and Dynamic Long PAVIs for Minimizing Ventricular Pacing

The common failure mechanism of extended PAVIs is that eventually the scheduled VP must occur when the iAVI exceeds the PAVI. Thus, the guarantee of AV synchrony on every cardiac cycle in the conventional dual chamber platform fundamentally contradicts the goal of suppressing all unnecessary ventricular pacing. Failure of long static and dynamic PAVIs to suppress unwanted ventricular stimulation can be explained by five factors: (1) baseline iAVI, (2) frequency of atrial pacing, (3) effect of rate response, (4) effect of autonomic tone on AV conduction, and (5) dual chamber timing cycle rules.

The pacemaker AP-VS interval begins with the emission of the atrial pacing stimulus and ends with right ventricular sensing. This interval is composed of atrial capture latency, intra(right)-atrial conduction time, AV conduction system time (primarily AV nodal), and latency in ventricular sensing. The right-sided AP-VS interval begins with right atrial capture and is identical to the pacemaker AP-VS after subtraction of the atrial capture latency time. Atrioventricular intervals (AVIs) during atrial sensing are similarly composed with the difference that atrial sensing latency replaces atrial capture latency during pacemaker AS-VS intervals.

The baseline iAVI is a marker for iAVI extensions during atrial pacing, rate response, and autonomic stress.[25] AVIs during atrial sensing are always shorter than AVIs initiated by atrial pacing at any heart rate (Fig 4.6). The increase in AVIs during atrial pacing is accounted for by atrial capture latency, intra(right)-atrial conduction time and AV nodal conduction, none of which can be quantified on a beat-to-beat basis by patient or within the study population. Atrial capture latencies are reported in the range of 30 to 50 ms[26] but may exceed 200 ms in unusual circumstances.[27] Atrial capture latencies and intra-atrial conduction times remain generally constant across heart rates assuming a stable site of atrial activation.[26] Therefore, increases in AV conduction time during atrial pacing are most likely entirely due to decremental AV nodal conduction at increasing pacing rates or differential AV nodal inputs relative to sinus rhythm. Atrial pacing results in a rightward shift in AVI histograms compared to sinus rhythm. This effect is exaggerated during rate responsive pacing (Fig 4.6). In either situation of atrial sensing or pacing, AVIs display evidence of autonomic sensitivity, typically in a diurnal pattern with longer AS-VS and AP-VS intervals occurring during sleep (Fig 4.7). There is also greater variation in AVIs during sleep versus waking hours, suggesting the autonomic condition is more dynamic during sleep. These observations suggest that the largest part of increases in AV conduction time during atrial pacing is accounted for by AV nodal delay, which is subject to exogenous (i.e., autonomic) influences.

Long PAVIs impose substantial penalties on conventional dual chamber pacing operation. These can be broadly grouped as (1) timing cycle conflicts and (2) proarrhythmia (Table 4.4). Because the TARP is the sum of the PAVI and the postventricular atrial refractory period (PVARP), long PAVIs force a reduced upper rate limit (URL). This can be addressed by automatic shortening of the PVARP and then the PAVI at increasing sinus or sensor-modulated rates (Fig 4.8). The consequence is an increase in Cum%VP at higher heart rates. Additionally, mandatory shortening of the PVARP dur-

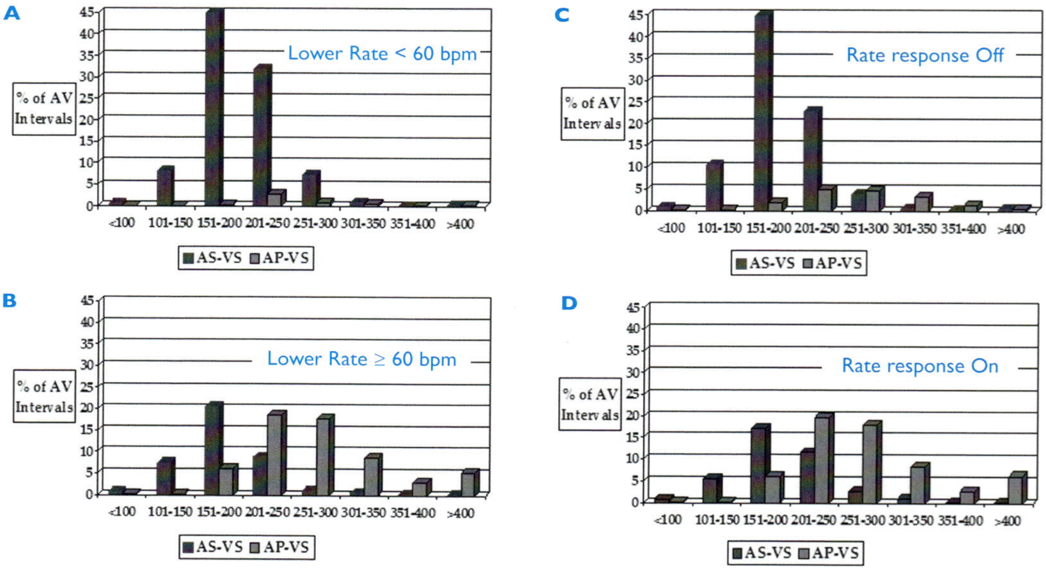

Fig 4.6 Effect of lower rate and rate response on AVIs during AAIR pacing. **A**: Lower rate < 60 bpm. **B**: Lower rate ≥ 60 bpm. Rate response Off in all comparisons. **C**: Rate response Off. **D**: Rate response On.[25]

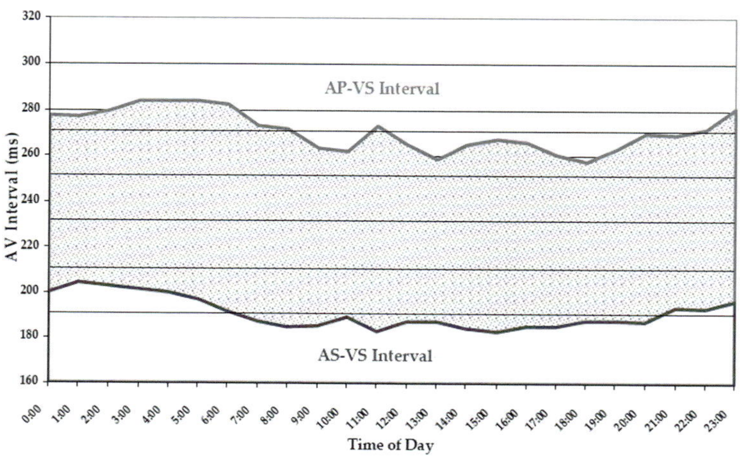

Fig 4.7 (left) Effect of time of day on AVI behavior during AAIR pacing. Hatched area indicates point-by-point differences in AP-VS versus AS-VS intervals (ms).[25]

Timing Cycle Conflicts

1. Upper Rate Behavior
   - Restricted upper tracking rate
   - Shortening of PVARP, SAV and PAV at high sinus rates (↑Cum%VP, ↑Risk of ELT)
2. AF Recognition
   - Under-detection of atrial premature depolarizations
   - Mode-switching delays, oscillations, or failure
3. ICD Tachycardia detection programming conflicts
   - Upper pacing rate ↔ lower VT detection rate conflict

Proarrhythmia

1. Endless Loop Arrhythmias
   - Classic pacemaker-mediated tachycardia (ELT)
   - AV desynchronization arrhythmia (AVDA)
2. Ventricular Proarrhythmia
   - Premature ventricular stimuli closely coupled to native ventricular activation or ventricular premature depolarizations initiating VT/VF

Table 4.4 Limitations and risks of long pAVIs during conventional dual chamber pacing.

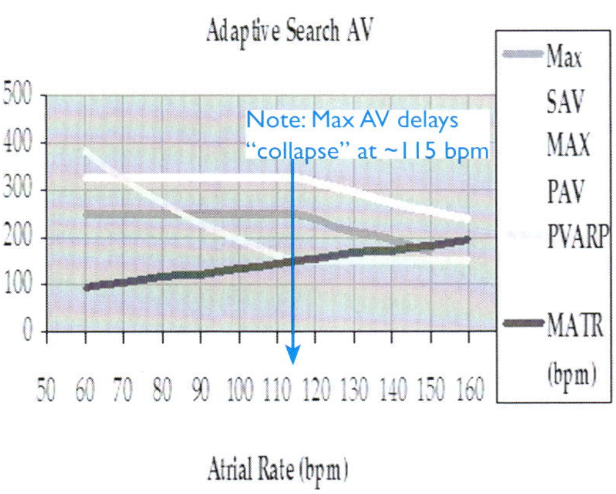

Fig 4.8 Effect of dual chamber timing rules during upper rate behavior on pacemaker AVIs (assumes nominal 120 ms SAV, 150 ms PAV, 110 max AVI offset).

ing automatic PAVI extensions increases the risk of pacemaker-mediated tachycardia (see following). Long PAVIs shorten the atrial sensing window, resulting in underdetection of atrial premature depolarizations and competitive atrial pacing, particularly at high sinus rates. Reduced atrial sensing windows increase the probability of delayed or failed AF response algorithms.

Risks of Fixed and Dynamic Long PAVIs for Minimizing Ventricular Pacing

Long PAVIs introduce unique programming conflicts in ICD platforms because bradycardia pacing is not permitted in or near a tachycardia detection zone. The reason for this is that inviolable cross-chamber blanking periods evoked by atrial and ventricular pacing outputs may result in VT detection delays or failures (Fig 4.9). The probability of this increased when: (1) pacing rate encroaches on the VT detection rate and (2) PAVI approximates VT cycle length. Longer AVIs increase the probability that the emission of atrial and ventricular pacing stimuli will syn-

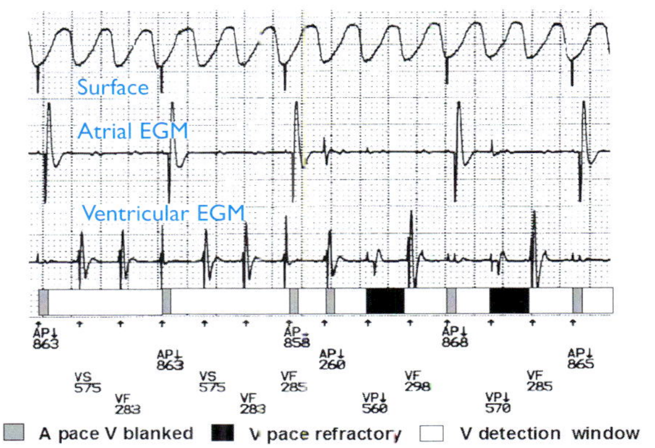

Fig 4.9 VT detection failure due to cross-chamber blanking. The first VT event is not sensed because it occurs during the cross-chamber blanking period invoked by AP/863 stimulus. The second VT event (VS/575) is sensed outside pacing refractory periods but the VT cycle length is misreported as 575 ms because the immediate preceding VT event was not sensed The third VT event (VF/283) is sensed and the cycle length calculated based on VS/575 falls in the VF detection zone. The fourth VT event is blanked by AP/863. The next two VT events (VS/575, VF/283) are sensed with cycle length timing as described previously. The next VT event (VF/285) is sensed immediately prior to AP/858. The next VT event is blanked by AP/260, which is delivered early due to Rate Smoothing operation. The next VT event is blanked by the ventricular refractory period initiated by the VP/560 stimulus. This process of cross-chamber blanking of ventricular events perpetuates, VT detection is never satisfied, and an external rescue shock was delivered. (Modified from Shivkumar et al.,[64] courtesy of Wiley and Sons, used with permission.)

chronize with consecutive VT events (i.e., PAVI 300 ms and VT cycle length 300 ms). It is for this reason that PAVIs are heavily constrained in ICD systems. To prevent VT detection failure during dual chamber pacing the VT detection interval must fit within the pacemaker VA interval (Fig 4.10). Progressive shortening of the VA interval at increasing heart rates occurs with long PAVIs. This requires either a sacrifice in the lower VT detection interval or a reduction in PAVI, which will increase Cum%VP.

Because patients targeted for dual chamber minimal ventricular pacing strategies have intact AV conduction, VPDs, or under certain circumstances VPs, may evoke retrograde atrial depolarizations initiating different forms of pacemaker-mediated endless loop arrhythmias. Long PAVIs may permit recovery of retrograde AV conduction prior to delivery of the scheduled VP. Retrograde conduction elicited by the VP elicits atrial events that fall outside the (shortened) PVARP that initiate and maintain classic ELT (Fig 4.11).[28] Retrograde atrial events that fall within the PVARP do not initiate a new AVI but may render the subsequent atrial pacing stimulus ineffectual if the coupling interval is shorter than the atrial functional refractory period (FRP). Perpetuation of this phenomenon results in an unusual form of ventriculoatrial synchrony without causing ELT. This has been referred to as "repetitive nonreentrant ventriculoatrial synchrony" or "AV desynchronization arrhythmia" (AVDA).[29] AVDA causes symptoms due to VA dissociation ("pacemaker syndrome") and may result in spurious mode-switching when repetitive atrial events in the PVARP are used for AT/AF evidence (Fig 4.12).[30] AVDA is typically initiated by VPDs during sensor-modulated rate responsive DDDR pacing. Sensor-modulated shortening of the atrial escape interval (AEI) increases the likelihood that the subsequent atrial pacing stimulus will fall in the atrial FRP.[29] Once initiated, AVDA persists until either VA conduction fails or atrial capture is restored by reprogramming a higher atrial output. More commonly, an initial rise in atrial pacing threshold at the onset of AVDA declines within several minutes and atrial capture is restored without reprogramming atrial output.[29] Most episodes of AVDA are nonsustained for this reason. Termination also occurs when slowing of the sensor-

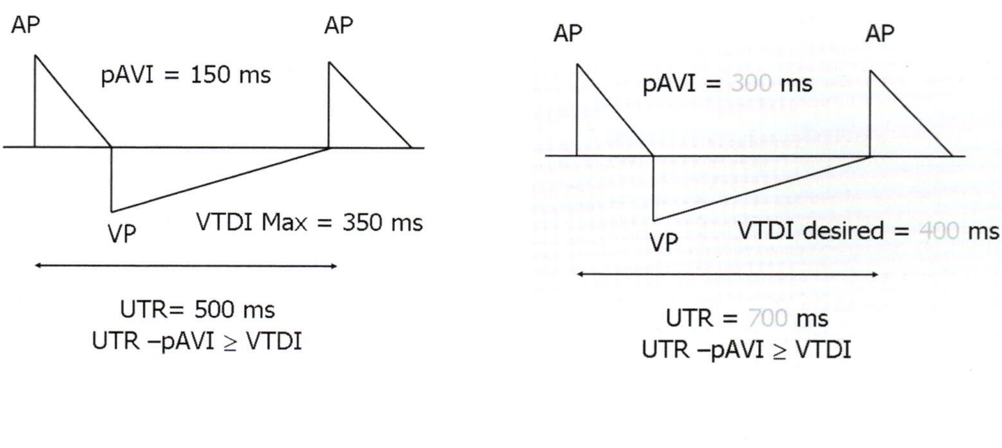

Fig 4.10 Interlock between PAVI, upper tracking rate (UTR), and VT detection interval (VTDI). **Left**: The programmed PAVI is 150 ms and the UTR is 500 ms. When operating at the upper sensor rate, the VA interval is 350 ms. Therefore, the VTDI cannot exceed 350 ms. **Right**: If the PAVI is increased to 300 ms while maintaining a VTDI of 400 ms, the UTR must be reduced to 700 ms.

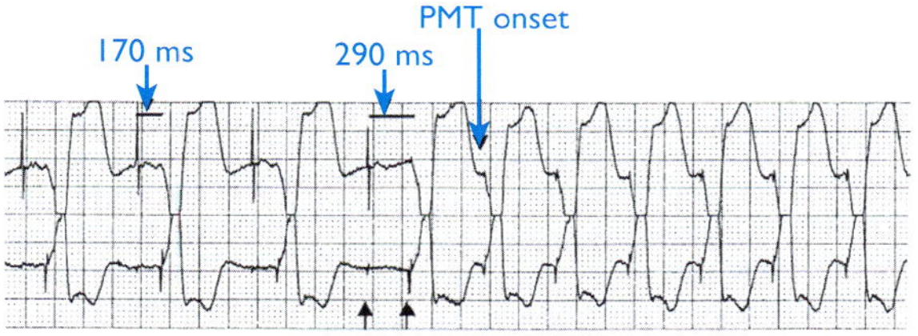

Fig 4.11 Endless loop tachycardia initiated by AICS. The PAVI is automatically increased from 170 to 290 ms, which is insufficient to prevent ventricular pacing. Slow antegrade AV nodal conduction elicited by the atrial pacing stimulus is followed by fast retrograde pathway elicited by the ventricular pacing stimulus (VA time 220 ms). VP (VA 220 ms). Retrograde atrial activation outside PVARP initiates classic PMT. (Reprinted by permission of Blackwell Publishing.)

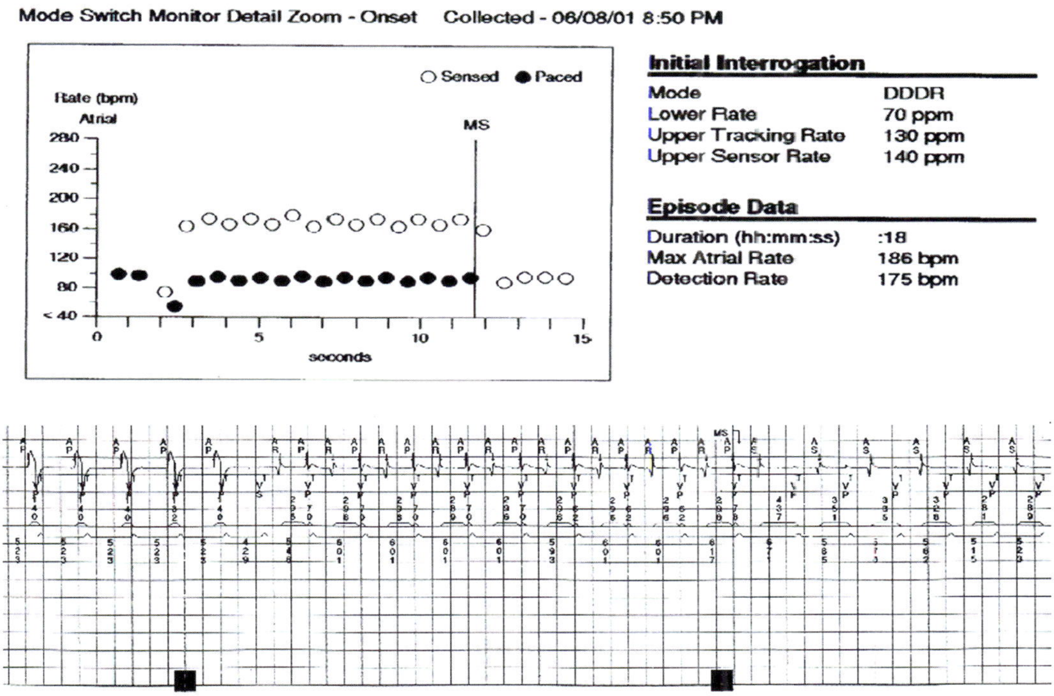

Fig 4.12 Spurious mode switching due to AVDA during DDDR pacing. **Top**: Mode Switch monitor detail. **Bottom**: Spontaneous AVDA causing spurious mode switch. Atrial EGM, event markers, timing intervals (top to bottom). MS denotes mode switch. The first 5 complexes show sensor modulated rate responsive DDDR pacing (AP-VP) with cycle length 523 ms. A late-coupled VPD, denoted as VS, occurs 429 ms after AP-VP5. This is followed 280 ms later by a retrograde atrial depolarization that falls in the PVARP (denoted as AR, atrial refractory). AP-VP6 follows the first retrograde atrial event. However, despite a coupling interval of 296 ms AP6 is ineffectual, presumably because it fell within the atrial FRP. Note absent evoked response on the local EGM indicating loss of capture following AP6 compared to AP1-5. The subsequent VP6 is followed 280 ms later by a retrograde atrial event with an identical local bipolar morphology as the first retrograde atrial event. This process (APineffectual - VP - retrograde AR) iterates for 9 consecutive cycles until mode switch occurs (denoted as MS) when the mean atrial interval (MAI) is shorter than the mode switch interval.

After mode switch, ventricular pacing (in the DDIR mode) continues to evoke retrograde atrial activation with identical timing relationship (VA time 280 ms) and local bipolar EGM morphology as prior to mode switch. Retrograde atrial events now fall outside the PVARP and are sensed (AS). Sensed atrial events in the DDIR mode initiate an AS-VP interval. The AS-VP interval lengthens in order to conform to the upper rate interval, which is equal to the lower rate interval in the DDI mode 65. In the last 6 beats, since the retrograde VP-AS time is constant, the subsequent AS-VP intervals vary slightly in order to conform to sensor modulation of the pacing rate.

modulated rate lengthens the AEI, eventually enabling an atrial pacing stimulus to fall outside the atrial FRP and restore capture. This terminates AVDA by either preventing retrograde VA conduction due to block in the AV node (assuming the programmed AV delay is not long) or causing the evoked retrograde impulse to fall in the atrial FRP.

The DDIR mode eliminates some of the timing cycle conflicts associated with long PAVIs, especially in ICD patients (Table 4.5). The DDIR mode was introduced in the late 1980s to address undesirable rapid ventricular pacing in response to AF in patients with SND and intact AV conduction. DDIR was initially relegated to obscurity by the subsequent introduction of mode switching in the DDDR mode. However, a clinical value of mode switching has not been proven[31] and the shortened PAVI range required for optimal AT/AF recognition and mode switching operation results in a high frequency of forced ventricular pacing, which increases the risk of AF.[3,10] Consequently, interest in the DDIR mode to provide functional atrial pacing support for SND has been renewed. The DDIR mode is best described not by what it does, but what it does not do compared to DDDR.[27] DDIR does not synchronize ventricular pacing to intrinsic atrial activity. This eliminates the upper tracking limit timing cycle conflicts as there is no sensed AVI, and permits long PAVIs without the possibility of URL tracking during AT/AF, unlike DDDR. Short AF sensing windows are irrelevant because mode switching is unnecessary. The programmed PAVI is only relevant in conjunction with atrial pacing, and it therefore eliminates unnecessary ventricular fusion or pseudofusion in the presence of sensed normal sinus rhythm. Competitive atrial pacing during sensor modulation may precipitate AF, similar to DDDR, and can be mitigated with a noncompetitive atrial pacing algorithm. A unique limitation imposed by the DDIR mode is that it is operationally VVIR during breakdowns in AV conduction if the sinus rate exceeds the programmed lower rate or sensor-indicated rate (Fig 4.13). AVDA during DDIR pacing has similar onset and offset mechanisms as during DDDR pacing. However, because there is no atrial tracking in the DDIR mode, the ventricular rate during AVDA is determined by the programmed lower rate or sensor-indicated rate (Fig 4.14).

Ventricular proarrhythmia is a potentially lethal consequence of long PAVIs to suppress ventricular pacing. The trigger for premature stimulation in the VRP in the dual chamber mode is (1) true or (2) functional undersensing of a VPD in the PAVI.[32] Functional undersensing occurs when a VPD falls within the short absolute ventricular blanking period initiated by an atrial-paced event. The scheduled VP then falls during the repolarization phase of the VPD. The probability of capture increases

	DDDR	DDIR
Advantages		
AV synchrony during AVB	Yes	No
Functional AAIR in absence of AVB	Possible	Possible
Limitations		
Reduced pump function, diastolic MR during VP at long AVI	Yes	Yes
Upper rate limitations	Yes	Not applicable
Mode switching delays	Yes	Not applicable
Endless loop arrhythmias	Yes	Yes
ICD tachy detection conflicts	Yes	Yes

Table 4.5 Dual chamber modes with long fixed AVIs.

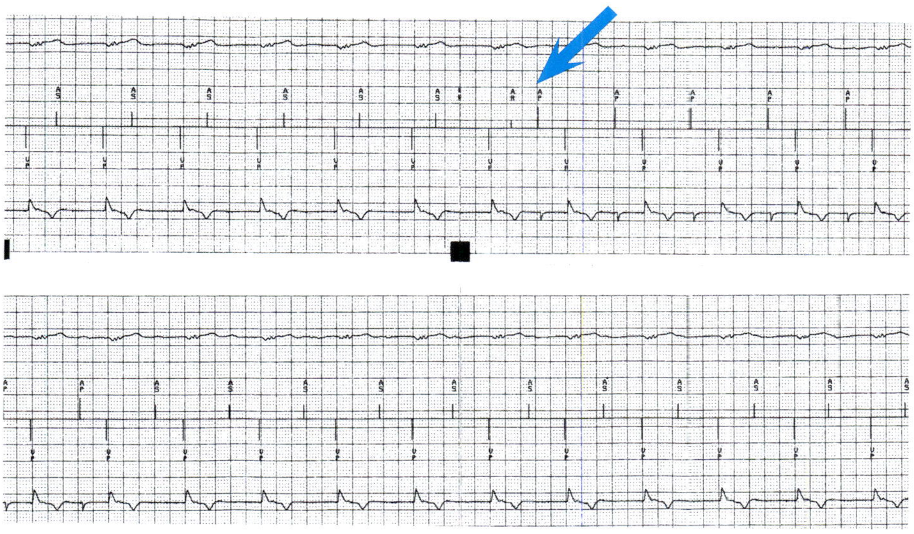

Fig 4.13 Functional VVI pacing during AV block in the DDIR mode. Dual chamber ICD, DD R mode, lower programmed rate limit 60 bpm, PAVI 350 ms. AV conduction has failed and atrial tracking is absent in the DDI mode. Ventricular pacing is isorhythmically dissociated from sinus rhythm. Eventually a sinus beat falls in the PVARP and is marked as a refractory event (AR, arrow). An AP is therefore released at the pacemaker AEI. Ventricular pacing is synchronized to atrial pacing at the extended PAVI assuming AV conduction does not pre-empt the scheduled VP. When the sinus rate supercedes the lower pacing rate, functional VVI pacing returns (lower strip).

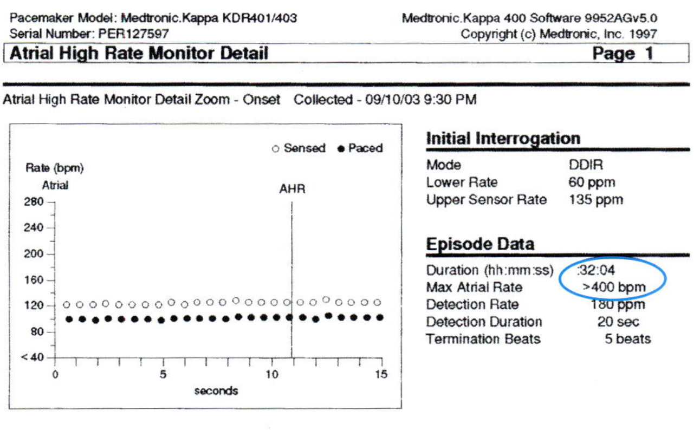

Fig 4.14 AVDA during DDIR pacing. The PAVI is 350 ms. **Top**: Atrial high-rate monitor detail. Note oscillating atrial paced and sensed events. **Bottom**: Stored electrogram. Each VP results in retrograde atrial activation that falls in the PVARP (AR). The scheduled AP is closely coupled to the AR event due to the long PAVI. The AP is ineffectual because it falls in the atrial FRP. Consequently, atrial capture does not occur and the subsequent scheduled VP at the long PAVI elicits retrograde conduction. The process continues until either (1) retrograde conduction fails; (2) retrograde conduction slows and the atrial event falls outside the PVARP, is sensed, and initiates classic ELT; (3) the sensor-indicated rate declines, displacing the scheduled AP beyond the FRP for the retrograde atrial event, resulting in atrial capture, which terminates AVDA by blocking retrograde AV nodal conduction or suppressing the scheduled VP.

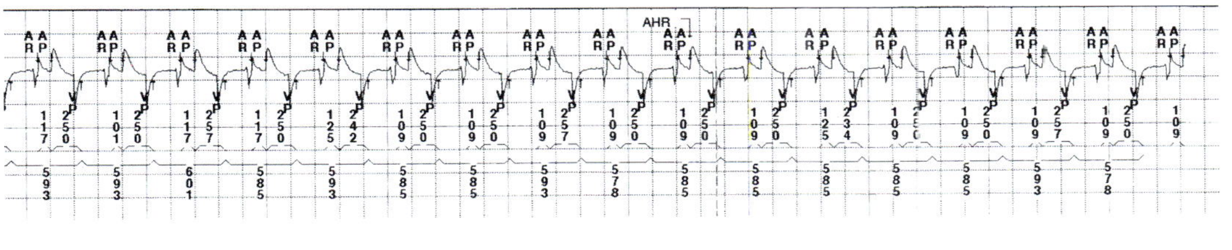

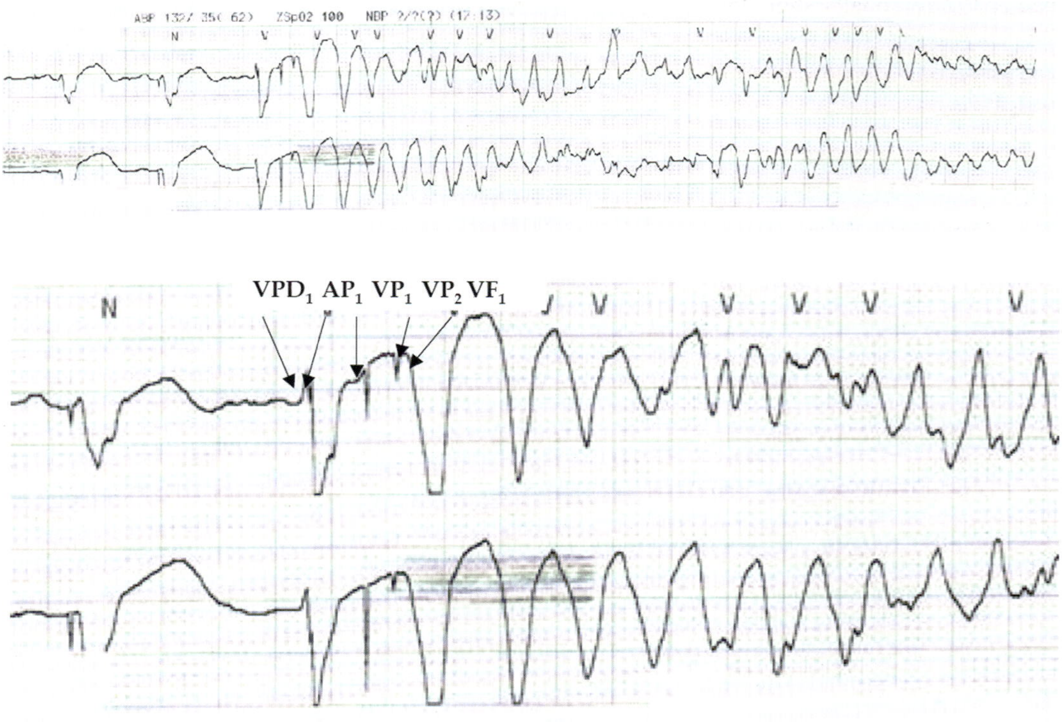

Fig 4.15 Ventricular proarrhythmia during ventricular autoCapture operation. **Top**: Dual chamber pacing is interrupted by ventricular fibrillation (VF) immediately preceded by closely coupled double ventricular pacing stimuli (VPs) following a ventricular premature depolarization (VPD). VF terminated after ≈ 90 s of chest compressions. **Bottom**: Analysis of VF onset using electronic calipers. A VPD occurs nearly simultaneously with an atrial-paced event (AP, note pacing stimulus on downstroke of VPD). However, the VP (VP1) is delivered at the programmed AVD 200 ms after AP, indicating that the VPD is not sensed. The first VP (VP1) therefore occurs ≈ 245 ms after the VPD onset. Because the ventricular muscle is refractory, capture does not occur. Therefore, a high output (4.5 V) backup bipolar pacing stimulus (VP2) is delivered 100 ms later, ≈ 345 ms after VPD onset, which initiates VF. The stimulus to QRS interval between VP2 and the first beat of VF (VF1) is ≈ 24 ms, which is identical to the stimulus to QRS interval for prior VP beats, implying that VP2 resulted in capture.

with longer AVDs, which may displace the pacing stimulus outside the ventricular effective refractory period (VERP). Ventricular capture outside the VERP may initiate VF (Fig 4.15).

AV Interval Intermittently Operational

Newer atrial-based dual chamber pacing modes have been developed to aggressively exploit intrinsic AV conduction, even when severely impaired, in order to minimize ventricular pacing. The common architecture of these modes is automatic switching between single chamber atrial and dual chamber pacing operation based on continuously updating, real-time assessment of atrial rhythm and AV conduction status. These modes permit unrestrained iAVIs and intermittent AV uncoupling (AV-UC; cycles devoid of ventricular activity) and therefore represent a significant departure from conventional dual chamber pacing. Because the PAVI is nominally eliminated, the fundamental obstacle to minimizing ventricular pacing does not exist. However, the absence of the PAVI permits potentially undesirable long iAVIs (AV decoupling, AV-DC), particularly during atrial pacing.[25] Additionally, short-long-short (S-L-S) sequences induced by intermittent AV-UC may be associated with ventricular proarrhythmia in some susceptible patients.[33]

Medtronic: Managed Ventricular Pacing (Table 4.6, Figs. 4.16–25)

MVP is most closely described as an enhanced ADIR mode with mode switching to DDDR during periods of AV conduction failure. During normal operation only the atrium is paced (resembling AAIR), while the ventricle is monitored to verify intact AV conduction. AVIs are not restricted under any circumstance but are influenced by the intrinsic atrial rate, sensor rate, and AV conduction behavior. VS events simply need to occur prior to the next atrial (sensed or paced) event. The operational definition of AV conduction failure is a single A-A interval without an intervening VS event. Single A-A cycles without a VS event are permitted, mimicking normal human AV nodal Wenckebach behavior. A single VP is delivered on the cycle following an A-A cycle without a VS. Higher level AV conduction failure (< 2 VS events for 4 atrial events) causes mode switch to DDDR to prevent ventricular asystole. Tests for recovery of AV conduction are scheduled at geometrically progressing time intervals beginning at 1 minute after DDDR mode switch. Ventricular pacing is withheld for 1 cycle; if a VS event is observed, the operating mode returns to AAIR. Detection of AF triggers mode switch to DDIR. MVP switches to DDDR for 1-minute postshock. A conduction check is scheduled after 1 minute of DDDR operation; if AVB is detected, normal MVP progressive AV conduction check search intervals (2, 4, 8 … minutes) occur until AV conduction resumes.

There is no dedicated diagnostic for MVP operation presently. Because ventricular pacing is influenced by AV conduction status and atrial rhythm status, MVP performance can be deduced from pacing event counters and

	MVP	AAIsafeR 1 and 2
Nominal maximum AVI	None	iAVI=350 ms, pAVI=450 ms (6 consecutive)
Criteria for AAI → DDD switch	2 of 4 A-A intervals without VS	1. 6 consecutive long AVI cycles (AS-VS > 350 ms or AP-VS > 450 ms; programmable) 2. 3 AS/AP events without VS in 12 consecutive cycles 3. 2 consecutive AS events without VS 4. Back-up ventricular safety pace for pauses (2 ,3, 4 seconds; programmable)
Response to AVB	Switch to DDDR at nominal AVIs	Switch to DDDR at nominal AVIs
Criteria for DDD → AAI switch	1 AS-VS cycle	12 consecutive AS/AP-VS cycles
Conduction Recovery Check	1 minute after AAI → DDD switch Doubles on each successive AV conduction failure 2 min, 4 min, etc. up to 16 hrs	Check after 100 DDD cycles, if not terminated first by 12 consecutive AS/AP-VS cycles
Criteria for permanent DDD	None	15 AAI → DDD switches over 24 hours 5 AAI → DDD switches over 3 consecutive days
Response to AT/AF	Switch to DDIR	Switch to DDIR

Table 4.6 MVP and AAIsafeR 1 and 2 Comparison.

device-recorded AF history. When AV conduction is intact, only the AS-VS and AP-VS counters are incremented. AV conduction breakdowns during sinus rhythm will increment the AS-VP and AP-VP counters. Ventricular pacing (in the DDIR mode) is also binned in the AS-VP counter. Therefore, if there is no device-recorded AF evidence, percent ventricular pacing in the AS-VP and AP-VP counters indicates total time of AV conduction failure.

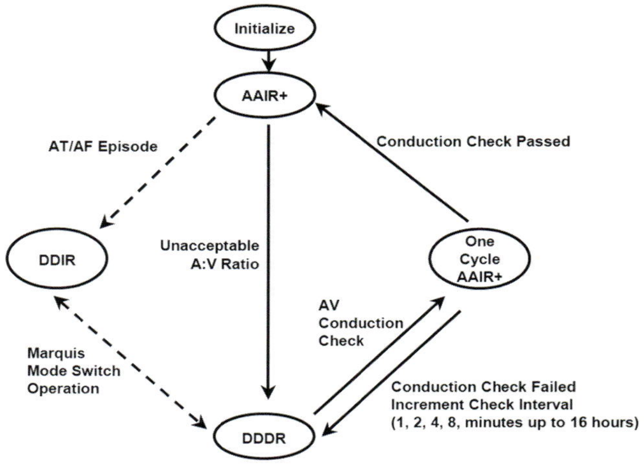

Fig 4.16 MVP operating scheme. During sinus rhythm, the operating mode is AAIR+. Functional atrial pacing is provided according to the programmed lower rate limit or sensor-indicated rate while AV conduction is continuously monitored. DDDR operation is triggered by AV conduction breakdowns. Conduction checks are scheduled at geometrically progressing time intervals by withholding a single scheduled VP. Recovery of AV conduction triggers return to AAIR+ mode. MVP is designed to work with Mode Switching. When Mode Switch is programmed On, it has priority. During an AT/AF episode, Mode Switch will force the mode to DDIR from either the AAIR+ or DDDR mode. After the AT/AF episode, Mode Switch will return the mode to DDDR. If the patient had AV conduction prior to the Mode Switch episode, a conduction check will occur to get back to AAIR+. Therefore, MVP continuously oscillates among three pacing modes based on cycle-to-cycle assessment of AV conduction status and atrial rhythm status.

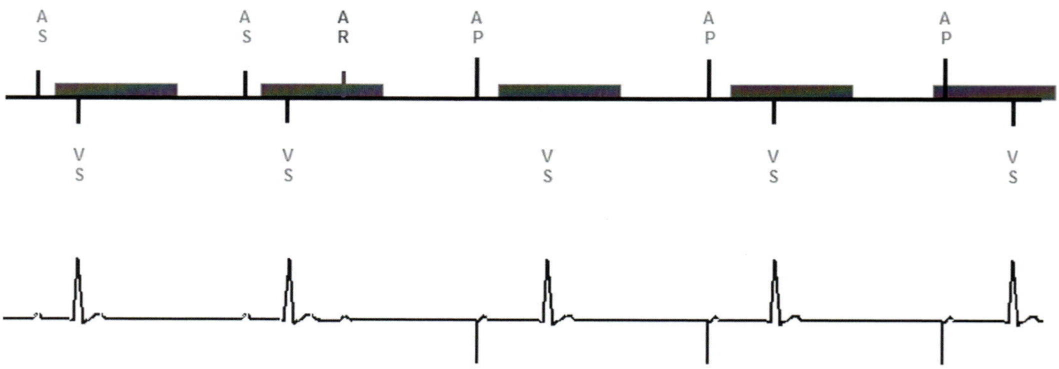

Fig 4.17 Dynamic atrial refractory period (ARP) during MVP. Dynamic ARP is 75% of the R-R median (PR Logic's measurement of the current heart rate). To prevent extremely long ARPs, the calculated value is limited by 600 ms. The R-R mean can lag behind a sudden increase in the pacing rate (eg, during Sensor Rate acceleration), so in these cases, ARP is 75% of the current pacing interval. The purpose of dynamic ARP is to avoid inappropriate DDDR mode switches in the presence of non-conducted APDs and also to ensure that the A-A escape interval is only reset after (true) sinus P waves. Note, non-conducted APD, denoted as "AR" event, does not satisfy AV conduction failure rule.

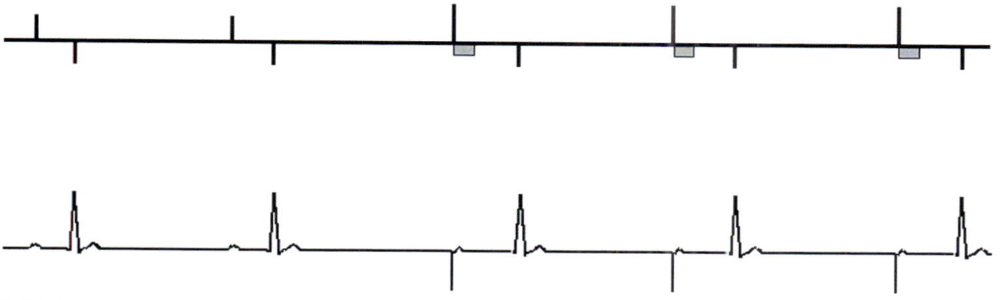

Fig 4.18 AAIR+ mode includes an 80-ms pseudoventricular blanking period after each atrial-paced event. Ventricular sensed events in the 80-ms window do not satisfy the AV conduction criteria (one VS event within each A-A interval). This provides crosstalk.

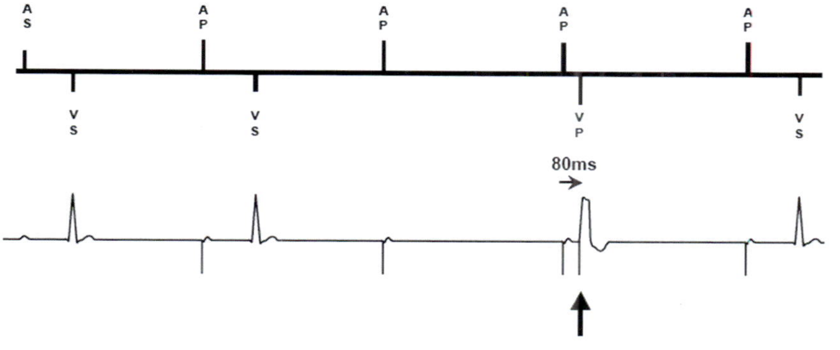

Fig 4.19 Single-cycle AV block response. A single backup VP occurs following an A-A interval without a VS event. The backup VP is scheduled 80 ms after the scheduled AP and is committed. This means that once the AP is released, the VP cannot be inhibited.

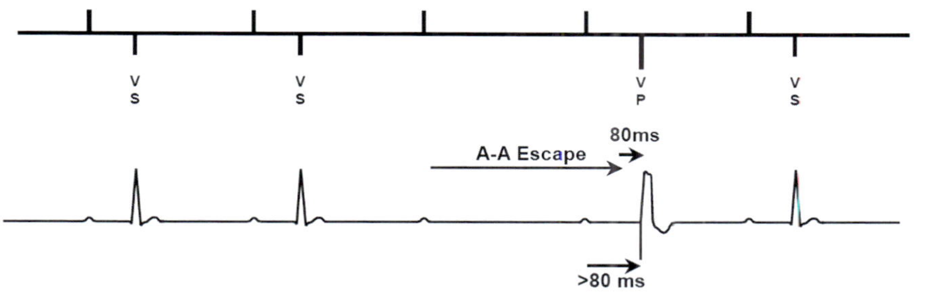

Fig 4.20 Single-cycle AV block response, continued. When the prevailing sinus rate exceeds the programmed atrial pacing rate (or sensor-indicated rate), the single backup VP does not occur 80 ms after the AS event. Rather, the backup VP occurs 80 ms after the inhibited AP (i.e., 80 ms after the escape A-A interval). For this case, the backup VP is not committed (i.e., it will be inhibited by a VS event).

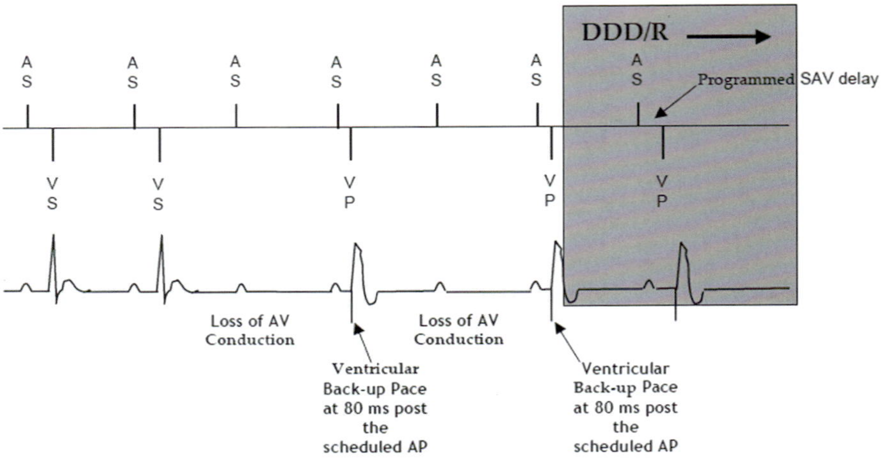

Fig 4.21 MVP: AV conduction criteria to switch from AAIR+ to DDDR. MVP switches from AAIR operation to DDDR operation when there is evidence of persistent loss of AV conduction. The criterion to switch is loss of AV conduction for 2 out of the last 4 pacing cycles (the four most recent A-A intervals). Immediately after the first A-A interval with no conducted VS, a backup VP is delivered 80 ms after the scheduled AP. A second A-A interval occurs with no conducted VS event. Again, the backup VP is delivered followed by a permanent switch to DDDR operation. Note: The PAVIs DDDR operation is the programmed PAVI values.

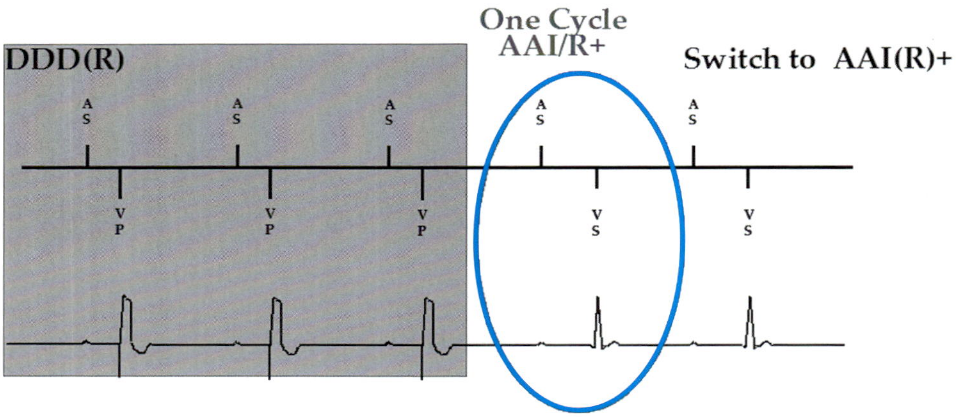

Fig 4.22 MVP: AV conduction check. After switching to DDDR operation, the device will periodically perform scheduled "conduction checks." These checks involve one atrial beat (AP or AS) and the device simply monitors for a conducted VS. If AV conduction occurs (VS event occurs), the mode switches back to AAIR operating mode with backup V-pacing. Otherwise, if no conducted VS occurs, the device continues to operate in DDDR. Scheduled conduction checks occur every 1, 2, 4, 8 minutes . . . up to every 16 hours. That is, after the first switch to DDDR the first conduction check is at 1 minute. If no VS found, the next check occurs 2 minutes later. If no VS found the next check occurs 4 minutes later, and so on. Conduction checks will continue to occur up to every 16 hours indefinitely. MVP is never suspended on the basis of failed AV conduction checks. Therefore, for patients with persistent AVB, one dropped ventricular beat will occur every 12 hours due to conduction checks.

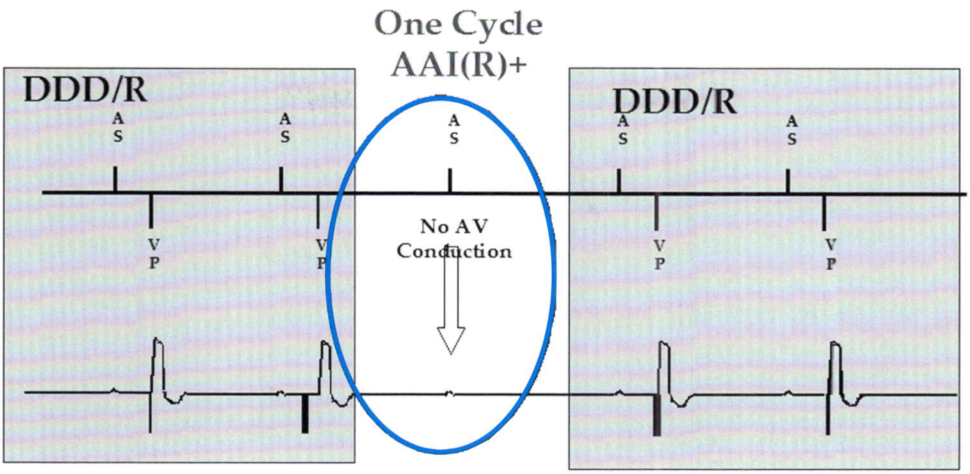

Fig 4.23 MVP: Failed AV conduction check. If no VS event occurs during a single cycle VP withhold, the mode returns to DDDR on the following cycle.

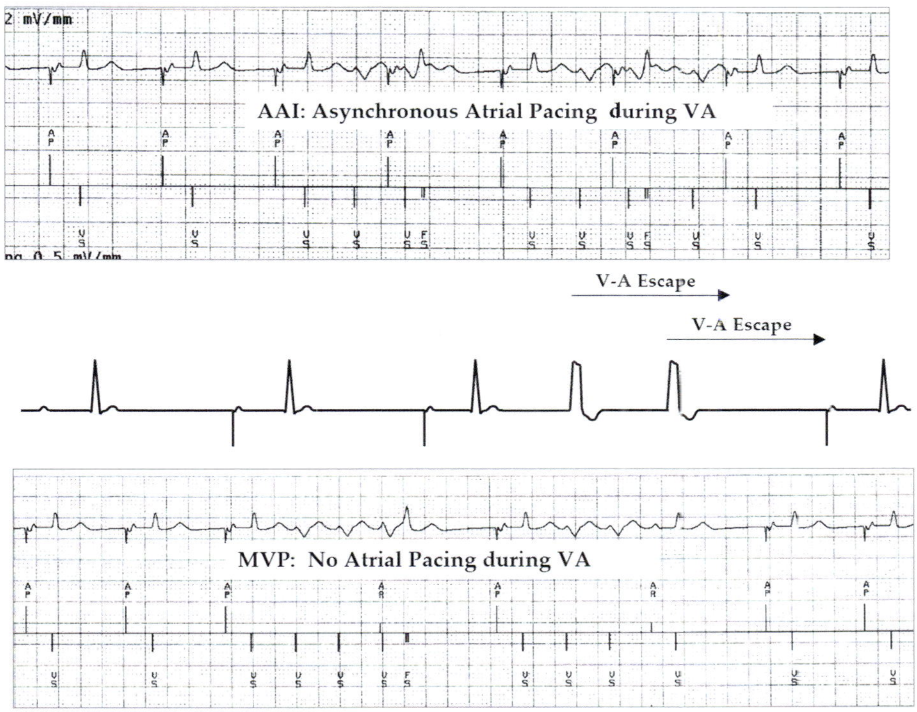

Fig 4.24 MVP: Special timing rules during ventricular arrhythmias. **Top**: In conventional AAIR operation, the AEIs continue to expire, resulting in asynchronous atrial pacing during VPDs and sustained VT or VF. Cross-chamber ventricular blanking during atrial pacing may delay or prevent VT detection (see text). **Middle**: During MVP, VPDs reset the V-A interval and cause the AEI to be re-calculated (which is similar to traditional DDDR timing rules). **Bottom**: Competitive atrial pacing is eliminated during MVP. Though this may appear to produce long A-A intervals, this is normal MVP timing operation.

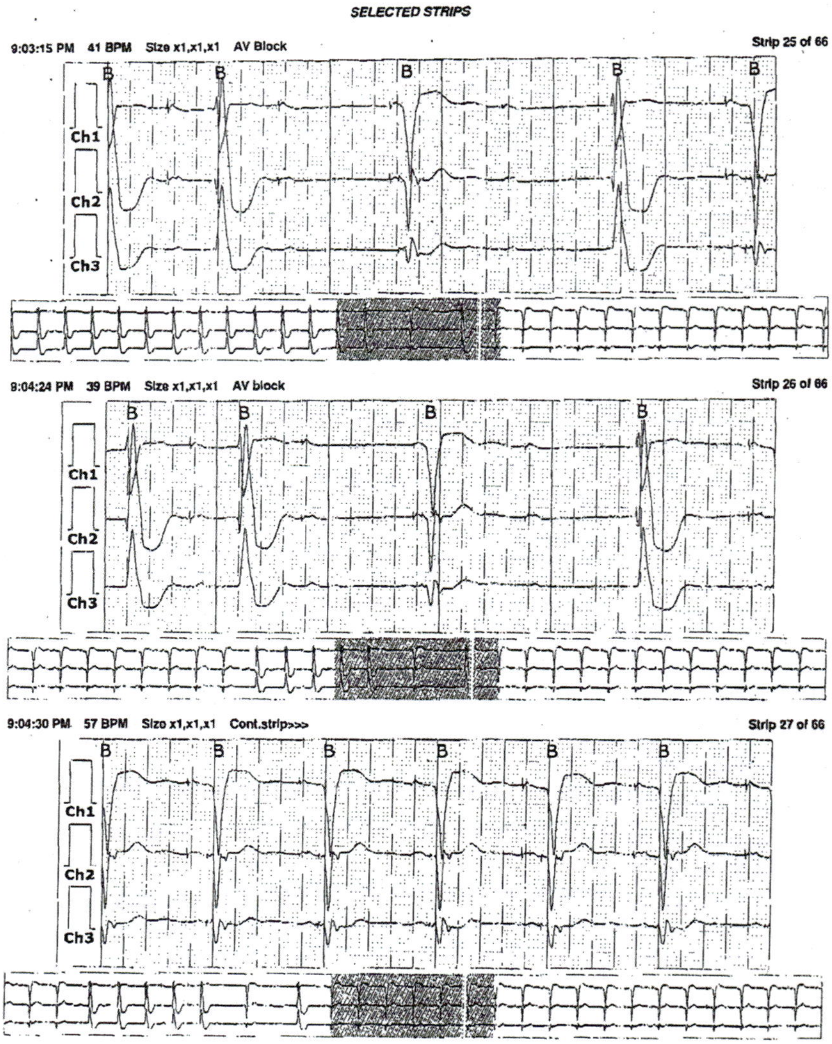

Fig 4.25 Ambulatory example of Wenckebach sequences and AAIR → DDDR switch during MVP.

ELA: AAIsafeR 1, 2 (Table 4.6, Figs. 4.26–4.29)
AAIsafeR (versions 1 and 2) is an enhanced ADIR mode similar in operational intent to MVP with several important differences.[34] First, multiple AV timing criteria are used to trigger DDDR switch. These address progressive AV conduction failure, summarized as follows: (1) consecutive cycles with long iAVIs (> 350–450 ms), or "first-degree AVB"; (2) X/Y A-A cycles without VS events, or "second-degree AVB"; (3) consecutive A-A cycles without VS events, or "third-degree AVB". Additionally, pauses (programmable at 2, 3, 4 s) trigger DDDR switch. Finally, in newer devices, VS events within the ventricular safety pacing window after 2 consecutive AS events will force DDDR switch. Switch from AAI → DDD occurs automatically if 12 consecutive VS events occur. Alternately, a test for recovery of AV conduction is initiated after 100 DDDR cycles by switching to AAIR and reapplying the AVB criteria. The algorithm is disabled until reprogramming if (1) > 5 AAI → DDD switches occur in each of 3 consecutive days

or (2) ≥ 15 AAI → DDD switches occur in 1 day. The purpose of this approach is to reduce symptomatic pauses in patients with evidence of extremely unreliable AV conduction.

Several enhancements were made to the original algorithm and refurbished as AAIsafeR2. The criteria for persistent AVB uses > 50% time in DDDR mode for disabling algorithm operation rather than the number of AAI ⟶ DDD switches in a specific time period. The long PAVI ("first-degree block") criteria for AAI ⟶ DDD switching can be disabled. AVB that occurs during exercise (indicated by sensor input) is not used to increment the persistent AVB time counter. Tests for recovery of AV conduction after a diagnosis of persistent AVB until 8 AM because autonomic conditions may facilitate spontaneous conduction.

Special timing rules are applied during atrial pacing and ventricular arrhythmia, similar to MVP. A 105-ms noise sampling period is applied after atrial and ventricular events to reduce cross-chamber oversensing without compromising atrial sensing. The AEI is reset by VPDs. Crosstalk response uses a ventricular safety pacing window following AP events, similar to the DDDR mode.

A dedicated diagnostic is provided for AAIsafeR. Complete statistics on AVIs, AVB types, and long-term daily trending are automatically stored and segregated by diurnal, nocturnal, rest, and exercise conditions. Pacing mode data is provided for DDDR, AAIR, and AAI → DDD switch percentages. Up to 7 stored electrograms triggered by AAI → DDD switches are also available.

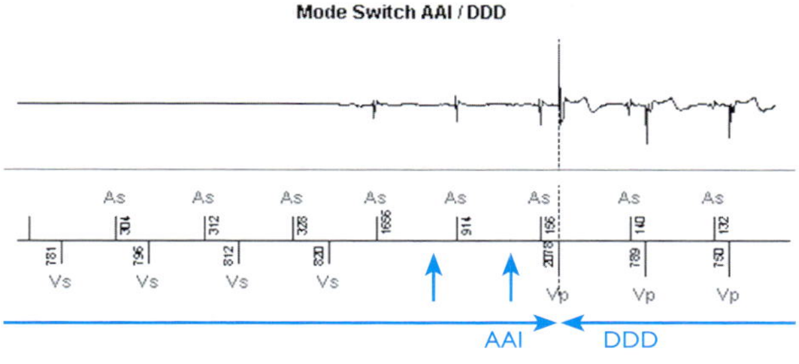

Fig 4.26 AAIsafeR2: AAI ⟶ DDD switch due to two consecutive nonconducted P waves.

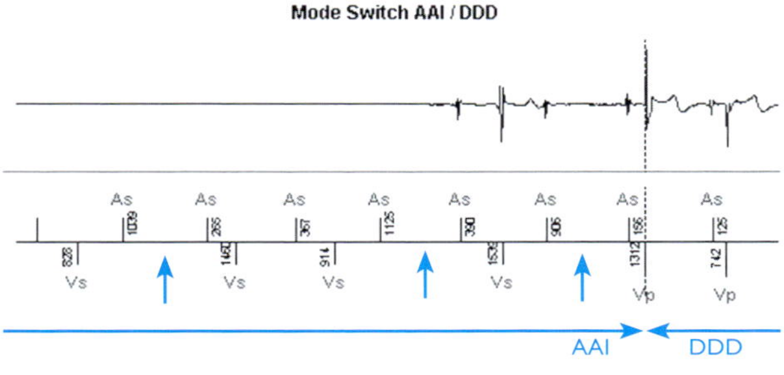

Fig 4.27 AAIsafeR2: AAI ⟶ DDD switch due to three nonconducted P waves out of any 12.

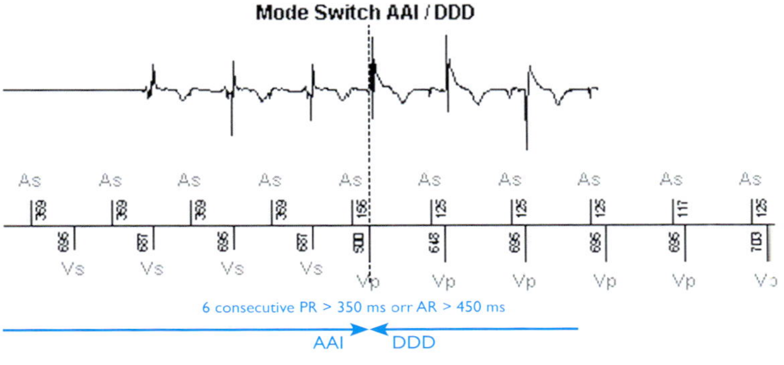

Fig 4.28 AAIsafeR2: AAI ⟶ DDD switch due to first-degree AVB.

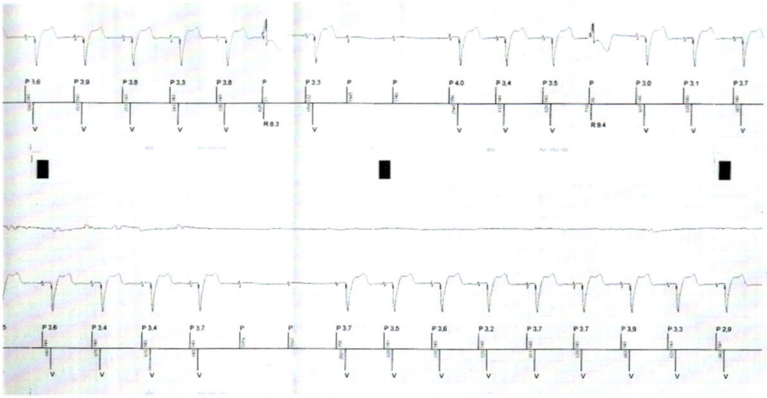

Fig 4.29 AAIsafeR2: Failed DDD → AAI switch due to persistent AVB. After 100 ventricular paced cycles in the DDD, mode switch to AAI occurs. Switch back to AAI occurs due to two consecutive nonconducted P waves.

Performance of Newer Dual Chamber Minimal Ventricular Pacing Algorithms

MVP

Two prospective randomized clinical trials have evaluated MVP performance in unselected ambulatory ICD patients. Cumulative percent ventricular pacing (Cum%VP) was significantly lower in MVP vs. DDDR (ranges 3.79 ± 16.3 to 4.1 ± 16.3 vs. 73.8 ± 32.5 to 80.6 ± 33.8, $p < 0.0001$). The median absolute and relative reductions in Cum%VP during MVP were 85.0 and 99.9, respectively. The large reduction in Cum%VP did not sacrifice atrial pacing support (Cum%AP), which was similar between MVP and DDDR (ranges 47.9 ± 37 to 48.7 ± 38.5 vs. 46.3 ± 36 to 47.3 ± 38.4). Backup DDDR pacing during MVP operation due to transient AVB occurred in ≥ 10% of pts (9.3 ± 7.4 [range 1–15] episodes/pt-day, duration 39.7 ± 156 minutes). At least 15% of AVIs during MVP operation exceeded 300 ms. During MVP overall time spent in AAIR was 89.6% (intrinsic conduction), DDDR 6.7% (intermittent AVB), and DDIR 3.7% (AF). No adverse events were attributed to MVP during short-term follow-up.[35,36] Importantly, the DDDR PAVIs were uniformly nominal or near-nominal, which guaranteed high Cum%VP. Systematic application of maximally allowable PAVIs in the DDDR group would have diminished the Cum%VP differential slightly.

MVP has also been compared with SAV+ for reducing Cum%VP in unselected pacemaker patients and by baseline AV conduction status (normal conduction, first-degree, second-degree, third-degree AVB).[37] SAV+ was applied with a nominal AV extension of 290 ms during atrial sensing and 320 ms during atrial pacing (maximum pAVI 600 ms, see Table 4.1). MVP resulted in a significantly lower Cum%VP than SAV+ in all AVB categories except for third degree (Fig 4.30): normal AV conduction (0.3 vs. 2.9, $p < 0.0001$), first-degree AVB (0.9% vs. 80.6%, $p < 0.0001$), second-degree AVB (37.6 vs. 99.3, $p < 0.002$), third-degree AVB (98.9 vs. 100, $p = 1.00$).

It is probably unlikely that the difference in Cum%VP between SAV+ and MVP for patients with normal AV conduction is clinically meaningful. Both groups achieved Cum%VP lower than observed in the superior treatment arm of SAVEPACe. Importantly, the greatest reduction in Cum%VP was observed in patients with first-degree AVB in which the lack of a PAVI during MVP provides a clearly superior outcome (Figs. 4.31 and 4.32). This reflects the fundamental weakness of the conventional dual chamber pacing system for minimizing Cum%VP. Eventually the PAVI will be exceeded by the iAVI and will guarantee ventricular pacing each time this condition is encountered.

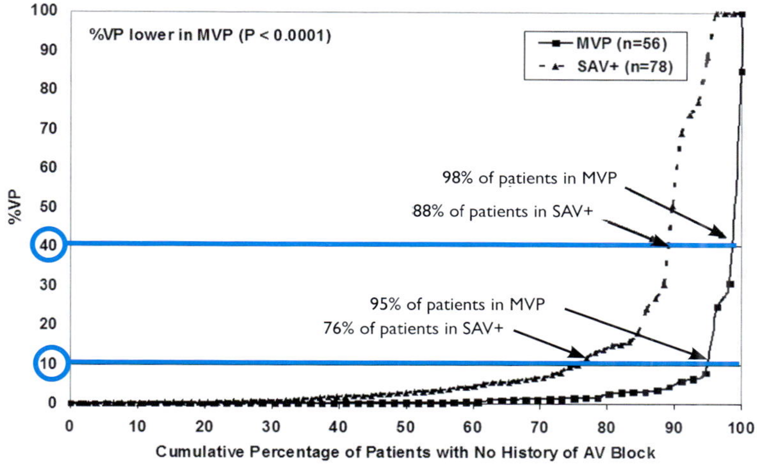

Fig 4.30 Cum%VP comparison between SAV+ vs. MVP among patients with no history of AVB. From these graphs, the percentage of patients that achieved different Cum%VP levels can be determined. The graphs include gridlines at 10% and 40% VP levels. The percentage of patients with less than 40% VP for both MVP and SAV+ are presented on each graph. (Courtesy of Todd Sheldon, MS, modified by M.O. Sweeney, MD.)

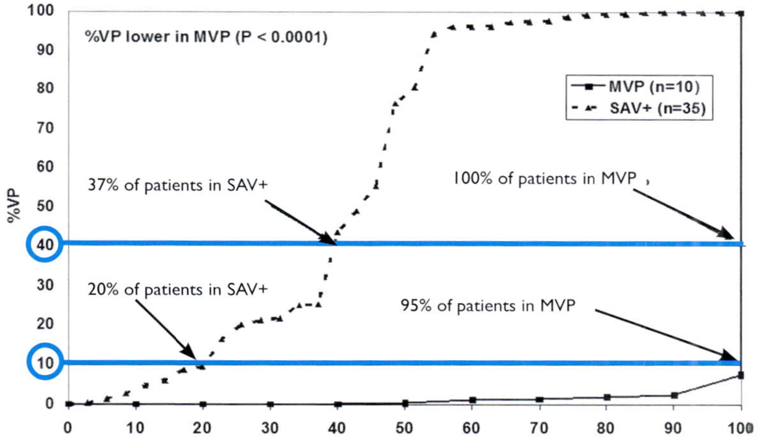

Fig 4.31 Cum%VP comparison between SAV+ vs. MVP for first-degree AVB. Same arrangements as Fig 4.30. (Courtesy of Todd Sheldon, MS, modified by M.O. Sweeney, MD.)

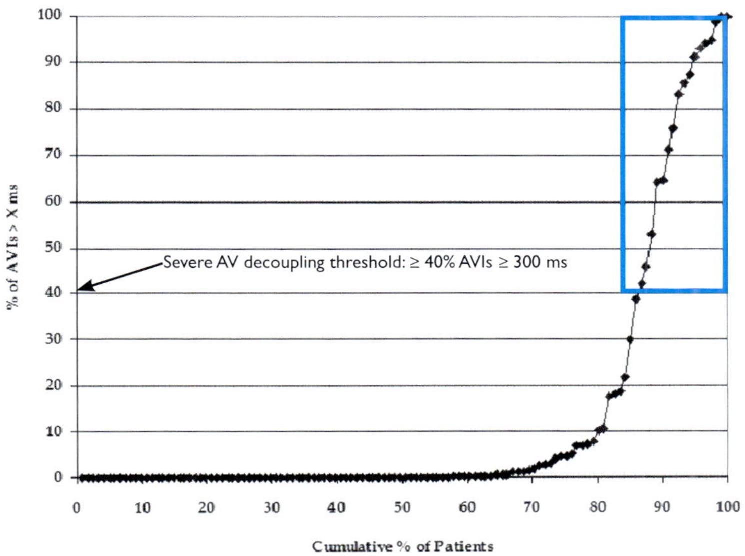

Fig 4.32 Frequency of severe AV decoupling during MVP. Plot of cumulative percent of patients (horizontal axis) by cumulative percent AVIs (vertical axis). Each point represents a single patient. Severe AV-DC (> 40% AVIs > 300 ms) is indicated by red box.

Similar reductions in Cum%VP have been reported with AAIsafeR. The Cum%VP was 9% ± 21% for AAIsafeR1 as compared to 95% ± 14% for DDDR at nominal pAVIs.[38] Similar results were demonstrated for AAIsafeR2.[34] Among patients with no or only transient AAI → DDD switches, the mean %VP was 0.13 ± 0.47. The mean %VP was significantly higher (41.8% ± 35.0%) among patients with persistent AAI → DDDR switches. "First-degree AVB" criterion accounted for 1% of AAI → DDDR, whereas mixed AVB types and "pauses" accounted for 81%.

Limitations and Risks of Newer Minimal Ventricular Pacing Strategies

AVIs are clinically relevant as surrogates for the timing of left-sided AV mechanical coupling (AV-C), which influences ventricular performance. Appropriately timed AV-C maintains a low mean atrial pressure (facilitating venous return), maximizes preload and pump function (Starling mechanism), and positions the mitral valve for closure during the isovolumetric phase of ventricular systole.

Newer dual chamber minimal ventricular pacing algorithms introduce two potential issues for clinical concern with the common mechanism of AV timing disruptions: (1) severely delayed AV coupling ("decoupling," AV-DC), transient breakdowns in AV conduction ("uncoupling," AV-UC) and V-A coupling (VA-C)[25]; and (2) ventricular proarrhythmia related to pauses terminated by isolated ventricular-paced beats (pacing-facilitated VT/VF).[33]

AV Timing Disruptions during Newer Dual Chamber Minimal Ventricular Pacing Algorithms

AV-C, AV-DC, VA-C, and AV-UC represent a time continuum of progressive prolongation of AV conduction time to the point failure. AV-DC (iAVI or PAVI > 220–230 ms) may induce diastolic mitral regurgitation in normal hearts[39] but its clinical significance is not established. Evidence from the Framingham study indicates that PR > 200 ms is associated with increased risks of AF and death.[40] Optimization of AV-C with dual chamber RVA pacing improved acute hemodynamics in some patients with low EF and long PR intervals,[41] but failed to improve outcomes in controlled trials presumably due to the offsetting negative effects of ventricular desynchronization.[42,43] AV-DC coexists with VA-C and may cause reversal of the left-sided AV timing sequence,[44] initiating adverse neuro-circulatory reflexes ("pseudo-pacemaker syndrome") during AAIR pacing.[45]

Detailed analysis of dynamic AVI behavior, quantification of AVIs under different patient and pacing conditions, and mechanisms of AV conduction breakdowns during MVP were described[25] in terms of (1) absolute magnitude of each timing interval in ms and (2) burden as % cardiac cycles during follow-up. Preserved AV-C was defined as the condition in which < 40% of all AVIs recorded during the study period were > 300 ms. Severely delayed AV coupling ("decoupling," AV-DC) was defined as the condition in which ≥ 40% of AVIs were > 300 ms. This threshold was based on the logic that most ICD systems permit a maximum PAVI of 300 ms, therefore AVIs > 300 ms would result in RVA pacing, and RVA pacing ≥ 40% of the time is associated with a 1.9–5.2 times increased risk of heart failure hospitalization compared to less pacing.[3-5]

Severe AV-DC occurred in 17 (14%) patients whereas AV-C was preserved in 104 (86%) (Fig 4.30). Among patients with preserved AV-C, 8/104 (7.7%) had 20%–40% AVIs > 300 ms, 16/104 (15.4%) had ≥ 1%–10% AVIs > 300 ms, and 80/104 (76.9%) had < 1% AVIs > 300 ms (Fig 4.32). Stepwise logistic regression identified only baseline iAVI (PR interval) (OR = 1.024, 95% CI 1.007–1.042; p = 0.005) and cumulative percentage atrial pacing (Cum%AP) (OR = 1.089, 95% CI 1.027–1.154; p = 0.004) as independent predictors of AV-DC (Fig 4.33). The interaction term PR and Cum%AP was not significant (p = 0.12), indicating that changes in PR did not affect AV-DC differently within levels of Cum%AP, and vice versa. AV-DC was associated with a higher requirement for backup DDDR pacing due to breakdowns in AV conduction (AV-UC). Patients with AV-DC had higher Cum%VP vs. all other patients (13.6 ± 28.3 vs. 1.2 ± 3.9, p = 0.023). Higher Cum%VP was due to AV-UC induced by rate responsive pacing in patients with long baseline PR intervals (> 240 ms) (Figs 4.34 and 4.35).

Only PR interval and Cum%AP predicted AV-DC. The relative risk of AV-DC increased by ≈ 2.4% for every 1 ms increase in PR and ≈ 9% for every 1% increase in Cum%AP. The increasing risk relationship between Cum%AP and AV-DC is explained by the effect of rate-related stress on normal and impaired AV conduction. Among patients with AV-DC during rate response On, ≈ 25% had PR ≥ 300 ms, whereas ≈ 75% had PR < 300 ms. Rate responsive worsened baseline AV-DC in the former group and induced AV-DC in the latter. More patients with AV-DC had rate response On, which increased Cum%AP and induced or worsened AV-DC during upward rate excur-

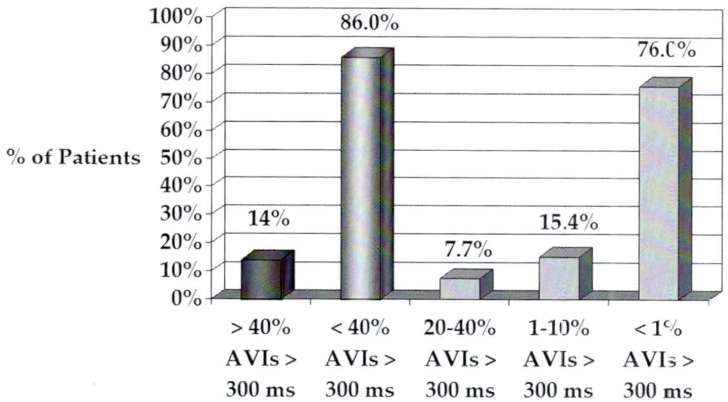

Fig 4.33 Distribution of AV decoupling frequency during enhanced AAIR pacing. Approximately 70% of patients had < 1% AVIs > 300 ms, ≈ 16% had 1%–40% AVIs > 300 ms, and 14% had > 40% AVIs > 300 ms.

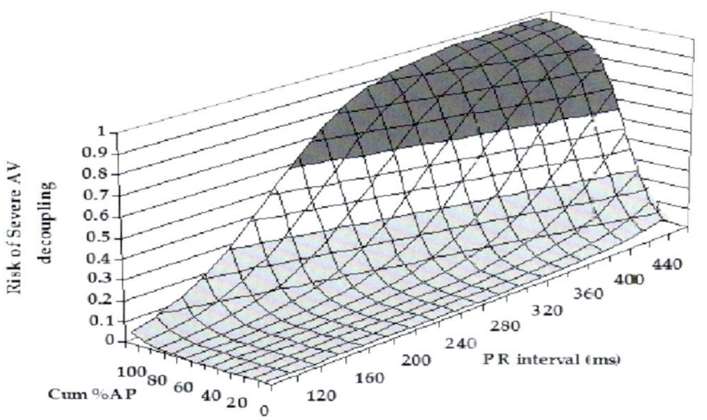

Fig 4.34 Predictors of AV Decoupling during MVP. Effects of increasing PR interval and Cum%AP on risk of severe AV-DC. The relative risk of severe AV-DC for any combination of PR interval and Cum%AP occurs at the intercept of their independent risk curves. The relative risk for PR=240 ms and Cum%AP=50 is 4.1%. Likewise, the relative risk for PR=300 ms and Cum%AP=50 is 15.2%; if Cum%AP increases to 90%, the relative risk is 84.4%. Shades of gray indicate approximate levels of risk (medium gray [bottom]: 0–30%, light gray [middle]: 30–60%, dark gray [top]: 60–100%).

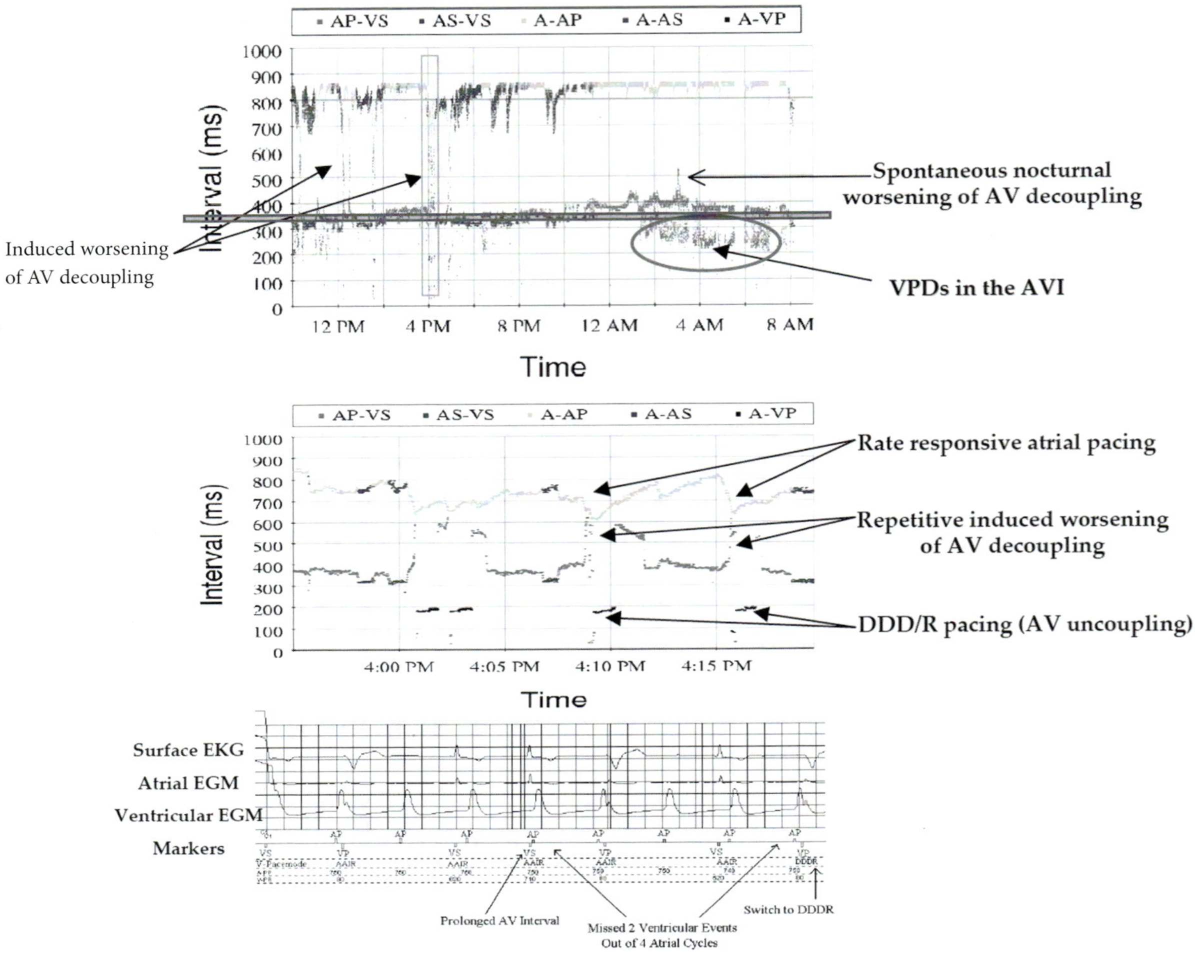

Fig 4.35 Transient AV decoupling during rate responsive pacing in MVP. Examples of spontaneous and induced worsening of severe AV decoupling in a representative patient with baseline PR > 300 ms. 24-hour A-A (AP or AS) intervals (upper) and AVIs (lower) are plotted on the y-axis and 24-hour time on the x-axis. **Top**: During waking hours (12 PM–10 PM) the majority of AVIs were > 300 ms. Rate responsive pacing up to 500 ms/120 bpm caused AVI extensions to ≈ 600 ms and loss of 1:1 conduction (AV uncoupling), triggering enhanced AAIR to DDDR switches (clustered AP-VP sequences at 4 PM). During sleeping hours (12 AM to 7 AM) sinus activity is suppressed and atrial pacing occurs at the lower rate (70 bpm) due to lack of sensor input. A spontaneous increase in AVIs to ≈ 530 ms despite no increase in atrial pacing rate occurs around 3 am, compatible with increased vagal tone. **Middle**: Higher resolution examination of repetitive induced AV uncoupling. Atrial pacing rate excursions (green) to ≈ 600 ms/100 bpm caused AVIs to abruptly increase from ≈ 325 → 600 ms (red), followed by conduction failure and DDDR pacing (black). **Bottom**: Very prolonged AVIs cause ventricular events to extend into the next atrial pacing cycle until AV conduction fails (4:2) which triggers mode switch to DDDR.

sions concealed within the comparison of mean ventricular rates.

This study demonstrated that (1) AV-DC occurred in 14% patients during MVP, whereas AV-C was preserved in 86%; (2) patients with AV-DC had a ≈ 10-fold increase in VA-C compared to those without AV-DC, and (3) AV-DC was associated with a ≈ 10-fold increase in Cum%VP due to spontaneous and pacing-induced breakdowns in AV conduction (AV-UC). Newer dual chamber minimal ventricular pacing algorithms prioritize an important timing relationship (ventricular synchrony) but may disrupt another (AV synchrony) in some patients by (1) permitting AV-DC (prolonged PR is not corrected) or (2) inducing AV-DC (unrestrained AVIs). Collectively, these disruptions to normal timing relationships may constitute an AV "desynchronopathy" which could have clinical implications during severe minimization of RVA pacing in some patients with low ejection fraction heart failure.

Ventricular Proarrhythmia during Newer Dual Chamber Minimal Ventricular Pacing Algorithms

Newer dual chamber minimal ventricular pacing algorithms permit one or more cycles without an intervening ventricular event and terminate pauses with ventricular pacing. Pauses terminated by isolated VPs in single chamber ICD systems have been implicated as a potential mechanism of ventricular proarrhythmia.[46,47] A similar possibility was compared during MVP and conventional pacing modes in ICD patients.[33]

VT/VF episodes initiated by short-long-short (S-L-S) sequences ("pauses") were classified as (1) pacing permitted (passively allowing longer pauses depending upon mode and lower rate) or (2) pacing facilitated (actively initiating and/or terminating pauses prematurely with single VPs) (Fig 4.36). If VPs did not participate in S-L-S generation the episode was designated as pacing permitted. If VPs participated in the

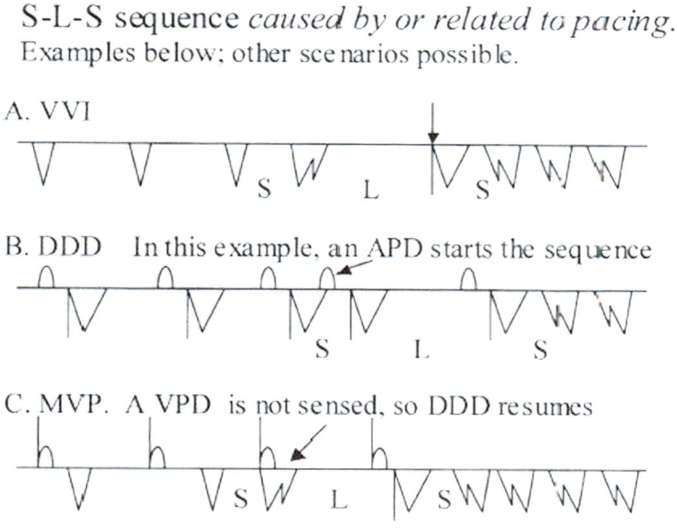

Fig 4.36 Schematic for pacing-facilitated VT/VF onset by pacing modes. (Copyright Elsevier, used with permission.)

S-L-S including the pause-terminating beat, the episode was designated as pacing facilitated. Episodes were categorized as S-L-S if the pauses were longer than the basic cycle length by ≥ 40 ms.[48]

The mechanism of S-L-S sequences preceding VT/VF onset differed by pacing mode (Fig 4.37). VVIR provides the simplest model for pacing facilitated S-L-S VT/VF because it requires only a single VPD and pause. The interaction between pacing system operation and S-L-S sequences is more complex in DDDR. Although single VPDs accounted for the majority of S-L-S initiations in DDDR, nearly 25% were

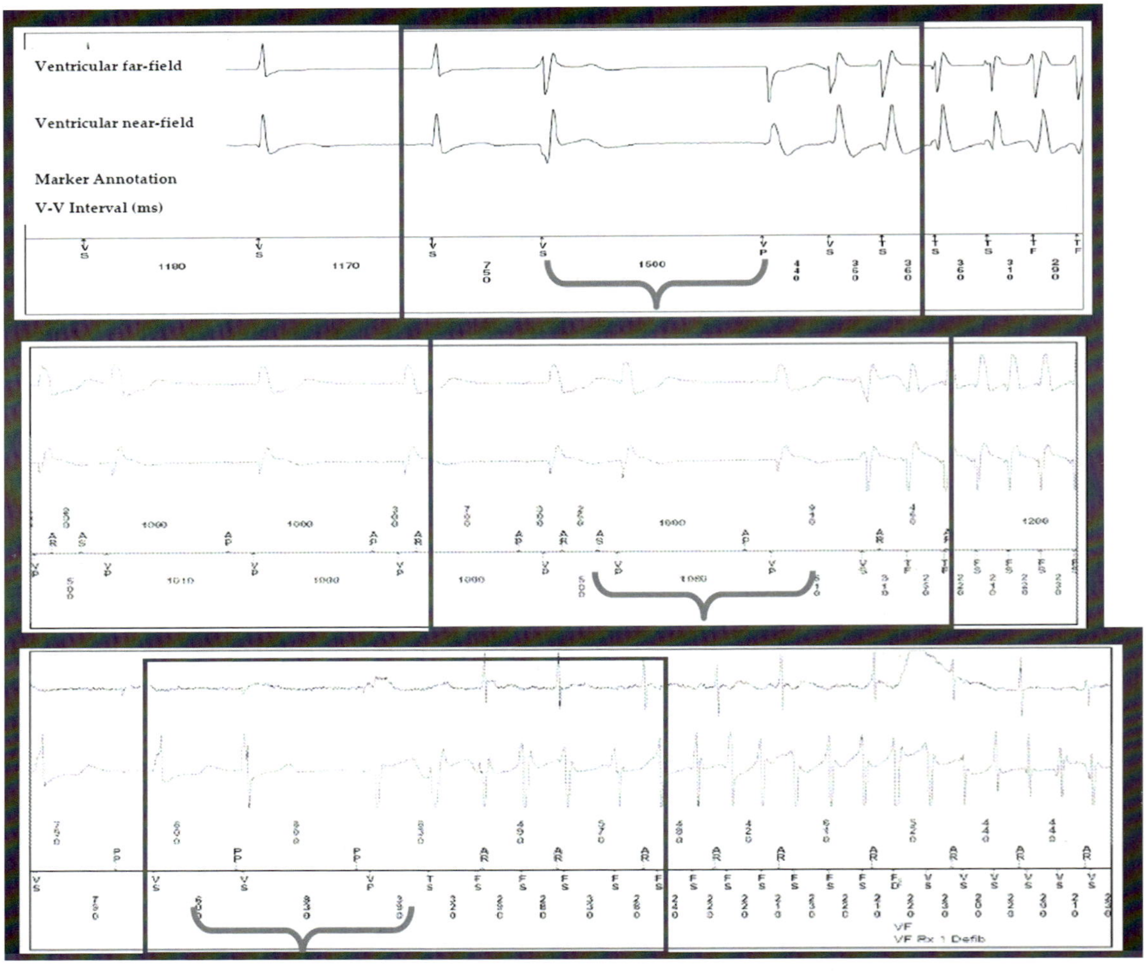

Fig 4.37 Pacing-facilitated S-L-S VT/VF by mode. **Top**: VVIR. For pacing facilitated S-L-S, sinus rhythm is interrupted by a single VPD (coupling interval 700 ms, asterisk) ("short"). A 1500-ms pause (bracket) ("long") is terminated by a single VP at the lower rate limit (40 bpm). A VPD (coupling interval 458 ms) ("short") after the VP anticipates VF. **Middle**: DDDR. For pacing facilitated S-L-S, the pacing rate approximates the lower programmed rate (1000 ms). Intermittent far-field R-wave oversensing (denoted as AR) occurs after VPs. An atrial premature beat 250 ms after far-field R wave (asterisk) is tracked and a synchronized VP occurs at the upper limit of 500 ms ("short"). A 1060-ms pause (bracket) ("long") follows due to normal lower rate behavior. A VPD (610 ms) ("short") after the final VP anticipates VF onset. **Bottom**: MVP. For pacing facilitated S-L-S, a VPD (600-ms interval, asterisk) ("short") occurs almost simultaneously with an AP (800-ms interval). The VPD is marked as a sensed event but because it falls in the 80-ms crosstalk window, is not considered a true ventricular event. The next AP (800 ms) fulfills the criteria for an A-A interval without an intervening VS event and a single VP is delivered ("long"). The pause (bracket) is only 830 ms because of rate modulation. An early-coupled VPD (390 ms) ("short") anticipates VT onset.

due to atrial tracking behavior. During MVP, the first short cycle was always due to VPDs. Long cycles followed VPDs that were incorrectly classified as electrical crosstalk because they occurred coincident with an atrial pace (AP) (92%) or due to VPDs with subsequent AV conduction failure (8%). Therefore, pacing facilitated S-L-S VT/VF during MVP requires the simultaneous occurrence of two unrelated events—a critically timed VPD coincident with an AP that triggers the S-L-S and is terminated with an unnecessary VP, or transient loss of AV conduction following a VPD.

Pacing facilitated S-L-S onsets accounted for 8.2%, 9.4%, and 14.8% of all VT/VF episodes during MVP, VVIR, and DDDR, respectively. Mean pause duration during pacing facilitated S-L-S VT/VF was 911 ± 322 ms (500–1760 ms). Pause duration was different among modes (VVIR 1180 ± 414 ms vs. MVP 865 ± 278 ms vs. DDDR 793 ± 172 ms; $p = 0.002$). Pause duration was shorter for DDDR vs. VVIR ($p < 0.001$), for MVP vs. VVIR ($p = 0.033$), but not for DDDR vs. MVP ($p = 0.607$)(Figs 4.36 and 4.37). Differences in pause duration were primarily due to lower rate programming. For VVIR, the lower rate was nominally 40 bpm whereas for DDDR and MVP lower rates were 60 bpm. Shorter pauses were seen during rate modulation. Because MVP permits single nonconducted atrial events, the maximum pause duration is twice the programmed lower rate interval. However, because S-L-S sequences during MVP were nearly always initiated by VPDs coincident with an AP event rather than a nonconducted atrial event, the resulting pauses were typically near the lower rate.

Pacing facilitated S-L-S VT/VF occurred in 3% to 5% of all patients and was the only form of VT/VF observed in ~1% to 2% of patients in any mode. Because ~ 80% of patients in the study population did not have a VT/VF episode, the percentage of pacing facilitated S-L-S that occurred in patients with VT/VF episodes was higher. Approximately 11% to 28% of patients with episodes had some pacing facilitated S-L-S VT/VF. Likewise, 4% to 10% of patients with episodes had pacing facilitated S-L-S as the sole onset sequence preceding VT/VF.

The main findings of this study are (1) pacing facilitated S-L-S VT/VF accounted for 8% to 15% of all VT/VF, (2) pacing facilitated S-L-S VT/VF was observed in 11% to 28% patients with VT/VF, (3) pacing facilitated S-L-S VT/VF was the *only* onset sequence in ~4% to 10% of patients with VT/VF, and (4) pacing facilitated S-L-S VT/VF is common to all pacing modes but is invoked in different ways specific to mode. Pacing facilitated S-L-S VT/VF may occur despite a very low frequency of single VPs. Therefore, pacing facilitated S-L-S VT/VF may occur even in patients who do not actively require bradycardia support. This analysis does not identify patients who may be susceptible to pacing facilitated S-L-S VT/VF and this may only be possible retrospectively.

Long-term Survival of Algorithms to Minimize Ventricular Pacing

The long-term (> 1–2 years) clinical performance of minimal ventricular pacing algorithms has not been reported. Potential constraints on the retention of atrial-based minimal ventricular pacing include (1) long term stability of AV conduction, (2) development of permanent AF, (2) clinical concerns regarding AV-DC.

Long-term Stability of AV Conduction in Sinus Node Dysfunction

Functional disturbances in AV conduction are common in SND and reflect histopathologic observations that SND is often the initial clinical manifestation of diffuse degenerative conduction system disease. However, detailed electrophysiology studies among patients with SND reveal that the majority (80%) of these conduction disturbances were confined to the AV junction (delayed and intermittent conduction during programmed atrial stimulation). Repeat electrophysiology study after 5 years revealed that conduction disturbances limited to the AV junction remained stable and did not predict a clinically important progression.[49]

Previous studies have demonstrated that intrinsic AV conduction remains stable during long-term follow-up in the majority of patients with SND.[50-55] Collected data from 28 different studies on atrial pacing for SND showed a median annual incidence of persistent AVB of 0.6% (0%–4.5%) with a total prevalence 2.1% (0%–11.9%). There was no significant difference in follow-up time between studies that showed a low, compared to a high incidence of AVB.[56] Variability in the reported incidence of persistent AVB likely relates to the exclusion of patients with bifascicular block or left bundle branch block in some studies with lower incidences[57] and inclusion in other studies with higher incidences.[55]

Another concern with the application of minimal ventricular pacing modes is the development of Type I second-degree AVB. Several studies suggest that this is unlikely to pose a significant clinical problem. Santini et al[7] measure the stability of the Wenckebach threshold in 135 of 339 patients with SND who received AAI pacemakers. By design, all patients who received AAI pacing systems had no AV conduction disturbances and baseline Wenckebach point > 140 bpm. During mean follow-up 5 years, Wenckebach threshold was unchanged in 111 (85%) and decreased in 12 (9.2%). However, amongst the 12 patients in whom the Wenckebach threshold declined, it remained > 100 bpm in 10 (7.5%) and < 100 bpm in only 2 (1.5%). None of the patients with a decline in Wenckebach threshold showed spontaneous Wenckebach behavior during atrial pacing at the base programmed rate of 70 bpm. Spontaneous second-degree AV block was observed in 7 (5%) patients—in 6 patients due to concomitant antiarrhythmic drug, in 1 patient due to carotid sinus hypersensitivity. Pacing mode was changed to DDD in 8 (6%) AAI paced patients—however, 3 were due to chronic AF and only 1 due to second-degree AVB.

Andersen et al[8] prospectively evaluated AV conduction and risk of developing AVB during long-term follow-up of 225 patients with SND. AV conduction, estimated as the PQ interval, the atrial stimulus-Q interval at atrial pacing rates of 100 and 120 bpm and the Wenckebach point, remained stable during long-term follow-up. In the VVI group, PQ increased during follow-up from 185 ± 32 ms at implantation to 199 ± 37 ms at last follow-up in 109 patients with sinus rhythm ($p < 0.001$). In 105 patients in the AAI group, PQ interval changed from 190 ± 30 to 191 ± 33 ($p < 0.65$). The increase in PQ interval from implantation to last follow-up was significantly higher in the VVI group (17 ± 36 ms) than in the atrial group (2 ± 34 ms) ($p = 0.002$). There was no significant difference between AAI and VVI groups in PQ interval at last follow-up. Stim-Q at 100 bpm increased a mean of 1 ± 42 ms to 245 ± 48 ms (100 patients) and Stim-Q at 120 bpm increased a mean of 9 ± 50 ms to 267 ± 54 ms (93 patients), neither of which were significant. The Wenckebach point remained stable in 60% patients during the follow-up period but changed in 40% of patients. Of 99 patients with Wenckebach point > 120 bpm at inclusion, 77 (78%) were unchanged, 14 (14%) dropped to 100–120 bpm, and 1 (1%) dropped to < 100 bpm. Of 9 patients with Wenckebach point 100–120 bpm at inclusion, 3 increased to > 120 bpm, 4 were unchanged, and 1 dropped to < 100 bpm. Only 2 patients had Wenckebach point < 100 bpm at enrollment. Overall, there was no significant difference between Wenckebach point at the time of implantation and that at last follow-up. None of the patients with Wenckebach point < 100 bpm were symptomatic, and none required pacemaker upgrade. Among the 34 patients in whom the Wenckebach point changed during follow-up, the change was associated with an alteration in medication in 16. Thus, the Wenckebach point is clinically stable in the majority of patients and does not predict progression to persistent AVB.

Brandt et al[55] studied the natural history of SND treated in 213 patients with atrial pacing for a median follow-up period of 60 months. High-grade AVB occurred in 8.5% (1.8% per year) and its incidence was much greater in patients with complete bundle branch block or bifascicular block (35%) than in patients with normal ventricular activation (6%). When patients with intraventricular conduction disturbances were excluded from analysis, the annualized incidence of high-grade AVB was 1.2%. The only significant predictor of high-grade AVB was the presence of ventricular conduction disturbance at baseline. Neither Wenckebach point not baseline PR interval were predictive of subsequent high-grade AVB. In fact, none of 8 patients with baseline PR interval > 220 ms developed AVB.

Emergence of Permanent Atrial Fibrillation

The development of permanent AF renders atrial pacing irrelevant and necessitates ventricular pacing if significant bradycardia exists. Brandt et al[55] observed a 7% incidence of permanent AF amongst 213 patients with SND during AAI pacing. The mean follow-up was 5 years, yielding a 1.4% annualized incidence of permanent AF. This was identical to that reported by Sutton[51] in a review of 410 SND patients treated with atrial pacing during a mean follow-up of 32.8 months. Andersen et al[57] observed permanent AF in 9/102 (8.8%) SND patients treated with AAI pacing versus 22/102 (21.6%) patients treated with VVI pacing. These figures were based on an intention-to-treat analysis. In fact, 3/9 patients assigned to AAI pacing actually received VVI pacing systems, therefore the true incidence of permanent AF among patients who actually received AAI pacing was 6/102 (5.9%). This yielded a 1.2% annualized incidence of permanent AF, also in alignment with the reports of Brandt et al[55] and Sutton.[51]

Summary

The survivability of atrial-based minimal ventricular pacing modes will be impacted by the natural history of conduction disturbances and AF in SND. The annual incidence of high-grade AVB and permanent AF are conservatively estimated at 2% each based on the studies presented earlier. Thus, excluding atrial lead malfunction, the survivability of atrial-based minimal ventricular pacing modes should be in the range of 96% per year.

Clinical Concerns regarding AV-DC during Dual Chamber Minimal Ventricular Pacing

There is no existing evidence that long AVIs during atrial-based minimal ventricular pacing modes among patients with SND are clinically adverse. In the Danish study,[57] the mean baseline PR was 180–190 ms, which is in the physiologically optimal range specified in studies of DDD pacing. Furthermore, the PQ interval was remarkably stable over 5 years follow-up among patients assigned to AAI pacing.[8] Dual chamber minimal ventricular pacing has been demonstrated to reduce the risk of developing permanent AF as compared to conventional dual chamber pacing in SND.[10]

It is possible that AV-DC permitted or induced by dual chamber minimal ventricular pacing algorithms may be adverse among patients with systolic heart failure. The DAVID II ICD trial demonstrated that AAI pacing at 70 bpm did not worsen outcomes compared to no pacing (VVI 40 bpm), even though ≈20% of patients had PR > 200 ms and Cum%AP was 50% at 24 months,[58] indicating AV-DC was present in some patients, however, patients with baseline PR > 230 ms were excluded from enrollment. Whether minimization of RVA pacing at the cost of AV-DC is worse than ventricular desynchronization when AV-C is intermittently maintained by RVA pacing is uncertain. There is one report of worse outcomes in some ICD patients with small versus modest amounts of RVA pacing,[59] but a more recent analysis suggests that high intrinsic heart rates may explain this observation.[60] Prospective clinical outcomes studies to examine the trade-off of part-time RVA pacing versus preserved AV-C under certain clinical conditions and their interactions with rate responsive pacing may be necessary.

References

1. Sweeney MO, Prinzen FW. Ventricular pump function and pacing: Physiological and clinical integration. *Circ Arrhythm Electrophysiol.* 2008;1(2):127–139.
2. The DAVID Trial Investigators. Dual-chamber pacing or ventricular backup pacing in patients with an implantable defibrillator: the Dual Chamber and VVI Implantable Defibrillator (DAVID) Trial. *JAMA.* 2002;288(24):3115–3123.
3. Sweeney MO, Hellkamp AS, Ellenbogen KA, et al. Adverse effect of ventricular pacing on heart failure and atrial fibrillation among patients with normal baseline QRS duration in a clinical trial of pacemaker therapy for sinus node dysfunction. *Circulation.* 2003;23:2932–2937.
4. Sharma AD, Rizo-Patron C, Hallstrom AP, et al., and the DAVID Investigators. Percent right ventricular pacing predicts outcomes in the DAVID Trial. *Heart Rhythm.* 2005;2:830–834.
5. Steinberg JS, Fischer A, Wang P, et al. The clinical implications of cumulative right ventricular pacing in the Multicenter Automatic Defibrillator Trial II. *J Cardiovasc Electrophysiol.* 2005;16(4):359–365.
6. Sweeney MO, Hellkamp AS. Heart failure during cardiac pacing. *Circulation.* 2006;113:2082–2088.
7. Santini M, Alexidou G, Ansalone G, Cacciatore G, Cini R, Turitto G. Relation of prognosis in sick sinus syndrome to age, conduction defects and modes of permanent cardiac pacing. *Am J Cardiol.* 1990;65:729–735.
8. Andersen HR, Nielsen JC, Thomsen PEB, et al. Atrioventricular conduction during long-term follow-up of patients with sick sinus syndrome. *Circulation.* 1998;98:1315–1321.
9. Lamas GA, Lee KL, Sweeney MO, et al., for the MOST Investigators. Ventricular pacing or dual chamber pacing for sinus node dysfunction. *N Engl J Med.* 2002;346:1854–1862.
10. Sweeney MO, Bank AJ, Nsah E, et al. Minimizing ventricular pacing to reduce atrial fibrillation in sinus-node disease. *N Engl J Med.* 2007;357(10):1000–1008.
11. Sweeney MO, Prinzen FW. A new paradigm for optimal ventricular pacing. *J Am Coll Cardiol.* 2006;47:282–288.
12. Andersen HR, Thuesen L, Bagger JP, Vesterlund T, Thomsen PEB. Prospective randomized trial of atrial versus ventricular pacing in sick sinus syndrome. *Lancet.* 1994;344:1523–1528.
13. Barold SS. Permanent single chamber atrial pacing is obsolete. *Pacing Clin Electrophysiol.* 2001;24:271–275.
14. Clarke KW, Connelly DT, Charles RG. Single chamber atrial pacing: an underused and cost-effective pacing modality in sinus node disease. *Heart.* 1998;80:387–389.
15. Kristensen L, Nielsen JC, Pedersen AK, Mortensen PT, Andersen HR. AV block and changes in pacing mode during long-term follow-up of 339 consecutive patients with sick sinus syndrome treated with AAI/AAIR pacemaker. *Pacing Clin Electrophysiol.* 2001;24(3):358–365.
16. Nielsen JC, Kristensen L, Andersen HR, Mortensen PT, Pedersen O, Pedersen AK. A randomized comparison of atrial and dual-chamber pacing in 177 consecutive patients with sick sinus syndrome: echocardiographic and clinical outcome. *J Am Coll Cardiol.* 2003;42:614–623.
17. Geelen P, Lorga-Filho A, Chauvin M, Wellens F, Brugada P. The value of DDD pacing in patients with an implantable cardioverter defibrillator. *Pacing Clin Electrophysiol.* 1997;20(1 Pt 2):177–181.
18. Higgins SL, Williams SK, Pak JP, Meyer DB. Indications for implantation of a dual-chamber pacemaker combined with an implantable cardioverter-defibrillator. *Am J Cardiol.* 1998;81(11):1360–1362.
19. Sweeney MO, Shea JB, Ellison KE. Upgrade of permanent pacemakers and single-chamber implantable cardioverter-defibrillators to pectoral dual-chamber implantable cardioverter-defibrillators: indications, surgical approach, and long-term clinical results. *Pacing Clin Electrophysiol.* 2002;25:1715–1723.
20. Janosik DL, Ellenbogen KA. Basic physiology of cardiac pacing and pacemaker syndrome. In: Ellenbogen KA, Kay GN, Wilkoff BL, eds. *Clinical Cardiac Pacing and Defibrillation.* 2nd ed. Philadelphia: W.B. Saunders; 2000:333–352.

21. Nielsen JC, Pedersen AK, Mortensen PT, Andersen HR. Programming a fixed long atrioventricular delay is not effective in preventing ventricular pacing in patients with sick sinus syndrome. *Europace.* 1999;1:113–120.
22. Nielsen JC, Pedersen AK, Mortensen PT, Thuesen L, Andersen HL. Programming a long AV delay does not prevent ventricular stimulation in patients with SSS and intact AV conduction. *Pacing Clin Electrophysiol.* 1997;20:1574.
23. Olshansky B, Day JD, Moore S, et al. Is dual-chamber programming inferior to single-chamber programming in an implantable cardioverter-defibrillator? Results of the INTRINSIC RV (Inhibition of Unnecessary RV Pacing with AVSH in ICDs) study. *Circulation* 2007;115(1):9–16.
24. Olshansky B, Day J, McGuire M, Stolen KQ, Pratt T. Optimization of right ventricular pacing among patients with dual-chamber ICDs. Paper presented at: Heart Failure Society of America 8th Annual Scientific Sessions, 2004; Toronto, Canada.
25. Sweeney MO, Ellenbogen KA, Tang ASL, Johnson J, Belk P, Sheldon T. Severe atrioventricular decoupling, uncoupling and ventriculoatrial coupling during enhanced atrial pacing: Incidence, mechanisms and implications for minimizing right ventricular pacing in ICD patients. *J Cardiovasc Electrophysiol.* 2008;19:1175–1180.
26. Ausubel K, Klementowicz P, Furman S. Interatrial conduction during cardiac pacing. *Pacing Clin Electrophysiol.* 1986;9(6 Pt 2):1026–1031.
27. Grant SC, Bennett DH. Atrial latency in a dual chambered pacing system causing inappropriate sequence of cardiac chamber activation. *Pacing Clin Electrophysiol.* 1992;15(1):116–118.
28. Dennis MJ, Sparks PB. Pacemaker mediated tachycardia as a complication of the autointrinsic conduction search function. *Pacing Clin Electrophysiol.* 2004;27(6p1):824–826.
29. Barold SS. Repetitive non-reentrant ventriculoatrial synchrony in dual-chamber pacing. In: Santini M, Pistolese M, Alliegro A, eds. *Progress in Clinical Pacing.* Amsterdam: Excerpta Medica; 1990:451–471.
30. Sweeney MO. Novel cause of spurious mode switching in dual chamber pacemakers: AV desynchronization arrhythmias. *J Cardiovasc Electrophysiol.* 2002;13:616–619.
31. Sweeney MO, Hellkamp AS, Ellenbogen KA, et al. Prospective randomized study of mode switching in a clinical trial of pacemaker therapy for sinus node dysfunction. *J Cardiovasc Electrophysiol.* 2004;15:153–160.
32. Sweeney MO, Porkolab FL. Ventricular fibrillation induced by double premature ventricular pacing stimuli in a dual-chamber pacemaker with AutoCapture. *Heart Rhythm.* 2009;6(3):429–432.
33. Sweeney MO, Ruetz LL, Belk P, Mullen TJ, Johnson JW, Sheldon T. Bradycardia pacing induced short-long-short sequences at the onset of ventricular tachyarrhythmias: a possible mechanism of proarrhythmia? *J Am Coll Cardiol.* 2007;50(7):614–622.
34. Frohlig G, Gras D, Victor J, et al. Use of a new cardiac pacing mode designed to eliminate unnecessary ventricular pacing. *Europace.* 2006;8:96–101.
35. Sweeney MO, Shea JB, Fox V, et al. Randomized trial of a new atrial-based minimal ventricular pacing mode in dual chamber implantable cardioverter-defibrillators: MVP. *Heart Rhythm.* 2004;1:160–167.
36. Sweeney MO, Ellenbogen KA, Betzold R, et al. Multicenter, prospective, randomized trial of a new atrial-based Managed Ventricular Pacing Mode (MVP) in dual chamber ICDs. *J Cardiovasc Electrophysiol.* 2005;16:1–7.
37. Purerfellner H, Brandt J, Israel C, et al. Comparison of two strategies to reduce ventricular pacing in pacemaker patients. *Pacing Clin Electrophysiol.* 2008;31(2):167–176.
38. Pioger G, Leny G, Nitzsche R, Ripart A. AAIsafeR limits ventricular pacing in unselected patients. *Pacing Clin Electrophysiol.* 2007;30(s1):S66–S70.
39. Ishikawa T, Kimura K, Miyazaki N, et al. Diastolic mitral regurgitation in patients with first-degree atrioventricular block. *Pacing Clin Electrophysiol.* 1992;15(11):1927–1931.
40. Cheng S, Keyes MJ, Larson MG, et al. Long-term outcomes in individuals with prolonged PR interval or first-degree atrioventricular block. *JAMA.* 2009;301(24):2571–2577.

41. Nishimura RA, Hayes DL, Holmes DR, Tajik AJ. Mechanism of hemodynamic improvement by dual-chamber pacing for severe left ventricular dysfunction: an acute doppler and catheterization study. *J Am Coll Cardiol.* 1995;25:281–288.
42. Gold MR, Feliciano Z, Gottlieb SS, Fisher ML. Dual-chamber pacing with a short atrioventricular delay in congestive heart failure: a randomized study. *J Am Coll Cardiol.* 1995;26(4):967–973.
43. Linde C, Gadler F, Edner M, Norlander R, Rosenqvist M, Ryden L. Results of atrioventricular synchronous pacing with optimized delay in patients with severe congestive heart failure. *Am J Cardiol.* 1995;75(14):919–923.
44. Hettrick DA, Mittelstadt JR, Kehl F, et al. Atrial pacing lead location alters the hemodynamic effects of atrial-ventricular delay in dogs with pacing induced cardiomyopathy. *Pacing Clin Electrophysiol.* 2003;26(4 Pt 1):853–861.
45. Mabo P, Pouillot C, Kermarrec A, LeLong B, Lebreton H, Daubert C. Lack of physiological adaptation of the atrioventricular interval to heart rate in patients chronically paced in the AAIR mode. *Pacing Clin Electrophysiol.* 1991;14(12):2133–2142.
46. Roelke M, Garan H, McGovern BA, Ruskin JN. Analysis of the initiation of spontaneous monomorphic ventricular tachycardia by stored intracardiac electrograms. *J Am Coll Cardiol.* 1994;23(1):117–122.
47. Himmrich E, Przibille O, Zellerhoff C, et al. Proarrhythmic effect of pacemaker stimulation in patients with implanted cardioverter-defibrillators. *Circulation.* 2003;108:192–197.
48. Viskin S, Fish R, Zeltser D, et al. Arrhythmias in the long QT syndrome: how often is torsade de pointes pause-dependent? *Heart.* 2000;83:661–666.
49. Vallin H, Edhag O. Associated conduction disturbances in patients with symptomatic sinus node disease. *Acta Med Scand.* 1981;210:263–270.
50. Hayes DL, Furman S. Stability of AV conduction in sick sinus syndrome patients with implanted atrial pacemakers. *Am Heart J.* 1984;107:644–647.
51. Sutton R, Kenny RA. The natural history of sick sinus syndrome. *Pacing Clin Electrophysiol.* 1986;9:1110–1114.
52. Rosenqvist M, Vallin H, Edhag O. Clinical and electrophysiologic course of sinus node disease: five-year follow-up study. *Am Heart J.* 1985;109:513–522.
53. Rosenqvist M, Brandt J, Schuller H. Atrial versus ventricular pacing in sinus node disease: a treatment comparison study. *Am Heart J.* 1986;111:292–297.
54. Rosenqvist M, Brandt J, Schuller H. Long-term pacing in sinus node disease: effects of stimulation mode on cardiovascular morbidity and mortality. *Am Heart J.* 1988;116:16–22.
55. Brandt J, Anderson H, Fahraeus T, Schuller H. Natural history of sick sinus syndrome treated with atrial pacing in 213 patients: implications for selection of stimulation mode. *J Am Coll Cardiol.* 1992;20:633–639.
56. Rosenqvist M, Obel IW. Atrial pacing and the risk for AV block: is there a time for change in attitude? *Pacing Clin Electrophysiol.* 1989;12:97–101.
57. Andersen HR, Nielsen JC, Rhomsen PEB, Mortensen PT, Vesterlund T, Pedersen AK. Long-term follow-up of patients from a randomized trial of atrial versus ventricular pacing for sick-sinus syndrome. *Lancet.* 1997;350:1210–1216.
58. Wilkoff B. The Dual Chamber and VVI Implantable Defibrillator Trial II (DAVID II). Paper presented at: Heart Rhythm Society Late-Breaking Clinical Trials, 2007; Denver, CO.
59. Olshansky B, Day JD, Lerew DR, Brown S, Stolen KQ. Eliminating right ventricular pacing may not be best for patients requiring implantable cardioverter-defibrillators. *Heart Rhythm.* 2007;4(7):886–891.
60. Ahmadi-Kashani M, Sbaity S, Stolen K, Brown S, Day J, Olshansky B. Heart rate predicts outcomes in an implantable defibrillator population. *Circulation.* 2007;116(16):II,535-a-2435.
61. Melzer C, Sowelam C, Sheldon TJ, et al. Reduction of right ventricular pacing in patients with sinus node dysfunction using an enhanced search AV algorithm. *Pacing Clin Electrophysiol.* 2005;28(6):521–527.
62. Deering TF, Wilensky M, Tondato F, Dan D,

Tyler J. Auto intrinsic conduction search algorithm: a prospective analysis. *Pacing Clin Electrophysiol.* 2003;26(4 (Part II)):1080. Abstract #1606.

63. Shivkumar K, Feliciano Z, Boyle NG, Wiener I. Intradevice interaction in a dual chamber implantable cardioverter defibrillator preventing ventricular tachyarrhythmia detection. *J Cardiovasc Electrophysiol.* 2000;11(11):1285–1288.

64. Barold SS, Falkoff MD, Ong LS, Heinle RA. All dual-chamber pacemakers function in the DDD mode. *Am Heart J.* 1988;115:1353.

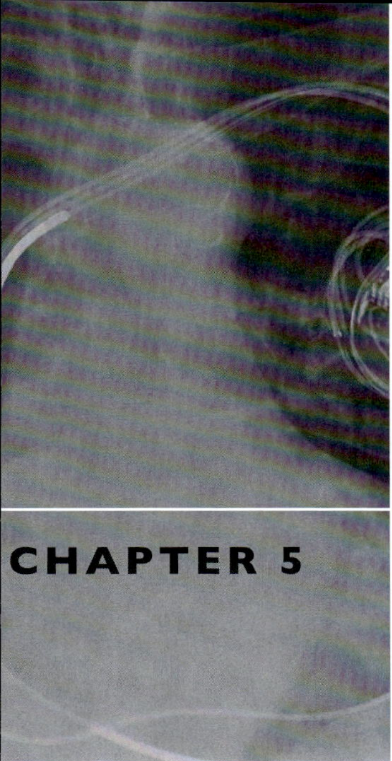

Normal Pacemaker Sensing, Abnormal Sensing, and Automatic Sensing

CHAPTER 5

Carsten W. Israel

Introduction

Sensing of the intrinsic cardiac activity is a prerequisite for appropriate pacemaker function because otherwise pacing can occur in the vulnerable phase, provoking arrhythmias or symptoms. In dual chamber pacing, inability to sense the atrial intrinsic activity can lead to asynchronous ventricular pacing with adverse clinical effects (eg, induction of pacemaker syndrome).

The pacemaker function of sensing is not trivial: Sensing of all "wanted" signals (P wave, R wave) has to be secured while "unwanted" signals (eg, myopotentials, T wave, QRS complex in the atrial channel, atrial stimuli in the ventricular channel) has to be avoided.

This chapter summarizes the technology that enables pacemakers to sense appropriately, events that lead to sensing failure (undersensing, oversensing), and pacemaker algorithms that are developed to automatically optimize sensing function.

Normal Sensing

The sensed signal is produced by the electrical activity of myocardium in proximity to the implanted lead. Electrical activity recorded via an intracardiac electrode is called an *electrogram*.

Electrogram Shape

Intracardiac electrograms have an appearance different from the surface electrocardiogram (ECG), A fixed pacemaker electrode records a near-field electrogram, which usually has the appearance of an "M" or "W" (Fig 5.1). This shape reflects the bipolar nature of the myocardial depolarization wavefront. The nearer the origin of the electrical signal is to the implanted electrode, the "sharper" and narrower

Pacemakers and Implantable Cardioverter Defibrillators: An Expert's Manual. © 2010 Amin Al-Ahmad, Kenneth A. Ellenbogen, Andrea Natale, and Paul J. Wang, eds. Cardiotext Publishing, ISBN: 978-0-9790164-6-2.

its appearance. If the electrode is not fixed to the myocardial wall (eg, sensing ring electrodes in VDD single lead systems, integrated bipolar sensing in ICD leads), the deflection is less sharp and the signal broader and reduced in amplitude. Similarly, if the origin of an intrinsic cardiac signal is far from the sensing electrode, for example a ventricular signal visible in the atrial electrogram, the deflection in the electrogram is broader and typically smaller in amplitude, called *far-field electrogram*.

The morphology of a sensed electrogram depends (apart from characteristics of the myocardium) on lead position, sensing polarity (unipolar, bipolar), other electrode characteristics (surface area, electrode material, fixed versus floating, bipolar ring spacing), and technical characteristics of the connected device (amplifier, band-pass filter, rectifier).

Lead Polarity and Bipole Spacing

In unipolar leads, the cathode at the lead tip senses against the anode formed by the device housing ("tip-to-can"). Thus, the unipolar sensing field is rather large and includes areas that overlay the pectoral muscle. Myopotential oversensing is therefore a frequent problem in unipolar sensing. Due to the limited ability of unipolar leads to discriminate between cardiac near-field and cardiac or non-cardiac far-field signals (such as far-field signals, Fig 5.2), the sensitivity in unipolar leads cannot be programmed to very sensitive values (maximum sensitivity usually 0.5 mV). Therefore, unipolar sensing is particularly not advisable in atrial leads that are unable to reliably distinguish atrial fibrillation from artifact.

Bipolar configurations use two different electrodes for sensing, such as the lead tip and a ring 1 to 3 cm proximal (tip-to-ring). Thus, bipolar electrodes can measure two electrograms simultaneously which register the myocardial depolarization wavefront with a time-shift (Fig 5.3A). Together with a differential amplifier, both electrograms can be subtracted from each other thus deleting signals that reach both electrodes simultaneously while augmenting signals that are sensed with a time-shift. This is particularly important in sensing with non-fixed, floating electrodes where the atrial signals are sensed by two full- or half-rings (Fig 5.3B).

In defibrillator leads, the ventricular coil electrode (with a much larger surface area) can be used for sensing instead of a dedicated ring electrode. This is referred to as integrated bipolar sensing and produces a bipolar electrogram that is in between a near- and far-field electrogram.

Pacemaker Sensing Circuit

The electrogram recorded by the implanted lead enters the pacemaker sensing circuit where it is amplified, filtered, and rectified.

After amplification, the sensed electrogram is filtered to facilitate discrimination between target signal (eg, P or R wave) and unwanted signals (myopotentials, T wave, far-field signals, Fig 5.1). Band-pass filters selectively amplify some frequencies of a sensed signal while attenuating others. In pacemakers, filters with cutoff frequencies of 20 (high pass) and 100 Hz (low

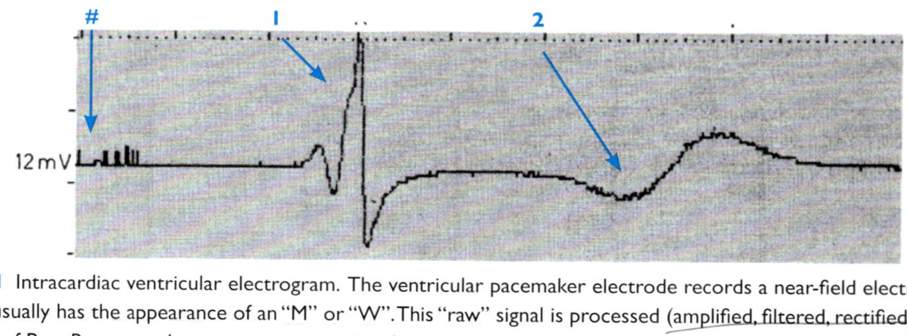

Fig 5.1 Intracardiac ventricular electrogram. The ventricular pacemaker electrode records a near-field electrogram which usually has the appearance of an "M" or "W". This "raw" signal is processed (amplified, filtered, rectified) to allow sensing of P or R wave and to prevent oversensing (eg, myopotentials, T wave). #, "noise"; 1, R wave; 2, T wave.

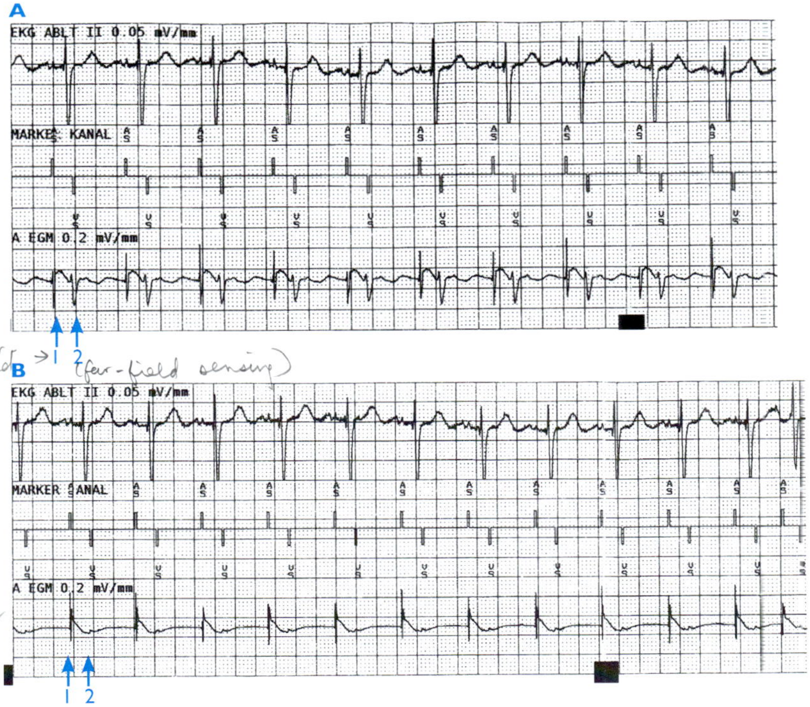

Fig 5.2 Unipolar and bipolar atrial sensing. Simultaneous registrations of surface ECG (lead II), marker annotations (middle), and intraatrial electrogram (A EGM). Paper speed 25 mm/s. **A**: Unipolar atrial electrogram. 1, P-wave signal: 2, far-field R-wave signal. The far-field signal is almost as big as the P wave. **B**: Same electrogram in bipolar sensing configuration. Ventricular far-field signals are still visible (2) but much smaller in amplitude.

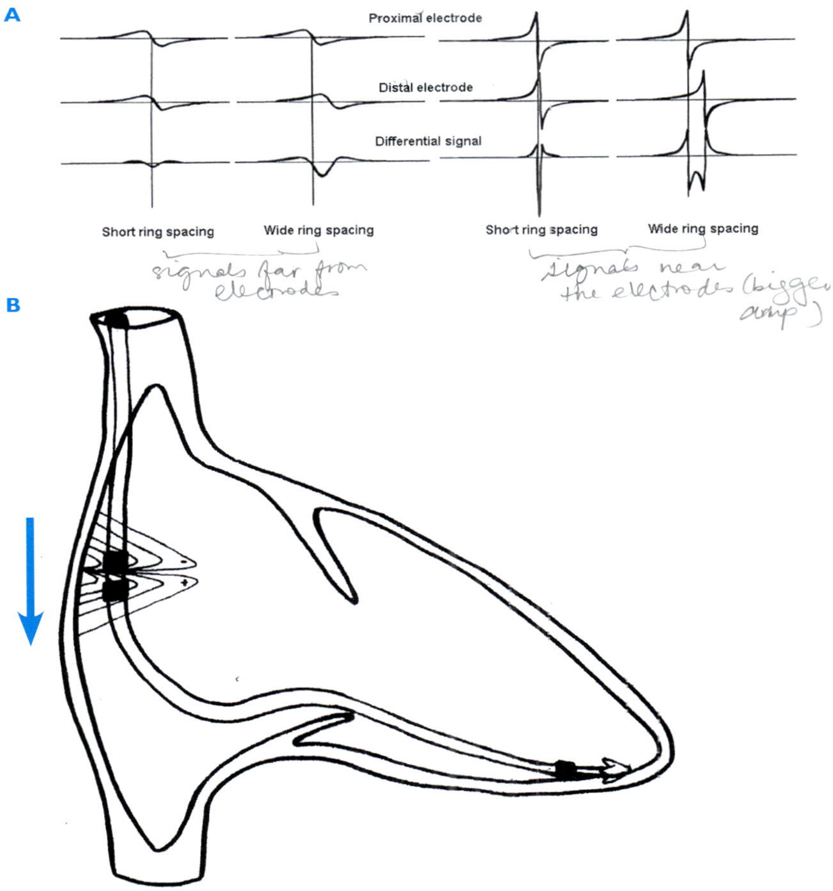

Fig 5.3 Atrial depolarization wavefront and bipolar VDD sensing. **A**: Differential signal in bipolar sensing of signals far from the electrodes (left) versus near to the electrodes (right). **B**: Propagation of the depolarization wavefront along the electrodes.

pass) are usually applied. This is highly effective in filtering out myopotentials (> 100 Hz) and T-wave potentials (< 10 Hz, Fig 5.4). However, also the amplitude of wanted signals can be reduced to some extent. Therefore, only filtered P-and R-wave amplitudes should be used when sensing is tested at lead implantation, otherwise P- and R-wave amplitudes may be insufficient for reliable sensing when filtered by the pacemaker. After filtering, the signal is rectified, thus the pacemaker defines the signal amplitude from baseline to signal maximum (Fig 5.5B).

The slew-rate (maximum slope of the intrinsic deflection, measured in V/s) provides an estimate of the frequency content and is thus a good predictor for the amplitude reduction of P and R waves after filtering: The sharper a cardiac signal, the less is filtered out.

Sensing at the Time of Implantation

At implantation, a sensed P and R wave has to be achieved that is sufficiently large for reliable sensing during the lifetime of the electrode. Some minimum values for sensing should therefore be regarded: A minimal P-wave amplitude of 2.0 mV (optimal) or 1.5 mV (acceptable), and a minimal R wave of 6 mV (acceptable) or 10 mV (optimal) should be confirmed. In unipolar leads, these values have to be respected more strictly

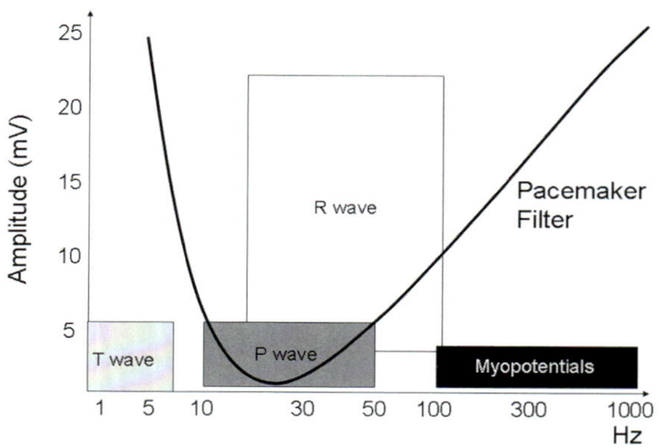

Fig 5.4 Frequency spectra of sensed signals and pacemaker filter. Sensed events with a frequency content inside the parable are augmented, outside the parable reduced.

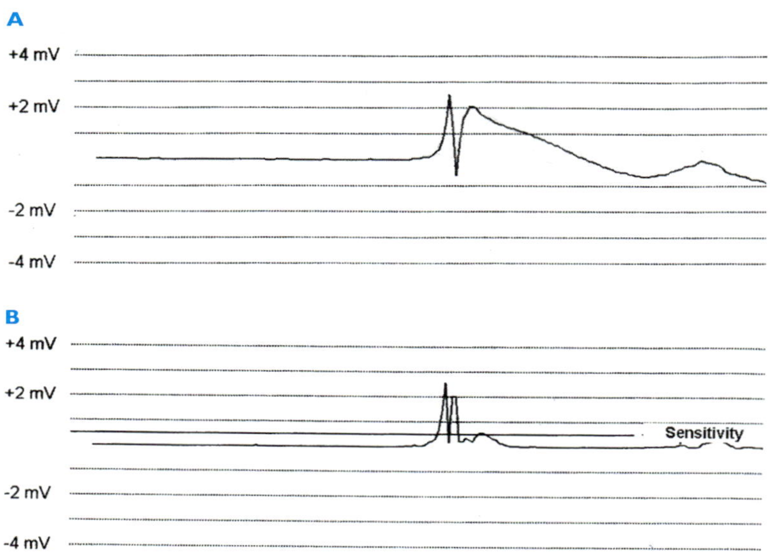

Fig 5.5 The unfiltered "raw" (**A**) versus the filtered and rectified (**B**) electrogram. This screw-in lead implanted in the atrium creates a sharp sensed signal together with a large acute injury current and a small ventricular far-field signal. The unfiltered (**A**) as well as the filtered (**B**) P-wave amplitude is sensed above 2 mV. Note that the filtered and rectified atrial electrogram (**B**) recorded at the same time as the unfiltered electrogram (**A**) shows almost no current injury and only a very small far-field signal.

because sensitivity cannot be programmed as high as in bipolar leads. P-and R-wave amplitudes measured by intraoperative pacing system analyzers have to be filtered (ideally with band-pass filters similar to the pacemaker that is going to be connected) to avoid a significant reduction after implantation. High values for slew-rates (atrium: > 0.3 V/s, ventricle: > 1.0 V/s) predict a small amplitude reduction after pacemaker connection.

An electrogram should be printed out after implantation to verify that the sensed signal represents a sensed P or R wave (Fig 5.5). Particularly after implantation of active-fixation leads, the screw-in process can provoke a so-called injury current (Fig 5.6). The presence of an injury current proves that the lead is screwed into the myocardium. However, the intraoperative pacing system analyzer may inadvertently measure the peak of the injury current instead of the P or R wave, and thus the sensed signal can be significantly smaller when the injury current has terminated. For this reason, intraoperative measurements should be repeated approximately 5 minutes after lead implantation. Sensing values should be stable (P-wave amplitude variations < 1 mV, R-wave amplitude variations < 2–3 mV) and amplitudes after screw-in should be larger than before, otherwise long-term sensing may be insufficient. At implant, the *smallest* sensed P and R wave should be sufficiently large to provide adequate sensing (ie, > 1.5–2.0 and > 6–10 mV, respectively).

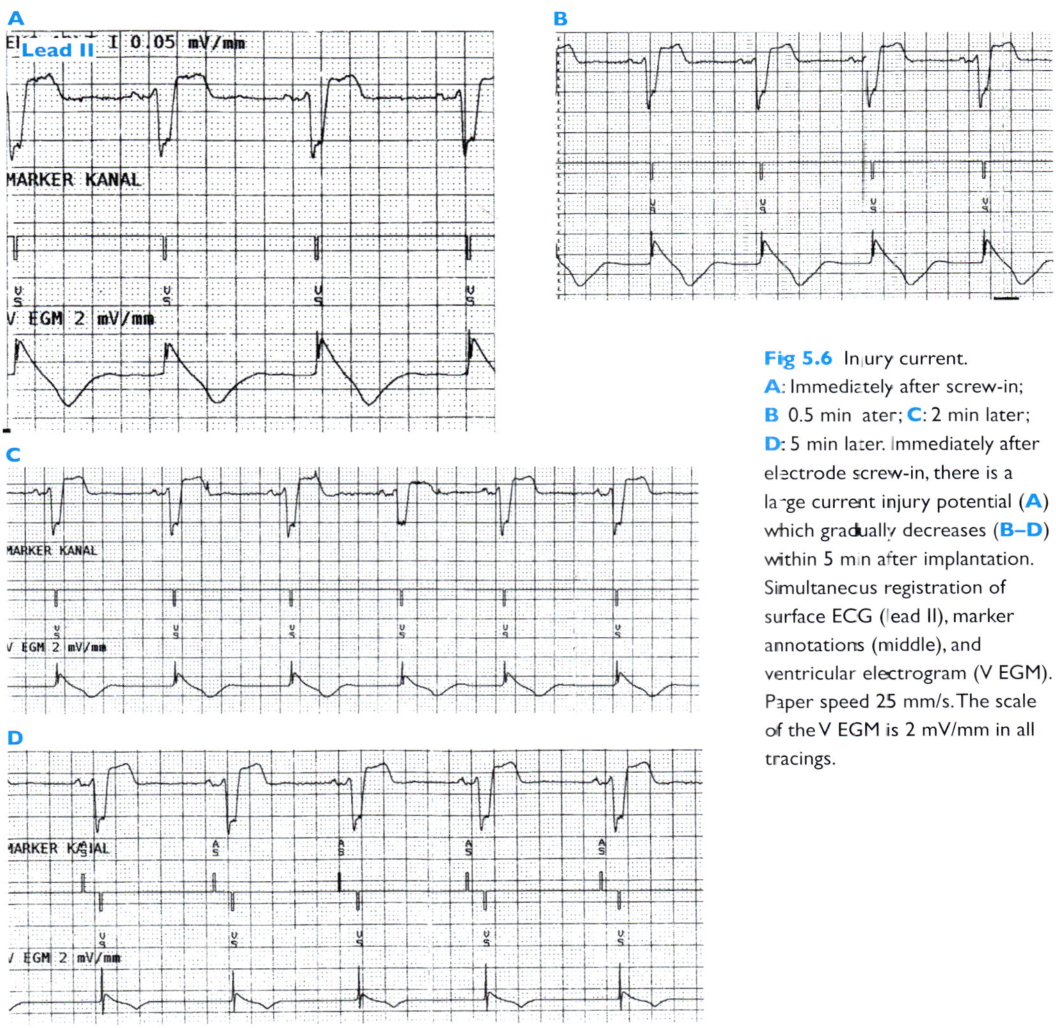

Fig 5.6 Injury current. **A**: Immediately after screw-in; **B** 0.5 min later; **C**: 2 min later; **D**: 5 min later. Immediately after electrode screw-in, there is a large current injury potential (**A**) which gradually decreases (**B–D**) within 5 min after implantation. Simultaneous registration of surface ECG (lead II), marker annotations (middle), and ventricular electrogram (V EGM). Paper speed 25 mm/s. The scale of the V EGM is 2 mV/mm in all tracings.

Sensing of Polarization Artifacts and Evoked Potentials

Depending on size and material, pacing causes more or less polarization, namely an accumulation of ions at the electrode-tissue interface, which creates an afterpotential artifact after a pacing stimulus. In high-polarization leads, this artifact is large and can prevent the reliable detection of the evoked response; therefore, it cannot be used alone to verify whether the pacing stimulus was effective. In low-polarization electrodes, the polarization artifact is small; therefore the pacemaker can verify the pacing efficacy and automatically optimize the pacing amplitude (Fig 5.7)[1].

Device Sensitivity Programming

After implantation, sensed P- and R-wave amplitudes have to be verified, and sensing polarity and sensitivity programmed accordingly. To ensure appropriate long-term ventricular sensing, the sensed cardiac signal should be at least twice as big as the sensing threshold (so-called 100% sensing safety margin). For example, if an R wave of 6 mV is sensed by the pacemaker, sensitivity should be programmed to 3.0 mV to make sure that even with amplitude variations the R wave will always be sensed. This is particularly important in unipolar leads where oversensing (eg, of myopotentials) is an issue.

In bipolar leads, it is possible to program a higher sensitivity. In fact, sensitivity in ICDs is usually programmed to 0.3 mV in the ventricle independently of the sensed R-wave amplitude to ensure sensing of ventricular fibrillation. Atrial sensitivity should be programmed to high values (eg, 0.2–0.3 mV) to ensure continuous detection of atrial fibrillation, which can be 300% to 400% smaller in amplitude than the P-wave amplitude. Because intermittent undersensing of atrial fibrillation can have disadvantageous consequences (lack of mode switching with irregular, fast tracking of atrial fibrillation, pacemaker-mediated tachycardia), programming of atrial sensitivity to lower values (eg, 0.5–0.75 mV) should be avoided. Atrial leads

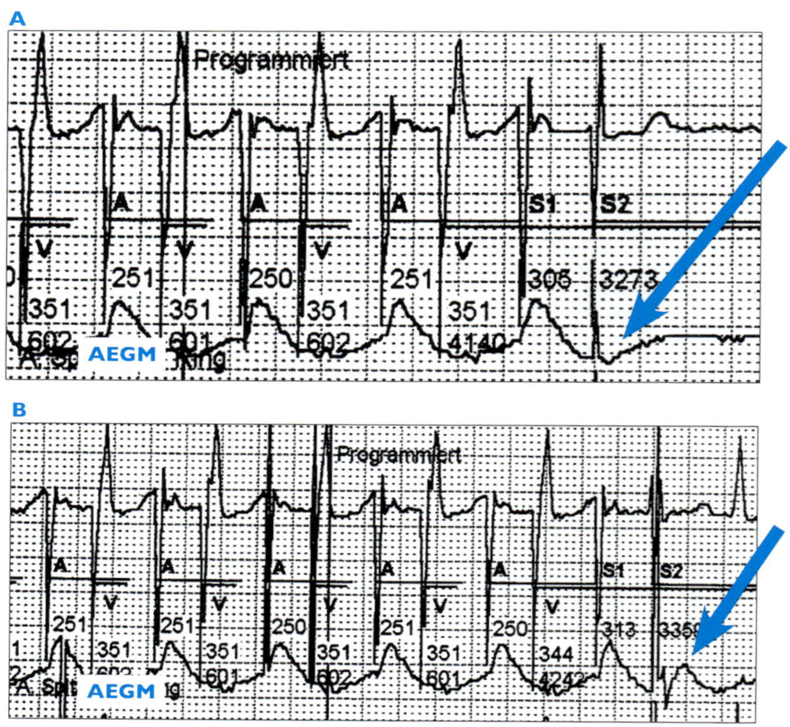

Fig 5.7 Electrograms with evoked response in low polarization leads. In this example of testing of the atrial refractory period, a coupled atrial extrastimulus (S2) is applied after a baseline stimulus (S1). In **A**, the extrastimulus S2 after 305 ms does not capture the atrium as can be seen from the atrial electrogram (AEGM) where the S2 stimulus is not followed by a positive potential (arrow) such as can be observed after all previous atrial stimuli (A and S1). In contrast, in **B** an atrial extrastimulus S2 at 313 ms is effective as documented by the evoked potential in the AEGM (arrow).

should be bipolar to allow this programming; unipolar atrial sensitivity programming is usually limited to 0.5 mV because higher sensitivity programming will cause myopotential oversensing (see following) with adverse side effects (inappropriate tracking of myopotentials, induction of endless loop tachycardia).

Particularly in unipolar atrial sensing, myopotential oversensing tests should be performed. Also for unipolar ventricular sensing, oversensing testing may apply in patients with AV block. If sensitivity is programmed to 2.0 mV or higher (ie, smaller threshold values), also diaphragmatic oversensing (coughing test) should be ruled out.

In biventricular pacemakers for cardiac resynchronization therapy, the sensing function is deactivated for the left ventricular lead in modern devices because it may cause ventricular double sensing.

Blanking and Refractory Periods

During some periods of the cardiac cycle, the atrial and/or ventricular channel cannot sense any signal, independent of its amplitude and programmed sensitivity. These time periods are called blanking periods. There are some short technical blanking periods (typically 30–50 ms) that are necessary to avoid detection of the stimulus itself in the paced or other channel. After an atrial stimulus, there is a postatrial atrial blanking (PAAB) and a postatrial ventricular blanking (PAVB) period. After a ventricular stimulus, there is a postventricular atrial blanking (PVAB) and a postventricular ventricular blanking period (PVVB, Fig 5.8). The PVAB is programmable and usually much longer than the other blanking periods because it has to protect the atrium from sensing ventricular far-field signals. Blanking periods are helpful to prevent oversensing independent of the programmed sensitivity. This is particularly important in the atrium where a bipolar sensitivity of 0.25 to 0.5 mV is required to reliably and consistently detect atrial fibrillation. To maintain this sensitivity, at the same time avoiding oversensing of ventricular far-field signals, programming the PVAB to a long value (eg, 100–150 ms) is highly effective. However, during blanking periods, intrinsic cardiac signals cannot be sensed. For this reason, ventricular blanking periods in ICDs are shorter and frequently non-programmable to avoid undersensing of ventricular fibrillation. In the atrium, programming the PVAB to long values (particularly to > 150 ms) may cause lack of detection of atrial flutter where every second flutter wave is not detected due to coincidence with the PVAB ("2:1 lock-in"). This can occur particularly if the AV delay is also blanked (in some pacemakers, the AV delay is automatically blanked whereas in others, only the initial part is blanked, see Fig 5.8) and programmed to

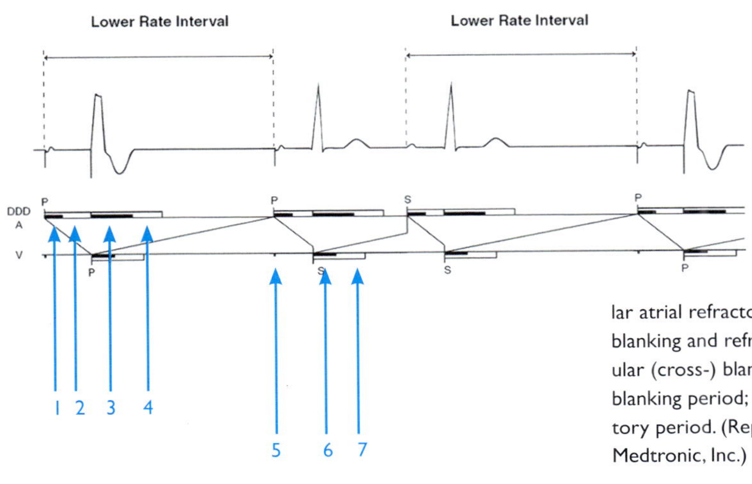

Fig 5.8 Blanking and refractory periods. Simulated surface ECG of DDD operation, atrial channel (A), ventricular channel (V). Blanking periods are expressed as black boxes, refractory periods as white boxes. 1–4, Atrial blanking and refractory periods. 1, Postatrial atrial blanking; 2, AV delay; 3, postventricular atrial blanking (PVAB); 4, postventricular atrial refractory period (PVARF). 5–7, Ventricular blanking and refractory periods. 5, Postatrial ventricular (cross-) blanking; 6, postventricular ventricular blanking period; 7, postventricular ventricular refractory period. (Reproduced with kind permission of Medtronic, Inc.)

long values. Undersensing caused by blanking periods is called functional undersensing and is discussed later.

In contrast to blanking periods, refractory periods allow sensing of atrial or ventricular intrinsic signals but they do not use these sensed events for timing of pacing. If an atrial event (or oversensed signal, eg, ventricular far-field signal) is sensed during the postventricular atrial refractory period (PVARP), it will not be triggered (Fig 5.9). This does not represent a form of undersensing but appropriately avoids triggering of nonphysiological signals or premature atrial beats which could cause endless loop tachycardia or a high ventricular rate. However, from the surface ECG this may look like undersensing of an atrial beat. Signals sensed during the PVARP cannot be triggered and do not reset atrial timing but are used to calculate the atrial rate. They are therefore used for automatic mode switching and can cause appropriate (caused by an atrial tachyarrhythmia) or inappropriate (caused by oversensing, eg, ventricular far-field signals) mode switching to nontracking or nontriggering mode. Therefore, prolonging the value of the PVARP does not prevent inappropriate mode switching due to ventricular far-field oversensing, instead the PVAB should be prolonged.

The ventricular refractory period (VRP) starts after a sensed or paced ventricular event and is designed to prevent ventricular oversensing of the paced QRS complex and the T wave.

Sensing over Time

Due to scar tissue formation around the lead tip, sensed intracardiac signals are typically slightly (< 10%) smaller 1 month after implantation and may further decrease slightly during their lifetime. Of note, the frequency content of P- and R-waves changes with the heart rate. Thus, cardiac signal amplitudes can be significantly smaller during exercise (Fig 5.10). Also, antiarrhythmic drugs of class I and III can reduce sensed signal amplitudes. Steroid elution of pacemaker leads can reduce the development of scar tissue after lead implantation and thus positively affect sensed signal amplitude.

Sensing Failure

Undersensing

If intrinsic cardiac signals are present, the lack of their detection by the device is called *undersensing*. Atrial undersensing can be caused by insufficient P-wave amplitudes and/or insufficient programming of the atrial sensitivity. At

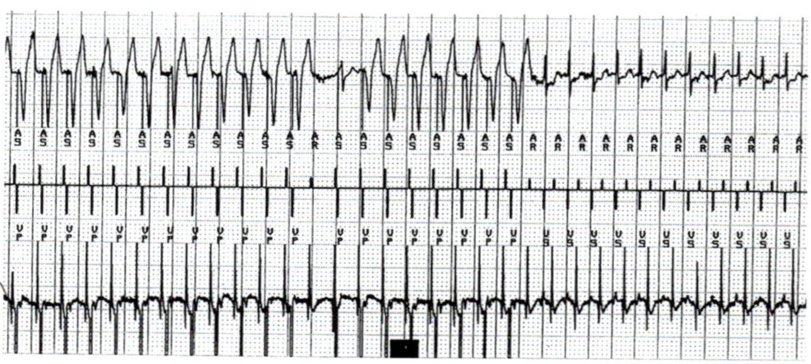

Fig 5.9 Atrial refractory sensing. During exercise, the atrial rate increases (ie, the atrial rate interval decreases) until it exceeds the maximum tracking rate (ie, the atrial rate interval is shorter than the total atrial refractory period). Thus, sinus beats fall into the postventricular atrial refractory period (PVARP, Fig 5.8) where they are sensed and annotated (AR, atrial refractory sensed signal) but not tracked. As a result, in this ECG sinus tachycardia is conducted intrinsically with AV block I°. Paper speed 12.5 mm/s, upper tracing: surface ECG, lead II; middle tracing: marker annotations (AS: atrial sensed event, VP: ventricular paced event, VS: ventricular sensed event); lower tracing, atrial electrogram.

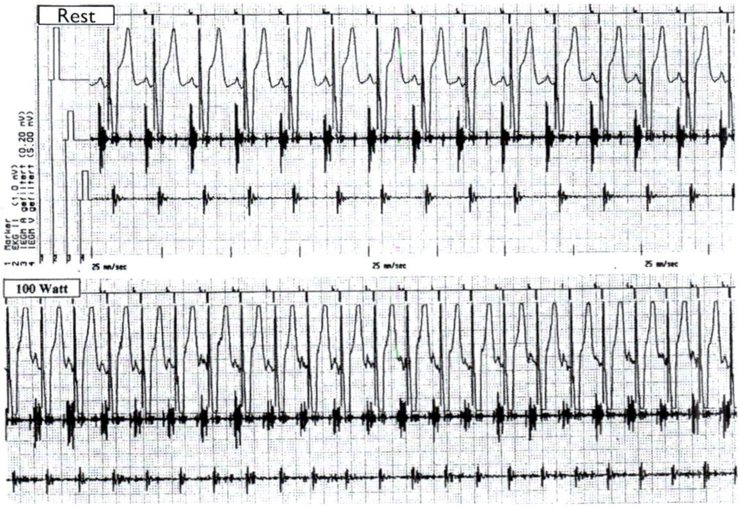

Fig 5.10 Reduction of the sensed P-wave amplitude during exercise. Simultaneous registration of marker annotations ("1," black symbols at the upper end), surface ECG ("2," lead II), atrial electrogram ("3," IEGM A), and ventricular electrogram ("4," IEGM V) at a paper speed of 25 mm/s. Note the amplitude of the atrial signal at rest (upper half) compared to exercise (100 watts, lower part).

implant, the sensed P-wave amplitude should be > 2 mV. The atrial sensitivity should not be programmed to 50% of the sensed P-wave amplitude because the latter can vary significantly (eg, during exercise, Fig. 5.10 or in atrial ectopic beats). Additionally, to reliably detect atrial fibrillation, atrial sensitivity should be programmed to 0.2 to 0.3 mV, independent from the P-wave amplitude because atrial fibrillation potentials can be much smaller (300%–400%) than the sinus P-wave amplitude, and highly variable. Examples of atrial undersensing of sinus rhythm and atrial fibrillation are shown in Figs 5.11 and 5.12. Undersensing of sinus rhythm can cause pacing in the atrial vulnerable period and induce atrial fibrillation. Undersensing of atrial fibrillation can lead to lack of mode switching because the (inappropriately) low sensed atrial rate does not meet mode switching criteria. In this case, the device will remain in triggering mode and may perform irregular and fast tracking of the fibrillation potentials that are detected.

Ventricular undersensing can occur whenever the sensed R-wave amplitude is below the sensing threshold (Fig 5.13). In unipolar ventricular sensing, sensitivity is usually programmed to 2.8 to 4.0 mV to avoid myopotential oversensing. Therefore, the sensed R-wave amplitude is required to be larger in unipolar ventricular leads at the time of implantation.

Of note, ventricular premature beats (VPBs) may originate far from the ventricular electrode and may have smaller sensed signal amplitudes leading to undersensing of VPBs while sinus beats are appropriately sensed.

Ventricular pacing at the time of spontaneous QRS complexes does not always represent ventricular undersensing, even if the ventricular pacing spike coincides with the descending limb or end of the R wave, particularly in patients with right bundle branch block (Fig 5.14). This pseudofusion is caused by the pacing lead only registering local electrical activity, such as in the right ventricular apex, which may occur late during the QRS complex.

Ventricular undersensing can lead to ventricular pacing despite the presence of an intrinsic ventricular rhythm. It may fall into the ventricular myocardial refractory period and be ineffective (Fig 5.15) despite an otherwise normal pacing function. Though it seems to be very rare, ventricular undersensing with pacing in the vulnerable period may induce ventricular fibrillation (Fig 5.16). If ventricular undersensing is detected, it therefore needs to be corrected, if possible by reprogramming ventricular sensitivity, otherwise by lead revision.

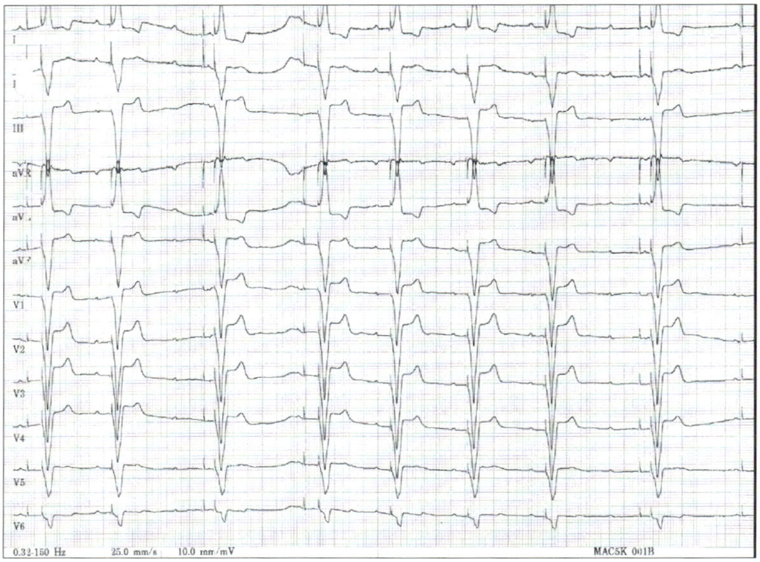

Fig 5.11 Intermittent undersensing of sinus rhythm. 12 lead ECG, paper speed 25 mm/s.

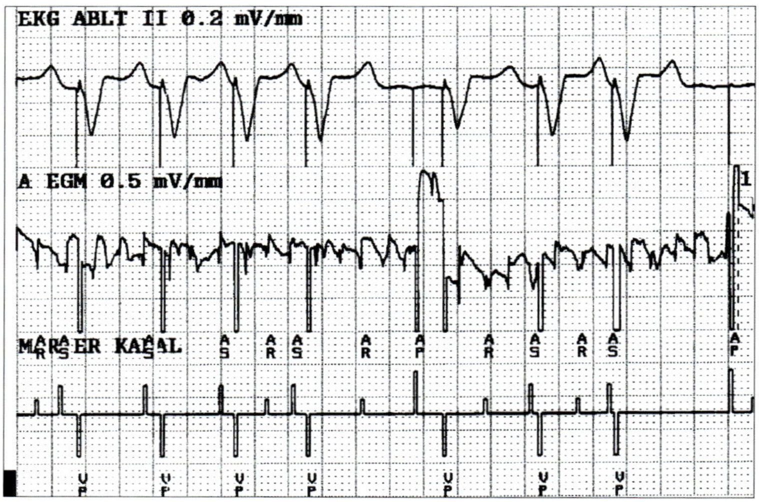

Fig 5.12 Intermittent undersensing of atrial fibrillation. Simultaneous recording of surface ECG (upper part, lead II), atrial electrogram (A EGM, middle), and marker annotations (below), paper speed 25 mm/s. The A EGM documents atrial fibrillation with a filtered amplitude of many fibrillation potentials smaller than the atrial sensitivity (0.5 mV). Therefore, atrial fibrillation is not detected (fibrillation potentials without marker annotation), in DDDR mode resulting in irregular and intermittently rapid tracking. In the middle of this tracing, only 1 out of 5 fibrillation potentials is sensed, but because it appears in the postventricular atrial refractory period (PVARP), an atrial pace follows. AP, atrial pacing; AR, atrial refractory sensing; AS: atrial sensing; VP, ventricular pacing.

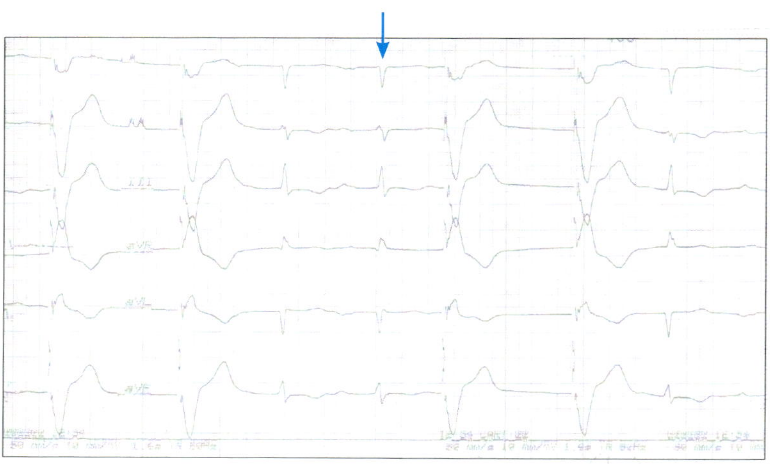

Fig 5.13 Intermittent ventricular undersensing. The fourth ventricular complex (arrow) is not sensed by the pacemaker, therefore premature ventricular pacing at a rate of approximately 120 bpm (500 ms after the undetected QRS) follows. Leads I, II, III, aVR, aVL, and aVF. Paper speed 50 mm/s.

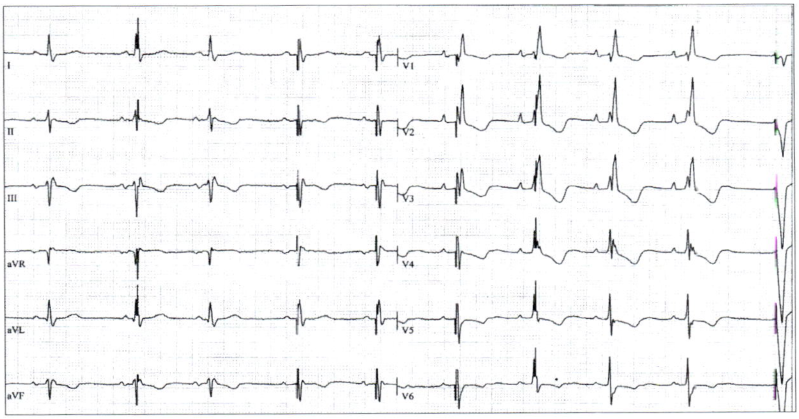

Fig 5.14 Ventricular pseudofusion in VVI pacing and right bundle branch block. Particularly in patients with right bundle branch block (RBBB), excitation may reach the right ventricular lead tip rather late, for example, at the time of the S wave. Therefore, pacing may occur in the R wave despite normal ventricular sensing, and cause pseudofusion (2nd, 4th, 5th, 6th, and 7th QRS). The last QRS represents ventricular pacing with capture in this patient with intermittent SA block. Paper speed 25 mm/s.

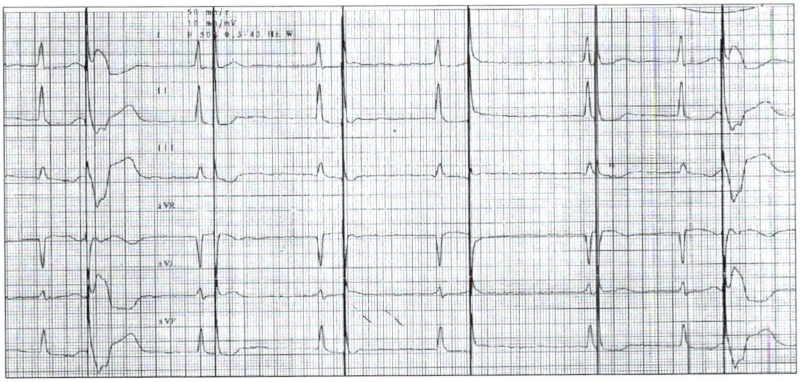

Fig 5.15 Ventricular undersensing and pacing in the refractory period. In this example of complete ventricular undersensing, ventricular pacing occurs immediately after the intrinsic QRS complex. Pacing is ineffective in most instances in this example. However, after the first and the last intrinsic QRS, pacing in the T wave is effective. There is a risk that T-wave pacing can trigger ventricular fibrillation. Extremity leads, paper speed 50 mm/s.

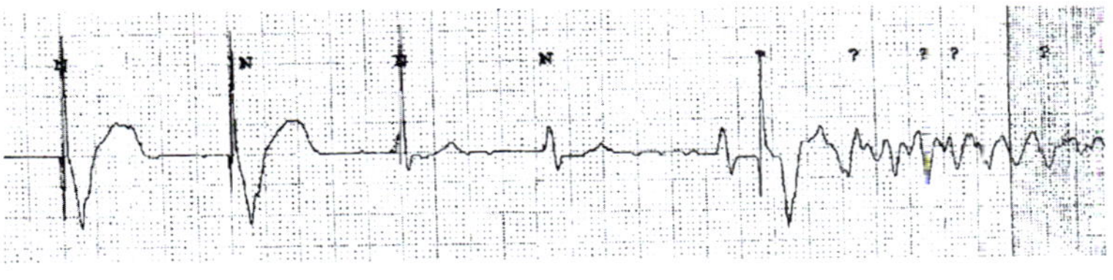

Fig 5.16 Ventricular undersensing and induction of ventricular fibrillation. In this patient with atrial fibrillation, intermittent AV block, and heart failure, there is intermittent undersensing of ventricular intrinsic activity. Pacing in the vulnerable phase induces ventricular fibrillation requiring defibrillation. Monitor printout, lead II, paper speed 25 mm/s.

Functional Undersensing

Whenever an intrinsic cardiac signal appears during a blanking period, it will not be sensed. This is referred to as functional undersensing, namely, the signal amplitude would be large enough to be sensed but due to timing, it is not detected by the device. Functional undersensing may occur in the atrium where it has specific clinical consequences in atrial flutter. In flutter with 240 bpm (= 250-ms cycle length) and a PVAB even as short as 100 ms, every second flutter wave will fall into the PVAB for AV delays programmed to 150 ms or longer (AV delay 150 + PVAB 100 = 250 ms). As a consequence, atrial flutter of 240 bpm may be detected as atrial tachycardia of only 120 bpm and tracked by a DDDR pacemaker (2:1 lock-in, Fig 5.17).

Ventricular functional undersensing may occur if an intrinsic QRS complex appears during or immediately after atrial pacing. The ventricular blanking period after atrial pacing (PAVB) is non-programmable and short (50 ms) in most devices. If an intrinsic QRS complex falls exactly into this period, it is completely undetected and ventricular pacing will occur after the programmed AV delay (Fig 5.18). If the paced AV delay is programmed to long values

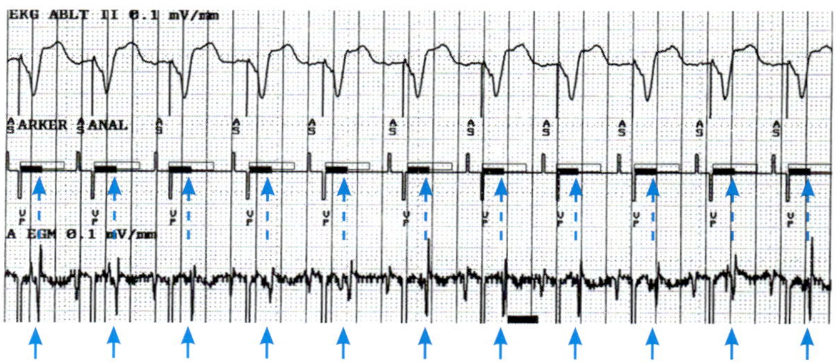

Fig 5.17 Atrial flutter 2:1 lock-in. Simultaneous registration of surface ECG (lead II), marker annotations with refractory/blanking periods, and atrial electrogram (A EGM) at 25 mm/s. In this example of atrial flutter, every second flutter potential appears during the postventricular atrial blanking time (PVAB, black boxes). Despite a large signal (see arrows to the A EGM), these flutter waves are not seen by the pacemaker.

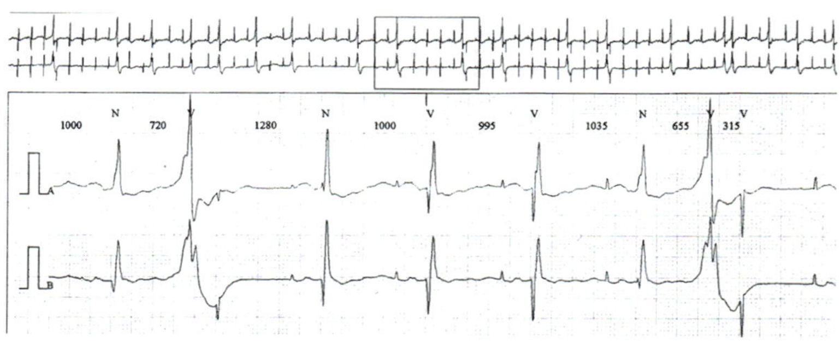

Fig 5.18 Functional ventricular undersensing. In this Holter tracing, two ventricular premature beats occur exactly at the moment of atrial pacing. The ventricular channel is blanked out (postatrial ventricular blanking, see Fig 5.8) and cannot sense this event. Therefore, ventricular pacing occurs when the paced AV delay times out, in this example, 300 ms after atrial pacing.

(eg, 250–300 ms), ventricular pacing may occur during the vulnerable phase.

If an intrinsic ventricular signal is sensed a little later (50–100 ms) after atrial pacing, it may fall into the window for safety pacing: The device assumes that atrial pacing cannot be conducted to the ventricle within 50 to 100 ms but may represent crosstalk (the atrial stimulus is sensed in the ventricle). In this situation, a ventricular safety pace is applied to prevent ventricular asystole due to crosstalk (Fig 5.19). The AV delay of safety pacing is fixed around 110 ms, independent of the programmed AV delay.

Functional ventricular undersensing can occur due to a premature ventricular beat at the same time as an atrial pace (Fig 5.18) or due to atrial undersensing (Fig 5.19). If a P wave or atrial fibrillation is not detected, atrial pacing may occur just at the time of intrinsic conduction of the unsensed atrial event to the ventricle.

Functional undersensing cannot be resolved by reprogramming atrial or ventricular sensitivity. In functional atrial undersensing of atrial flutter, the PVAB or sensed AV delay may be shortened or the maximum tracking rate reduced to < 120 bpm. Some devices provide specific algorithms (Blanked Flutter Search, Atrial Flutter Response[2]) that inhibit atrial tracking for one beat whenever an atrial cycle length < two times the total atrial blanking period (AV delay + PVAB) is detected. In ventricular functional undersensing, the atrial sensing function should be checked and reprogrammed if necessary.

Oversensing

Oversensing can be caused by: (1) cardiac intrinsic signals from the same chamber, (2) cardiac intrinsic signals from the other chamber, (3) pacing artifacts from the other chamber (afterpotentials), (4) myopotentials of near muscles, (5) electromagnetic interference, or (6) defects of the lead or the pacemaker generator. See Table 5.1. Oversensing is much more frequent in unipolar sensing. Particularly in the atrium where a high sensitivity is necessary to reliably detect atrial fibrillation, only bipolar leads should be implanted. Only bipolar leads can be connected to ICDs to allow sensing at a high sensitivity (necessary to reliably detect ventricular fibrillation) without oversensing.

Atrial oversensing

The atrium is more prone to oversensing because the atrial sensitivity has to be higher than the ventricular to detect P-wave and atrial fibrillation potentials. By far, the most important cause of atrial oversensing in bipolar sensing is oversensing of ventricular far-field signals

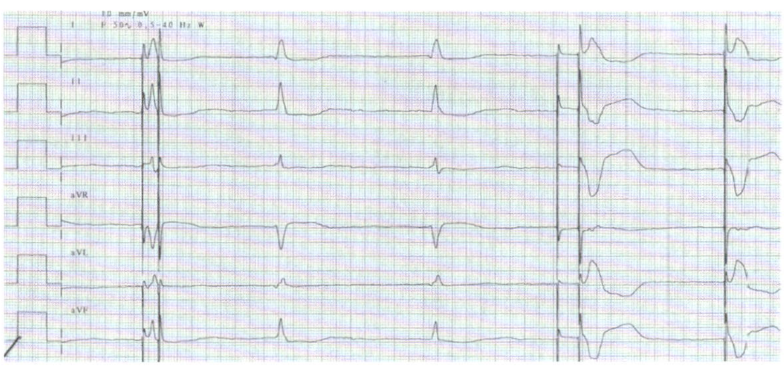

Fig 5.19 Ventricular safety pacing: Atrial fibrillation with intermittent undersensing. Surface ECG, extremity leads, paper speed 50 mm/s. Atrial fibrillation with intermittent undersensing leads to atrial pacing. Shortly after the atrial pace, spontaneous AV conduction occurs. The QRS complex is detected by the pacemaker 50 to 110 ms after atrial pacing which applies a safety pace to prevent ventricular asystole if this ventricular sensing would represent crosstalk, that is the atrial pace is sensed in the ventricle. This safety pace appears 110 ms after atrial pacing, independent of the programmed AV delay. The programmed AV delay of 150 ms is visible later in this tracing.

(Fig 5.20). It can best be prevented by sufficiently long postventricular atrial blanking periods (PVABs) while reduction of atrial sensitivity compromises detection of sinus P waves and atrial fibrillation. Only if ventricular far-field oversensing occurs in the terminal part of the AV delay (ie, ventricular far-field signals sensed in the atrium before the ventricle, Fig 5.21), does reprogramming atrial sensitivity become necessary.

Atrial Oversensing		
	Causes	**Consequences**
Ventricular far-field oversensing	QRS or T wave sensed outside the PVAB	Inappropriate MS
P-wave double counting	Local block	Inappropriate MS
Myopotentials	M. pectoralis	Inappropriate tracking with asynchronous ventricular pacing; endless loop tachycardia; inappropriate MS; noise reversion resulting in DOO or DVI pacing
Crosstalk	Ventricular pacing afterpotential	Inappropriate MS if PVAB not activated
Electromagnetic interference	All electronic sources	Same as myopotentials
Insulation failure	Outer insulation leakage	Same as myopotentials
Connection failure	Loose set-screw	Same as myopotentials
Electrode fracture	Overlapping conductor fragments	Same as myopotentials
Ventricular Oversensing		
	Causes	**Consequences**
Myopotentials	M. pectoralis; Diaphragm	Inhibition of a ventricular stimulus; asystole; noise reversion resulting in DOO or DVI pacing
QRS double counting	Short PVVB; very broad QRS in BBB	Inappropriate counter data
T wave	Large T wave ± high sensitivity (eg, due to small R wave)	Inappropriate counter data; inappropriate PVC reaction
P wave	Lead dislodgment/ malplacement; inappropriate ventricular sensitivity	Inhibition of a ventricular stimulus; asystole
Crosstalk	Atrial pacing afterpotential	Inhibition of a ventricular stimulus/ asystole if safety pacing not activated
Electromagnetic interference	All electronic sources	Same as myopotentials
Insulation failure	Outer insulation leakage	Same as myopotentials
Connection failure	Loose set-screw	Same as myopotentials
Electrode fracture	Overlapping conductor fragments	Same as myopotentials

Table 5.1 Potential Causes and Consequences of Oversensing in Pacemakers. BBB, bundle branch block; MS, mode switching; PVAB, postventricular atrial blanking; PVC, premature ventricular complex; PVVB, postventricular ventricular blanking.

In unipolar leads, myopotentials can also cause atrial oversensing (Fig 5.22). After implantation of unipolar leads, myopotential oversensing should be excluded by asking the patient to press both hands together (pectoral muscles) and coughing (diaphragm) and sensitivity reduced as long as oversensing can be provoked. However, myopotential oversensing potentials can be larger than P-wave potentials. As myopotential oversensing can frequently not be resolved in unipolar sensing, the use of unipolar leads is not advisable.

Rare causes of atrial oversensing are P-wave double sensing (Fig 5.23), electromagnetic interference (Fig 5.24, Table 5.2), connection failure (eg, loose set-screw), and insulation failure as well as incomplete lead fracture (Fig 5.25).

Atrial oversensing can lead to inappropriate inhibition of pacing in AAI and DDI modes. In DDDR mode, it may cause inappropriate tracking with fast and irregular, asynchronous ventricular pacing, and inappropriate mode switching to DDIR (reactions to electromagnetic interference, see Table 5.2). Asynchronous ventricular pacing, for example caused by myopotential oversensing, can induce endless loop tachycardia.

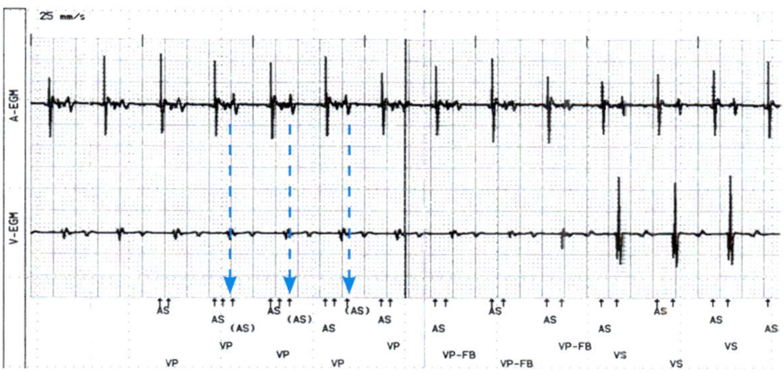

Fig 5.20 Oversensing of ventricular far-field signals in the atrium. Stored mode switching episode. The bipolar atrial electrogram (A-EGM) shows large potentials that represent P waves, annotated AS (atrial sensed events). At the time of ventricular pacing (annotation VP), there are small artifacts in the atrial channel. These are not sensed because they fall into the postventricular atrial blanking period (PVAB). However, shortly later, there are other, bigger potentials (3 dotted arrows) that are sensed in the refractory periods. [(AS), atrial refractory sensed signals] In this example, far-field oversensing leads to inappropriate mode switching: The black line marks the time at which criteria for detection of atrial tachyarrhythmia are fulfilled (sensed atrial rate > 170 bpm) and the device switches to DDIR mode, that is, atrial sensed events are no longer tracked. V-EGM, ventricular electrogram; VP, ventricular pacing; VP-FB, ventricular pacing in fallback mode; VS, ventricular sensing.

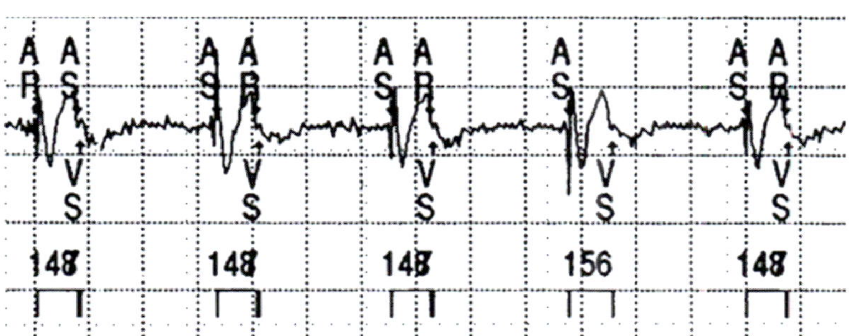

Fig 5.21 Oversensing of ventricular far-field signals in the atrium before the ventricle. Stored inappropriate atrial tachyarrhythmia detection due to ventricular far-field oversensing in the terminal portion of the AV delay before ventricular sensing. Annotations, refer to Figs. 5.9, 5.12, and 5.23.

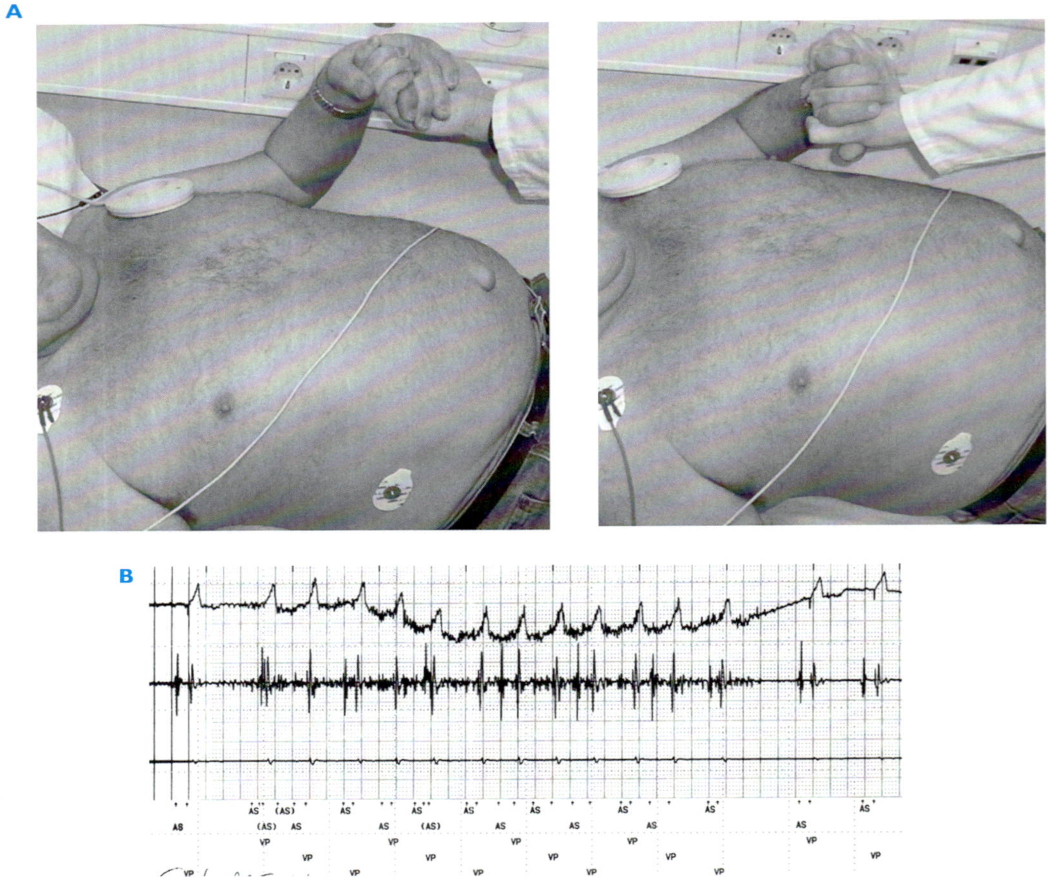

Fig 5.22 Myopotentials oversensing in a unipolar atrial lead. Activation of the pectoral muscle (arm pressing, see provocation test in **A**) leads to small myopotentials in the unipolar atrial channel that are sensed and tracked to the ventricle causing rapid and irregular ventricular pacing (**B**). Myopotential oversensing is virtually nonexistent in bipolar differential sensing.

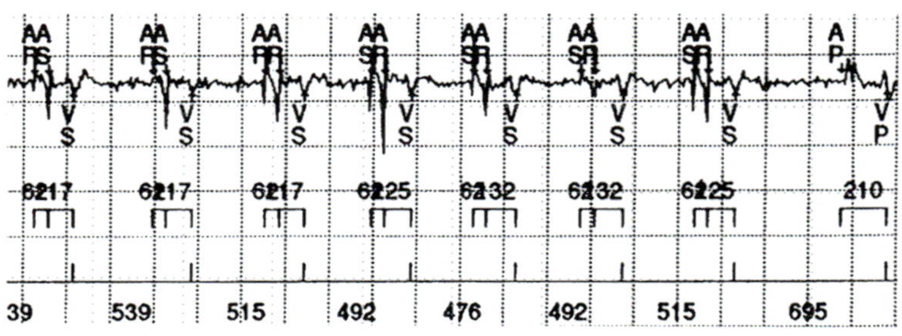

Fig 5.23 P-wave double counting. Stored episode of atrial tachyarrhythmia, inappropriately detected due to split atrial potentials during sinus tachycardia. Annotations are overlapping. AR, atrial refractory sensed; AS, atrial sensed; AP, atrial paced; VS, ventricular sensing; VP, ventricular pacing.

Far-field oversensing in the atrium: Testing and reprogramming

Inappropriate sensing of ventricular signals in the atrium is the most frequent oversensing problem in pacemakers, even with bipolar leads. In the BEATS study, approximately 80% of all inappropriate atrial tachyarrhythmia detections were due to ventricular far-field oversensing.[3] It may be prevented in bipolar leads by short ring spacing (eg, 1.1 mm as in lead model OptiSense 1999, St. Jude Medical, Sylmar, CA[4]). However, to prevent far-field oversensing, its presence should be checked after implantation (Table 5.3, Fig 5.26). At testing with maximum sensitivity,

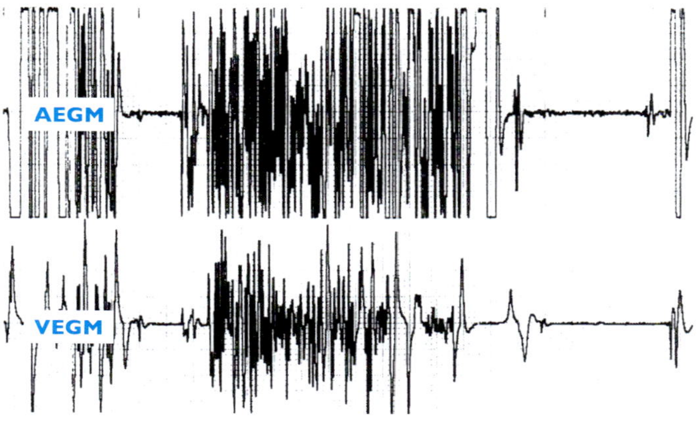

Fig 5.24 Electromagnetic interference. Stored episode of tachycardia (AEGM, atrial electrogram; VEGM, ventricular electrogram; paper speed 25 mm/s). These artifacts with a sharp beginning and end were caused by electrocautery during coronary bypass surgery.

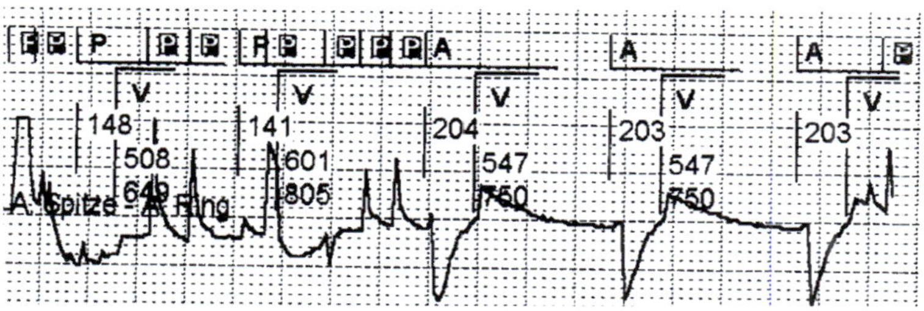

Fig 5.25 Inner insulation failure. In this old bipolar lead with a pacing impedance < 200 Ohms, inappropriate detection of atrial tachyarrhythmia occurred due to failure of the inner insulation. Typical for inner insulation failure, oversensing signals vary in amplitude from 0.2 to > 2.5 mV.

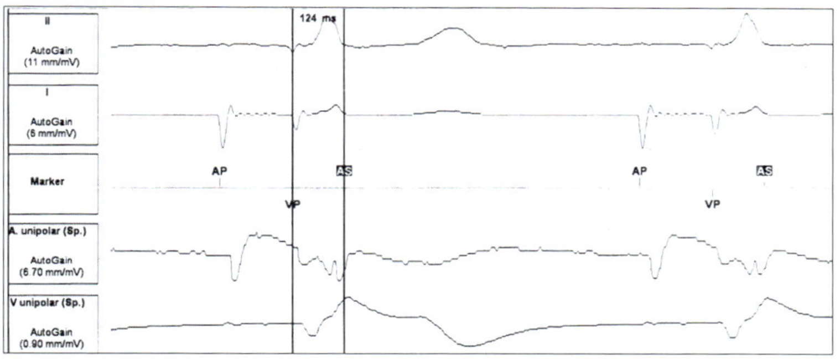

Fig 5.26 Ventricular far-field oversensing test in the atrium. After programming atrial bipolar sensitivity to 0.1 mV, the timing of ventricular far-field oversensing in the atrial channel becomes visible (marker "AS" in black box: atrial refractory sensed signal). Note that despite bipolar sensing, the atrial electrogram is programmed to unipolar ("A. unipolar") to facilitate visibility of the far-field signal. In this tracing with a paper speed of 100 mm/s, calipers measure an interval from ventricular pacing (VP) to refractory atrial sensing (AS) of 124 ms. Programming the postventricular atrial blanking (PVAB) period to 125 + 25 = 150 ms (and reprogramming bipolar atrial sensitivity to 0.2 mV) would be optimal to prevent ventricular far-field oversensing without compromising detection of atrial fibrillation. Printout of surface ECG (leads II and I), marker annotations (AP, atrial pacing), unipolar atrial electrogram, and unipolar ventricular electrogram (V unipolar).

Electromagnetic Fields
Home and private environment
Cellular telephones
Electronic article surveillance devices, metal detectors
Improperly grounded appliances in close contact to the body; some home appliances (e.g., electric razor), toy remote controls)
Work and industrial environment
High-voltage power lines
Transformers, welders, electric motors, induction furnaces
Medical environment
Magnetic resonance imaging
Electrosurgery
Defibrillation
Neurostimulation, transcutaneous electrical nerve stimulation
Radiofrequency catheter ablation, therapeutic diathermy
Ionizing radiation
Radiotherapy
Acoustic radiation
Lithotripsy
Potential Pacemaker Reactions
Pacemaker inhibition, asystole
Asynchronous pacing (VOO, DOO, DVI modes)
Atrial oversensing with inappropriate tracking and asynchronous ventricular pacing
Impaired telemetry
Reprogramming (power-on-reset)
Lead or device damage, loss of function
Inappropriate algorithm activation (sensor, mode switching, automatic capture detection, etc.)
Inappropriate memory data (atrial or ventricular tachycardia detection, etc.)

Table 5.2 Sources of Electromagnetic Interference and Potential Pacemaker Reactions

ventricular far-field oversensing can be sensed in almost all atrial bipolar leads, and its timing after ventricular pacing can be assessed.[5] Programming the PVAB period to a value 25 ms longer than the interval from ventricular pacing to the oversensed signal (Fig 5.26) is highly effective in preventing far-field oversensing, at the same time maintaining a high atrial sensitivity (eg, 0.2 mV) that does not compromise detection of atrial fibrillation.

Ventricular oversensing

Causes for ventricular oversensing are myopotential oversensing (in unipolar leads, Fig 5.27), electromagnetic interference (Table 5.2), T-wave oversensing, and hardware complications of the sensing circuit (eg, failure of inner/outer lead insulation, loose connection screw, partial electrode fracture). In rare cases, QRS double counting (particularly in bundle branch block and in the first generations of biventricular devices, Fig 5.28) and P wave far-field oversensing (Fig 5.29) have been reported. P-wave oversensing in the ventricular channel is usually associated with a lead position in proximity to the atrium.

Myopotential oversensing can lead to inhibition of ventricular pacing with potentially dangerous consequences in patients with AV block (Fig 5.27). Unipolar ventricular leads should therefore be programmed as insensitive as possible in these patients, for example, to 4.0 mV or an even higher sensing threshold. This requires sensed R-wave amplitudes > 8 mV to provide a 100% sensing safety margin. Similar to atrial sensing, bipolar sensing is also preferable in the ventricle due to the better rejection of oversensing without compromising sensing function.

Program maximum bipolar atrial sensitivity (eg, 0.1 mV)

↓

Program short AV delay to achieve ventricular pacing (eg, 100 ms)

↓

Record simultaneous ECG, marker annotations, atrial electrogram (if possible high resolution, paper speed 100 mm/s)

↓

Measure interval from marker for ventricular pacing to far-field signal in the atrium (if possible with calipers)

↓

Program the PVAB 25 ms longer than the measured interval from ventricular pace to far-field signal (minimum 100 ms, maximum 180 ms)

Table 5.3 Far-Field Ventricular Oversensing Testing

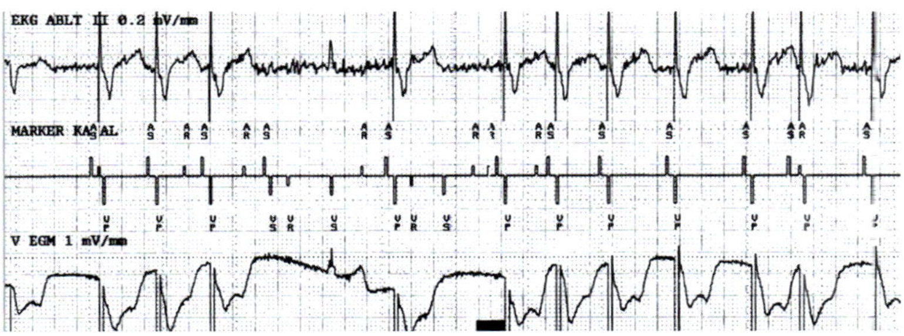

Fig 5.27 Myopotential oversensing in the ventricle. Pectoral muscle testing (arm pressing, see Fig 5.22) causes ventricular bradycardia due to ventricular oversensing together with atrial oversensing with rapid and irregular ventricular stimulation. Simultaneous recording of surface ECG (lead II), marker annotations, and ventricular electrogram (V EGM) at 25 mm/s.

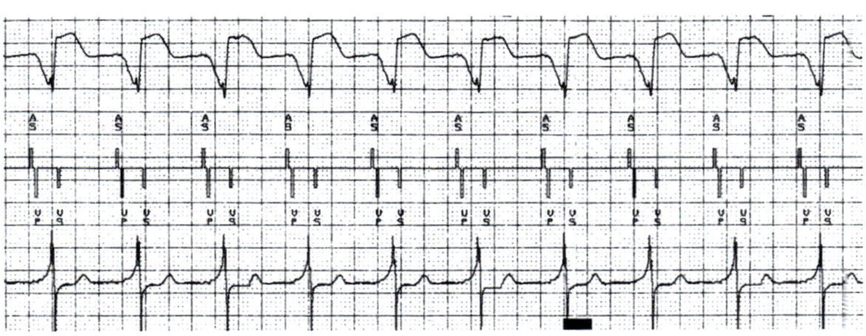

Fig 5.28 QRS double counting. Simultaneous recording of surface ECG (upper tracing, lead II), marker annotations (middle tracing), and ventricular electrogram (lower tracing) at 25 mm/s. AS, atrial sensing; VP, ventricular pacing; VS, ventricular sensing.

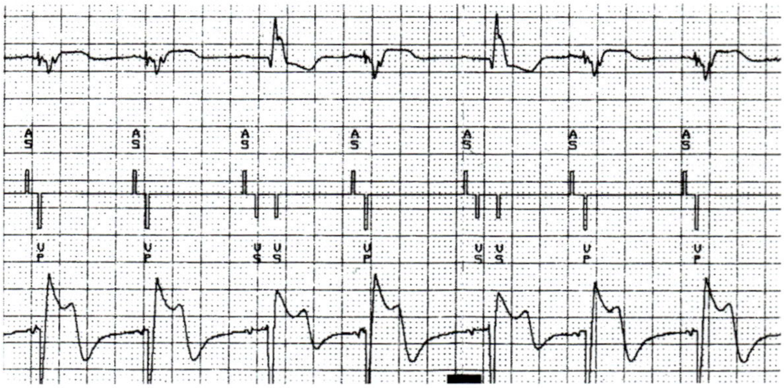

Fig 5.29 P wave far-field oversensing in the ventricle. Simultaneous recording of surface ECG (lead II), marker annotations, and ventricular electrogram at 25 mm/s. Of note, P wave oversensing in the ventricle prevents (bi-)ventricular pacing. AS, atrial sensing; VP, ventricular pacing; VS, ventricular sensing.

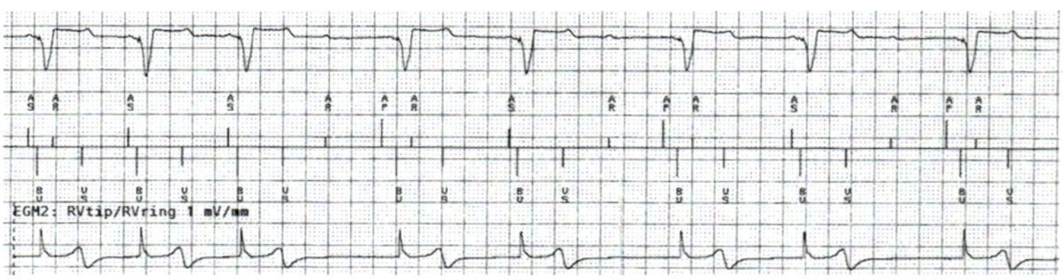

Fig 5.30 T wave oversensing in the ventricle. Simultaneous recording of surface ECG (lead II), marker annotations, and ventricular electrogram (EGM2) at 25 mm/s. T wave oversensing (visible through the marker annotation "VS" in this patient with AV block III°) starts a prolonged postventricular atrial refractory period (PVARP), referred to as PVC reaction given that for the device, any ventricular sensed event not preceded by an atrial event is a premature ventricular complex (PVC). Due to the long post-PVC PVARP, sinus P waves are refractory sensed (AR) and not conducted.

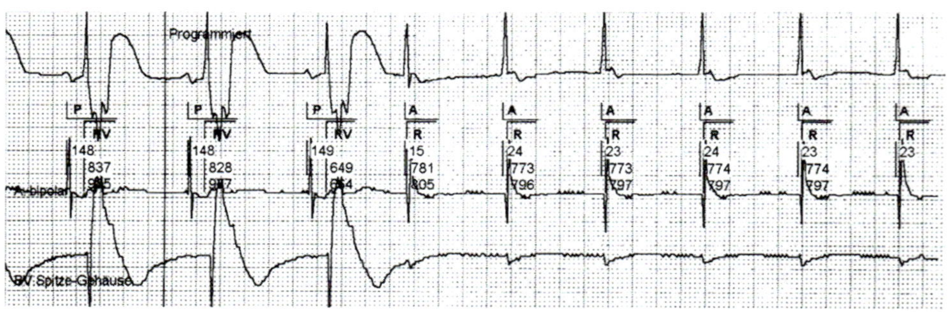

Fig 5.31 Crosstalk. Simultaneous recording of surface ECG (lead II), marker and cycle length annotations, atrial (A bipolar), and ventricular electrogram (RV tip to ring) at 25 mm/s. After atrial pacing (marker "A"), a very small artifact is visible in the unipolar ventricular electrogram which is annotated with "R" (ventricular sensed event) 15 to 24 ms after atrial pacing. In this device, the postatrial ventricular blanking period (PAVB) and ventricular safety pacing are deactivated during testing; in this case, atrial threshold testing. As a result, there is prolonged asystole in a patient with AV block III°.

T-wave oversensing may reset the PVARP (PVARP extension after premature ventricular beat, Fig 5.30) and ventricular timing. It requires reduction of ventricular sensitivity or reprogramming of automatic sensitivity adjustment functions (see later).

Crosstalk

Sensing of the atrial stimulus in the ventricle is referred to as crosstalk in the stricter sense (Fig 5.31). It is caused by atrial pacing artifacts that are visible in the ventricle and persist beyond PAVB (typically 30–50 ms, usually non-programmable). Crosstalk may lead to ventricular asystole and can thus be life threatening (Fig 5.31). To avoid crosstalk, most modern pacemakers are nominally programmed with activation of ventricular safety pacing. If ventricular activity is sensed shortly (eg, 50–110 ms) after atrial pacing, the device assumes a nonphysiologic signal and provides immediate ventricular pacing. Ventricular safety pacing can be identified in the surface ECG by an AV time after atrial pacing of 110 ms, independent of the programmed AV delay. Crosstalk can sometimes be avoided by reducing the atrial output or ventricular sensitivity.

Sensing Amplifier Saturation, Noise Reversion

In the phenomenon of paradoxical undersensing, undersensing appears if the sensitivity is increased. For instance, reprogramming the atrial sensitivity from 0.5 to 0.2 mV may cause undersensing. In this case, the atrial channel detects signals immediately (eg, within 60 ms) after preceding signals. Each detected signal starts a retriggerable refractory period. If these retriggerable refractory periods add up to a complete cardiac cycle, the device assumes "continuous" sensing as in an electromagnetic field and can switch to DOO or DVI mode (Fig 5.32).

Additionally, some devices can define repetitive signals with a non-physiological short cycle length as (electromagnetic) noise and perform switch to OOO (in ICDs), DOO, or DVI mode (Fig 5.33).

Electromagnetic Interference

Multiple sources of electromagnetic interference (EMI) may influence pacemaker sensing during everyday life, at work, and in a medical environment (Table 5.2[6,7]). Although most electrical appliances (eg, computers, television, hearing aids, electrical toothbrush, etc.) generally do not cause pacemaker sensing errors, this is not true for all electronic devices that are improperly grounded and come in contact or close proximity to the patient. However, with the introduction of feed-through filters (Fig 5.34), there is virtually no risk of electromagnetic interference by GSM mobile phones.

Pacemaker reactions to EMI are numerous and include errors in sensing and pacing performance, errors in interrogation and telemetry (phantom interference), inappropriate memory data, device reprogramming (power-

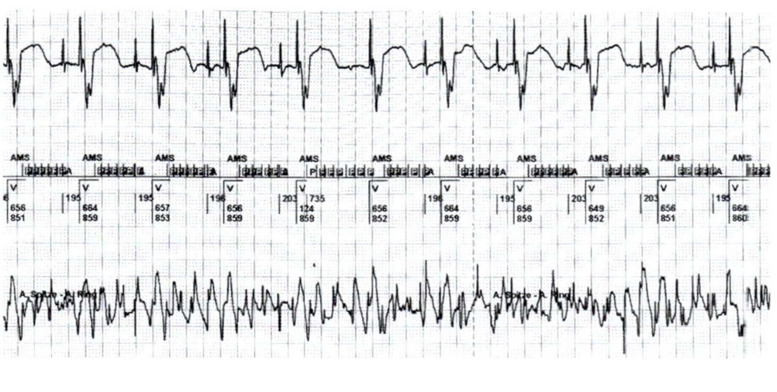

Fig 5.32 Amplifier saturation. At an atrial sensitivity of 0.2 mV, atrial fibrillation potentials are sensed almost continuously. Each sensed event retriggers another refractory period (white "P" in black box). Therefore, the device effectively paces in the DVI mode. A, atrial pacing; black "P" on white background, atrial sensing; V, ventricular pacing.

on-reset, Table 5.2), or permanent damage to pacemaker or lead hardware. The potential risk of EMI depends on the indication for pacing: in permanent AV block III°, ventricular pacing inhibition due to EMI can be life threatening. Asynchronous stimulation (eg, VOO, DVI, or DOO mode) due to reprogramming (noise or magnet mode), inadequate atrial tracking, or inappropriate algorithm reaction may be symptomatic and may trigger atrial or ventricular arrhythmias.

Automatic Sensing Algorithms

In new pacemaker systems, automatic algorithms attempt to maintain a safety margin between the sensed atrial or ventricular signal amplitude and the programmed sensitivity threshold. Because the intrinsic signals may vary after implantation (chronic signal reduction, impact of exercise, heart rate increase, respiration, drugs, electrolytes, etc.), sensing may become less reliable with a fixed sensi-

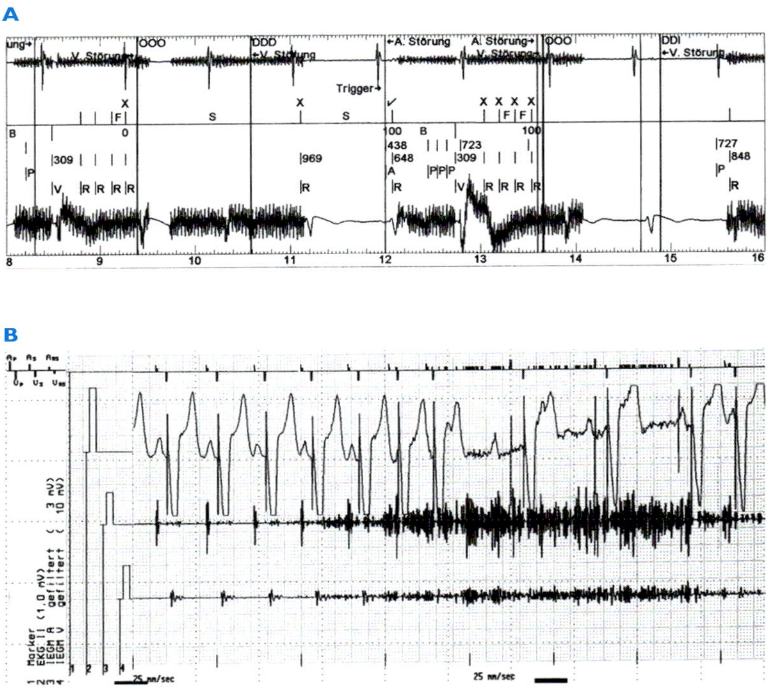

Fig 5.33 Noise reversion. **A**, ICD reverting from DDD to OOO mode in response to electromagnetic interference from a drilling machine. **B**, Myopotential oversensing in the atrium leading to noise reaction and DVI mode.

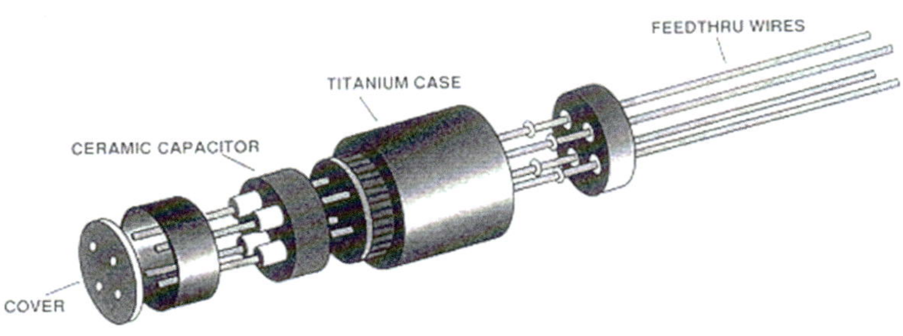

Fig. 5.34 Feed-through filter. This four-pole filter prevents electromagnetic noise from GSM mobile phones to enter the sensing circuit. (Reproduced with kind permission of St. Jude Medical, Inc.)

tivity threshold that is only adjusted every 12 months during an outpatient visit. Particularly during periods of paroxysmal atrial fibrillation, a temporary higher atrial sensitivity may improve continuous detection. Companies have different automatic sensing algorithms that are presented in the following. The term *automatic sensitivity adjustment* is used as a generic name and not as a specific algorithm of any company in this context.

Biotronik Automatic Sensitivity Adjustment

In devices by Biotronik (Berlin, Germany), automatic sensitivity adjustment algorithms start a Detection Blanking Time (DBT; atrium: 100 ms, ventricle: 120 ms) during which the maximum positive or negative peak amplitude is registered as soon as an intrinsic event is sensed (Fig 5.35). After expiration of this DBT period, the sensitivity threshold is set to 50% of the sensed signal amplitude for 80 ms (atrium) and 125 ms (ventricle). Thereafter, the sensitivity threshold is set to 25% of the sensed signal. If no intrinsic signals are sensed for 1 s, bipolar sensitivity is increased to its maximum (atrial 0.2 mV, ventricle 2.0 mV). This stepwise increase in sensitivity aims at preventing double sensing while maintaining sufficient reliability to sense the next intrinsic event, even if sensed amplitudes vary significantly. Return to maximum sensitivity is implemented particularly to avoid undersensing of atrial fibrillation.

After pacing, the atrial (ventricular) sensitivity threshold is reset for a period of 120 ms to 2 mV (ventricle: 200 ms at 5 mV), then to half of this initial value for 160 ms (atrium) and 250 ms (ventricle), thereafter to a quarter of the initial value for 80 ms (atrium) and 125 ms (ventricle), finally to its minimum (atrial bipolar 0.2 mV, ventricle 2.0 mV). The period of low sensitivity is longer after pacing compared to sensing to account for the delay between pacing and evoked potentials. In this algorithm, evoked signals should not be sensed because they would bias the sensed amplitude and in turn could influence sensitivity.

Boston Scientific Auto Sense

The Auto Sense algorithm automatically adjusts the atrial and/or ventricular sensitivity threshold to a percentage of the amplitude of the last sensed event. The sensitivity threshold is updated beat to beat. Sensitivity threshold settings depend on the preceding cardiac event (pacing or sensing) and the presence of myopotential or environmental noise (Fig 5.36).

If the algorithm detects an intrinsic event, it adjusts the sensing threshold on the basis of a smoothed average of the preceding intrinsic events. If the underlying rhythm is paced, the algorithm slowly increases the sensitivity, becoming more sensitive each cycle until a maximum is reached (0.25 mV in the atrium, 1.5 mV in the ventricle).

For ventricular sensing, the sensitivity is adjusted in multiple steps. First, the device establishes an average intrinsic R-wave amplitude based on previously sensed events. This average accounts for 75% of the smoothed average intrinsic R-wave amplitude. Secondly, sensing of an intrinsic R-wave accounts for 25% of the smoothed intrinsic average, and both values together establish the current smoothed average R-wave amplitude. Thirdly, baseline noise is measured during the last 50 ms of the ventricular refractory period of each cycle. The ventricular sensitivity threshold (range is 1.5–6.0 mV) is automatically adjusted to one third of the difference between the smoothed average R wave and the measured baseline noise. The maximum sensed R-wave amplitude is limited to 9 mV. For example, if an R wave of 8 mV and a noise level (T wave or other) of 2 mV during the terminal ventricular refractory period are detected, the difference is 8 – 2 = 6 mV, and sensitivity threshold is set to one third of 6 mV, that is, 2 mV.

In the atrium, the Auto Sense algorithm adjusts the sensitivity level to half of the difference between P-wave amplitude and baseline noise. Similar to ventricular measurements, previously measured atrial events account for 75%, an intrinsic P wave sensed immediately before the respective cycle for 25% of the smoothed

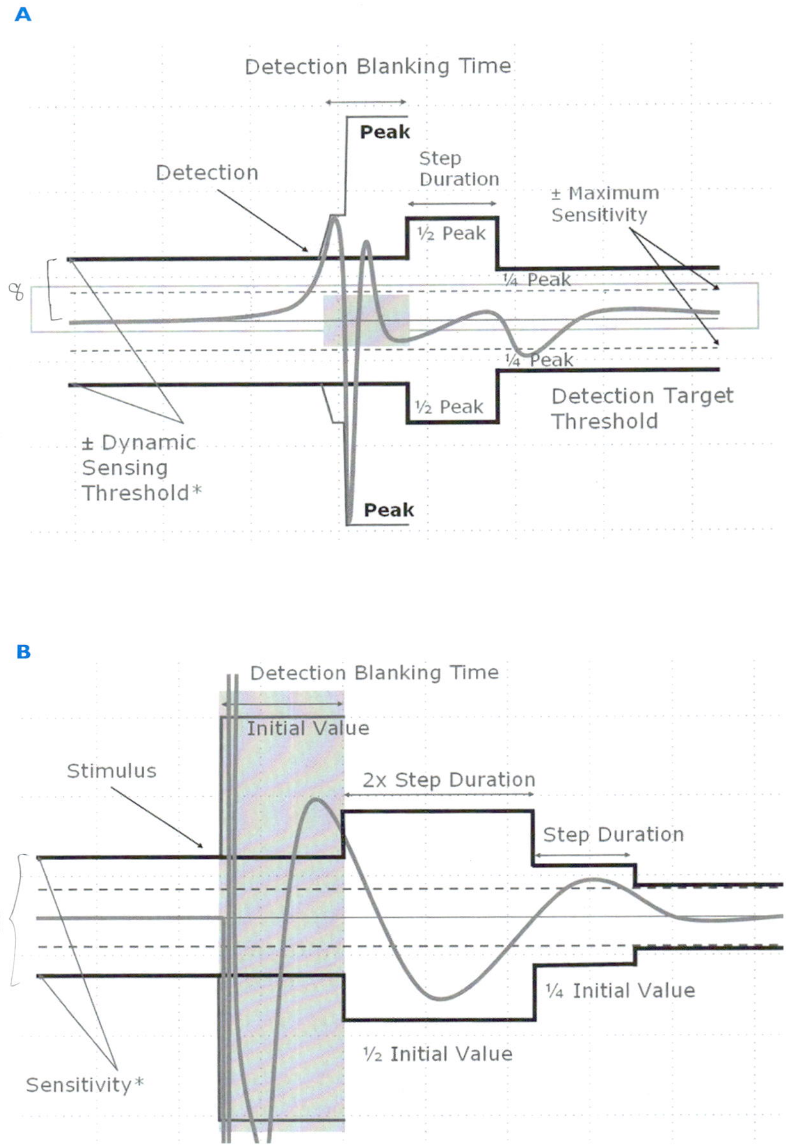

Fig 5.35 Automatic sensing in Biotronik devices. **A**: Sensing of an intrinsic event triggers a "Detection Blanking Time" (DBT; atrium: 100 ms, ventricle: 120 ms) during which only the peak-to-peak amplitude is considered. After expiration of this period, a "Step Duration" of 80 ms (atrium) or 125 ms (ventricle) provides a sensitivity threshold of 50% of the sensed signal amplitude. After this period, sensitivity threshold is set to 25% of the sensed signal. If no intrinsic signals are sensed for 1 s, sensitivity is increased to its maximum (atrial bipolar 0.2 mV, ventricle 2.0 mV). **B**: After pacing, the atrial and ventricular sensitivity threshold is reset during a DBT of 120 ms (atrium) and 200 ms (ventricle) to an initial value of 2 respective of 5 mV. After expiration of the DBT, the sensitivity is set to half of the initial value for twice the step duration (atrium: 2 × 80 ms, ventricle 2 × 125 ms), after expiration of this period to a quarter of the initial value for one step duration, then to its maximum (atrial bipolar 0.2 mV, ventricle 2.0 mV). *Calculated from the preceding sensed event. (Reproduced with kind permission of Biotronik.)

intrinsic average. The device limits the maximum measured noise level to 1.75 mV. The atrial sensitivity range is 0.25 to 3.5 mV, sensing of P-wave amplitudes is limited to 4 mV.

Medtronic Sensing Assurance

The Sensing Assurance algorithm in devices by Medtronic, Inc. automatically adjusts atrial and ventricular sensitivity within defined limits to maintain an optimal sensing safety margin (Fig 5.37). The amplitude of each atrial or ventricular event sensed outside a refractory period is compared to the current sensitivity threshold. The latter is then eventually reset to achieve preset target sensing margins. The sensed P-wave amplitude should be equal to 4 to 5.6 times the programmed bipolar atrial sensitivity (2.8 to 4 times in unipolar atrial sensing). The sensed R-wave amplitude should be equal to 2.8 to 4 times the ventricular sensitivity threshold. Events sensed within a refractory period, premature beats, continuous interference, etc. are excluded, all other sensed events are used to calculate a running average. Sensed events falling below the target sensing margin (low events) are assigned a negative value, and those sensed above the target sensing margin (high events) are assigned a positive value. When the accumulated value of the events exceeds the upper or lower limits of a counter, the pacemaker adjusts the sensitivity threshold. Adjustment to a more sensitive threshold if 17 low amplitudes are detected, adjustment to a less sensitive threshold if 36 high amplitudes are detected.

Sensitivity adjustment is more gradual if low and high events occur together or if there is intermittent pacing. If < 60% of events are large (or small), or if the pacing-to-sensing ratio is

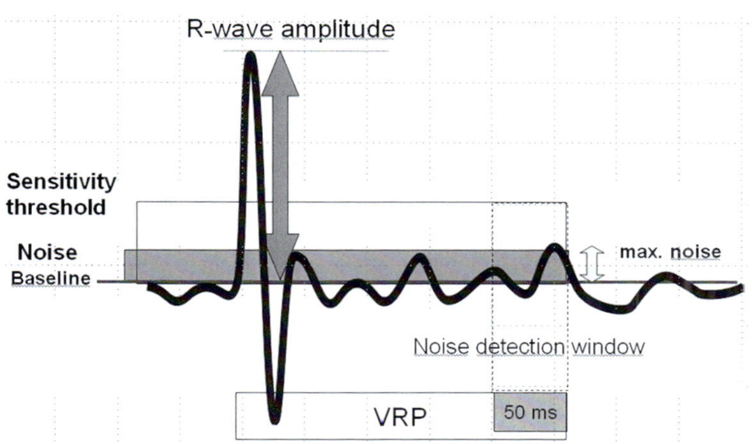

Fig 5.36 Autosensing in Boston Scientific systems. VRP, ventricular refractory period. (Reproduced with kind permission of Boston Scientific Corp.)

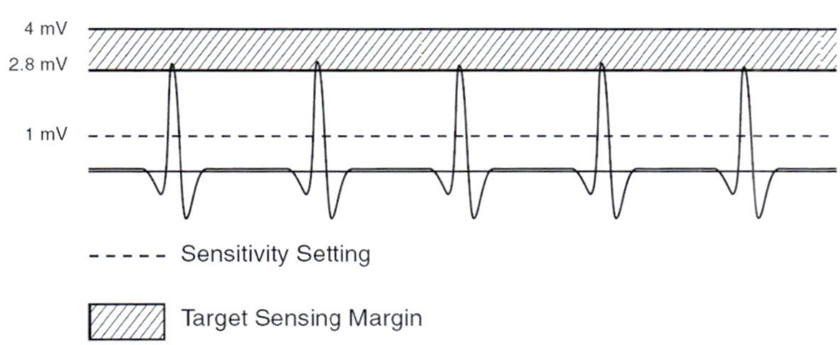

Fig 5.37 Sensing Assurance. In order to maintain a safety margin of 3:1, all sensed events below a preset value will increase the "low amplitude" counter by 1. If this counter reaches a value of 17, sensitivity will be automatically increased. (Reproduced with kind permission of Medtronic, Inc.)

> 5:1, no sensitivity adjustment is performed. Pacemaker-defined premature ventricular complexes (PVCs) will cause ventricular sensitivity adjustments that are slower than those for non-PVC, nonrefractory senses. During periods when the pacing percentage is near 100%, the pacemaker adjusts the sensitivity threshold toward the long-term average. Also if persistent undersensing or persistent noise reversion pacing (due to continuous interference, see earlier) occurs, sensitivity threshold is adjusted toward the long-term average. In the VDD mode, sensitivity is increased if no atrial sensing is present for several pacing cycles.

While the Sensing Assurance algorithm is active, the sensitivity settings have to be programmed in a prespecified range (atrial 0.18–0.5 mV, ventricle 2.0–5.6 mV) and ventricular safety pacing (VSP) must be activated.

Data on automatic sensitivity threshold adjustments are collected by the memory function of the devices and the minimum and maximum sensitivity setting is recorded for periods of 7 days.

Medtronic Automatic Sensitivity Adjustment

Similar to implantable defibrillators, the EnRhythm pacemaker automatically adjusts atrial and ventricular sensitivity thresholds following sensed and paced events to reduce the incidence of far-field R-wave oversensing in the atrium and T-wave oversensing in the ventricle, at the same time maintaining a very high maximum sensitivity.

In this algorithm, sensitivity threshold decays exponentially to its programmed settings during one cardiac cycle, beginning at the electrogram peak or at the end of the blanking period (Fig 5.38, Table 5.4). Thus, two thirds of the cardiac cycle provide sensing at the maximum sensitivity whereas periods with high probability of oversensing (eg, after a ventricular event in the atrium) have a sensitivity threshold up to eight times the maximum sensitivity.

St. Jude Medical SenseAbility

Similar to the automatic sensitivity adjustment algorithm in Medtronic EnRhythm devices, the SenseAbility algorithm by St. Jude Medical (Sylmar, CA) offers sensitivity adjustment within a cardiac cycle with the key parameters initial threshold, decay (± delay), maximum sensitivity, and refractory periods. SenseAbility uses the filtered, digitally rectified signal (Fig 5.5B).

Devices reset the sensitivity threshold at each cardiac cycle with a "threshold start" after an atrial or ventricular sensed or paced

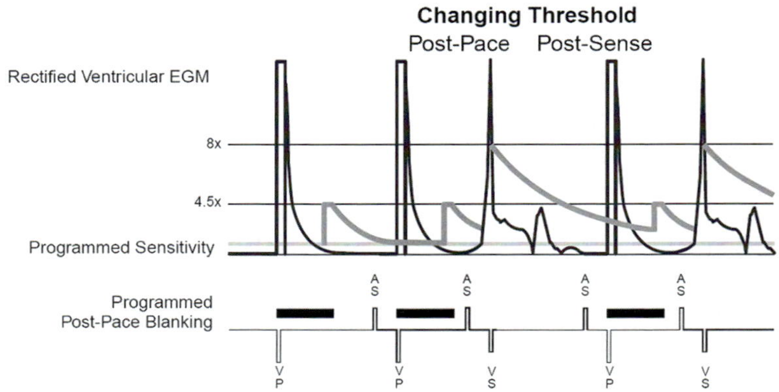

Fig 5.38 Automatic sensitivity adjustment. In Medtronic EnRhythm devices, the atrial and ventricular sensitivity changes after paced and sensed events up to a maximum threshold value that decays toward the (minimum) programmed sensitivity threshold. AS, Atrial sensed; VP, ventricular paced, VS, ventricular sensed. (Reproduced with kind permission of Medtronic, Inc.)

A

Adjustment of Atrial Sensitivity			
Preceding Event	Adjustment*	Duration	Decay Constant
Atrial sensed event	75% of EGM peak*	10 ms	100 ms
Atrial paced event	Minimum adjusted value	10 ms	100 ms
Ventricular event preceded by atrial sensed event	75% of EGM peak*	120 ms	100 ms
Ventricular event not preceded by atrial sensed event	Minimum adjusted value	120 ms	100 ms
Adjustment of Ventricular Sensitivity			
Preceding Event	Adjustment*	Duration	Decay Constant
Atrial sensed event	As programmed	Perpetual	None
Atrial paced event	As programmed	Perpetual	None
Ventricular sensed event	75% of EGM peak*	None	450 ms
Ventricular paced event	4.5 times programmed value*	None	450 ms

B

Programmed atrial sensitivity	0.15 mV	0.3 mV	0.45 mV	0.6– .5 mV	2.1 mV
Minimum adjusted threshold	0.9 mV	1.2 mV	1.35 mV	1.8 mV	2.1 mV

Table 5.4 Automatic Sensitivity Adjustment in Medtronic EnRhythm Pacemaker Systems. **A**: Atrial and ventricular sensitivity adjustment. **B**: Minimum adjusted atrial sensitivity thresholds.

*Sensitivity threshold limits are minimum programmed value response eight times the programmed value.

event (Fig 5.39). This initial sensitivity threshold is a programmable percentage of the peak amplitude (nominally set to 62.5%). The peak amplitude is the maximum amplitude detected during a "sensed refractory period" which has a programmable duration (93, 125, or 157 ms in the atrium, 125 or 157 ms in the ventricle). The value of the peak amplitude is stored and used for the next "threshold start." After "threshold start," the sensitivity threshold linearly decreases (Fig 5.39). There is a programmable "decay delay" that delays the time before the linear decay occurs. The sensitivity threshold decreases until the programmable maximum sensitivity is reached or until the next event is sensed.

This algorithm attempts to avoid oversensing even if a high sensitivity is programmed to avoid undersensing. It is programmable in several different ways whenever oversensing occurs, such as increase of the initial sensitivity threshold or activation of a delay before the sensitivity threshold decreases. If undersensing occurs, opposite programming (decrease of the initial sensitivity threshold, deactivation of a decay delay) is possible. There is also the option of an automatic post-pacing decay delay in patients with high heart rates or a high percentage of (sensor-driven) pacing.

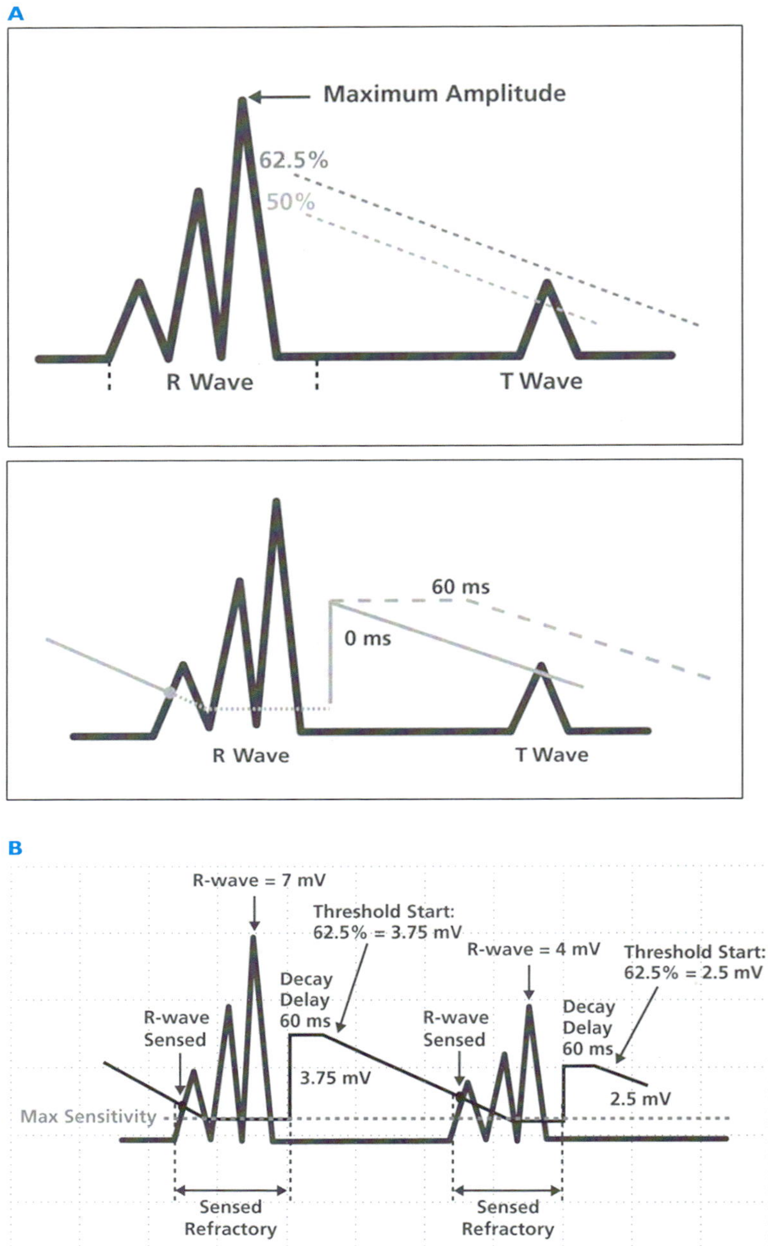

Fig. 5.39 SenseAbility automatic algorithm performance. **A**: Possibilities to prevent T-wave oversensing (or far-field R wave oversensing) by reprogramming the initial sensitivity threshold from 50% of the sensed signal amplitude to 62.5% (upper panel) or programming a decay delay of 60 ms (lower panel). **B**: Algorithm performance during 2 sensed ventricular cycles. (Reproduced with kind permission of St. Jude Medical, Inc.)

References

1. Lau C, Cameron DA, Nishimura SC, et al. A cardiac evoked response algorithm providing threshold tracking: a North American multicenter study. Clinical Investigators of the Microny-Regency Clinical Evaluation Study. *Pacing Clin Electrophysiol.* 2000;23:953–959.
2. Barold SS, Israel CW, Herweg B. Mode switching of dual chamber pacemakers from activation of a blanked flutter search algorithm by a single atrial event. *Pacing Clin Electrophysiol.* 2005;28:917–920.
3. Israel CW, Neubauer H, Olbrich HG, et al. Incidence of atrial tachyarrhythmias in pacemaker patients: Results from the Balanced Evaluation of Atrial Tachyarrhythmias in Stimulated patients (BEATS) study. *Pacing Clin Electrophysiol.* 2006;29:582–588.
4. De Groot JR, Schroeder-Tanka JM, Visser J, Willems AR, De Voogt WG. Clinical results of far-field R-wave reduction with a short tip-ring electrode. *Pacing Clin Electrophysiol.* 2008;31:1554–1559.
5. Kolb C, Wille B, Maurer D, et al. Management of far-field R wave sensing for the avoidance of inappropriate mode switch in dual chamber pacemakers: results of the FFS-test study. *J Cardiovasc Electrophysiol.* 2006;17:992–997.
6. Pinski SL, Trohman RG. Interference in implanted cardiac devices, Part I. *Pacing Clin Electrophysiol.* 2002;25:1367–1381.
7. Pinski SL, Trohman RG. Interference in implanted cardiac devices, part II. *Pacing Clin Electrophysiol.* 2002;25:1496–1509.

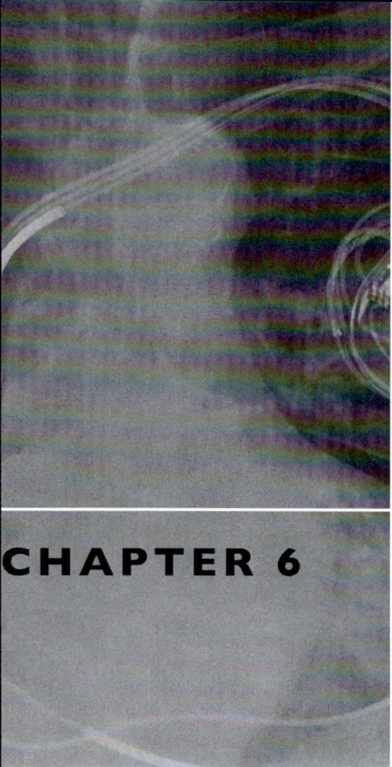

Pacemakers and Atrial Arrhythmias

Detection and Treatment

CHAPTER 6

David S. Kwon and Byron K. Lee

Introduction

Atrial arrhythmias have the potential to cause changes in heart rate that may result in significant symptoms for patients. Older-generation pacemakers were not adept at detecting these atrial arrhythmias and would often exacerbate the swings in heart rate. Fortunately, modern pacemakers have a multitude of features with which they may approach atrial arrhythmias. These improved devices aid the clinician in detecting atrial arrhythmias and provide useful information to help diagnose the type of atrial arrhythmia. Furthermore, newer pacemakers have features that maintain physiologic heart rates when atrial arrhythmias occur, thus protecting patients from potentially disturbing heart rate changes.

This chapter focuses on how pacemakers manage atrial arrhythmias, including the detection and treatment options for these arrhythmias. Significant beneficial features of specific pacemakers will also be discussed. The basics of pacemaker design and function, including pacing and sensing algorithms, have been discussed in previous chapters and will not be reviewed except where directly relevant to atrial arrhythmia detection and treatment.

Atrial Arrhythmias Definition

There are several types of atrial arrhythmias that can disturb heart rate or trigger the pacemaker to pace abnormally fast. The more common of atrial arrhythmias are atrial tachycardia, atrial flutter, and atrial fibrillation, but the list of supraventricular tachycardias also includes reentrant arrhythmias, either within the AV node (AV Nodal Reentrant Tachycardia) or involving an extranodal circuit (Atrial Ventricular Reciprocating Tachycardia).

Pacemakers and Implantable Cardioverter Defibrillators: An Expert's Manual. © 2010 Amin Al-Ahmad, Kenneth A. Ellenbogen, Andrea Natale, and Paul J. Wang, eds. Cardiotext Publishing, ISBN: 978-0-9790164-6-2.

Initial Interrogation

Much information regarding atrial arrhythmias may be gleaned from the basic device interrogation report. For patients in normal sinus rhythm, atrial heart rate histograms should display a smooth distribution of heart rates, reflecting normal cardiovascular physiology. Patients with atrial tachyarrhythmias, such as atrial flutter, may have a histogram that reveals a period of rapid heart rate at a distinct AA interval. If several distinct atrial rates are seen, the patient may have more than one type of atrial tachyarrhythmia. Alternatively, if patients have periods of high atrial rates with scattered AA intervals, paroxysmal atrial fibrillation is likely (see Fig 6.1).

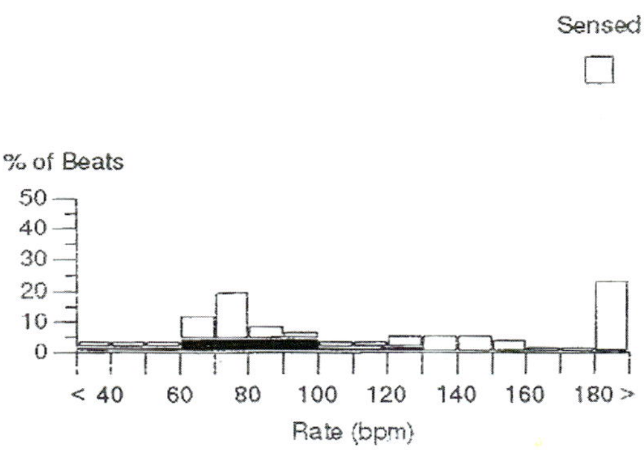

Fig 6.1 Atrial rate histogram. PPM interrogation reveals varied atrial high rates, suggestive of atrial arrhythmia.

As expected, single chamber devices (ventricular only) are more limited in their ability to diagnose and treat atrial arrhythmias. Nevertheless, careful interpretation can still yield much information. For example, intermittent episodes of high ventricular rates that are irregularly irregular are strongly supportive of paroxysmal atrial fibrillation. Polymorphic ventricular tachycardia or ventricular fibrillation can also cause irregularly irregular ventricular rates and could be confused with atrial fibrillation. However, polymorphic ventricular tachycardia and ventricular fibrillation are much rarer and are usually accompanied by a distinctly ominous clinical scenario.

Another critical piece of information gained from the initial interrogation is the time spent in atrial tachyarrhythmia or atrial fibrillation, referred to as the AT/AF burden (see Fig 6.2). This diagnostic parameter reveals the amount of time the patient has an atrial rate above a predefined threshold, usually set around 180 bpm. Be aware that for young patients, sinus rhythm may easily reach this threshold rate. Therefore, the AT/AF burden reading will be misleading for these patients and the rate cutoff should be increased.

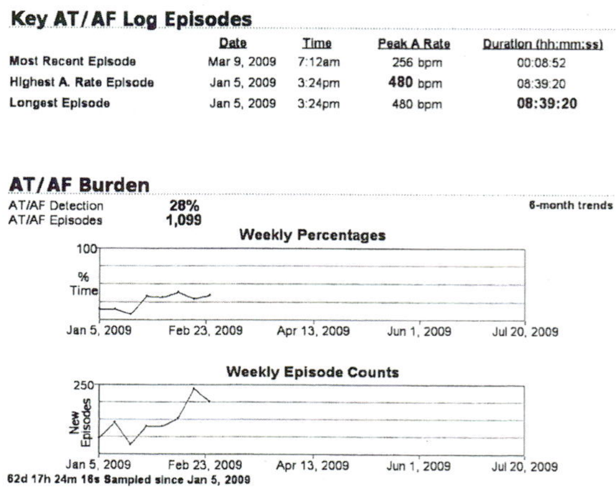

Fig 6.2 AT/AF burden reveals the number of atrial arrhythmia episodes and the time spent in atrial arrhythmia.

Basic Arrhythmia Counting Features

As mentioned, the AT/AF burden is defined by programmed rate cutoffs, or detection intervals. However, for correct counting, the device must detect atrial depolarization accurately. Thus, the sensitivity feature may need to be adjusted depending on the P-wave measurement and on a given arrhythmia for which detection is desired. For example, the atrial sensitivity setting (mV) may need to be lowered to fully detect all fibrillation waves if they are of low amplitude, thus allowing for proper mode switching (discussed later). However, caution must be taken when adjusting atrial sensitivity in order to prevent far-field R-wave or T-wave sensing. Although there are other programming methods to distinguish such confounding electrical signals, attention must be given to each specific patient's programming in order to achieve the highest specificity and sensitivity of detection.

Clinicians should realize that individual devices may offer some unique programmable parameters that are seldom adjusted but which may be useful for particular patients. For example, a parameter that may be programmed is the number of ventricular beats required to initiate atrial tachyarrhythmia detection algorithms and also the number of ventricular beats required to redetect after therapy is given for an atrial arrhythmia. Once the minimum detection protocol has been triggered, the pacemaker will scan within each V-V interval for any and all atrial signals to determine the appropriate response. Each specific pacemaker may also have secondary criteria that must be met before therapy is delivered. For example, an AV conduction ratio ≥ 2:1 may be required. Another potential secondary criterion is for an episode duration of < 48 hours. Consequently, the multitude of detection features allows the clinician to tailor therapy for each patient's particular needs.

The pacemaker's response to an atrial arrhythmia may be initiated at any point once the arrhythmia has been detected. The extent of a particular episode and the cumulative duration of all episodes are recorded by the pacemaker and are simply reflected by the duration of AT/AF as a percentage of time. Accurately understanding the burden of atrial arrhythmias may be essential in determining diagnosis and treatment plans for the patient.

Automatic Mode Switching

For atrial arrhythmias that meet the AT/AF cutoffs, automatic mode switching (AMS) is the usual device response (see Fig 6.3). The change of programming mode allows for more organized ventricular pacing in a non-tracking mode (eg, VVI or DDI). While mode switched, the pacemaker is constantly scanning atrial electrograms to see whether the atrial arrhythmia has terminated. Once termination is detected by the device, the pacemaker switches back to its original pacing mode.

Some pacemakers are programmed to perform atrial overdrive pacing following a return to the original pacing mode after a mode switch event. The rate of overdrive pacing may be equal to the lower rate limit or faster and has been proposed as a method to prevent arrhythmia recurrence in the immediate postarrhythmia period. Maximizing atrial pacing may result in electrical concordance in the atrium and, thus,

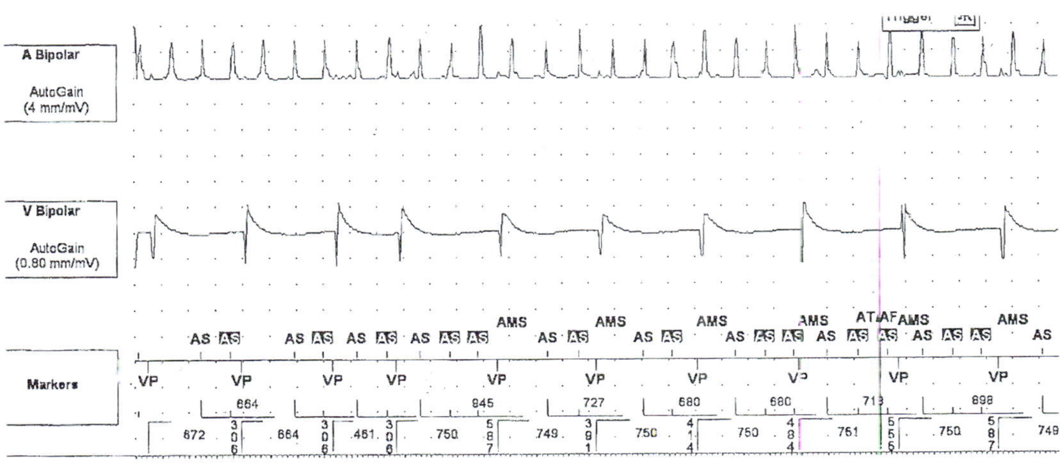

Fig 6.3 Automatic mode switch. Atrial arrhythmia detection results in automatic mode switching to a VVI nontracking pacing mode.

reduce episodes of atrial arrhythmia; however, studies have revealed mixed benefit of atrial pacing for the suppression of atrial arrhythmias. Several of these studies are highlighted later in *Atrial Arrhythmia Prevention*.

Difference between AT and AF

Although pacemakers tend to group all atrial tachyarrhythmias including atrial fibrillation together as AT/AF events, it can be clinically very important to distinguish between the types of atrial tachyarrhythmia. If the patient is having atrial fibrillation or atrial flutter, anticoagulation or antiplatelet agents may be necessary. The detection AA intervals may be helpful because atrial fibrillation and atrial flutter usually have much faster atrial rates and, thereby, shorter AA intervals. However, there is some overlap of these intervals, accounting for coarse atrial fibrillation or slower atrial flutter and the occasional other atrial tachyarrhythmia with high atrial rates. Atrial signals falling within either of these regions may be further distinguished by the regularity of atrial signals; irregularly irregular electrograms are more consistent with atrial fibrillation. The rapid atrial arrhythmias with a more regular atrial electrogram are unlikely to be atrial fibrillation. The mechanism of the atrial tachyarrhythmia may be revealed by close examination of the intracardiac electrograms, particularly with attention to the onset and termination.

In Fig 6.4, the intracardiac electrogram shows an A on V tachycardia with a cycle length (CL) of 355. Because the V-A time is < 70 ms, AV node reentrant tachycardia (AVRT) is ruled out. In AVRT, the V and A are sequential and, therefore, the V-A time should be > 70 ms. The tachycardia terminates with a premature atrial contraction (PAC) that does not advance the

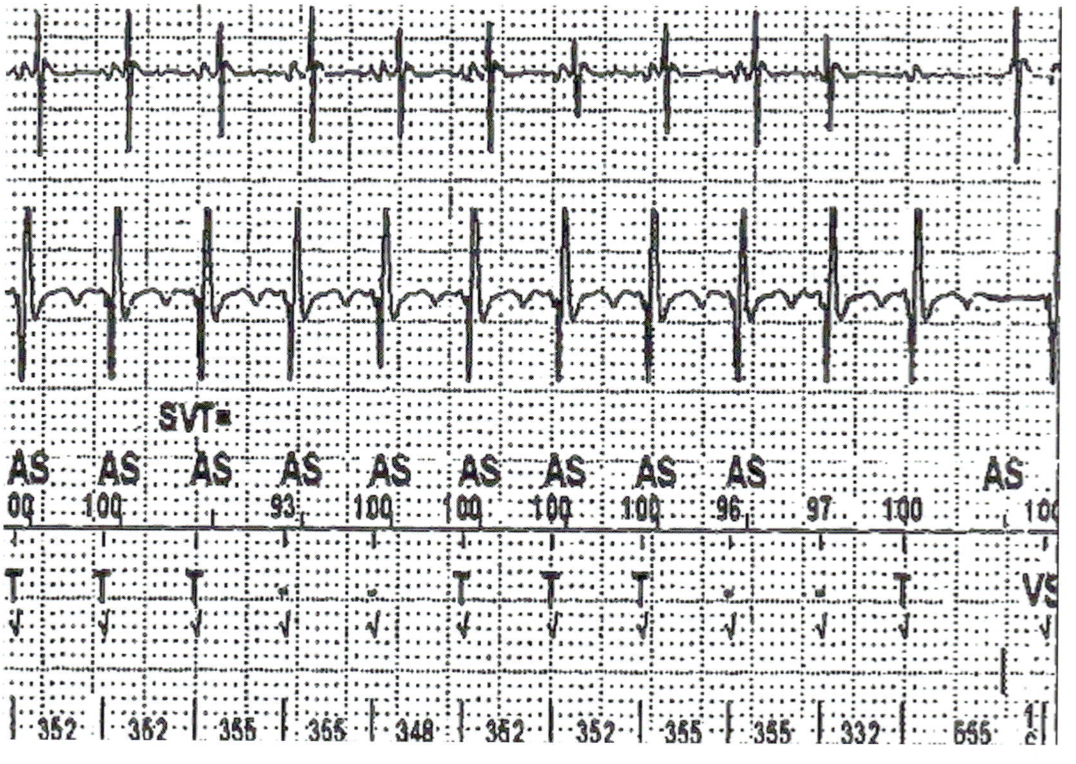

Fig 6.4 A on V tachycardia (AVNRT) terminates with a premature atrial contraction. The premature atrial contraction does not pull in the next V, strongly suggesting that the atrial arrhythmia is AVNRT.

next V. This fortuitous diagnostic event makes atrial tachycardia also unlikely because the next V would be expected to be early, unless the PAC happens to be delayed in the AV node by the exact amount of time that the PAC is early. This reasoning, similar to what occurs in a basic electrophysiology study for the diagnosis of supraventricular tachycardias, suggests that the atrial tachyarrhythmia is most likely AV nodal reentrant tachycardia (AVNRT). In AVNRT, a PAC frequently breaks the tachycardia without bringing in the next V, as was seen here. This patient subsequently had an electrophysiologic (EP) study where AVNRT was found and successfully ablated.

Atrial Arrhythmia Prevention

Concepts regarding cardiac pacing have been integral to an understanding of atrial arrhythmogenesis and treatment with pacemakers. Certainly, the majority of patients who require pacemakers, those with sinus node dysfunction or AV block, are generally older. Not only does this population have a higher risk of developing conduction system disease, but older patients also have a higher prevalence of atrial arrhythmias, notably atrial fibrillation. Studies by Andersen et al[5] and Lamas et al[6] revealed that pacing was associated with a lower incidence of atrial fibrillation. In fact, Andersen reported not only a benefit in reducing atrial fibrillation, but also a reduction in thromboembolic events and heart failure from their 8-year follow-up study. It is not entirely clear, however, whether the benefit in atrial fibrillation reduction with AAI or DDD pacing may be due to creating an electrical syncytium in the atrium or whether the detrimental effects of VVI pacing may manifest in the atrium as atrial fibrillation. Although larger studies supported this benefit for atrial fibrillation reduction (eg, CTOPP[7] and MOST[8]), other studies, in turn, such as by Gillis et al[9] have concluded no benefit from pacing. Interestingly, in follow up to the DAVID trial (Dual Chamber And VVI Implantable Defibrillator),[10] which demonstrated an increased hospitalization and mortality with DDDR pacing in heart failure compared to VVI back-up pacing, DAVID II[11] compared atrial pacing with ventricular back-up pacing and found no difference in the amount of atrial fibrillation between the two groups. Therefore, it is still unclear whether pacing truly reduces atrial fibrillation. It may be that the benefit is minimal and therefore, it could only be demonstrated in some trials.

There has also been some evidence that pacing the atria in more than one location simultaneously or pacing at the atrial septum can reduce atrial fibrillation. The Dual-Site Atrial Pacing to Prevent Atrial Fibrillation trial (DAP-PAF)[12] demonstrated that overdrive dual-site right atrial pacing (80 ppm) and overdrive high right atrial single-site pacing (80 ppm) were both able to extend the time to AF recurrence when compared to support pacing (DDI, VDI) at a low rate. However, event-free survival from AF tended to be longer with overdrive dual-site right atrial pacing compared to overdrive right atrial pacing. Furthermore, the Atrial Septal Pacing Clinical Efficacy trial (ASPECT)[13] evaluated atrial arrhythmia pacing prevention algorithms from a septal versus right atrial appendage pacing site. The trial's conclusion was that although atrial pacing prevention algorithms were able to decrease the burden of atrial premature beats, there was no significant benefit to overall AT/AF burden with septal pacing.

Another interesting trial, the Atrial Dynamic Overdrive Pacing Trial (ADOPT)[14] examined the St. Jude Medical AF Suppression Algorithm, which attempts to suppress atrial fibrillation by maintaining a paced rhythm in patients with sinus node dysfunction. The device will automatically increase the pacing rate when the native rhythm emerges and periodically reduce the rate to search for intrinsic atrial activity. This study showed a 25% reduction in AF burden (the percentage of days in which patient-activated recordings indicated AF). However, the absolute reductions in AF burden were minimal at best: only 1.2% at 1 month (3.2% vs. 4.4%) and 0.7% at 6 months (1.4% vs. 1.7%). Once again, these results are consistent with other reports indicating a marginal or no benefit of pace prevention algorithms.

Overall, incorporating atrial pace prevention programming to reduce AT/AF burden has had limited benefit in larger studies; however, as has been stressed earlier, each patient's particular arrhythmia characteristics must be considered. Pacing algorithms for arrhythmia prevention may be more beneficial in subsets of patients, which are yet to be clearly defined. Also, the benefit of a pacemaker extends beyond pacing alone, as medical therapy may be more effectively titrated with the safety of backup pacing.

Atrial Arrhythmia Treatment with Anti-Tachycardia Pacing (ATP)

Analogous to ventricular anti-tachycardia pacing (ATP), atrial ATP is another option for treatment of atrial arrhythmias. Atrial ATP pacemakers and defibrillators had been removed from the U.S. market previously due to concerns that the device could inadvertently trigger dangerous ventricular tachyarrhythmias; however, with more sophisticated detection and treatment algorithms, they have returned to the arsenal of atrial arrhythmia therapy. Most programming features common to ventricular algorithms are also available for atrial ATP. Specifically, these programmable options include burst therapy, ramp therapy, amplitude and pulse width of each atrial paced beat, and the number and sequence of treatment episodes. Typically, a ventricular backup pacing mode is available but its use depends on individual programming. Atrial ATP is given in an asynchronous mode, AOO, and may be highly effective in terminating atrial arrhythmias.

Much of the investigation into atrial ATP has centered on atrial tachycardia, as this rhythm may precede and, thereby, cause degeneration to AF. Gillis et al[15] distinguished AT/AF episode frequency versus burden by revealing that although patients may not have a decrease in the frequency of atrial arrhythmia episodes, the duration of these episodes may decrease with successful ATP therapy. Thus, clinical benefit may be accomplished by reducing the number of episodes or the overall duration of episodes.

Not all studies have been convincingly supportive of atrial ATP use. Lee et al[16] reported no reduction in either AT/AF burden or frequency with pace prevention and termination therapies for atrial arrhythmias when compared to conventional pacing. However, they admitted that their prospective randomized study of 3 months' follow-up may not have permitted sufficient time for a difference to manifest. More recently in the Prevention Or Termination trial (POT),[17] neither atrial fibrillation burden nor frequency was reduced when atrial ATP therapy was added to a preventive pacing algorithm (PPA).

A word of caution must be given for atrial ATP therapies. Prior to testing and programming atrial ATP, the atrial lead must be relatively secure. If the atrial lead drops into the ventricle, there is potential to induce ventricular tachyarrhythmias with extremely rapid pacing. Therefore, the atrial lead should be allowed to mature before therapy is programmed, generally at least 1 month after implantation. Furthermore, another potential issue is that the placement of the atrial lead tip may not be optimal for atrial ATP, such as atrial lead tip placement in the lower atrium with output that can be sensed on the ventricular lead, otherwise known as crosstalk. For pacemakers, crosstalk will be noted as ventricular high rate episodes or ventricular bigeminy, depending on the heart rate. However, a potentially harmful situation may occur in defibrillators, as crosstalk may result in ventricular high rates that fall into one of the defibrillator's tachyarrhythmia therapy zones and result in inappropriate ventricular ATP or defibrillation therapy. Alternatively, ventricular sensing of atrial depolarizations may inappropriately inhibit ventricular pacing function. The disastrous potential in a patient with AV block is evident.

Thus, from multiple studies, it is observed that, overall, pace prevention and treatment strategies have inconsistent benefits on atrial arrhythmia reduction, with regard to burden of arrhythmia and symptoms. But as varied as are atrial arrhythmias for patients, therapy must be individualized for each patient's needs and therapeutic responses. Potentially, there are some patients who derive more benefit than others with these pacing therapies. The astute clinician should be familiar with these advanced device options in order to help the occasional patients with difficult to treat atrial arrhythmias.

Atrial Defibrillation

The ultimate atrial arrhythmia therapy is cardioversion back to the normal sinus rhythm. There are ICDs that were designed to shock patients with atrial tachyarrhythmias as well as ventricular tachyarrhythmias. With the Medtronic Jewel AF ICD, Friedman et al[18] described a reduction in AT/AF burden with atrial defibrillation therapy. Similarly, approved in 2001, the Medtronic GEM III AT ICD system offers atrial defibrillation therapy in addition to standard ATP and preventive pacing algorithm. Wellens et al[19] nicely demonstrated that an "Atrioverter" was specific and effective treatment for atrial fibrillation. However, in that 1998 study of 51 patients with drug refractory recurrent AF, a notable complication of the atrial defibrillation devices was atrial perforation by the atrial defibrillation lead, likely due to increased weight and stiffness. In the future, with advances in lead technology, such complications may be reduced.

Rate Smoothing Therapy

Rate smoothing is yet another feature of pacemakers that may be beneficial in the setting of atrial tachyarrhythmias. This feature attempts to modulate the pacemaker's response to abrupt changes in heart rate due to atrial or ventricular arrhythmias, including single premature beats. Rate-smoothing algorithms attempt to minimize the symptoms associated with these types of arrhythmias, and programming operates between the lower rate limit and the maximum track rate, expressed as a percentage change from the applicable preceding RR interval. Synchronization between atrial and ventricular chambers then depends on the programmed AV delay time. In the rate responsive mode, rate smoothing will be bound by the maximum sinus rate or the maximum tracking rate, whereas in the non-rate responsive mode, the upper limit of rate smoothing is determined by the maximum tracking rate alone.

Rate Drop Response

Another feature of modern dual chamber pacemakers is the Rate Drop Response. The clinical usefulness of this pacing feature is most clearly demonstrated in the situation of vasovagal syncope. It is rapid backup pacing in order to prevent the symptoms associated with prolonged episodes of excess vagal stimulation or any other circumstance in which a patient may experience an occasional significant fall in heart rate. The rate of heart rate decline that triggers the rate drop response is programmable. Once triggered, pacing ensues at an elevated rate and will be provided for a programmed duration. As the programmed pacing duration expires, the pacemaker will gradually reduce the pacing rate until either an intrinsic rate is detected or until the lower rate limit is reached. Alternatively, during the elevated pacing period, should the pacemaker sense several consecutive intrinsic atrial events, the intervention period is then terminated. Rate drop response therapy may be programmed in the DDI mode when AV conduction is competent or in the DDD mode for those patients with partial or complete AV block. In 2002, Kapoor[20–22] summarized the benefit of such rate drop response treatment methods for syncope, reporting an 85% relative risk reduction for recurrent syncope. Unfortunately, when the rate drop response feature is active, mode switch response, rate adaptive and sensor varying PVARP, and atrial preference pacing are not possible.

PVAB and PVARP

It is important to remember that the detection and treatment algorithms for atrial arrhythmias depend critically on the postventricular atrial blanking period (PVAB) and the postventricular atrial refractory period (PVARP). These intervals are integral to the pacemaker's ability to accurately detect the atrial arrhythmias. A simple example occurs in atrial flutter, in which timing intervals may mask the arrhythmia (see Fig 6.5). The first critical timing period is the postventricular atrial blanking period (PVAB). The PVAB is essentially a null period in which any signals on the atrial channel are not counted and do not result in a corresponding ventricular response. Therefore, if some of the atrial signals land in the PVAB interval, they will be missed and the device may not detect that the patient is in an atrial arrhythmia.[23] The postventricular atrial refractory period (PVARP) is similar to the PVAB, but longer, and represents atrial refractoriness during which an extra atrial signal will be counted toward arrhythmia diagnosis, but not tracked by the ventricle. The PVARP encompasses the PVAB period and, when added to the AV interval, comprises the total atrial refractory period (TARP), which thereby determines the upper rate limit (URL). For patients with known atrial arrhythmias, sometimes the PVAB and the PVARP can be programmed specifically to avoid missing any true atrial signals.

PVAB Excludes Confounders

The "blinding" of the device to atrial signals during the PVAB period serves a critical purpose. The PVAB prevents the device from sensing confounding signals such as far-field sensing of R waves, retrograde P waves, or even electrical noise. Notably, electrical noise generally occurs at a different frequency such that noise reduction algorithms effectively distinguish this potential confounder. It is often the PVAB that prevents far-field R-wave sensing and retrograde P waves from inappropriately signaling the device to mode switch and initiate atrial arrhythmia therapy.

Atrial Arrhythmias within PVARP

Signals that fall within the remaining PVARP are generally not tracked but may be counted in the pacemaker's mode switching algorithm for AT/AF, thus allowing for automatic mode switching. The Guidant Pulsar pacemakers

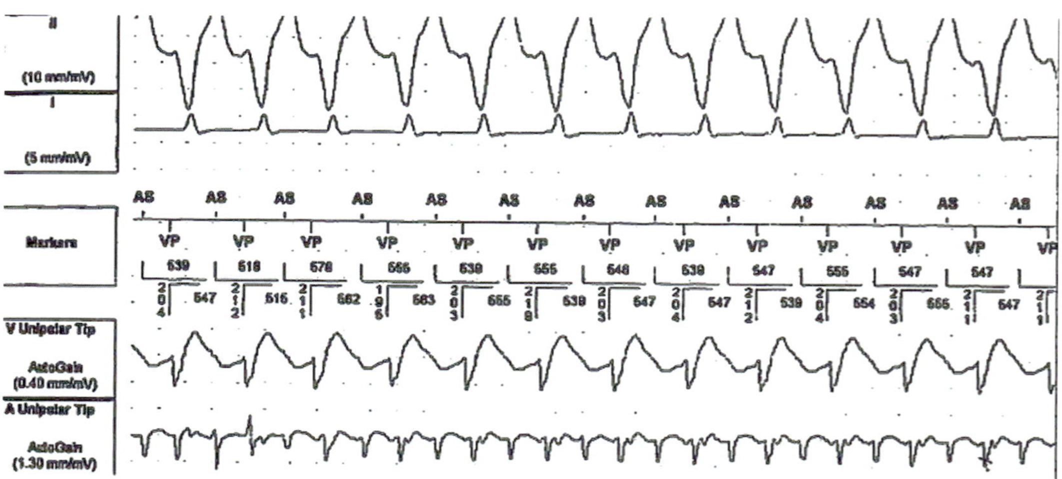

Fig 6.5 Intracardiac atrial flutter. Example of 2:1 atrial flutter that is not detected by the PPM because every other flutter wave falls within the postventricular atrial blanking period (PVAB).

detect atrial arrhythmias by Atrial Flutter Response (AFR) programming. An atrial event within the PVARP initiates a secondary timing cycle (AFR window), in which additional atrial events are not tracked but which trigger subsequent AFR windows. If the detected atrial activity is faster than the programmed AT/AF cutoff rate, mode switching is triggered, and the ventricle will pace at the lower rate limit or the sensor-indicated rate. Should an atrial-pacing event have been deferred due to the PVARP and AFR windows, a paced atrial event may then occur once all the windows have expired and as long as it is consistent with the AV delay and the lower rate limit.

In contrast, the Medtronic Kappa system operates with a Blanked Flutter Search algorithm. Eight consecutive atrial events must have a cycle length less than twice the sum of the PVAB and the AV Delay (AVD). In addition, twice the sensed atrial rate must be greater than the programmed tachycardia detection rate. When these conditions are fulfilled, the pacemaker will automatically extend the PVARP for one beat and calculate the atrial rate. If the atrial rate is greater than the tachycardia detection rate, mode switching will be triggered.

Of course, these two detection systems are not infallible and have their respective limitations. The Guidant Pulsar AFR system depends on atrial-sensed events within the PVARP. Should events fall into the PVAB interval, the AFR windows will not be triggered. A limitation of the Medtronic Kappa Blanked Flutter Search occurs in sinus tachycardia. As the device scans and counts atrial events, periodically a ventricular-paced event will be missed. Alternatively, inappropriate mode switching may be triggered with an inopportune premature atrial beat that occurs within the extended PVARP.

Summary

Effectively discriminating atrial tachyarrhythmias will ultimately lead to more appropriate patient treatment. Modern pacemakers have straightforward algorithms to accurately detect atrial tachyarrhythmias, primarily based on atrial rate and regularity. Treatment options attempt to protect the patient from rapid arrhythmias typically by changing the pacing mode. In large measure, these features for detection and therapy are beneficial and can work automatically. However, the clinician must be properly trained at interpreting the information derived from the device in order to dictate the best overall therapeutic course, including the initiation of anticoagulation, further programming modifications, or even referral for catheter ablation of arrhythmia. We must reiterate and emphasize the usefulness of the initial interrogation report and how careful interpretation may guide programming optimization.

References

1. Ellenbogen KA, Wood MA, eds. Cardiac Pacing and ICDs. 5th Ed. Williston: Blackwell Publishing, 2008.
2. *The Boston Scientific CRM Compass, Technical Guide to Boston Scientific Cardiac Rhythm Management Products*. St Paul: Boston Scientific Corp, 2007.
3. *Medtronic AT500 DDDRP Pacing System Reference Guide*. Minneapolis: Medtronic, Inc., 2000.
4. *Merlin Patient Care System*. St. Jude Medical Cardiac Rhythm Management Division. Minneapolis: St. Jude Medical, Inc., 2007.
5. Andersen HR, Nielsen JC, Thomsen PE, et al. Long-term follow-up of patients from a randomized trial of atrial versus ventricular pacing for sick-sinus syndrome. *Lancet* 1997;350:1210–1216.
6. Lamas GA, Orav EJ, Stambler BS, et al. Quality of life and clinical outcomes in elderly patients treated with ventricular pacing as compared with dual-chamber pacing. Pacemaker Selection in the Elderly Investigators. *N Engl J Med.* 1998;338:1097–1104.
7. Connolly SJ, Kerr CR, Gent M, et al. Effects of physiologic pacing versus ventricular pacing on the risk of stroke and death due to cardiovascular causes. Canadian Trial of Physiologic Pacing Investigators. *N Engl J Med.* 342:1385–1391.

8. Lamas GA, Lee KL, Sweeney MO, et al. Mode selection trial in sinus-node dysfunction. Ventricular pacing or dual-chamber pacing for sinus-node dysfunction. *N Engl J Med.* 346:1854–1862.
9. Gillis AM, Morck M, Exner DV, et al. Impact of atrial antitachycardia pacing and atrial pace prevention therapies on atrial fibrillation burden over long-term follow-up. *Europace.* 2009 (epub ahead of print).
10. Wilkoff BL, Dual Chamber and VVI Implantable Defibrillator trial investigators. The Dual Chamber and VVI Implantable Defibrillator (DAVID) Trial: rationale, design, results, clinical implications and lessons for future trials. *Cardiol Electrophysiol Rev.* 2003;7:468–472.
11. Wilkoff BL, Kudenchuk PJ, Buxton AE, et al. The DAVID (Dual Chamber and VVI Implantable Defibrillator) II Trial. *J Am Coll Cardiol.* 2009;53:872–880.
12. Saksena S, Prakash A, Ziegler P, et al. Improved suppression of recurrent atrial fibrillation with dual-site right atrial pacing and antiarrhythmic drug therapy. *J Am Coll Cardiol.* 2002;40:1140–1150.
13. Padeletti L, Purerfellner H, Adler SW, et al. Combined efficacy of atrial septal lead placement and atrial pacing algorithms for prevention of paroxysmal atrial tachyarrhythmia. *J Cardiovasc Electrophysiol.* 2003;14:1189–1195.
14. Carlson MD, Ip J, Messenger J, et al. A new pacemaker algorithm for the treatment of atrial fibrillation: results of the Atrial Dynamic Overdrive Pacing Trial (ADOPT). *J Am Coll Cardiol.* 2003;42:627–633.
15. Gillis AM, Koehler J, Morck M, Mehra R, Hettrick DA. High atrial antitachycardia pacing therapy efficacy is associated with a reduction in atrial tachyarrhythmia burden in a subset of patients with sinus node dysfunction and paroxysmal atrial fibrillation. *Heart Rhythm.* 2005;2:791–796.
16. Lee MA, Weachter R, Pollak S, et al. The effect of atrial pacing therapies on atrial tachyarrhythmia burden and frequency. *J Am Coll Cardiol.* 2003;41:1926–1932.
17. Mont L, Ruiz-Granell R, Martinez JG, et al. Impact of anti-tachycardia pacing on atrial fibrillation burden when added on top of prevention pacing algorithms: results of the Prevention or Termination (POT) trial. *Europace.* 2008;10:28–34.
18. Friedman PA, Dijkman B, Warman EN, et al. Atrial therapies reduce atrial arrhythmia burden in defibrillator patients. *Circulation.* 2001;104:1023–1028.
19. Wellens HJ, Lau C-P, Luderitz B, et al. Atrioverter: an implantable device for the treatment of atrial fibrillation. *Circulation.* 1998;98:1651–1656.
20. Kapoor WN: Current evaluation and management of syncope. *Circulation.* 2002;106:1606–1609.
21. Connolly SJ, Sheldon R, Roberts RS, Gent M. The North American Vasovagal Pacemaker Study (VPS). A randomized trial of permanent cardiac pacing for the prevention of vasovagal syncope. *J Am Coll Cardiol.* 1999;33:16–20.
22. Sutton R, Brignole M, Menozzi C, et al. Dual-chamber pacing in the treatment of neurally mediated tilt-positive cardioinhibitory syncope: pacemaker versus no therapy: a multicenter randomized study. The Vasovagal Syncope International Study (VASIS) Investigators. *Circulation.* 2000;102:294–299.
23. Goethals M, Timmermans W, Geelen P, Backers J, Brugada P. Mode switching failure during atrial flutter: the "2:1 lock-in" phenomenon. *Europace.* 2003;5:95–102.
24. Platonov M, Gillis AM: Pacing therapies for atrial fibrillation. In: Kusumoto FM, Goldschlager NF, eds. *Cardiac Pacing for the Clinician.* 2nd Ed. New York: Springer Science+Business Media, LLC, 2008:453–470.

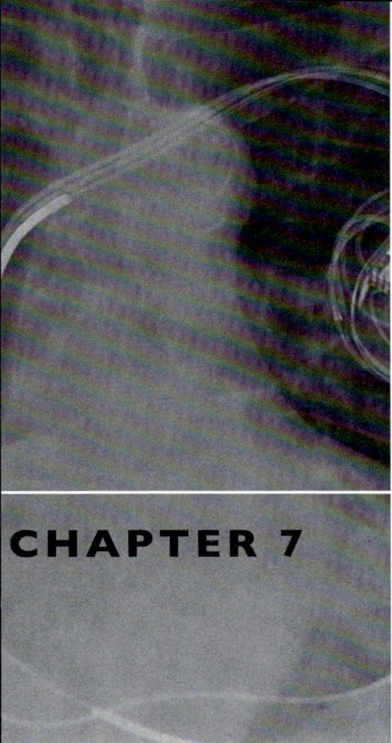

Miscellaneous Pacing Algorithms

CHAPTER 7

George H. Crossley and Robert Andrew Pickett

Pacemaker Mediated Tachycardia

Pacemaker mediated tachycardia (PMT) is a term that has sometimes been used to refer to any tachycardia caused by some interaction of the pacing system with the patient.[1] This might include conduction of atrial arrhythmias, tracking of myopotentials, tracking noise, or inappropriate rate response. It has been used more classically, though, to refer to an endless loop tachycardia where a ventricular event is conducted retrogradely to the atrium, sensed there and then the dual chamber pacemaker paces in the ventricle. This situation is addressed here.

PMT can be induced by any event where a ventricular depolarization occurs in a dual chamber pacemaker without a preceding atrial depolarization and there is retrograde conduction of that event to the atrium. The classic causes are (1) a premature ventricular contraction (PVC), (2) having loss of atrial capture, (3) the presence of a long first-degree AV block, and (4) atrial undersensing or oversensing. The rate of the PMT is usually rapid, but can be slower if there is a long retrograde conduction time. Algorithms have been developed to prevent this significant clinical problem.

In Medtronic pacemakers and ICDs PMT is detected when there are 8 consecutive ventricular paced events followed by sensed atrial events with a VA interval of < 400 ms. The pulse generator then queries the rate responsive sensor to determine whether there is significant activity and the rhythm is likely sinus tachycardia. If the sensor rate is at or below the activities of daily living (ADL) rate, PMT is diagnosed. If the sensor rate is above the ADL rate, sinus tachycardia is diagnosed, the PMT algorithm is not activated, and the algorithm continues to run. When PMT is diagnosed, the pulse generator intervenes by extending the PVARP to 400 ms after the ninth event. This terminates the

Pacemakers and Implantable Cardioverter Defibrillators: An Expert's Manual. © 2010 Amin Al-Ahmad, Kenneth A. Ellenbogen, Andrea Natale, and Paul J. Wang, eds. Cardiotext Publishing, ISBN: 978-0-9790164-6-2.

endless loop tachycardia. After activation, the algorithm is suspended for 90 s. It is important to realize that a patient with sinus tachycardia at rest could have this algorithm activated every 90 s. This situation would only be noticeable if the patient had heart block and marked sinus tachycardia at rest. Such would be the case in a chronotropically competent patient with heart block who is sedated and being given stimulant drugs such as dobutamine or epinephrine.

St. Jude Medical takes a different approach. There are two different algorithms in their devices. For both of these algorithms there is a single programmable parameter: the PMT detect rate. This rate can be programmed between 90 bpm and the maximum track rate. First, there is a scheme named "10 beats > PMT." If the pulse generator detects a series of 10 beats sensed in the atrium and paced in the ventricle at a rate higher than the PMT detect rate, it resets the PVARP to 480 ms for one cycle. As a result, the pulse generator fails to respond to the retrograde P wave. Following this detection, there is an atrial alert period of 330 ms. After activation, the algorithm is suspended for 256 ms. Activation occurs when the pulse generator senses 8 consecutive ventricular-paced events followed by atrial-sensed events at or above the PMT detect rate. In response to that detection the sensed AV delay is modified. If the interval between the sensed atrial event and the paced ventricular event is > 99 ms, the sensed AV interval is shortened by 50 ms for one beat. If that interval is < 100 ms the sensed AV interval is increased by 50 ms. Then the next interval from the ventricular pace to the atrial sense is measured. If this interval is within 16 ms of the mean of the previous 8 intervals, the pulse generator suspends its ventricular output for one cycle and delivers an atrial impulse 330 ms after the sensed atrial event. The algorithm is then suspended for 256 cycles. Both of these algorithms are suspended during mode switching and during magnet application.

In Boston Scientific devices, PMT is detected if there are 16 consecutive events sensed in the atrium and paced in the ventricle at the maximum tracking rate and where there is < 32 ms variation in the VA interval. If PMT is diagnosed, the PVARP is extended to 500 ms for one interval. There is no "time-out" in the Boston Scientific devices. The algorithm resumes immediately.

Rate Drop Pacing

The role of pacing in the treatment of neurocardiogenic syncope is not as well established as it is for sinus node dysfunction and AV block. It is recognized that almost all neurally mediated syncope has both a vasodepressor and a cardioinhibitor component. It was recognized early that simply having demand pacing at a usual rest rate (50–70 bpm) was often not enough to inhibit syncope. Rate drop pacing is an algorithm that was developed for the treatment of neurally mediated syncope. The concept is to identify the onset of syncope and to provide for a heart rapid rate for a period of time, thus treating the cardioinhibitory component and partially compensating for the vasodepressor component with an increased rate. The genesis of this algorithm was early anecdotal data suggesting that simply pacing at a routine rate (60–70 bpm) was insufficient to interrupt syncope.

Clinical trials of this algorithm have been interesting. The initial sizable trial was a nonblinded study that demonstrated a strongly positive effect.[2] This trial was planned to involve 284 patients. However, the data safety and monitoring board closed the study after the first interim analysis with only 54 patients enrolled due to a huge benefit in the treatment group. The incidence of syncope at one year was 18.5% in the patients with a pacemaker and 59.7% in the patients without a pacemaker. It is certainly possible that there was a strong placebo effect. This study prompted a second trial (VPS-II) that was in fact blinded to the patient.[3] All patients had a rate drop pacemaker implanted and the algorithm was randomly turned On or Off for the first 6 months. There were 100 patients in this study. This trial revealed that there was no difference in the outcome between the group with the algorithm active and the algorithm passive.

The inclusion criteria for VPS-II were problematic though. A history of recurrent syncope and a tilt test with a trough heart rate × blood pressure product of < 6000/min × mm Hg was required. Therefore a patient could be included in this study if at the time of syncope the heart rate was 60 and the systolic blood pressure was 99 mm Hg. It was seen in the trial that the mean trough heart rate on the qualifying tilt table test was 56 bpm in the treatment group and 53 bpm in the placebo group.

This author contends that the appropriate conclusion for this study was that patients who don't need pacemakers are not helped by pacing. Based upon this study the general opinion developed that pacing was not first line therapy for syncope. Other studies, involving patients with profound syncope have been more positive.[4] Our center and others have had a very different result in patients with major cardioinhibitory response to syncope. We have implanted rate drop pacemakers in more than 50 patients over the last 10 years who have had a history of recurrent severe syncope and a tilt test with cardioinhibitory syncope (asystole > 5 s). Almost all of these patients had injuries due to falls prior to the pacemaker implantation. In his limited population, there have been excellent clinical responses, with a marked reduction in incidence and severity of syncope and no injuries due to syncope.

Algorithm

The first vendor to develop such an algorithm was Medtronic. Their Rate Drop Response is described here. There are three different modes of this algorithm. In one (Drop detect) the detection is based upon the heart rate falling through a window that has a programmable heart rate change (Drop size) over a programmable number of beats (Detection window) (Fig 7.1). The heart rate must also fall to or below a programmable drop rate. Also, a simpler algorithm (Low rate detect) is available that specifies a lower rate only (Fig 7.2). If the heart rate falls to that rate for a programmable number of beats then the intervention is triggered. In the third iteration, both of these features are programmed On.

Programmable Parameter	Possible Values (nominal)
Rate drop response	Off, Drop, Low Rate, Both (Off)
Drop size	10–50 bpm (25)
Drop rate	30–100 bpm (50)
Detect window	10–15 sec (25)
Intervention rate	60–180 bpm (100)
Intervention duration	1–15 min (10 min)

The response is to pace at a programmable rate (nominal is 100 bpm) for a programmable amount of time. The heart rate then decays at approximately 5 bpm every minute until either the lower rate or the intrinsic rate is reached, whichever is higher.

It is worth noting that the Medtronic automatic mode switch algorithm cannot be programmed to On once the Rate Drop Response algorithm is programmed On. This may limit the utility of this algorithm in individuals who have frequent atrial tachyarrhythmias and need to have the mode switch feature activated.

The Boston Scientific algorithm is called Sudden Brady Response. This is triggered when there is (1) atrial sensing for the detect interval, and (2) the heart rate drops by 10 bpm and there is pacing for a programmable number of beats at the lower rate limit. When therapy is initiated, pacing occurs at the sensor-indicated rate plus the rate offset.

Programmable Parameter	Possible Values (nominal)
Sudden Brady Response	On or Off (Off)
Detect time	1–15 min (5 min)
Number of beats	1–8 beats (4 beats)
Therapy duration	1–15 min (10 min)
Therapy rate offset	5–40 bpm (5 bpm)

The name of the St. Jude Medical equivalent of the rate drop response is Advanced Hysteresis. This algorithm is similar to the Medtronic Low

Rate detect algorithm. It is activated by reaching a low rate for a programmable number of beats.

Programmable Parameter	Possible Values (nominal)
Cycle count	1–16 cycles (1 cycle)
Intervention duration	1–10 min (3 min)
Intervention rate	Off, intrinsic + 10–120 bpm (Off)
Recovery time	Fast, Medium, Slow, Very Slow (Medium)

Crosstalk Prevention

Failure to pace due to output inhibition can have disastrous consequences for a pacemaker-dependent patient. This can result from crosstalk, which is defined as the sensing of atrial pacing output on the ventricular sensing channel. By sensing the output, the ventricular channel detects a sensed beat and withholds ventricular pacing. This can potentially develop in any dual chamber platform, both in pacemakers and in ICDs.

Crosstalk is more likely to occur in settings of high output pacing in the atrium, a very sensitive ventricular setting, rapid rates of atrial activity, shorter ventricular blanking times, and unipolar pacing. When traditional reprogramming, such as lowering atrial lead output or safely changing ventricular sensing parameters, is not able to eliminate the issue, the pacing platform may rely on an algorithm to help eliminate the condition.

One such algorithm to prevent failure of output is ventricular safety standby present in St. Jude Medical systems. When the feature is programmed On, the pacemaker creates a second timing window after the ventricular blanking period called the crosstalk detection window. The device watches for ventricular sensing that may occur during the detection

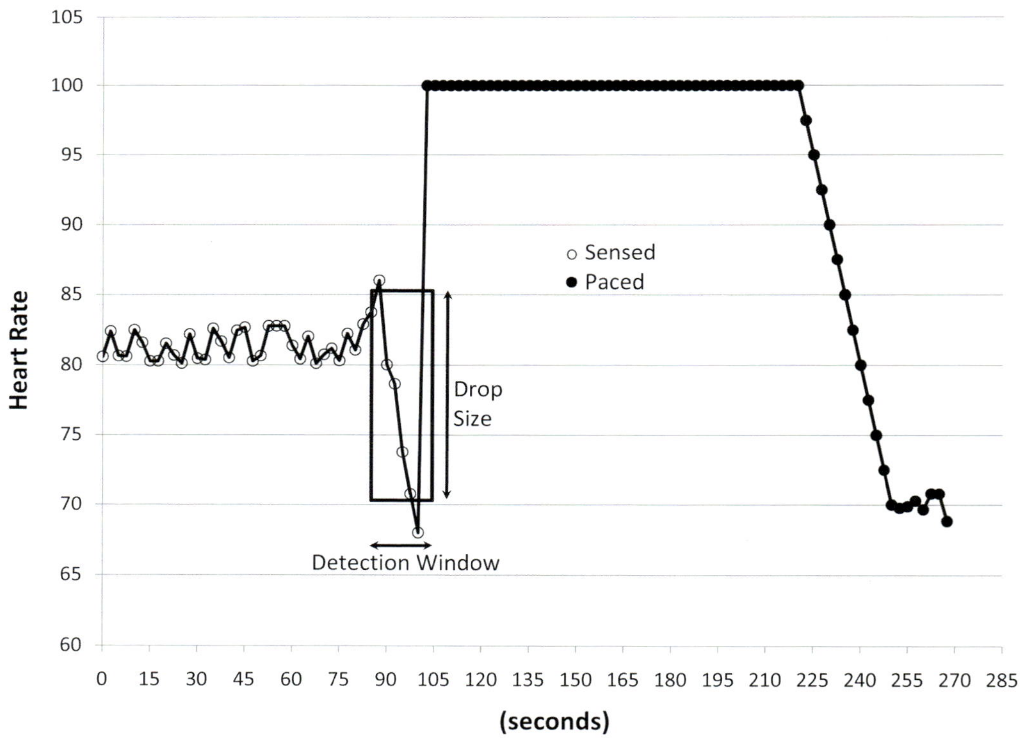

Fig 7.1 In the drop detect algorithm, the heart rate must fall through a window that has a height defined by a change in heart rate and a duration defined as time. The pacemaker then paces at a prescribed rate and decays over time.

window, and if an event is detected, a ventricular pulse is delivered 120 ms after detection of the cardiac signal. If a signal is detected after the end of the window, the pacemaker assumes it is a spontaneous ventricular signal and withholds ventricular pacing.

In Medtronic pacing platforms, ventricular safety pacing[5] is a timing-based feature that utilizes a 110-ms window from the atrial depolarization. If a signal is detected in this window, a paced ventricular beat is delivered. If the detected signal is actually a ventricular depolarization, the safety paced beat will fall within the refractory period of the tissue and produce no effect. If the detected signal within the window is not a ventricular event, the paced beat delivered at the end of the 110-ms window will cause ventricular capture.

Another possibility for interruption of or inhibition of ventricular pacing output is noise. Noise can be due to internal components, such as a lead fracture or device header issue, or it can be due to external factors such as electrocautery in the operating room setting.

A feature found in St. Jude Medical devices is noise response[6] which normally operates in the setting of electromagnetic interference that is in the range of 400 cycles per minute (Hertz). In the event noise is detected on a pacing channel, a noise sampling period of 150 ms is initiated. The 150-ms window is divided into 75 ms of absolute refractory period and 75 ms of relative refractory period. If the noise abates during the relative period, normal pacing resumes. If the noise continues to the end of the relative period, the device reverts to asynchronous pacing at either the lower rate pacing or at the programmed sensor rate until the noise stops. When the noise resolves, pacing reverts to normal programmed parameters.

In Medtronic pacing platforms, noise reversion[5] is the continuous sensing during atrial

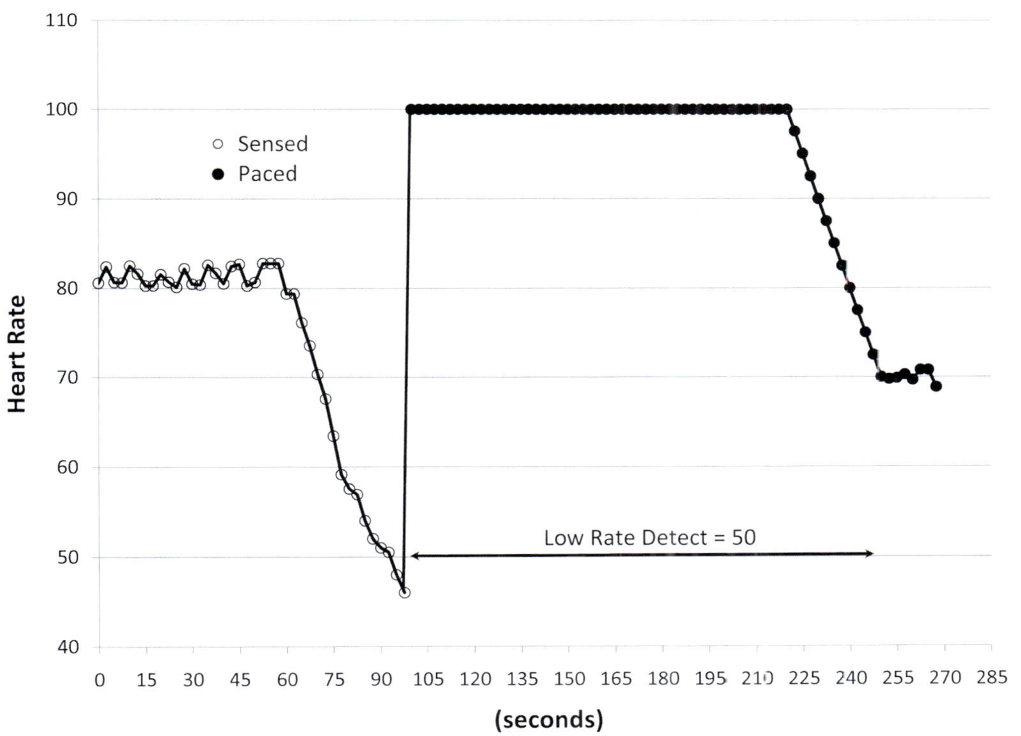

Fig 7.2 In the lower rate algorithm, the heart rate must reach a low rate for a programmed number of intervals. The pacemaker then paces at a prescribed rate and decays over time.

and ventricular refractory periods for noise. When noise is detected, on either channel, the refractory period on the corresponding channel is reset. By prolonging the refractory period, sensing can continue to occur, but the device classifies the event as refractory. This prevents the device from acting upon the sensed episode and resetting pacing intervals. Rather than switching to asynchronous pacing, the refractory periods are continuously reset until either the noise resolves or lower rate pacing/sensor rate is met. Once the lower rate pacing time is met, pacing is delivered without interruption.

In Boston Scientific devices, the noise response[7] works along the same lines with a few differences. When noise is detected, a noise window of 40 to 55 ms, depending on the platform, will start, and if the noise continues, the noise window continues until the timeout for lower rate pacing is met. At this point asynchronous pacing (either VOO or DOO depending on baseline programming) starts and continues until the noise resolves. During device interrogation the markers AP-Ns or VP-Ns will be displayed in response to the channel that had the abnormal electrical signal.

Magnet Mode

The application of a magnet over a device can result in different responses depending upon whether it is an ICD or a pacemaker.

In a pacemaker, the placement of a magnet over the generator results in asynchronous pacing at a predetermined rate. This is especially useful for determining battery status, because the rate is consistent until elective replacement indicator (ERI). Once ERI is met, the asynchronous magnet rate drops to a different rate. In Medtronic pacemakers, for example, the magnet rate with a normally functioning battery is 85 bpm, and the rate drops to 65 bpm when ERI is met.[5]

In ICDs, magnets are used for a different purpose, which is the suspension of tachyarrhythmia detection. Brady pacing is not affected in an ICD system. Magnets can be used to prevent inappropriate therapies from being delivered in the case of noise (ie, a broken lead) or incessant arrhythmias (eg, sinus tachycardia or atrial tachycardia). Depending on the manufacturer, the response to magnets may be programmable.

In many Boston Scientific ICD systems, the Enable Magnet Use feature can be programmed On or Off.[7] With the feature On, the magnet can be placed over the device giving an audible tone. Depending on the family of device in question, the tone can start as a tone that is synchronized to the R waves. After 30 s, if the tone becomes continuous, the tachyarrhythmia therapy delivery is permanently deactivated. If the tone remains synchronous to the R waves, the tachyarrhythmia therapy is suspended only while the magnet is in place. If the magnet placed over the device is immediately one continuous tone, the tachyarrhythmia therapies are already Off. In some devices, or depending on specific programmed parameters, a programmer must be used to turn therapies On. In other systems, by keeping the magnet over the device for 30 s, the continuous tone can become synchronous indicating that tachyarrhythmia therapies are again reactivated with the removal of the magnet.

In the St. Jude Medical family of ICD/CRT-D, the Magnet Response[6] feature can be programmed to the On setting to allow the suspension of therapy delivery by placement of a magnet over the generator. It can also be programmed to the Ignore setting which allows the system to delivery therapy regardless of the presence of a magnet. Again, there is no effect on Brady pacing in the high-power platforms.

In Medtronic high-powered devices, the magnet response is consistent with other companies. By placing the magnet over the device, an audible tone is heard and tachyarrhythmia therapies are suspended as long as the magnet is in place. Brady pacing is not affected. By removing the magnet, therapies can again be delivered.

References

1. Ellenbogen KA, Kay GN, Lau CP, Wilkoff BL, eds. *Clinical Cardiac Pacing, Defibrillation, and Resynchronization Therapy.* 3rd ed. Philadelphia, PA: Saunders Elsevier; 2007.
2. Connolly SJ, Sheldon R, Roberts RS, Gent M. The North American Vasovagal Pacemaker Study (VPS). A randomized trial of permanent cardiac pacing for the prevention of vasovagal syncope.[see comment]. *J Am Coll Cardiol.* 1999 January;33(1):16–20.
3. Connolly SJ, Sheldon R, Thorpe KE, et al. I. Pacemaker therapy for prevention of syncope in patients with recurrent severe vasovagal syncope: Second Vasovagal Pacemaker Study (VPS II): a randomized trial.[see comment]. *JAMA.* 2003 May 7;289(17):2224–2229.
4. Benditt DG, Sutton R, Gammage MD, et al. Clinical experience with Thera DR rate-drop response pacing algorithm in carotid sinus syndrome and vasovagal syncope. The International Rate-Drop Investigators Group. *Pacing Clin Electrophysiol.* 1997 March;20(3:Pt 2):t–9.
5. *Adapta / Versa / Sensia Pacemaker Reference Guide.* Medtronic, Inc.; 2009.
6. *St. Jude Bradycardia References Manual.* St. Jude Medical; 2009.
7. *The Boston Scientific CRM Compass.* Boston Scientific; 2009.

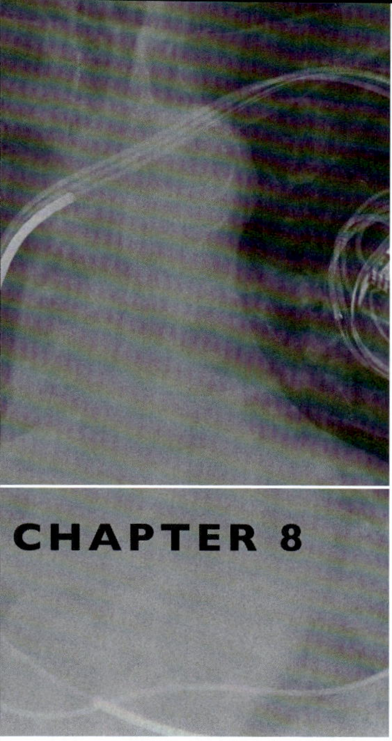

CHAPTER 8

Automatic Threshold Measuring Algorithms

Marco V. Perez, Henry H. Hsia, Paul C. Zei, Mintu P. Turakhia, Paul J. Wang, and Amin Al-Ahmad

Introduction

The ability of pacemakers to reliably and automatically assess whether or not pacing stimuli result in successful myocardial capture and depolarization has been a goal since the initial use of implantable devices. The primary clinical goals of automatic verification of capture (AVC) are to conserve battery life by allowing lower pacing outputs to be programmed over the long term, provide immediate backup pacing at high output if failure to capture is detected, and to achieve the safety of maintaining capture. With AVC, a pacemaker is able to periodically assess for changes in thresholds and to automatically adjust pacing output slightly above threshold as opposed to a traditional two-fold safety margin. There are several methods of AVC, which are discussed later.

In the immediate post-implant period and the chronic setting, thresholds may change for a variety of reasons. With older leads, pacing thresholds would rise dramatically over the course of 2 to 8 weeks during lead maturation, as the inflammatory and fibrotic process that followed lead implantation evolved. The maturation process with modern drug-eluting leads is faster and has a less pronounced effect on threshold. Most leads reach steady-state threshold values by 10 weeks. There are, however, a number of medications and disease conditions that can contribute to a rise in myocardial thresholds. Chronic amiodarone use leads to a modest rise in ventricular threshold of, on average, approximately 1 Volt. However, class Ia and Ic antiarrhythmic agents such as propafenone and flecainide[1] can cause up to a two-fold rise in thresholds. Conditions that cause myocardial remodeling, such as diffuse cardiomyopathy or focal myocardial infarction, can also lead to large increases in myocardial thresholds. Sudden spikes in thresholds during acute illnesses,

Pacemakers and Implantable Cardioverter Defibrillators: An Expert's Manual. © 2010 Amin Al-Ahmad, Kenneth A. Ellenbogen, Andrea Natale, and Paul J. Wang, eds. Cardiotext Publishing, ISBN: 978-0-9790164-6-2.

particularly in epicardial leads, have also been reported and can lead to failure to capture.[2]

Because of threshold fluctuation after lead maturation, a safety margin has traditionally been used to ensure that relatively small rises in thresholds will not lead to loss of myocardial capture. Traditionally, this output safety window was empirically programmed at least twice the threshold voltage, or three times the threshold pulse width. The disadvantage of this excess output energy is a faster rate of battery depletion. One purpose of AVC is that by automatically assessing thresholds on a regular basis, output can be safely maintained at a marginal level above threshold with emergency backup pacing if needed. Saving battery life allows for greater time between generator changes and further miniaturization of devices with smaller batteries.

Automatic Verification of Capture Techniques

The idea that the pacemaker itself could assess whether or not it successfully depolarized the myocardium after delivering a pacing stimulus was first introduced in the early 1970s.[3,4] It was not until 1994 that Pacesetter, later acquired by St. Jude Medical, introduced AutoCapture, the first clinically available AVC algorithm. Today, most pacemakers from the major manufacturers use one of various techniques and algorithms to automatically assess capture.

Evoked Response

The most widely used method for assessing capture automatically is the measurement of the myocardial evoked response (ER). After a pacing stimulus is delivered, positively charged ions cover the negatively charged pole of the lead and result in local lead-myocardial polarization, regardless of myocardial capture (Fig 8.1A). These ions then disperse at varying rates, depending on the makeup of the lead. Polarization results in a deflection that is sensed immediately after the pacing stimulus. This signal usually decays over the course of 10 to 15 ms (Fig 8.1B). ER is the deflection that represents true myocardial depolarization and is usually sensed over the first 60 ms following the pacing stimulus. The critical factor for most AVC is distinguishing ER from polarization signals (Fig 8.1C). Polarization, however, can be of high amplitude and prolonged, thereby obscuring the ER.

To better distinguish the ER from polarization, several techniques, both software- and hardware-based, have been developed. A blanking window of about 15 ms immediately after the pacing stimulus (Fig 8.1C) is programmed to ignore most of the post-pacing stimulation local polarization signal, while the period between 20 ms and 100 ms is usually programmed to detect the myocardial ER. Another technique often used is to create an independent pace/sense (IPS) configuration. For example, pacing is programmed unipolar (tip to can), whereas sensing is programmed bipolar (tip to ring).[5] However, IPS requires the use of bipolar leads and increases the risk of far-field sensing in other chambers. The use of low-polarization leads is a technologic advance that has made ER detection more feasible. Most of the newer leads are coated with titanium-nitrite, which helps minimize the polarization artifact.

Another method for improving ER detection is the adjustment of the pacing output circuitry with reduced coupling capacitor (RCC) technology which can produce a faster decay of the polarization artifact.[6] However, this technique is limited by a relatively low maximum voltage output that can be used. An additional strategy is to improve signal-to-noise ratio by subtracting the polarization signal from the paced ER. To accomplish this, pacing during the myocardial refractory period is performed and the polarization signal is recorded. This signal is then subtracted from a subsequent paced beat and the difference is recorded as the ER.

Most devices that offer detection of AVC propose a combination of these techniques for the most accurate reading of the ER. Although some devices strictly require the use of low-polarization leads, other devices use alternative technologies such as RCC or IPS and are more

Figure 8.1 (A–C) Evoked response.

A

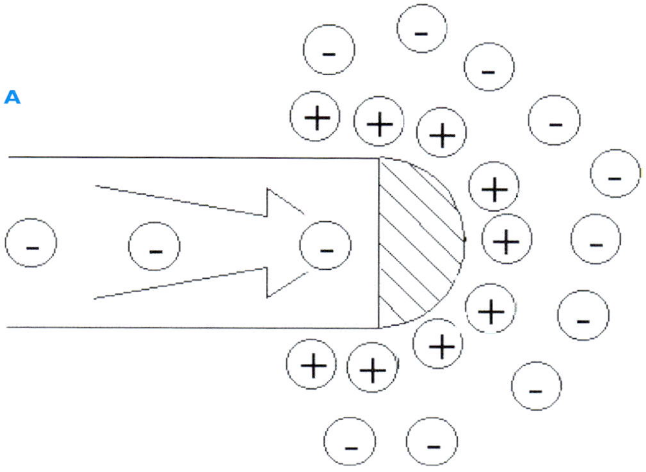

Figure 8.1A Polarized lead.
Positively charged ions surround the lead tip and produce a positively charged layer on the electrode called polarization. (Reproduced with permission of Medtronic, Inc.)

Figure 8.1B Evoked response.
The top tracing demonstrates the initial pacing pulse followed by the lead polarization signal and finally the evoked response which represents myocardial depolarization. The bottom tracing demonstrates the pacing and polarization signals without myocardial depolarization. This is then followed by a large output safety pulse. (Reprinted with permission from St. Jude.)

B

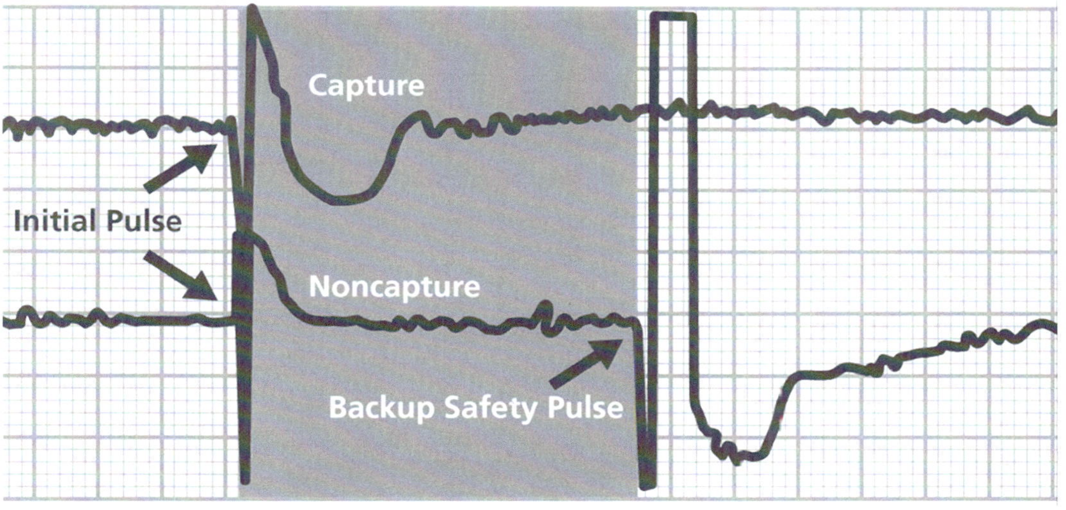

Figure 8.1C Detecting the evoked response.
The first 10-20 ms (closed) are usually blanked to ignore polarization. The ensuing 14-100 ms (open) are programmed to detect ER. If no ER is detected, a backup safety pulse is delivered at a fixed interval. Reprinted with permission from St. Jude.

C

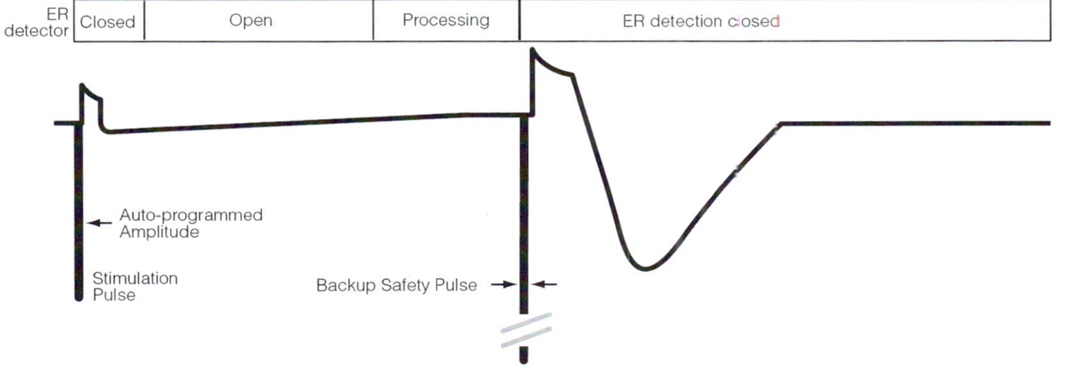

permissive of the lead type used. Lead compatibility is discussed in more detail later.

Physiologic Response

Although measurement of ER is the most common technique used to assess AVC, alternative techniques that are based on a more global response to pacing have been developed and are used predominantly with right atrial and left ventricular pacing. This is particularly important in the atrium as the myocardial ER signals can be much lower than those from the ventricle due to its smaller mass.

In patients with intrinsic atrioventricular (AV) conduction, atrial pacing should be followed by ventricular depolarization. Atrial capture can therefore be assessed in patients with dual chamber devices by analyzing sensing in the ventricle. This would, of course, not be possible in patients with any AV conduction disturbance during atrial pacing. An alternative approach is the assessment of suppression of intrinsic sinus activity with atrial pacing. If the sinus node is not reset with atrial pacing, then atrial capture is unlikely.

Left ventricular leads in cardiac resynchronization devices have unique properties that make AVC challenging. Output optimization is crucial in these devices as the goal is nearly complete pacing and battery life tends to be shorter. Although newer LV leads are bipolar, most existing leads are unipolar, making the ER more difficult to interpret. One technique that has been developed assesses left ventricular capture by sensing depolarization in the right ventricular lead. The conduction time between the two leads is usually constant and can be used to obviate the need for ER detection.

Algorithms for Threshold Testing

The specific algorithms used to perform threshold tests, adjust pacing output, and deliver emergent backup pacing when needed, vary from one manufacturer to the next (Table 8.1). Although the algorithms are similar, knowing the differences enables better troubleshooting and assessing whether automatic threshold testing is appropriate. Inappropriate programming can lead to unnecessarily high rises in pacing output and hence earlier battery depletion. Before reviewing the details of each device's algorithm, the characteristics of these algorithms and their importance will be discussed.

Algorithm Characteristics

Method for AVC: Accurate verification of capture is essential for automated threshold testing. As discussed earlier, most algorithms use measurement of ER, however, some atrial and left ventricular algorithms employ a physiologic response to determine capture.

Lead compatibility: Before the threshold algorithms are evoked, one must check for lead requirements. Although most modern leads are low-polarization, bipolar, and compatible with appropriate ER detection algorithms, older leads may be incompatible.

Initial verification: Some devices require manual verification that the ER signal is well above the background noise after a pacing spike before the threshold algorithm can be turned on. Other devices perform this check automatically and may turn the feature Off if the signal-to-noise ratio is not adequate.

Beat-to-Beat capture assessment: Some devices check for capture after every beat. This allows for real-time emergency backup pacing if necessary (Fig 8.2) and can trigger a recheck of the pacing threshold or an automatic increase in pacing output. Other manufacturers argue that thresholds rarely change abruptly and continuous capture assessment unnecessarily consumes additional energy. If fusion or pseudofusion occurs, where an intrinsic depolarization occurs simultaneously with a paced beat, the device could erroneously underdetect capture, which could then unnecessarily prompt an increase in output. Some algorithms delay the sensed/paced AV interval following a beat that failed

Algorithm	AVC Method	Lead Requirements	Initial Verification	Beat to Beat Verification	Threshold Testing Triggers	Programmability
St. Jude						
Ventricular Autocapture	Vent. ER	Bipolar* Low polarization	Automated High signal to noise**	Yes	Scheduled Interval Loss of capture Magnet/ Programmer Ventricular noise	Threshold testing frequency 8 or 24h. ER Sensitivity Sensed/paced AV delay during threshold testing Backup pace uni/ bipolar
ACap Confirm	Atrial ER	Bipolar Low polarization	Automated High signal to noise	No	Scheduled Interval One hour after scheduled test, if capture was not successful	Threshold testing frequency 8 or 24h. Monitoring mode Backup pace uni/ bipolar
Boston Scientific						
Automatic Capture Verification	Vent. ER	Uni or bipolar	Leads must meet typical implant criteria	Yes	Scheduled every 21 hours Loss of capture Initially turned on	Only On and Off
Medtronic						
Right Ventricular Capture Management	Vent. ER	Uni or bipolar	Not specified	No	1:00 A.M. on internal clock	Monitoring mode Output safety margin Lead maturation time Output lower limit
Atrial Capture Management	Physiologic response	Any lead	Stable sinus rate or stable 1:1 AV conduction	No	1:00 A.M. on internal clock	Monitoring mode Output safety margin Lead maturation time Output lower limit
Left Ventricular Capture Management	Physiologic response	Any lead	Stable LV to RV conduction time RV sensed before LV on a-pacing	No	1:00 A.M. on internal clock	Monitoring mode Output safety margin Lead maturation time Output lower limit Output upper limit
Biotronik						
Automatic Capture control	Vent. ER	Low polarization recommended	Signal quality check (see text)	Yes	Scheduled interval twice daily Loss of capture	Monitoring mode Output safety margin Output lower limit Output upper limit
ELA						
Ventricular Autothreshold	Vent. ER	Low polarization recommended	Not specified	No	Scheduled interval every 6 hours Pacing mode changes Magnet mode	Monitoring mode Output lower limit

Table 8.1 Algorithms by Manufacturer. *With newer device models, bipolar leads are not necessary.

to capture in order to minimize fusion, a technique called pseudofusion avoidance (Fig 8.3).

Threshold testing: In essence, threshold algorithms decrease the pacing output until verification of capture is lost. How the output varies, how often thresholds are routinely checked and what situations trigger threshold checks are different among the various algorithms. There are also certain conditions, such as persistent intrinsic conduction or excessive noise, under which some algorithms will not attempt to check thresholds. There is usually a maximum threshold above which the device determines that capture is either not occurring or is not being detected adequately. An inappropriately high threshold assessment can lead to output settings that are higher than necessary and hence shorten battery life.

Response to threshold test: Most algorithms will program the pacing output slightly above the automated threshold, leaving a small "safety margin." Algorithms that check for capture beat by beat and can provide backup pacing (Fig 8.2) tend to leave a smaller safety margin than algorithms that only check thresholds intermittently. A complex set of rules governs the minimum and maximum output that can be set.

Programmability: Some devices offer greater flexibility in programming the threshold testing algorithm than others. The frequency of threshold checks and maximum output, for example, can be programmed in some devices.

Specific Algorithms

St. Jude Medical: Ventricular AutoCapture

Method for AVC: Measurement of ventricular ER. After a pacing pulse, there is a blanking period of 14 ms, followed by an Evoked Response Detection Window between 46 and 72 ms long. Ventricular output is programmed to unipolar and ventricular sensing is programmed to bipolar.

Lead compatibility: With most models, bipolar low-polarization leads are necessary. With newer devices (such as Zephyr), any low-polarization lead is sufficient.

Initial setup: To properly initialize AutoCapture, the device must be able to pace the patient consistently. If AV conduction is too short or if ventricular rates are too high, AutoCapture may not be turned on. The Ventricular ER Sensitivity test will measure ER, suggest ER-sensitivity settings, calculate ER-sensitivity safety margin, and recommend whether or not Ventricular AutoCapture should be turned On (Fig 8.4). To recommend use of AutoCapture, the test must find a ratio of at least 1.7:1 between the suggested ER sensitivity (about half of the average ER) and the underlying lead polarization noise. Failure to run the sensitivity test will lead to auto-programming of a high ER sensitivity and underdetection of ER, with subsequent pacing in a high output mode. In the newer models, the Ventricular AutoCapture Setup test will be performed and AutoCapture will either be recom-

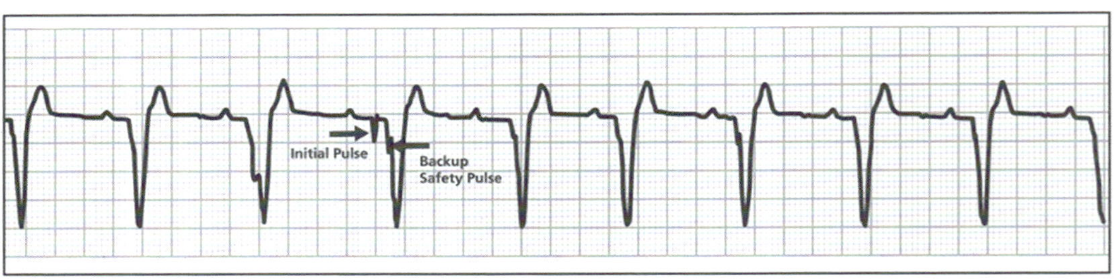

Figure 8.2. Backup safety pulse. In the fourth beat, the initial pacing pulse failed to capture, and was therefore followed immediately by a backup safety pulse. (Reprinted with permission from St. Jude.)

mended or not, however detailed information about the ER sensitivity and safety margins will not be reported. Finally, Ventricular Lead Type must be programmed to "Unipolar/Bipolar" or "Single-Pass VDD."

Beat-to-Beat capture verification: Present.

Response to failed capture: A backup safety pulse with an output of 4.5 or 5.0 V at the programmed pulse width, approximately 80 to 100 ms after the initial pulse, will be delivered. Loss of capture will cause a 100-ms AV delay in the subsequent beats (Fig 8.3). If two consecutive beats fail to capture, then a scan for the minimal output necessary for capture (Ventricular Loss of Capture Recovery) is begun: The output of the next beat is increased by 0.25 V. If capture is still not verified, then the output of the following beats is increased sequentially by 0.125 V to a maximum of 3.875 V. Once capture is verified, a threshold search is begun. If maximum out-

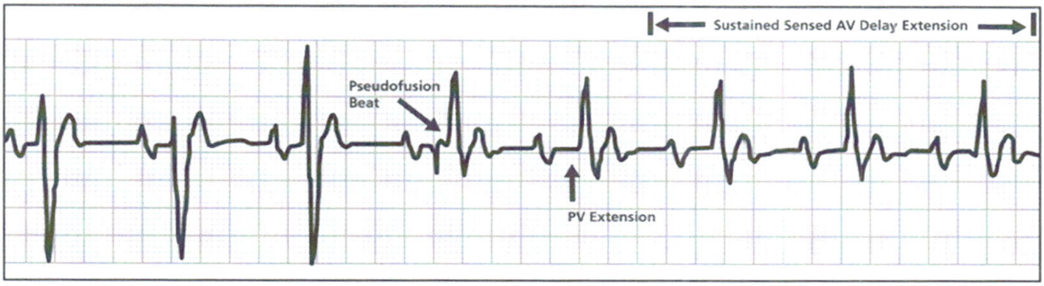

Figure 8.3 Pseudofusion avoidance. Following a pacing impulse where capture is not detected due to fusion and a backup beat is given, the following cycle undergoes an AV delay that permits intrinsic conduction to proceed. If intrinsic conduction is present, pacing is no longer required and repeated fusion is avoided. (Reprinted with permission from St. Jude.)

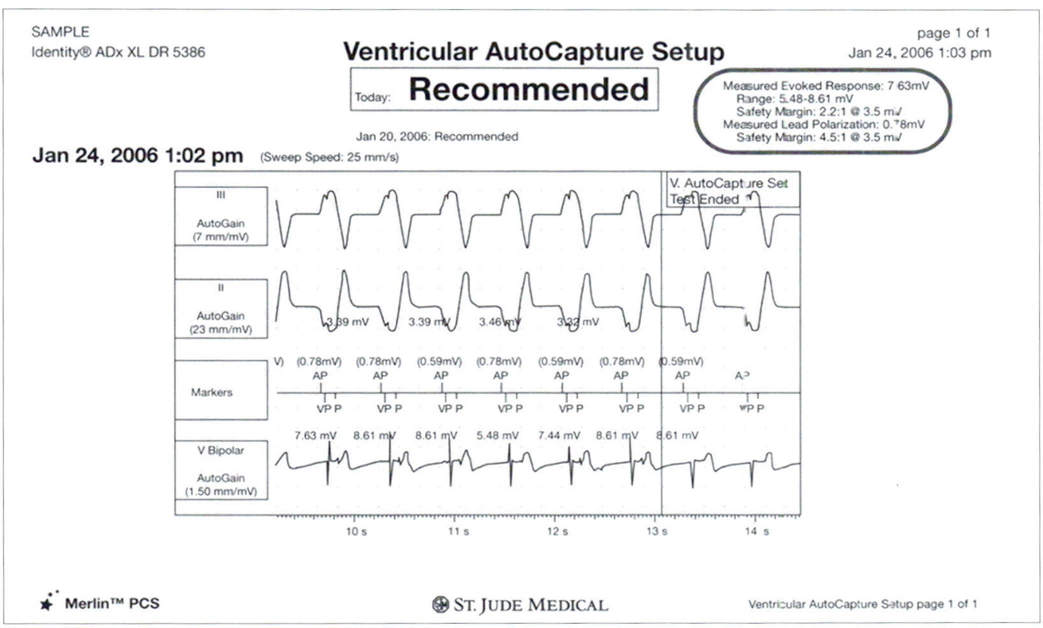

Figure 8.4 ER sensitivity test. The average measured evoked response was 7.63mV. The Suggested ER sensitivity was 3.5mV (providing a safety margin of 2.2:1). The ratio between the suggested ER sensitivity and lead polarization was 4.5:1, which was well above the 1.7:1 ratio required. Ventricular Autocapture was therefore recommended. (Reprinted with permission from St. Jude.)

put is reached without capture, then the device switches to a high output mode with an output of 4.5 to 5.0 V at the programmed pulse width (at least 0.5 ms) for 128 cycles, followed by a threshold search.

Threshold testing: Several situations can trigger threshold testing: (1) following capture recovery after two consecutive beats with loss of capture, (2) scheduled interval, (3) after removal of program wand or magnet, (4) manually triggered Ventricular AutoCapture, and (5) termination of ventricular noise response (a high output mode that is entered if ventricular noise is detected). Upon initiation of the threshold testing protocol, the sensed/paced AV delay is shortened to a preprogrammed interval to avoid fusion and the device decreases the pulse amplitude by 0.25 V. If capture is confirmed, the pulse amplitude is successively lowered by 0.25 V. Once capture is lost over two consecutive cycles, the pulse amplitude is increased by 0.125 V until capture over two consecutive cycles is confirmed, thereby confirming capture threshold. The amplitude is then set at 0.25 V above the capture threshold. If the search algorithm fails to verify capture close to 0.0 V, then the device is set to high output mode and threshold testing is restarted after 128 cycles.

Programmability: Ventricular AutoCapture can be programmed On or Off. Threshold testing can be scheduled every 8 or 24 hours. The ER sensitivity can be chosen from a set of values determined by the ER sensitivity test. The sensed/paced AV delay during threshold testing or capture recovery can be programmed to 50/25 ms, 100/70 ms, or 120/100 ms. The nominal setting is 50/25 ms, which helps minimize fusion. The ventricular backup pulse can be programmed to unipolar or bipolar.

St. Jude Medical: ACap Confirm

Method for AVC: Measurement of bipolar atrial ER during a short detection window following an atrial test pulse.

Lead compatibility: Bipolar, low-polarization leads only.

Initial setup: The ACap Confirm Setup test must be performed prior to turning On ACap Confirm. The test will measure ER, calculate ER sensitivity, and recommend whether ACap Confirm should be turned On. Atrial Pulse Configuration must be set to "Bipolar" and Atrial Lead Type must be programmed to "Unipolar/Bipolar" or "Bipolar."

Beat-to-Beat capture assessment: Not present.

Response to failed capture: Backup pulse is set to 5.0 V at the programmed pulse width (minimum of 0.5 ms), 40 ms after the initial pulse. The AV delay is set to a maximum of 120 ms.

Threshold testing: Threshold testing is triggered by a scheduled interval, manual trigger, or 1 hour after threshold testing fails to verify capture. The threshold testing algorithm is as follows: Atrial pulse amplitude is decreased in steps of 0.25 V until three loss-of-capture beats occur. The amplitude is then increased in 0.125 V steps until two capture beats are identified. If the threshold is less than 2.85 V, the programmed pacing amplitude is set using a safety margin of approximately 1.7:1. If the threshold is greater than 2.875 V, the amplitude is set at 5.0 V. If capture is not confirmed, then the device enters a high output mode with output at 5.0 V at the programmed pulse width (minimum of 0.5 ms).

Programmability: ACap can be turned to an On, Off, or Monitor mode. In monitor mode, thresholds are checked as programmed and recorded, but the programmed pacing output is not changed. Threshold testing can be scheduled every 8 or 24 hours. The atrial backup pulse can be programmed to unipolar or bipolar.

Boston Scientific: Automatic Capture Verification (ACV)

Method for ACV: Measurement of the ventricular ER.

Lead compatibility: Unipolar or bipolar leads are compatible.

Initial setup: ACV is recommended if the leads meet typical implant criteria: ventricular threshold between 0.1 and 3.0 V at 0.4 ms, lead impedance between 100 and 2500 Ω, and intrinsic amplitude of > 5 mV. A commanded threshold test must be run before turning on beat-to-beat capture verification.

Beat-to-Beat capture assessment: Present.

Response to failed capture: A backup safety pulse between 3.5 and 4.5 V, depending on the measured threshold, is delivered within 100 ms if capture is not detected. The following beat will have an extended AV interval of 64 ms. Threshold testing will be triggered.

Threshold testing: Testing is triggered when (1) the ACV algorithm is initially turned On, (2) manually commanded, (3) scheduled every 21 hours, or (4) loss of capture is detected. Threshold testing is performed as follows: Paced AV delay changes to 60 ms and sensed AV is diminished by 30 ms; the ventricular rate may be increased in single chamber devices to ensure ventricular pacing. Pacing amplitude begins with 3.5 V at 0.4 ms and the amplitude is gradually diminished until 2 out of 4 beats fail to capture. The programmed output is then set at ventricular threshold plus 0.5 V. If thresholds cannot be measured, then high output pacing will begin at twice the previous threshold, between a minimum of 3.5 V and a maximum of 5.0 V. If thresholds cannot be measured because of noise, then threshold testing is attempted every hour thereafter. Threshold testing will also be performed every 21 hours.

Programmability: Automatic Capture Verification can be turned On or Off.

Medtronic: Right Ventricular Capture Management (RVCM)

Method for AVC: Measurement of ventricular ER.

Lead compatibility: Unipolar or bipolar. Most Medtronic leads are low polarization leads.

Beat-to-Beat capture assessment: Not present.

Threshold testing: Threshold testing is performed every day at 1:00 AM based on the device's internal clock. Testing begins at an output of 0.125 V lower than the last measured threshold at a fixed pulse width of 0.4 ms and the amplitude is decreased by 0.125 V until loss of capture is confirmed. The device then increases the output by 0.125 V until the same amplitude demonstrates capture three times in succession. The target pacing output is then set at the threshold multiplied by the RV Amplitude Safety Margin, which is a programmable factor chosen by the user. The greater the factor, the larger the safety margin. The device then reduces the programmed amplitude by 0.25 V every other day until it reaches the target amplitude. If the target is higher than the programmed amplitude, the adjustment is made immediately. The pulse width is reset at the previously programmed value. During lead maturation, the period immediately after implant, the minimum amplitude is 3.5 V and pulse width is 0.4 ms. The amplitude is adjusted to a high output state of 5.0 V at 1.0 ms if the threshold is determined to be > 2.5 V or the target amplitude is > 5.0 V.

Programmability: RVCM can be set to an Off, Adaptive, or Monitor mode. In the adaptive mode, pacing outputs are automatically adjusted based on automatic threshold measurements; in the monitor mode, thresholds are recorded but outputs are not adjusted. The Ventricular Amplitude Safety Margin, which determines by what factor the threshold is multiplied to determine pacing output after a threshold test, is also programmable. The lead maturation period is nominally 120 days but can be reprogrammed. A lower limit for the pacing amplitude can be programmed.

Medtronic: Atrial Capture Management (ACM)

Method for AVC: Capture is verified by physiologic responses. If the sinus rate is stable at < 87 bpm, then the Atrial Chamber Reset (ACR) is used: ACR evaluates capture based on the presence of a sensed atrial event after delivery of a premature paced beat. If an atrial event is seen during the atrial refractory period following a premature atrial paced beat, then loss of capture is verified (Fig 8.5). If stable 1:1 conduction is present, then the AV Conduction method is chosen: overdrive atrial pacing is followed by a short atrial paced (coupling) interval that is then immediately followed by a backup, high output atrial pace. The timing of the ventricular-sensed event that follows determines atrial capture (Fig 8.6).

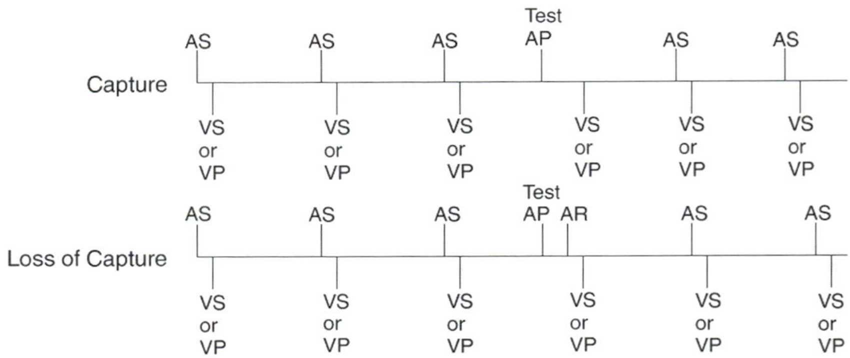

Figure 8.5 Medtronic atrial chamber reset. Method of AVC in the Medtronic Atrial Capture Management algorithm. If an atrial event is seen during the atrial refractory period following a premature atrial paced beat, then loss of capture is verified. (Reproduced with permission of Medtronic, Inc.)

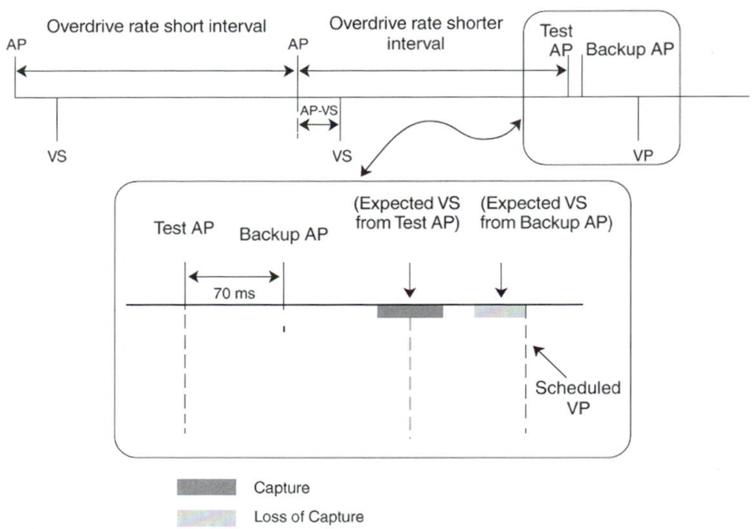

Figure 8.6 Medtronic AV conduction method. Method of AVC in the Medtronic AV Conduction algorithm. Overdrive atrial pacing is followed by a short atrial (coupling) interval which is then followed by a backup high output atrial pace. Assuming AV conduction time remains constant, if a ventricular sensed event is seen in the "Expected VS from Test AP" zone, then capture is verified. If the event is seen in the backup zone, then loss of capture is recorded. (Reproduced with permission of Medtronic, Inc.)

Lead compatibility: Any lead.

Beat-to-Beat capture assessment: Not present.

Threshold testing: Threshold testing in ACM follows the same algorithm as the Medtronic RVCM algorithm.

Programmability: The programmable options are the same as the corresponding options in the Medtronic RVCM.

Medtronic: Left Ventricular Capture Management (LVCM)

Method for AVC: Capture is verified by detecting LV to RV conduction. Before threshold testing, the device delivers eight left ventricular-only paced beats and measures the LV to RV conduction times. If conduction times are consistent during four consecutive beats, verification of capture can be performed. Next, atrial pacing with a prolonged AV delay is performed and if RV sensing occurs before LV pacing, then LVCM cannot be performed; LVCM requires that RV sensing be detected from LV pacing, not from AV conduction.

Lead compatibility: Any LV lead.

Beat-to-Beat capture assessment: Not present.

Threshold testing: Threshold testing in LVCM follows the same algorithm as the corresponding RVCM algorithm.

Programmability: The programmable options are the same as the corresponding options in the Medtronic RVCM. In addition, a maximum output can be programmed to help avoid diaphragmatic stimulation.

Biotronik: Automatic Capture Control (ACC)

Method for AVC: Measurement of ventricular ER. After a pacing pulse, there is a blanking period of 20 ms, followed by an ER evaluation over the next 60 ms. The sensed/paced AV delay is shortened to 15/50 ms to ensure ventricular pacing.

Lead compatibility: Any lead, but low polarization lead recommended.

Initial setup: Before capture verification is turned On, a signal quality check must be passed. Ventricular pacing is delivered at the maximum programmable output (up to 6.4 V), and if there is failure to capture, ACC is turned Off. Next, five pulses with double stimulation (one pacing pulse followed by a second pacing pulse at 100 ms) at maximum output are delivered. The polarization artifact is measured in the second, refractory pulse and if higher than a certain limit, ACC is disabled. If the first quality check fails, the device is programmed to a maximum predetermined output. If the first quality check is successful, but three subsequent quality checks fail, then the device is automatically programmed to the maximum predetermined output plus a safety margin of up to 1.2 V after disabling ACC.

Beat-to-Beat capture assessment: Present.

Response to failed capture: A safety backup pulse is delivered at the existing amplitude with the pulse width extended to 1.0 ms, within 130 ms of a noncaptured pulse. To minimize fusion, the AV is delayed in the subsequent beat and then returns to the normal AV delay in the third beat. If loss of capture is detected in three consecutive beats with these varying AV delays, a signal quality check is reinitiated and the threshold search algorithm is started.

Threshold testing: Threshold testing is activated by loss of capture during beat-to-beat analysis, or twice during daily programmed intervals. Threshold testing begins at the maximum programmed output. The amplitude then decrements until loss of capture is noted. Thresholds are ultimately determined to a resolution of 0.1 V and the output is programmed to the threshold plus the programmed safety margin.

Programmability: ACC can be set to On, Off, or Monitor. In the monitor mode, thresholds are checked but pacing outputs are not reprogrammed based on threshold measurements. Maximum output can be programmed up to 6.4 V. The ventricular output safety margin can be programmed between 0.3 V through 1.2 V. The minimum amplitude can also be programmed.

ELA: Ventricular Autothreshold

Method for AVC: Measurement of ER during the first 63 ms following a paced beat.

Lead compatibility: Unipolar or bipolar. Low polarization lead recommended.

Beat-to-Beat capture assessment: No.

Threshold testing: Testing is performed when (a) there is a manual change in the ventricular pacing function, (b) magnet mode, (c) manual trigger, (d) scheduled interval of every 6 hours, or (e) lead measurements are made. To begin threshold testing, the AV delay is shortened by 63 ms to avoid fusion. Pacing output is set to 1.95 V and is decreased to 0.15 V gradually until loss of capture is noted. The programmed pacing output is then changed to twice the determined threshold. If the threshold test fails to identify the threshold, the pacing output is set to 5 V.

Programmability: Autothreshold can be set to Off, Auto, and, as with other algorithms, Monitor only. The minimum pulse amplitude can be selected between 2.5 and 3.5 V. The programmable pulse widths are limited to values between 0.1 and 0.5 ms.

Clinical Outcomes

St. Jude Medical's AutoCapture is the oldest and best-studied AVC algorithm. Multiple studies, including an early multicenter study,[7] have confirmed the efficacy and safety of this AVC algorithm with near complete lack of adverse events. There was minimal need for backup pacing and a near total lack of failure to capture with backup pacing when the patients were followed with external monitors.

The greatest benefit from using AVC remains the promise of extended battery life and the need for potentially fewer procedures to change the generator. When compared to the traditional empirical setting with the pacing output at twice the manually measured threshold, conservative estimates are that AVC can provide an 8- to 12-month savings in battery life (Fig 8.7).[8] This effect is more pronounced in patients with thresholds higher than 2.0 V at 0.5 ms; however, it is not as significant in patients with low thresholds closer to 0.5 V at 0.5 ms. Individual patients who have sudden and significant rises in pacing thresholds stand to benefit considerably.

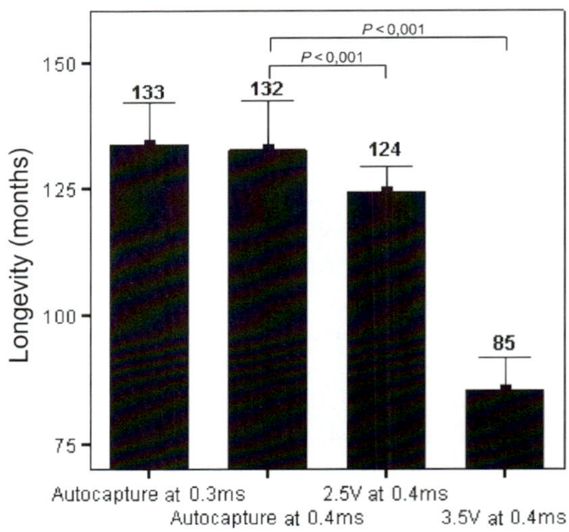

Figure 8.7 Projections of device longevity. Projections of device longevity for different programming based on threshold data measured at 13–14 months of follow-up. (Reprinted with permission from Boriani et al.)

Limitations

Although AVC has clear benefits, primarily related to prolonged battery life and minimized need for generator changes, a few limitations must be considered. There remains a small percentage (approximately 5%–10%) of patients in whom ER cannot easily be measured[9] and in whom AVC either cannot be programmed or leads to either ER oversensing or undersensing.

Early battery depletion from ER undersensing is one of the more commonly encountered side effects of AVC. If ER is undersensed, then most algorithms discussed earlier will record failure to capture at relatively high outputs and will switch to a high output mode. This output is usually much higher than the output that would otherwise have been programmed manually and ironically will lead to quicker drain on battery life. More worrisome, but less commonly seen, ER oversensing can lead to failure to provide backup pacing. This can lead to an underestimated threshold and a programmed output below the true capture threshold. The widespread use of modern bipolar, low polarization leads is helping eliminate many of the traditional difficulties with ER sensing.

The increasing complexity of these algorithms can also lead to diagnostic dilemmas. A case was reported where failure to capture at an intrinsic atrial rate near the maximum tracking rate resulted in pacing alternans.[10] Of greater concern are life-threatening arrhythmias that have been reported with AVC. In one report,[11] a premature ventricular contraction (PVC) occurred simultaneously with an atrial-paced event, resulting in the blanking by the device of the PVC. After the programmed paced AV delay, a ventricular signal was delivered and was correctly detected as failure to capture. The high-output backup paced beat was then delivered 340 ms after the initial PVC. Because this occurred on the T wave, ventricular fibrillation was induced (see fig 4.15 on page 94). Although exceedingly rare and likely dependent on particular patient characteristics, these scenarios will require refinement of the backup pacing algorithms.

References

1. Hellestrand KJ, Burnett PJ, Milne JR, et al. Effect of the antiarrhythmic agent flecainide acetate on acute and chronic pacing thresholds. *Pacing Clin Electrophysiol.* 1983;6(5 Pt 1):892–899.
2. Shepard RB, Kim J, Colvin EC, et al. Pacing threshold spikes months and years after implant. *Pacing Clin Electrophysiol.* 1991:14(11 Pt 2):1835–1841.
3. Funke HD. [Threshold pacemaker—a new principle of myocardial electric stimulation]. *Z Kreislaufforsch.* 1972;61(9):853–862.
4. Preston TA, Bowers DL. The automatic threshold tracking pacemaker. *Med Instrum.* 1974;8(6):322–325.
5. Luria D, Gurevitz O, Bar D, et al. Use of automatic threshold tracking function with non-low polarization leads: risk for algorithm malfunction. *Pacing Clin Electrophysiol.* 2004;27(4):453–459.
6. Sperzel J, Neuzner J, Schwarz T, et al. Reduction of pacing output coupling capacitance for sensing the evoked response. *Pacing Clin Electrophysiol.* 2001;24(9 Pt 1):1377–1382.
7. Clarke M, Liu B, Schüller H, et al. Automatic adjustment of pacemaker stimulation output correlated with continuously monitored capture thresholds: a multicenter study. European Microny Study Group. *Pacing Clin Electrophysiol.* 1998;21(8): 1567–1575.
8. Boriani G, Rusconi L, Biffi M, et al. Role of ventricular AutoCapture function in increasing longevity of DDDR pacemakers: a prospective study. *Europace.* 2006;8(3):216–220.
9. Ribeiro AL, Rincón LG, Oliveira BG, et al. Automatic adjustment of pacing output in the clinical setting. *Am Heart J.* 2004;147(1):127–131.
10. Chun HJ, Cock K, Wang PJ, et al. Pacemaker alternans terminated by telemetry wand: what is the mechanism? *Heart Rhythm.* 2008;5(7): 1080–1082.
11. Sweeney MO, Porkolab FL. Ventricular fibrillation induced by double premature ventricular pacing stimuli in a dual-chamber pacemaker with AutoCapture. *Heart Rhythm.* 2009;6(3): 429–432.

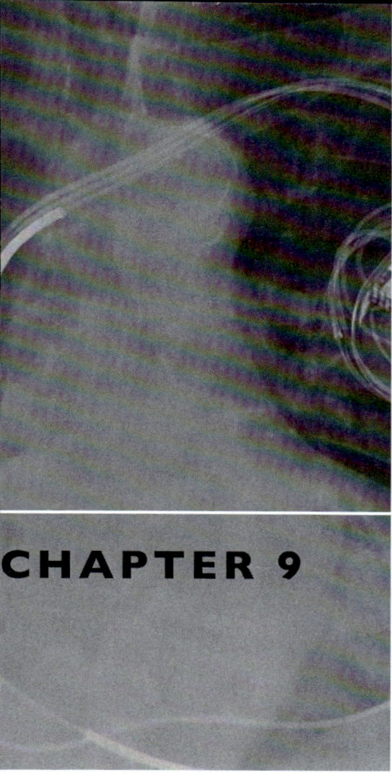

Sensor-Driven Pacing

CHAPTER 9

Chu-Pak Lau, Chung-Wah Siu, and Hung Fat Tse

Introduction

Sinus node chronotropic incompetence may occur in up to 30% of patients with sinus node disease. In addition, patients with a slow ventricular response in atrial fibrillation may have inadequate heart rates during activity. Implantable sensors for cardiac pacing were therefore developed as alternatives to allow a pacing system to respond to exercise and nonexercise requirements. Sensors are now a programmable option of almost all bradycardia pacemakers. In addition, sensors are used for purposes other than rate augmentation—such as detection of ventricular capture and monitoring heart failure, sleep disordered breathing, and hemodynamic or ischemic status.

In this chapter, the physiological basis of sensor-driven pacing and the clinical applications of currently available sensors in implantable devices are discussed. The chronotropic incompetence especially in diseased state such as heart failure will be defined. Recent studies on sensor-driven pacing modes (VVIR, DDDR, AAIR; septal and biventricular rate adaptive pacing), and their clinical benefits are reviewed.

Physiological Basis of Sensor-Driven Pacing

Atrioventricular (AV) synchrony enhances cardiac output by augmenting the stroke volume by 20% to 30% during exercise. However, this increase is relatively small compared with the three- to fourfold increase achieved by an increase in rate. The relative contribution of AV synchrony and rate increase in patients with complete AV block was studied in dual chamber (DDD) and a rate matched ventricular pacing (VVI) mode.[1] At rest, the cardiac output during DDD pacing was 18% higher compared

Pacemakers and Implantable Cardioverter Defibrillators: An Expert's Manual. © 2010 Amin Al-Ahmad, Kenneth A. Ellenbogen, Andrea Natale, and Paul J. Wang, eds. Cardiotext Publishing, ISBN: 978-0-9790164-6-2.

with VVI pacing as a result of increase in stroke volume, and the left ventricular (LV) filling pressure was also lower. However during exercise, the net cardiac output was only 8% higher during DDD pacing compared with VVI pacing at an identical rate. An equivalent exercise capacity was reported in another study,[2] and both DDD and rate matched VVI were superior to fixed rate VVI pacing during exercise. Cardiac output was similar at near maximal exercise between the two modes, but at lower workload levels, cardiac output was maintained by an increased arteriovenous oxygen saturation difference and arterial lactate level. In addition, systolic and mean blood pressures were lower when exercise was performed without AV synchrony. These findings suggest rate response is the primary driver for exercise cardiac hemodynamics although maintaining AV synchrony remains important.

Exercise Response in Heart Failure

In a patient with heart failure, LV filling pressures are elevated, and the heart is working at the flat portion of the Frank-Starling curve. An increase in heart rate is the only means to increase cardiac output. In a study of 22 patients with poor LV function and implanted rate adaptive pacemakers,[3] the benefit of rate adaptation was higher in those with poorer LV function.

In a study of patients with implanted cardiac resynchronization therapy (CRT) devices,[4] chronotropic incompetence defined as maximum heart rate < 70% age predicated maximum was found to be present in 70% of heart failure patients. In this group of patients, sensor-driven CRT pacing improved maximum oxygen consumption and work capacity compared with CRT pacing without rate adaption. This increment is independent of the shortening of AV interval shortening during exercise. Taken together, these data suggest that rate modulation plays a critical role in some patients with impaired LV function who required pacing therapy, even in patients with CRT.

Heart Rate Modulation for Nonexercise Needs

Exercise is only one of the many physiologic requirements for variation in heart rate. A number of other physiological events can lead to increases or fluctuations in heart rate. An appropriate compensatory heart rate response is especially important in pathophysiological conditions such as anemia, acute blood loss, or other causes of hypovolemia, and during febrile illness. Mental stress or emotional upset leads to an increase in heart rate. The sinus rate increases with upright posture when cardiac output decreases. Isometric exercise also results in an increase in cardiac output and heart rate in most people. The changes in heart rate that occurs during various physiologic maneuvers (eg, Valsalva maneuver) and baroreceptor reflexes may also be potentially important. The potential benefit, if any, of sensor-driven pacing in these physiological conditions has not been well studied.

Ideal Sensor Characteristics

Based on the physiology of the normal sinus node, a sensor system to overcome chronotropic incompetence needs to be sensitive to both exercise and nonexercise needs. It should be specific so that rate changes inappropriate for metabolic demands are avoided. Finally, rate modulation should occur at an appropriate response time and the magnitude of its response should be proportional to the level of exercise load. Technically, a sensor should be easy to implement (preferably with a standard pacer and lead system), be stable in the body's internal environment, and avoid significant increases in pacemaker battery consumption.

Classification of Sensors

In a sensor-driven pacing system, a sensor (or a combination of sensors) must first detect a physical or physiologic parameter that is related to metabolic demand (Fig 9.1). Second, the rate-modulating circuit in the pulse generator must have an algorithm that relates changes in the sensed parameter to a change in pacing rate. Third, because the relationship between the magnitude of the physical or physiologic change and the desired heart rate response differs among patients, physician input is usually necessary to adjust the "algorithm" (generally by programming one or more rate responsive variables). Most sensors operate in open loop algorithm: the induced rate changes do not induce a negative feedback on the sensor parameter. In a closed loop sensor, the induced hemodynamic changes will reduce the level of the sensed parameter that is responsible for the initial rate adaptation (a negative feedback loop), and theoretically, very little programming is required in such a system.

Technical Classification

A practical classification is to categorize sensors according to the technical methods used to measure the sensed parameter (Table 9.1). Body movements during exercise result in changes in acceleration forces that are transmitted to the pacemaker. Sensors capable of measuring the acceleration or vibration forces in the pulse generator are broadly referred to as *activity* sensors. Technically, detection of body movement can be achieved using a piezoelectric crystal, an accelerometer, a tilt switch, or an inductive sensor. Each of these devices transduces motion of the body either directly into a voltage or indirectly into measurable changes in the electrical resistance of a piezoresistive crystal. Activity sensing is the most widely used control parameter in rate adaptive pacing because of its ease of implementation and its compatibility with standard unipolar and bipolar pacing leads, both in atrial and ventricular stimulations.

Impedance is a measurement of the resistivity to an injected electric current across a tissue. The impedance principle has been used extensively for measuring respiratory parameters and parameters associated with ventricular contractility, such as relative stroke volume or the pre-ejection interval. The simplicity of impedance has enabled it to be used with pacing leads. The pulse generator casing is used as one electrode for the measurement of impedance in

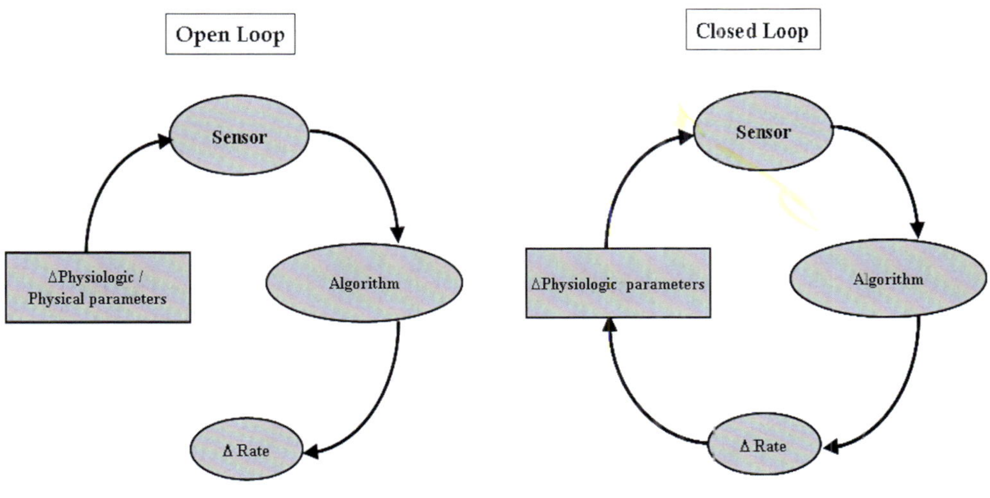

Fig 9.1 Open and closed loop sensor-driven pacing. Open loop: The physiologic or physical change detected by the sensor is converted to a change in rate using an algorithm. The resultant rate change does not have a negative feedback effect on the physiologic/physical parameter. Closed loop: The physiologic change detected by the sensor is converted to a change in rate using an algorithm. The resultant rate change induces a change in the physiologic parameter in the opposite direction, thereby establishing a negative feedback loop.

most of these pacing systems, and the pacing lead constitutes one or more of the impedance electrodes and can be used to detect relative changes in either ventilatory mechanics such as respiration rate or minute ventilation (MV). When used in a unipolar configuration at the right ventricular (RV) lead, impedance measurements have been used to assess ventricular contractility in the so-called closed loop stimulation (CLS) sensor.

The *intracardiac ventricular electrogram* resulting from a supra-threshold pacing stimulus has been used to provide several parameters that can guide rate modulation. The total du-

Methods	Physiologic Parameter	Examples Models	Manufacturers
Vibration / acceleration sensing	Body movement	Sigma, Kappa, EnRhythm	Medtronic Inc. Vitatron
		Talent Miniswing, Neway	ELA-Sorin
		Insignia, Pulsar Max, Discovery	Boston Scientific
		Actos, Protos, Philos	Biotronik
		Identity, Integrity, Affinity	St. Jude Medical
Impedance sensing	Minute ventilation	Kappa 400	Medtronic Inc.
		Talent	ELA-Sorin
		Insignia, Pulsar Max	Boston Scientific
	Ventricular inotropic parameter	Protos, Inos	Biotronik
Ventricular evoked response	Evoked QT interval*	Diamond, Clarity, Selection AF	Vitatron
Special sensors on pacing electrode	**Physical Parameters** 1. Central venous temperature 2. dP/dt 3. Right ventricular pressure 4. Pulmonary arterial pressure 5. Peak endocardial acceleration **Chemical Parameters** 1. pH 2. Mixed venous oxygen saturation 3. Catecholamine	Chronicle† BEST-Living system	Medtronic Inc. ELA-Sorin

Table 9.1 Major Classes of Sensors Used in Implanted Devices, Classified according to Method of Technical Realization. *Manufacturers and their locations:* Biotronik, GmbH & Co., Berlin, Germany; Boston Scientific, St. Paul, MN; ELA-Sorin, Rougemont, France; Medtronic Inc., Minneapolis, MN. *Currently no longer available in the market. † For hemodynamic monitoring only.

ration of depolarization and repolarization can be estimated by the interval from the pacing stimulus to the intracardiac T wave (the QT or stimulus-T interval). This parameter is sensitive to changes in heart rate and circulating catecholamines and can be derived from the paced intracardiac electrogram with conventional pacing electrodes. This was incorporated into a QT sensing pacemaker, making use of the advantage of the shortening of QT interval during exercise and stress.[5]

The last group of sensors is those incorporated into the pacing lead. Examples of these specialized leads include thermistors (used to measure blood temperature), piezoelectric crystals (used to measure pulmonary artery or RV pressure), optical sensors (used to measure mixed venous oxygen level), and accelerometers at the tip of pacing leads. Some of these sensors measure highly physiologic parameters. For example, mixed venous oxygen saturation is closely related to oxygen consumption during exercise. Physical activities increase cardiac output and oxygen extraction from the blood, and a widening of the tissue arteriovenous oxygen difference occurs if the cardiac output does not match the requirements of increased tissue oxygen consumption. The fall in oxygen saturation will trigger an increase in rate that will improve cardiac output and increase the oxygen saturation. Theoretically a closed loop system, although technical complexity limits its use for sensor-driven pacing.

Using an accelerometer incorporated at the tip of a unipolar ventricular electrode, the contractile state can be assessed indirectly from the endocardial vibration generated during isovolumic contraction of the heart, a parameter known as *peak endocardial acceleration* (PEA). PEA is significantly increased by emotional stress, exercise, and inotropic stimulation.

Over the years, many of the aforementioned sensors have been tested and implemented in implantable devices. There are significant differences in rate response characteristics among sensors, notably between their sensitivity and specificity (Table 9.2). Activity, MV, and CLS are the most common sensors in pacing today. Amongst these, the activity sensor is always used as a default sensor because of its reliability and ease of implementation. Its lack of proportionality has not been found to be a major clinical disadvantage. Sensors in special leads have generally been limited because of their uncertain long-term reliability and pacemaker compatibility during subsequent generator replacement.

	Speed	Proportionality	Specificity	Sensitivity	Reliability refers to technical and clinical realization
Activity	High	Low	Low	Low	High
Minute ventilation	Moderate	High	Moderate	Low	Moderate
QT	Low	Moderate	Moderate	Moderate	Low
PEA	Moderate	Moderate	Moderate	High	Moderate
CLS	Moderate	Moderate	Moderate	High	Moderate

Table 9.2 Relative Performance of Different Sensors. Reliability refers to technical and clinical realization for rate adaptive pacing. Abbreviations: CLS, closed loop stimulation; PEA, peak endocardial acceleration.

Current Sensor-Driven Pacemakers

Activity Sensing and Accelerometer-based Pacemakers

Activity sensing is the most widely used sensor, alone or in combination. As activity-based pacemakers are operationally simple and do not require a special sensor outside the pulse generator casing, they work with any type of pacing lead, have excellent long-term stability, are highly reliable, and are implanted like an ordinary pacemaker. Although they may not be excellent proportional sensors, they react promptly to the start and end of physical exercise. The first activity sensors were piezoelectric crystals that responded mostly to the frequency of vibrations transmitted to the pulse generator, and their response was more variable depending on the pulse generator and the pocket. Subsequent activity sensors are accelerometers that detect body accelerations and have less interpatient variability and better proportionality (Fig 9.2).

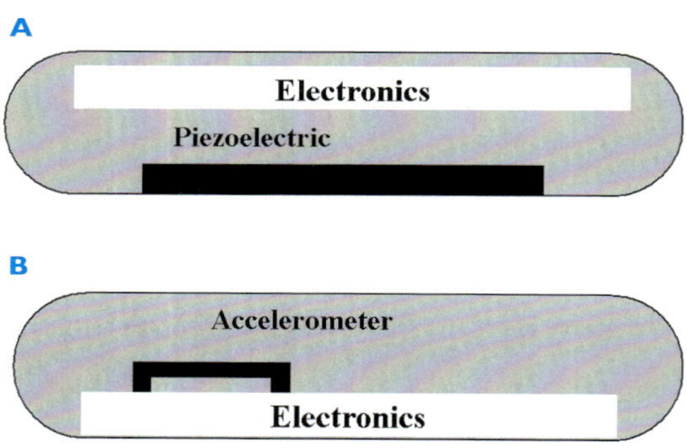

Fig 9.2 Schematic representation of two different designs of activity sensors shown as a cross-section of a pacemaker. **A**: The piezoelectric sensor is bound to the inside surface of the pacemaker case. Vibration is sensed through tissue contact. The mechanical forces are transmitted by the surrounding connective tissue, fatty tissue, and muscles. The extent of contact and the coupling mass of the mechanical forces can vary considerably between patient and maturation of the pacemaker pocket. **B**: The accelerometer is mounted on the pacemaker hybrid circuitry and thus the seismic mass of the accelerometer is fixed. Therefore, measured accelerations are independent of surrounding tissue and patient physical properties.

Current devices

Medtronic activity sensing devices (Kappa 700, 900, 400, EnPulse, and EnRhythm) The Activitrax and Thera devices were the first generation activity-sensing system using a piezoelectric crystal bonded to the inside of the pacemaker casing to detect activity. Activity levels that exceed a programmable threshold are counted, and the number of counts exceeding a programmable threshold is used to determine the rate response. The physician adjusts the overall rate response by programming the activity threshold and the rate response slope. Typically this instrumentation allows a good response from the lower rate to about 100 bpm during daily activities. A proportionate response to higher levels of activity may be more difficult to achieve, and will depend on the patient and the programming setting. These devices were highly clinically effective when first introduced.

In the Kappa (700 and 900), EnPulse, and EnRhythm series, a "beam accelerometer" is attached to the circuit board to detect movement in the anteroposterior plane. Instead of a fixed threshold, a "rolling threshold" is used to provide a count of activity that is dependent not only on the frequency of counts that cross the threshold, but also on the strength of these counts. This rolling threshold in effect minimizes the detection of low-intensity and high-frequency accelerations such as those occurring during a car ride, but allows high-intensity signals during physical activities to be detected.

The sensor-driven rate is adjusted by the use of Activity of Daily Living (ADL) and Exertion Response (ER) programming (Fig 9.3). The physician determines the lower rate limit (LRL), the ADL rate, and the sensor-driven upper rate limit (SURL). When sensor-driven pacing is first initiated at the nominal setting of ADL response of 3 (out of 5), counts between 12 and 20 will also give the ADL rate, during which the rate response will be stable. When counts are $>$ 20, ER will occur to the maximum programmed SURL. The flat portion of the response curve corresponds to 25% of the total counts. Adjustment of the ADL and ER to a more sensitive setting will decrease the number of counts to reach between

ADL rate and SURL, and shorten the ADL portion of the response curve.

The actual number of counts to affect a rate response is not fixed, but is different among patients. Rather, an ADL response of 3 implies that the patient will spend up to 30 minute/day at sensor rate at or above the ADL. This is achieved by adjusting the rate/count relationship to achieve this percentage of rate response. Similarly, an ER response of 3 means that the patient will be spending about 20 minutes/week at the higher rates (eg, between 105 and 120 per minute). Thus, in effect, the physician is adjusting the target rate profile for a patient by altering the ADL and ER, based on the medical condition of the patient and his/her activities. This is termed rate profile optimization, which typically adjusts itself to the optimal rate profile in steps over days to months.

St. Jude Medical activity sensing devices (Affinity, Integrity, Identity, and Vitality) These activity devices use an Omnisense accelerometer bonded to the circuit board, and are sensitive to accelerations that occur in the anteroposterior axis. Activity counts above a programmable threshold (1 = most sensitive, 7 = least sensitive) will be integrated and translated to a rate response using a rate response slope (1 = least sensitive, 16 = most sensitive).

The threshold level can be adjusted manually or automatically (AUTO). In the AUTO setting, the device measures the sensor activity level over the preceding 18 hours to determine the threshold parameter. The AUTO threshold can be adjusted manually using AUTO threshold offset. Similarly, the slope of response can be calibrated manually or automatically. In the slope AUTO adjustment, the device records the activity variance occurring above the threshold over the last 7 days, to form a resting level against which acceleration change will effect rate response. The slope is adjusted to achieve a rate response such that almost 1% heart rate occurs beyond 23% of heart rate reserve. Typically the slope adjusts by a factor of 2 each week. In the event that the patient is immobile for the last week as indicated by the small activ-

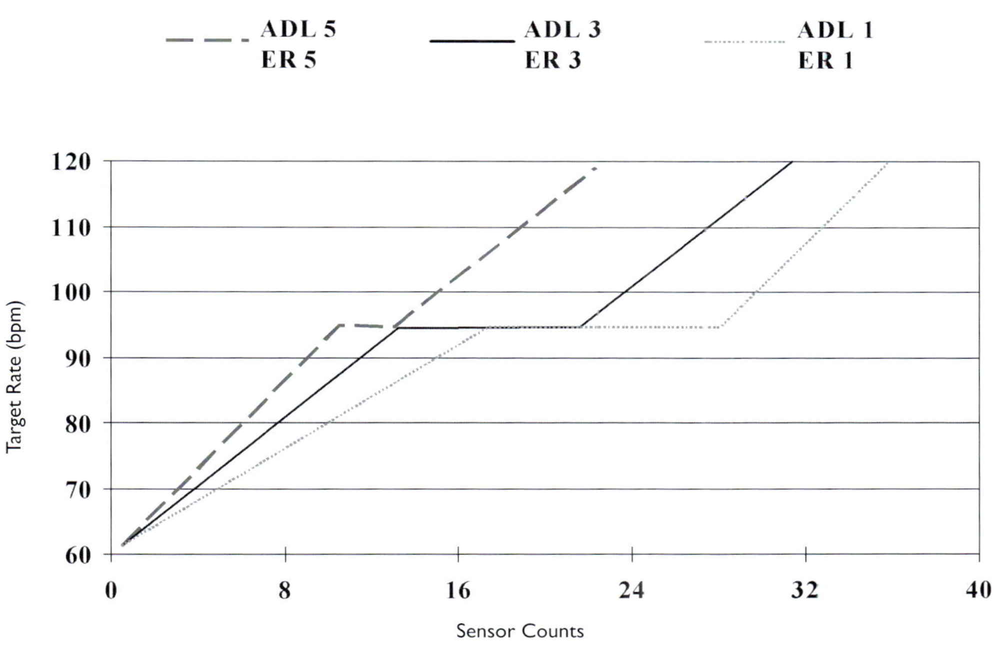

Fig 9.3 Triphasic rate-responsive curve of the Medtronic accelerometer activity-sensing pacemakers. The ADL and ER determine the rate response to an ordinary exertion level and peak exercise, respectively. Abbreviations: ADL, activity of daily living response; ER, exertion response.

ity variance, the slope setting will be held constant. This will avoid undue rate response when the patient resumes activity. In addition, rapid manual slope adjustment can be achieved by instructing the patient to perform an exercise at a prescribed slope. The Prediction Model will attempt to suggest an alternative slope based on the detected rate response. In addition, the onset and recovery kinetics are separately programmable. The device also features a rest rate set below the LRL. The rest rate is attained when the acceleration sensor does not register significant counts (the activity variance level) over an extended period of time, thus implying the patient is resting or asleep.

Boston Scientific activity sensing devices (Insignia and Pulsar Max) An accelerometer mounted in the circuit board is used to detect anteroposterior acceleration. Apart from LRL and URL, four other parameters are used to determine the rate response: Response factor (1 = least sensitive, 16 = most sensitive); Activity threshold (very low, low, medium-low, medium-high, high, and very high); reaction time; and recovery time. Programming can be affected either manually or automatically using the Automatic Response Factor. In this method, the physician uses the Expert Ease feature in the programmer to decide the LRL, SURL, and the Sensor Rate Target, based on the patient's age, gender, exercise frequency, and target heart rate during exercise derived from a population average. After inputting these parameters, an initial nominal slope such as 8 (1–16) is programmed. The Automatic Response Factor will track the maximum sensor rate each day for a week, and the average of this maximum will be compared to the Sensor Rate Target. The response factor will then be scaled to either effect a more aggressive or conservative response, depending on whether the average rate falls below or exceeds the "Sensor Rate Target" by 5 bpm, respectively.

Other activity sensors ELA-Sorin has introduced a gravitational sensor that is used either alone (Swing) or in combination with PEA sensor (MiniLiving). The gravitational sensor utilizes the vibrations from a mercury ball to measure body activity. ELA has an accelerometer activity sensor (Opus G) that uses a half-bridge variable capacitance accelerometer.

The accelerometer senses anteroposterior axis at a frequency range of 0.6 to 6 Hz, and samples acceleration signals every 1.56 seconds. The device can be programmed manually or automatically using the "Autocalibration." The level of acceleration at rest is reset daily based on the lowest mean acceleration of 64 consecutive measurements. The maximum mean acceleration of 8 consecutive accelerations is used to match the programmed upper sensor rate.

Clinical results

Clinical studies have convincingly demonstrated that activity-based pacing systems offer the potential for greater exercise capacity and fewer related symptoms than do VVI pacemakers. In an early clinical study of a piezoelectric vibration-based sensor pacemaker, Benditt et al[6] compared exercise tolerance during VVI and VVIR pacing using cardiopulmonary treadmill exercise tests. Sensor pacing prolonged exercise duration by 35% and led to similar increments in peak oxygen consumption and oxygen consumption at anaerobic threshold. Activity sensor-driven pacing also reduced the patient's perception of exertion at comparable exercise levels, and the benefit was sustained when exercise testing was repeated after an average of 5 months of follow-up. Furthermore, at the time of follow-up exercise testing, reversion of the pacing system to a VVI mode resulted in prompt deterioration of both observed oxygen consumption and exercise duration. The VVIR mode was compared to DDD pacing in crossover studies,[7–8] and no significant difference between the DDD and VVIR modes were found with respect to symptom scores, maximal exercise performance (treadmill), or plasma concentrations of epinephrine, norepinephrine, and atrial natriuretic peptide.

The efficacy of automatic Rate Profile Optimization over time has been investigated.[9] Eleven patients with the Kappa 700 pacemakers performed treadmill testing at 1 month,

1 year, and 2 years after implantation. Based on the sinus profile at follow-up, the investigators found that the use of a more aggressive slope was needed to match the sinus rate profile. This required the change of ADL response from 3 to 4 and ER from 3 to 4 at 1 year, and the change of activity threshold from medium/low to low at 2 years. These adjustments enabled better approximation of pacing rate to sinus rate during treadmill exercise. Exercise capacity was maintained during the 2 years of study. Absence of activity counts as detected by an accelerometer has been used to determine the rest rate,[10] without affecting the overall appropriate rate response.

Limitations of activity sensing devices

Activity sensing may give inappropriate heart rate responses when subjected to environmental vibrations, such as those induced by the movement of a motor vehicle over rough terrain or those resulting from air travel or the use of appliances or machinery. The piezoelectric vibrational sensor also responds to the application of static pressure on the pulse generator, which may be important when the patient lies prone. This false-positive response to pressure is no longer a problem with pacemakers that incorporate an accelerometer.

The effects of various means of locomotion on pacing rate were assessed for different activity-based pacemakers.[11] Three different activity-based pacing systems (peak counting algorithm, integration type, and accelerometers) were strapped to the chests of volunteers. Bicycling on the street resulted in higher pacing rates than did stationary bicycling for each type of pacemaker, although none of the pacemakers reached the heart rate achieved by the normal sinus node. During driving, the pacemakers increased the pacing rate, although the intrinsic sinus rate continued to be higher. In passively riding passengers, the pacemakers tended to produce a higher pacing rate than that of the normal sinus node. Independent of the sensor, activity-initiated rate response is dependent on the manner in which activity is being carried out, rather than on the exercise workload, and proportionality is generally limited.[12] They may manifest paradoxically slower heart rates during walking uphill than during walking downhill. Non–exercise-related stresses such as emotional changes will not be detected, which limited the sensor sensitivity.

Minute Ventilation (MV) Sensing

Although a respiratory rate-sensing pacemaker had been in use as early as 1983, it was limited by the need of an auxiliary subcutaneous electrode and easy interference by arm movement because of unipolar impedance sensing.[13] All subsequent generations of respiratory sensor detect MV for rate adaptation. The advantage of this sensor is that no additional hardware (except for a bipolar pacing lead in either the right atrium or ventricle) is required. It is proportional and responds at a reasonable speed. It entails some battery usage but is not excessive.

Medtronic Kappa 400 The Medtronic MV pacer is marketed as a dual sensor device. The MV component requires a bipolar lead. Subthreshold 30-μV biphasic pulses at 1 ms are injected between the electrode (either atrial or ventricular) and pacemaker case at 16 Hz, and the resulting impedance measured between the lead tip and the case. Changes in MV are measured as MV counts over a 32-second short-term moving average to avoid transient events such as coughing and speech that affect impedance. The short-term average is compared over an 18-hour long-term average to effect a change.

Medtronic Kappa 400 has been evaluated using symptom-limited treadmill exercise testing.[14] All patients had cardiopulmonary gaseous analysis in conjunction with simultaneous recording of MV-induced impedance changes. The calibration between them during resting, supine, sitting, and the type of exercise (bicycle or treadmill) were made. The impedance-derived MV was smaller for sitting versus supine position, for shallow versus slow breathing, and for bicycle versus treadmill exercise, possibly due to change in chest cage geometry. Correlation coefficients of the best fit line for measured and device-based MV were high (> 0.9 in first, second, and third order polynomial equations).[15] Furthermore, the calibration between measured MV and impedance MV changes over time (between 1 week and 1 month). However, the changes were not correlative. This has implication in the need of continual automatic adaptation and the potential use of the sensor for MV monitoring.

Boston Scientific MV devices (Pulsar Max and Insignia) In the Boston Scientific devices, MV is available in conjunction with an accelerometer sensor, although the rate adaptive function can be used either alone or blended with the accelerometer. MV collected by either the atrial or ventricular lead (programmable) over 24 hours will be used as an average against which future changes in MV is compared for a rate response. The minimum time for achieving a baseline is 4 minutes (thus 4 → On). A linear response curve is used, and a total of 16 response factors can be chosen below the judged pacing rate for anaerobic threshold. This rate is also programmable. In between the pacing rate for anaerobic threshold and the maximum predicted heart rate, a gentler High Rate Response can be programmed. The adaptation can be made faster by activating the 4-minute Walk within 30-minute option, in which the subject is instructed to exercise to achieve the maximal MV change.

Telemetered MV impedance signal from a Boston Scientific MV device has been compared with measured MV in 20 patients.[16] Respiratory rate was accurately measured by the device during hyperventilation, with difference < 0.2 breath/minute. During 10-minute cycle ergometry at 50 W, the correlation between MV measured directly and that by the device was 0.99. Large individual variations between the measured and impedance MV slope exist, requiring individual rate response curves adjustment.

ELA-Sorin MV Devices (Chorus, Talent, Opus, Symphony, Rhapsody) The automatic slope algorithm in the Chorus determines the resting and maximum MV values on a daily basis. If MV over 128 cycles remains below the 24-hour MV average, the lower rate will decrease to the LRL. The device calculates the exercise MV signal by looking for the maximal MV signal and recalculates this value every eighth cycle. The exercise MV value is increased or decreased in 6% intervals. The mean resting and exercise MV values are used to adjust the rate-response slope automatically over the range of values from 1 to 15 in steps of 1. The response of the Talent DR (ELA Medical) during the exercise was compared in 81 patients. The correlation coefficient between the sensor rate- and programmer-derived sensor rate was 0.983 ± 0.005, and a linear relationship was observed between the heart rate reserve and MV reserve.[17]

Clinical experience of MV sensor pacemakers

MV is an indirect but reliable marker of metabolic demands, and in the first generation of MV pacer (Meta MV, Telectronics Pacing Systems), the rate response was proportional to the level of exertion and correlated with the sinus response.[18,19] Compared with VVI pacing, MV-driven VVIR pacing increased exercise capacity by 33%,[19] and maximal oxygen consumption and cardiac output are significantly better. In one study on 10 patients with the first version of MV driven-VVIR pacing, pacing rate was highly correlated with measured MV (r = 0.89), respiratory quotient (r = 0.89), VCO_2 (r = 0.87), tidal volume (r = 0.87), VO_2 (r = 0.84), and respiratory rate (r = 0.84). Maximum oxygen consumption also increased from 13.4 ± 3.4 to 16.3 ± 4.1 ml/kg per minute (P = 0.0004) using MV-driven pacing over VVI pacing.

Improvement in symptoms was also documented in the VVIR mode.[19] MV sensor has good long-term stability, and sensor programming is relatively simple, and the rate response was appropriate during daily activities. Compared to activity pacing, MV is significantly better in achieving a near-normal pacing rate—workload relationship, whereas activity sensing tends to overpace at low level of exercise and underpace at the peak exercise and in the recovery period.

Limitations

As expected with all impedance system, MV sensor is liable to be interfered by electromagnetic interference, arm swinging, coughing, and hyperventilation.[13] Artificial ventilation will induce a nonphysiological rate so that MV sensor needs to be disabled in this setting, such as during general anesthesia and in intubated patients. The use of MV devices in patients with lung disease and heart failure remains controversial. Because of filtering of cardiac component, MV sensor does not accurately reflect rate adaptation at high respiratory rate, which occurs commonly in children. A bipolar ventricular lead is needed for MV sensing. The battery current for MV sensing may take up about 2% of the total current of a dual chamber pacemaker.

It is possible for some sense amplifiers to sense the small impedance pulses unless some preventive steps are taken. In some products, a blanking period of about 1 ms is applied to the amplifiers to "blind" them to these pulses. In other cases, special balancing of the pulse is carried out, achieving the same objective.

Sensing of the impedance pulses by a surface ECG monitor is always a possibility and depends on the sensitivity of the ECG machine. The pulse width and the balancing of the impedance pulse influence this possibility.

Frequencies above a few kilohertz, such as generated by electrocautery and electrosurgery are detected by the rate-response circuitry and could drive a pacemaker to its maximum rate, and it is recommended to inactivate the rate-response function whenever electrosurgery is to be used. Respiration is also potentially influenced by phonation and coughing, which do not have direct relevance to change in cardiac output.

Unipolar Ventricular Impedance ("Closed-Loop Stimulation" CLS Sensor)

Cardiac contractility of the ventricle will increase during catecholamine stimulation, as occurs during exercise and emotional stresses. In the absence of an adequate rate response, exercise will induce a higher contractility that will decrease when rate response is adequate, thus establishing a negative feedback loop and a new steady contractility state. On the other hand, pacing rate increases per se can increase contractility, the so-called Treppe effect, although this has not been important in clinical practice. This parameter can be derived from a standard pacing lead, and has the potential to monitor heart function and catecholamine state.

Sensor and algorithm

The CLS sensor is based on unipolar impedance at the tip of a pacing lead.[20] Subthreshold pulses of automatically selected outputs (ranging from 100 to 400 μA), biphasic duration of 46 ms are emitted 50 to 300 ms after a sensed or paced ventricular event. During diastole (immediately after a Vp or Vs), there is significant amount of blood around the electrode tip, and the impedance is low. On the other hand, as contraction occurs, the walls surrounding the electrode tip get closer, and impedance rises (Fig 9.4A). A baseline waveform will occur dependent on the conduction state of the heart: AsVs, AsVp, ApVs, ApVp. Baseline CLS waveforms will only be acquired when the associated accelerometer indicates no activity, and a waveform will be discarded within 48 hours if not referenced. An average template of the baseline CLS waveform will take 2 to 3 days to optimize.

As contractility increases during exercise, unipolar impedance will change. The time integrated difference between the exercise and baseline impedance waveform is converted to a pacing rate using an Auto Response Factor, until SURL is reached for the first time. This Auto Response Factor is continually adaptive and is patient specific. Thereafter the response is determined by a programmable Exertion

Threshold Rate (ETR) (very low, low, medium, high, and very high) (Fig 9.4B). The ETR, acting through the Auto Response Factor, will determine that 80% of the heart rate will occur below the ETR and 20% above the ETR. A young and active individual will probably require a higher ETR than an inactive sedentary individual. Again, the type of rate profile attained will be determined by the cardiac condition, the patient's physical state, and the patient-specific Auto Response Factor, even though the same ETR is programmed.

While not strictly a dual sensor pacemaker, the incorporated accelerometer performs an On-Off function to decide on the acquisition of baseline CLS waveform and the CLS-driven response. Full CLS-driven rate according to the programmed ETR will be allowed only if the accelerometer registers exercise, otherwise only a 20 bpm rate above the LRL is allowed to enable nonexercise rate increase. In case of neurocardiogenic syncope, this rate-limiting algorithm can be inactivated for full sensor-driven response, as occurring during a syncopal episode.

Biotronik CLS devices (Inos, Protos) Acute measurement of CLS parameter (previously known as ventricular inotropic index) was taken in 82

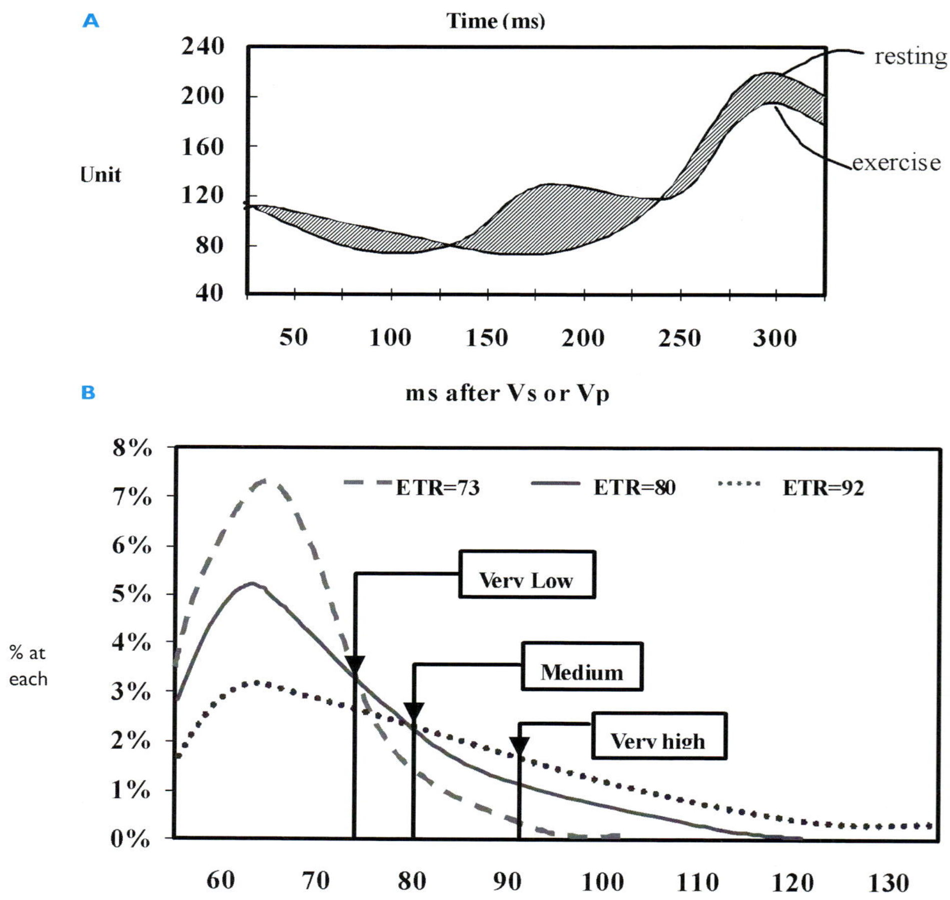

Fig 9.4 A: Changes in closed loop stimulation (CLS) during exercise. The hatched area represents reference between baseline and exercise CLS voltage. The area is converted to a rate using the exertion threshold rate (ETR). **B**: The rate profile at different programmed level with the lower rate set at 60 bpm. Setting an ETR of 80 bpm (medium) will result in 80% of rate occurring below 80 bpm.

patients with chronically implanted unipolar ventricular leads at the time of pulse generator replacement.[20] A wide fluctuation of baseline impedance was observed (500–1500 Ω), whereas CLS fluctuated by about 4 to 25 Ω, with a good correlation between CLS and the baseline impedance. A clinical study involving 205 patients was performed to evaluate the CLS pacemaker.[21] A significant proportion of these patients were young subjects with complete AV block due to Chagas' disease. Satisfactory rate modulation was reported in 93% of patients. In the remaining 7% of patients, rate adaptation could not be achieved because of such factors as poor exercise tolerance, severe myocardial dysfunction, or intermittent AV conduction. In a multicenter study[22] that included 178 VVIR (Biotronik Neos-PEP) and 84 DDDR devices (Biotronik Diplos-PEP and Inos DR), physiologic rate adaptation was possible in 93% and 96% of patients with these devices, respectively. Apart from exercise rate response, this study also involved mental stress testing using color-word matching and the infusion of inotropic agents. A moderate level of rate response was documented in some patients with CLS pacemakers during these nonexercise challenges over accelerometer-based pacing. Studies are underway to determine the benefit of CLS sensor pacing that occurs during mental stresses on cognitive function.[23]

There is interest in the use of this sensor to detect posture. Passive upright tilt, which deplete intravascular volume, will increase the inotropic state of the heart. In a multicenter study entitled INotropy Controlled pacing in Vasovagal SYncope (INVASY),[24] 50 patients with severe vasovagal syncope and positive head-up tilt test were randomized between DDD-CLS and DDI mode at 40 bpm. Seven of nine patients in the DDI arm-experienced syncope in 1 year, whereas only 4 of 41 patients in the DDD-CLS arm had presyncope. The authors suggested the efficacy of this approach, although a placebo effect of pacing was suspected to occur in 22% of patients. In 131 patients with chronotropic incompetence, CLS pacing resulted in a higher pacing rate compared with accelerometer sensor, but no difference in 6 minutes walking distances.[25] However, twice as many patients preferred the CLS mode. The use of CLS in the left ventricle as in a CRT device for monitoring would be of interest. So that alternative sensor-driven pacing can be chosen if needed.

Advantages and limitations

CLS appears to be an interesting sensor to measure contractility of the heart and can be achieved using a conventional ventricular pacing electrode. The demand on pacing energy is acceptable. As a contractility sensor, it is sensitive not only to exercise but also to nonexercise requirements, and it may therefore be used for monitoring cardiac contractility for non–rate augmentation purposes. CLS can only be used in a pacing mode that incorporates a ventricular lead. It is likely that CLS is affected by RV ischemia or cardioactive medications. These may influence rate adaptation with this sensor, although automatic adjustment may permit long-term function. A small proportion of patients are not suitable for CLS sensors because of severely impaired RV function, although it may be possible to identify such patients preoperatively.

Peak Endocardial Acceleration (PEA)

Sensor and algorithm

The contractile state of the heart can be identified by the maximal velocity of shortening of unloaded myocardial contractile elements, and this can be measured with a catheter tip accelerometer attached to the ventricular wall. The PEA represents the endocardial vibration measured by the accelerometer in the right ventricle during isovolumetric contraction phase of the ventricles. This signal is in close relationship to the intensity of the first heart sound. This sensor, developed by ELA-Sorin, is termed the BEST sensor (Biomechanical Endocardial Sorin Transducer). This microaccelerometer consists of an acceleration sensor built into an undeformable capsule located on the tip of a standard unipolar ventricular pacing lead. The lead is placed against the RV wall so as to be sensitive to its acceleration and insensitive to the pressure of blood and myocardium (Fig 9.5A). This system has a frequency response up to 1 kHz and a sensitivity of 5 mV/G (1 G = 9.8 m/s per second). In preliminary animal experience using an external system and an implantable radiotelemetry system, the PEA was reported not to be affected by heart rate but significantly increased by emotional stress, exercise stress testing, and inotropic stimulation.[26] The PEA signal changes in parallel to the maximal LV dp/dt and appears to measure the global LV contractile performance rather than the regional mechanical function. The PEA signal that occurs at 150 ms after the R wave corresponds to the isovolumetric contraction phase of the left ventricle (PEA-I).[27] A smaller signal also occurs in the 100-ms period after the T wave, the so-called PEA-2, which corresponds to the isovolumetric LV relaxation. PEA-2 is related to peak negative dp/dt (r = 0.92) and aortic diastolic pressure (r = 0.91).[27] For the future application in hemodynamic monitoring the PEA sensor has been incorporated into a RA lead (sonR sensor). Preliminary results suggest the sonR sensor to be similar to the RV PEA signal and suggest that it may be feasible to use it in a CRT-D setting.[28]

The BEST sensor rate adaptive pacemakers (Sorin BEST-Living Systems: MiniLiving D and S) These devices use a dedicated unipolar ventricular pace/sense lead, which is IS1 compatible. Together with the two electrodes for PEA signals, a tripolar connector is necessary. These devices also incorporate an activity sensor using the vibration from a mercury ball (Gravitational sensor). In the PEA mode, continuous PEA signal collected over time is used as a reference, against which the change in PEA is compared. A linear pacing rate to PEA signal rate adaptive curve is used to control the rate response.

In the dual sensor mode, the combined output from both sensors is used to drive the rate to a middle level, further rate increase will be effected with PEA sensor alone. In addition, prolonged absence (about 45 minutes) of signals from both the gravitational and PEA sensor will allow the base rate to decrease to the programmable rest rate. On the other hand, once the sensors were active, approach to rate response will be rapid.

Clinical results

A multicenter study has shown a good correlation between the sinus rate and PEA sensor-indicated rate during daily life activities and submaximal stress test.[26,29] Similar results were

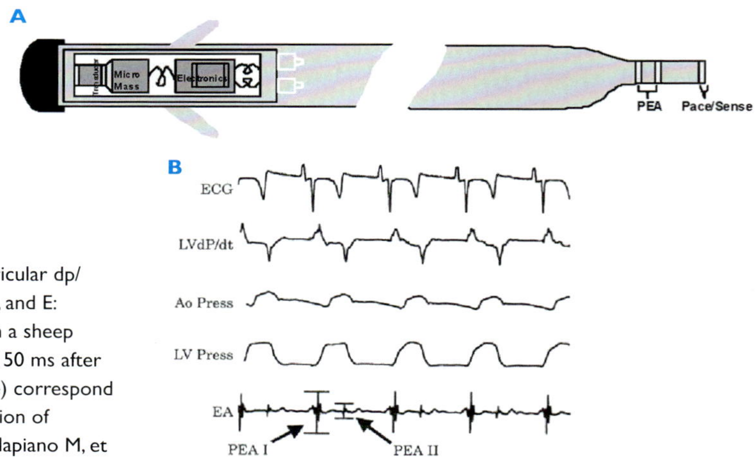

Fig 9.5 **A**: The Biomechanical Endocardial ELA-Sorin Transducer (BEST) sensor (ELA-Sorin) consists of a microaccelerometer located inside a rigid capsule at the tip of a standard ventricular pacing lead. This is connected to a triple-header of the device. Abbreviation: PEA, peak endocardial acceleration.
B: Electrocardiographic (ECG), left ventricular dp/dt (LV dp/dt), aortic pressure (Ao press), and E: accelerometer tracing (EA) recordings in a sheep heart with the BEST sensor. The PEA-I (150 ms after R wave) and PEA-II (100 ms after T wave) correspond to isovolumetric contraction and relaxation of ventricle. (From Plicchi G, Mercelli E, Parlapiano M, et al. PEA I and PEA II based implantable haemodynamic monitor: Preclinical studies in sheep. *Europace*. 2002;4:49).

also obtained in patients being tested during electrophysiological studies by using an external system, and the changes in PEA were found to be linearly related to the RV dp/dt during dobutamine infusion. PEA signals have been used to monitor hemodynamic function and for programming the AV interval. In 13 patients with end-stage heart failure implanted with a DDD-PEA device with customized lead arrangement,[30] PEA level during RV, LV, and biventricular pacing were compared. Both LV and biventricular pacing increased stroke volume compared with RV pacing (+21% and +37% respectively), and mean PEA changes over a 15-minute duration were also higher (+43% and +38% respectively). In addition, there appears to be a minimum PEA level at the optimal AV interval, and this has shown some promise to automatically detect the optimum AV interval in a dual chamber device.[31] An increase in PEA during head-up tilting has been observed, and the use of PEA-driven overdrive pacing in patients with vasovagal syncope has been reported.[32] Patients randomized to DDDR have a reduced frequency of syncope compared with DDI pacing. In patients with CRT, the PEA correctly identified the optimal AV interval.[33] These data suggest the potential use of PEA sensor for hemodynamic monitoring.

Advantages and limitations

PEA is a proportional sensor that shows good correlation to workload especially at the higher ranges. The PEA sensor is limited by the need for a specialized lead, and it remains a concern on its longer-term stability and the use of this lead at the time of a pacemaker replacement when a standard header pacemaker is used. Currently, the PEA sensor is being developed for hemodynamic monitoring.

Current Combined Sensor Devices

Experience with sensors have suggested that fast-responding sensors such as activity are not proportional at higher levels of workload, whereas a proportional sensor is usually slow in response. Furthermore, a single sensor may be limited by insensitivity to nonexercise stress, and is liable to be interfered with by nonphysiological causes. Thus, it is logical to enhance their rate response profile by combining two or more sensors.

There are two principles of sensor combination, *sensor blending* and *sensor cross-checking*. Sensor blending involves combining sensor-driven rates from individual sensors in a certain ratio. This can be the "faster win" method in which the higher rate is chosen as the dual sensor rate, or ratios of the individual rates are added together to compile the ultimate rate response. Sensor cross-checking enhances the specificity of each sensor. If a more-specific sensor registers no exercise or physiological stresses, changes in the other less-specific sensor will be ignored or its response attenuated. In some situations sensor blending and cross-checking may not be cleared out, but occurs in combination to derive the rate adaptation. The instrumentation of current dual sensor devices is summarized in Table 3. Details of the combined CLS and activity and PEA and activity devices have been presented previously.

Current devices

Medtronic Kappa 400 A piezoelectric sensor is used for activity sensing, and MV is sensed from a bipolar ventricular lead. Differential sensor blending is used. Up to the ADL rate, activity input predominates, whereas MV-driven pacing will predominant at the SURL. Activity and MV sensors are checked against one another. In the absence of piezoelectric sensor indicating exercise, MV pacing will only reach the ADL rate, and vice versa. Pacing above the ADL rate will occur only when both MV and activity signify exercise.

The dual sensor rate response has been reported to be reliable for both maximal and submaximal activities, and resistant to nonphysiological interference.[34] Compared with MV sensor alone, dual sensor mode reduces oxygen deficiency acquired during exercise by enhancing the initial rate response.[35] Rate

Manu-facturer	Models	Sensors	Algorithms	Cross-checking	Automaticity
Medtronic	Kappa 400	ACT= piezoelectric MV = impedance	Blending : ≤ ADL Range : ACT + MV; ADL-ER range : mainly ACT	ACT (0) and MV (+) : up to ADL rate; ACT (+) and MV (0) : up to ADL rate	"Rate Profile Optimization"
Boston Scientific	Pulsar Max Insignia	ACT = accelerometer MV = impedance	Blending : Low heart rate : ACT 80%, MV 20%; High heart rate : ACT 40% MV 60%	ACT (0) and MV (+) and MV (0) : limited rate	"AutoLife style"
ELA-Sorin	Chorus Talent Symphony Rhapsody	ACT = accelerometer MV = impedance	No Blending : MV-determined rate response if ACT indicates exercise	ACT (+) and MV (0) : initial limited rate response; ACT (0) and MV (+) : rate recovery	Automatic matching MV sensor to LRL and SURL
Biotronik GmBH	Inos Protos	CLS = uniporlar ventricular impedance ACT = accelerometer	No blending : No ACT rate contribution. Rate response determined by CLS only	ACT (0) and CLS (+) : limited rate response; ACT (+) and CLS (0) : no rate response	"Auto Response Factor" adjusts CLS data to reach rate distribution determined by the programmed "Exertion Threshold Rate"

Table 9.3 Types of Dual-Sensor Pacemakers in Current Use. Abbreviations: ACT, activity sensor; ADL, activity of daily living; CLS, closed loop stimulation sensor; LRL, lower rate limit; MV, minute ventilation sensor; SURL, sensor upper rate limit.

Profile Optimization was found to be a useful method for rate adaptive programming, and comparable to manual programming,[36] and may be superior to the use of accelerometer alone for rate optimization.[9]

Boston Scientific Insignia, Pulsar Max An accelerometer activity sensor is integrated with the MV sensor. A differential sensor-blending algorithm is utilized. At low heart rate, blended sensor rate is contributed in approximately 80% by the accelerometer, and 20% by MV sensor. This ratio changes to 40% versus 60% near the SURL. In addition, if the MV-indicated rate is higher than the accelerometer rate, the dual sensor rate will follow the MV level.

In one study,[37] 120 patients with Insignia were randomized in the accelerometer single sensor, MV single sensor and dual sensor modes, each for a 3-month period. Using the implanted Activity Log to determine the mean percentage and intensity of activity, quality of life (QOL) and NYHA classes were assessed at the end of each period. Overall, either type of single sensor DDDR mode improved Activity Log, QOL, and NYHA scores compared with DDD pacing, but there was no difference between the two sensors. Dual sensor mode also did not add additional benefit. This study may be limited by the prolonged triple crossover design, but does suggest the clinical differences between sensors and their combinations to effect a better adaptation is likely to be small. A study[38] that incorporated 1256 patients with chronotropic incompetence found that the blended sensor improved metabolic-chronotropic slope more than the activity sensor alone. However, apart for improved physical activity time and energy expenditure, there was no difference in measurable QOL between the blended sensor and the activity-only mode.

ELA-Sorin dual sensor devices (Chorus, Talent, Symphony, Rhapsody) An accelerometer and a MV sensor are combined in these devices. Sensor blending and cross-checking are both operative to effect rate adaptation during exercise (Fig 9.6). When the accelerometer is active but MV has not increased, as may occur at the beginning of exercise, rate response occurs according to a fixed activity response curve to a limited rate. When MV increases, rate response follows the MV sensor-driven rate. Persistent absence of accelerometer signal will be considered as cessation of exercise, and this will decrease the pacing rate in a recovery curve to the LRL even though MV remains higher than baseline.

A report from the multicenter study[39] that involved 81 patients have been reported. In patients who underwent exercise stress testing at 1 month of follow-up, the sensor-driven rate was found to be well correlated to the sinus rate ($r = 0.92 \pm 0.07$, P=0.001), with the slope of linearity of 1.0 ± 0.2. Using metabolic reserve to relate to heart rate reserve, a slope of 1.1 ± 0.2 was obtained, suggesting a close relationship between the dual sensor rate and the metabolic workload.

When should a dual sensor device be used? The previous discussion suggests that dual sensor devices are effective in enhancing rate response profile, although the added clinical benefit over single sensor has yet to be established. Situations in which a dual sensor device may be superior to single sensor are detailed in Box 9.1 on the following page.

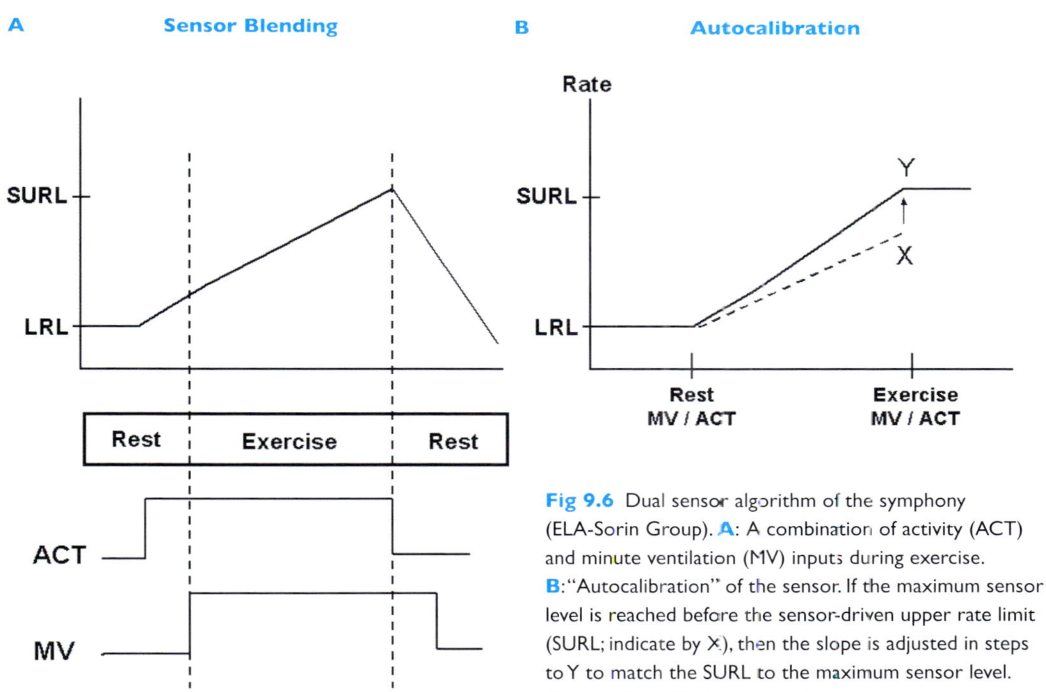

Fig 9.6 Dual sensor algorithm of the symphony (ELA-Sorin Group). **A**: A combination of activity (ACT) and minute ventilation (MV) inputs during exercise. **B**:"Autocalibration" of the sensor. If the maximum sensor level is reached before the sensor-driven upper rate limit (SURL; indicate by X), then the slope is adjusted in steps to Y to match the SURL to the maximum sensor level. Abbreviation: LRL, lower rate limit.

1. High exercise heart rate preferred
   (eg, young athletic individuals may require a minute ventilation sensor)

2. Avoidance of undue rate acceleration
   (eg, working in a vibrational environment may require a sensor to cross check an activity sensor)

3. Need for non-exercise rate response
   (eg, Vasovagal syncope)
   Stress response

4. Hemodynamic or other monitoring

Box 9.1 Situations When a Dual Sensor Device Is Preferable.

Clinical Benefits of Sensor-Driven Pacing

There remains controversy about the clinical benefits of sensor-driven pacing, especially the lack of symptomatic benefit observed in some comparative studies. Factors that may effect such comparisons include (1) definition of chronotropic incompetence, (2) programming of sensor (extent of rate adaptation), (3) patient populations including their comorbidities, (4) pacing modes, and (5) site of ventricular pacing (Box 9.2). Some of these factors are discussed next.

Patient-related Issues

- Degree of chronotropic incompetence
- Left ventricular function
- Sinus versus atrial fibrillation
- Age and co-morbidities

Device-related Issues

- Sensor type
- Site of ventricular lead(s)
- Rate adaptive pacing mode

Programming issues

- Sensor programming
- Lower and upper rate
- Percentage of ventricular pacing

Methods of measurements

- Protocol: cross over or parallel arm
- Exercise
- Symptoms
- Quality of life

Box 9.2 Factors Affecting Clinical Benefit of Sensor-Driven Pacing.

Chronotropic Incompetence

Factors contributing to chronotropic incompetence (CI) are sometimes obvious: age, coronary artery disease, sinus node dysfunction, and cardioactive medications. However, what constitutes CI remains a matter of uncertainty. It can vary between 9% and 84% depending on the definition used.[38] Based on cardiac mortality, CI defined as inability to reach 85% maximum age predicted heart rate will identify 2.2 times as many individuals with increased cardiac mortality. A more-sensitive definition of CI in the Framingham Cohort suggested inability to achieve 80% heart rate reserve at maximum exercise increased the prediction of cardiac mortality compared with 85% maximum age predicted heart rate.[41]

From the pacemaker patient perspective, CI should be defined as a level at which its reversal by a sensor will impact better exercise capacity and QOL. There is less data, although it is generally accepted that inability to reach a rate > 100 bpm is severe CI.[42] The metabolic–chronotropic relationship may be a scientific way to classify CI at peak and each level of exercise, with a slope value of the plot of heart rate reserve to metabolic reserve < 0.8 identifying CI.[43] Luke et al[44] also used maximum predicted rate < 70% as an indication of CI. A large study including 547 patients performed exercise testing for defining CI at 1 month after implantation.[38] The definition of CI used in this study is the ability to complete ≥ 3 stages of chronotropic assessment exercise protocol (CAEP) and a perceived exertion scale of ≥ 16. CI is defined as a heart rate reserve < 80% of metabolic reserve at each stage of the CAEP exercise test, and if > 50% of these stages were incompetent, CI is defined. Based on this study, 34% of these patients were CI. The study further assessed the prevalence of CI using different definitions in the same cohort according to the aforementioned definition, and found that the incidence is similar to using maximum predicted heart rate < 70% as CI. The other definitions tend to be more sensitive and identify 70% to 80% recipients as CI (Fig 9.7). This study does not address whether rate adaptation improves exercise or QOL. However, those patients suffering from CI have a lower QOL (physical and mental component) than those who are chronotropic competent. There was an increase in physical activity time and Kilocalories expanded per week compared to baseline DDD at 1 month, with a tendency for higher levels for the dual sensors that single activity sensor, [Mean change for activity score from baseline to 6 months: activity sensor = 1.45 ± 17.12, dual sensor = 2.69 ± 15.3, and energy expenditure change: activity sensor 359 ± 367, dual sensor 716 ± 3810] Kcal. These data suggest that a more stringent criterion for CI may identify a group of pacemaker recipients who are more symptomatic, and may benefit from sensor-driven pacing, although the benefit of rate adaptation remain controversial on large-scale studies.

Upper Rate Limit

Peak heart rate based on age has been traditionally defined as (220 − age)/minute. While this is a useful guide for exercise prescription for physical training, its application to pacemaker recipients remains controversial. Kindermann et al[45] exercised 49 patients with conventional DDD pacemaker using cardiopulmonary exercise results and Doppler

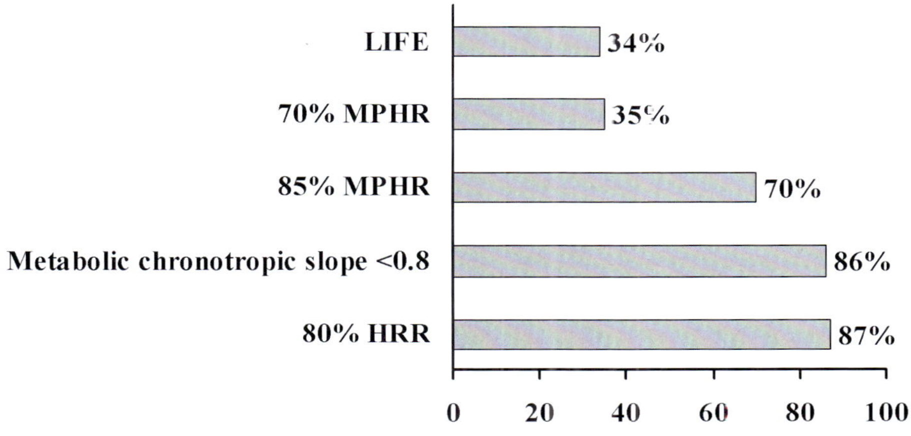

Fig 9.7 Prevalence of chronotropic incompetence in a group of 547 pacemaker recipients during maximum exercise according to published criteria. See LIFE study for definition. Redrawn from data of Coman J et al. *PACE.* 2008;31:1433–1442. Abbreviations: HRR, heart rate reserve; MPHR, maximum age predicted heart rate.

echocardiography to define the optimal URL. They found that in patients with normal heart function (EF ≥ 55%), the URL was 86% of the maximum predicted heart rate. In those with impaired heart function (EF ≤ 45%), a 75% maximum predicted heart was optimal, beyond which heart rate increase caused a fall in cardiac output. This may be related to decreased ventricular compliance and other factors such as ischemia at higher heart rate. Of interest, the rate-related contractility augmentation appeared to be attenuated with RV pacing. In 22 patients with heart failure and wide QRS complex, Vollmann et al[46] found that biventricular pacing restored the rate-related contractility when pacing at 80 to 140/minute, whereas the change in RV pacing was minimal, and the changes during LV only pacing were intermediate. Thus the site of ventricular pacing is also important to determining the URL.

Rate Adaptive Pacing Modes

VVIR versus VVI

This first pacing mode introduced was VVIR pacing. This mode was most extensively studied, and often applies to patients who had complete CI, such as in patients with complete AV block. Independent of the sensor type, and the level of rate response that ranged from 51% to 104%, a 26% to 33% exercise capacity increase was observed over VVI pacing[47] (Fig 9.8). In addition, VVIR pacing has been shown to improve all but one aspect of QOL.[48]

AAIR versus AAI/VVI

An uncommon pacing mode used is AAIR pacing. This pacing mode has the theoretical advantage of preserving native AV conduction and avoiding ventricular pacing altogether. A disadvantage includes progression of AV conduction disease even in patients with normal AV conduction at baseline. In addition, besides conduction capacity, the speed of AV conduction may be an issue, as lack of AV adaptation during an appropriate sensor-driven atrial rate will prolong PR interval, thereby causing the R wave to fall on the subsequent P wave, resulting in AV dyssynchrony or even simultaneous AV contraction. This has been reported to result in pacemaker syndrome.[49] One of the first studies[50] on AAIR pacing had compared AAIR, DDDR, and VVIR mode in patients with intact intrinsic AV conduction (1:1 AV ≥ 100/minute, and atrial to R ≤ 220 ms). VVIR pacing had worse QOL compared to AAIR pacing. Patients had more palpitation and depression despite a lower level of ventricular pacing compared to DDDR mode (39 ± 7 vs. 64 ± 11%). There was no difference between AAIR and DDDR mode. All patients had normal LV function to begin with, and may have obscured minor difference

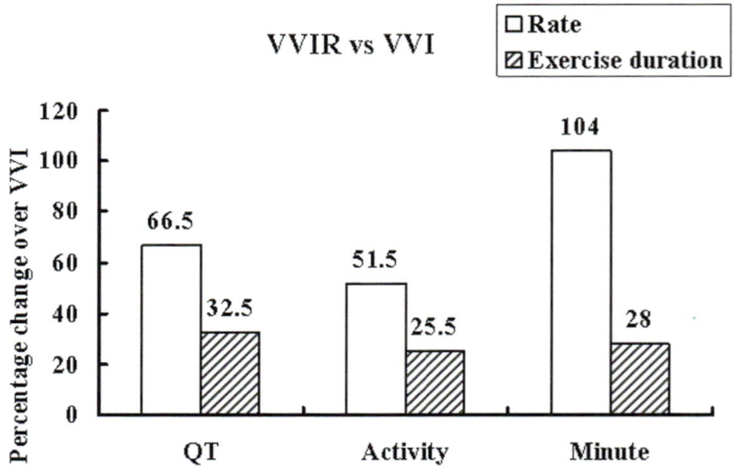

Fig 9.8 Reported studies of rate and exercise augmentation by VVIR over VVI pacing for some sensors. Changes are expressed as a percentage of the parameters achieved during exercise in the VVI mode.

between modes. In one study,[51] AAIR pacing that increased heart rate to 142/minutes did not increase exercise oxygen uptake versus VVI backup at 40/minute. The study was limited by the high intrinsic rhythm maximum rate of 130/minute even without rate adaptation. However it underscores the need of biventricular pacing to improve cardiopulmonary performance during exercise in heart failure patients. It would be of interest to see whether new pacing modes that incorporate minimal ventricular pacing but use atrial rate adaptation can improve exercise capacity, over conventional DDR device.

DDDR versus DDD

Much controversy surrounds the potential benefit of DDDR versus DDD pacing. In a small cohort of 10 patients, DDDR improved exercise capacity over DDD pacing in those with severe chronotropic incompetence.[42] However, in a trial including 873 patients,[52] despite an increase in heart rate from 101.1 ± 21.1 to 113.3 ± 19.6/bpm at 6 months, there was no difference in exercise capacity between the two pacing modes. Over 90% of beats in the two modes were ventricularly paced, and a potential reason for lack of benefit may be related to deleterious effect of RV apical pacing. In a small study, Van Hamel et al[53] compared DDDR to DDD mode in 99 patients with either AV block or sinus node disease, and showed no difference between DDDR and DDD in terms of QOL, despite a significantly higher atrial pacing rate in the sensor-driven arm. Again, this study documented a high percentage of RV pacing in both sinus node patients (87.9%) and AV block patients (96.8%).

Ventricular Pacing Site

The role of sensor-driven pacing in CRT/CRT-D has been discussed for patients with heart failure.[4] Observations have shown that RV apical pacing may be associated with impaired ventricular function in the long term, especially in patients with depressed ejection fraction who do not require pacing.[54] Thus the benefit of rate increase might be limited by the deleterious effect of RV apical pacing. RV septal pacing by inducing a narrower QRS complex, has been shown to improve LV function.[55] However, the role of VVIR (septal) has not been studied.

A study[55] of 12 patients with a high level of AV block (8 of 12 had permanent AF) in the VVIR mode received an upgrade from chronic RV apical to RV septal VVIR pacing. This showed, over a course of 18 months, a significant increase in ejection fraction (55.2% ± 2.6% to 60.4% ± 2.9%), and improvement in 6-minute walking distance (Fig 9.9). In a controlled group with simple pacemaker upgrade and remaining in RV apical VVIR pacing, there was no change in LV function. This study suggests that the potentially harmful effect on LV function by VVIR pacing can be ameliorated with septal VVIR pacing.

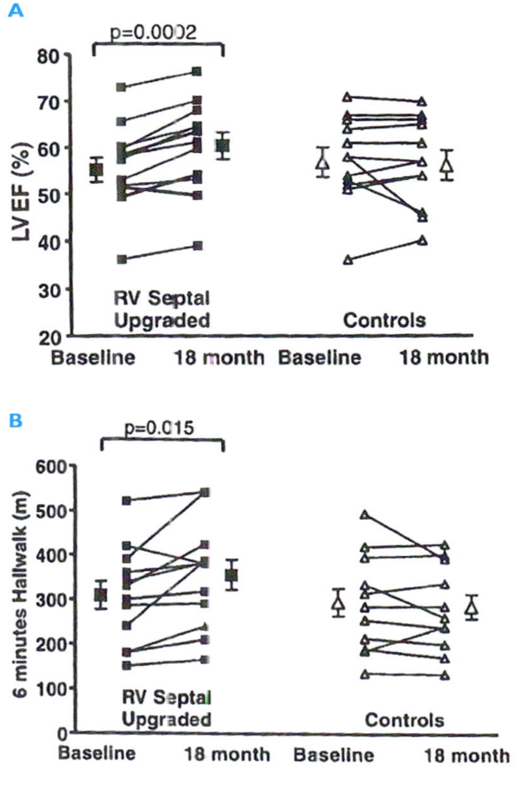

Fig 9.9 Septally paced VVIR versus apically paced VVIR. Changes in LVEF (**A**) and 6-minute walking distance (**B**) in those VVIR septal-paced (upgrade) versus continuation of RVA pacing.

Conclusion

There is little doubt that sensor-driven pacing is going to be an integral part of almost all bradycardia devices. Activity sensing, despite its theoretical disadvantage, is universally used, followed by the CLS and MV sensors. The clinical benefit of dual sensor over single sensor is likely to be small, but may be useful for certain patient cohorts. The lack of observed clinical benefit of sensor-driven pacing in DDDR mode may be related to the definition of CI, excessive RV apical pacing, and the site(s) of pacing used. Further studies will be needed to clarify the best cardiac chamber stimulation to be paced by sensor-driven pacing.

References

1. Karlof I. Haemodynamic effect of atrial triggered versus fixed rate pacing at rest and during exercise in complete heart block. *Acta Med Scand.* 1975;197:195–206.
2. Fananapazir L, Bennett DH, Monks P. Atrial synchronized ventricular pacing: contribution of the chronotropic response to improved exercise performance. *PACE.* 1983;6:601–608.
3. Lau CP, Camm AJ. Role of left ventricular function and Doppler derived variables in predicting hemodynamic benefits of rate-responsive pacing. *Am J Cardiol.* 1988;62:906–911.
4. Tse HF, Siu CW, Lee KLF, et al. The incremental benefit of rate-adaptive pacing on exercise performance during cardiac resynchronization therapy. *J Am Coll Cardiol.* 2005;46:2292–2297.
5. Rickards AF, Norman J. Relation between QT interval and heart rate: new design of physiologically adaptive cardiac pacemaker. *Br Heart J.* 1981;45:56–61.
6. Benditt DG, Mianulli M, Fetter J, et al. Single-chamber cardiac pacing with activity-initiated chronotropic response: evaluation by cardiopulmonary exercise testing. *Circulation.* 1987;75:184–191.
7. Menozzi C, Brignole M, Moracchini PV, et al. Intrapatient comparison between chronic VVIR and DDD pacing in patients affected by high-degree AV block without heart failure. *PACE.* 1990;13:1816–1822.
8. Oldroyd KG, Rae AP, Carter R, et al. Double-blind crossover comparison of the effects of dual-chamber pacing (DDD) and ventricular rate-adaptive (VVIR) pacing on neuroendocrine variables, exercise performance, and symptoms in complete heart block. *Br Heart J.* 1991;65:188–193.
9. Schuster P, Faerestrand S, Ohm OJ, Schouten V. Proportionality of rate response to metabolic workload provided by a rate adaptive pacemaker with automatic rate profile optimization. *Europace.* 2005;7:54–59.
10. Duru F, Block KE, Weilenmann D, et al. Clinical evaluation of a pacemaker algorithm that adjusts the pacing rate during sleep using activity variance. *PACE.* 2000;23:1509–1515.
11. Matula M, Alt E, Fotuhi P, et al. Rate adaptation of activity pacemakers under various types of means of locomotion. *Eur J Cardiac Pacing Electrophysiol.* 1992;2:49.
12. Lau CP, Mehta D, Toff WD, et al. Limitations of rate response of an activity-sensing rate-responsive pacemaker to different forms of activity. *PACE.* 1998;11:141–150.
13. Lau CP, Ward DE, Camm AJ. Single-chamber cardiac pacing with two forms of respiration-controlled rate-responsive pacemaker. *Chest.* 1989;95:352–358.
14. Duru F, Radicke D, Wilkoff BL, et al. Influence of posture, breathing pattern, and type of exercise on minute ventilation estimation by a pacemaker transthoracic impedance sensor. *PACE.* 2000;23:1767–1771.
15. Cole CR, Jensen DN, Cho Y, et al. Correlation of impedance minute ventilation with measured minute ventilation in a rate responsive pacemaker. *PACE.* 2001;24:989–993.
16. Simon R, Ni Q, Willems R, et al. Comparison of impedance minute ventilation and direct measured minute ventilation in a rate adaptive pacemaker. *PACE.* 2003;26:2127–2133.
17. Bonnet JL, Geroux L, Cazeau S, on behalf of the French Talent Dr Pacemaker Investigators. Evaluation of a dual sensor rate responsive pacing system based on a new concept. *PACE.* 1998;25:2198–2203.

18. Mond HG, Kertes PJ. Rate responsive pacing using a minute ventilation sensor. *PACE.* 1988;11:1866–1874.
19. Lau CP, Antoniou A, Ward DE, et al. Initial clinical experience with a minute ventilation sensing rate modulated pacemaker: improvements in exercise capacity and symptomatology. *PACE.* 1998;11:1815–1822.
20. Schaldach M, Hutten H. Intracardiac impedance to determine sympathetic activity in rate responsive pacing. *PACE.* 1992;15:1778–1786.
21. Pichlmaier AM, Braile D, Ebner E, et al. Autonomic nervous system controlled closed loop cardiac pacing. *PACE.* 1992;15:1787–1791.
22. Witte J, Reibis R, Pichlmaier AM, et al. ANS-controlled rate-adaptive pacing: clinical evaluation. *Eur J Cardiac Pacing Electrophysiol.* 1996;6:53–59.
23. Wiegand U, Nuernberg M, Maier SK, et al. The COGNITION study rationale and design: influence of closed loop stimulation on cognitive performance in pacemaker patients. *PACE.* 2008;31:709–713.
24. Occhetta E, Bortnik M, Audoglio R, et al. Closed loop stimulation in prevention of vasovagal syncope. Inotropy controlled pacing in vasovagal syncope (INVASY): a multicenter randomised, single blind, controlled study. *Europace.* 2004;6:538–547.
25. Coenen M, Malinowski K, Spitzer W, et al. Closed loop stimulation and accelerometer-based rate adaptation: Results of the PROVIDE study. *Europace.* 2008;10:327–333.
26. Clementy J. Dual chamber rate responsive pacing system driven by contractility: final assessment after 1-year follow-up. The European PEA Clinical Investigation Group. *PACE.* 1998;21:2192–2197.
27. Plicchi G, Marcelli E, Parlapiano M, et al. PEA I and PEA II based implantable haemodynamic monitor: pre clinical studies in sheep. *Europace.* 2002;4:49–54.
28. Gras D, Kubler L, Ritter P, et al. Recording of peak endocardial acceleration in the atrium. *Pacing Clin Electrophysiol.* 2009;32 Suppl 1:S240–246.
29. Langenfeld H, Krein A, Kirstein M, et al. Peak endocardial acceleration-based clinical testing of the "BEST" DDDR pacemaker. European PEA Clinical Investigation Group. *PACE.* 1998;21:2187–2191.
30. Bordachar P, Garrigue S, Reuter S, et al. Hemodynamic assessment of right, left and biventricular pacing by peak endocardial acceleration and echocardiography in patients with end-stage heart failure. *PACE.* 2000; 23: 1726–1730.
31. Leung SK, Lau CP, Lau CT. Automatic optimization of resting a peak endocardial acceleration sensor: validation with Doppler echocardiography and direct cardiac output measurements. *PACE.* 2000;23:1762–1766.
32. Deharo JC, Brunetto A, Bellocci F, et al. DDDR pacing driven by contractility versus DDI pacing in vasovagal syncope: a multicenter, randomized study. *PACE.* 2003;26:447–450.
33. Delnoy PP, Marcelli E, Oudeluttikhuis H, et al. Validation of a peak endocardial acceleration-based algorithm to optimize cardiac resynchronization: early clinical results. *Europace.* 2008;10:801–808.
34. Leung SK, Lau CP, Tang MO, et al. New integrated sensor pacemaker: comparison of the rate responses between an integrated minute ventilation and activity sensor and single sensor modes during exercise and daily activities and non-physiological interference. *PACE.* 1996;19:1664–1671.
35. Leung SK, Lau CP, Tang MO. Cardiac output is a sensitive indicator of difference in exercise performance between single and dual sensor pacemakers. *PACE.* 1998;21:35–41.
36. Leung SK, Lau CP, Tang MO, et al. An integrated dual sensor system automaticity optimized by target rate histogram. *PACE.* 1998;21:1559–1566.
37. Pieragnoli P, Colella A, Moro E, et al. Blended dual sensor does not give additional benefits to single sensor in DDDR PM patients: results from the DUSISLOG study *Heart Rhythm.* 2005;2:S40–S41.
38. Coman J, Freedman R, Koplan BA, et al. A blended sensor restores chronotropic response more favorably than an accelerometer alone in pacemaker patients: the LIFE study results. *PACE.* 2008;31:1433–1442.
39. Bonnet JL, Geroux L, Cazean S. Evaluation of dual sensor rate responsive pacing system based

on a new concept. French Talent DR Pacemaker Investigators. *PACE.* 1998;21:2198–2203.

40. Lauer MS, Okin PM, Larson MG, et al. Impaired heart rate response to graded exercise. Prognostic implications of chronotropic incompetence in the Framingham heart study. *Circulation.* 1996;93:1520–1526.
41. Azarbal B, Hayes SW, Lewin HC, et al. The incremental prognostic value of percentage of heart rate reserve achieved over myocardial perfusion single-photon emission computed tomography in the prediction of cardiac death and all cause mortality: superiority over 85% of maximal age-predicted heart rate. *J Am Coll Cardiol.* 2004;44:423–430.
42. Protor EE, Leman RB, Mann DL, et al. Single versus dual chamber sensor-driven pacing: comparison of cardiac outputs. *Am Heart J.* 1991;122:728–732.
43. Corbelli R, Masterson M, Wilkoff BL. Chronotropic response to exercise in patients with atrial fibrillation. *PACE.* 1990;13:179–187.
44. Lukl J, Doupal V, Sovova E, et al. Incidence and significance of chronotropic incompetence in patients with indications for primary pacemaker implantation or pacemaker replacement. *PACE.* 1999;22:1284–1291.
45. Kindermann M, Schwaab B, Finkler N, et al. Defining the optimum upper heart rate limit during exercise: a study in pacemaker patients with heart failure. *Eur Heart J.* 2002;23:1301–1308.
46. Vollmann D, Luthje L, Schott P, et al. Biventricular pacing improves the blunted force-frequency relation present during univentricular pacing in patients with heart failure and conduction delay. *Circulation.* 2006;113:953–956.
47. Lau CP. Comparative hemodynamic studies between different pacing modes. In: Lau CP. *Rate Adaptive Cardiac Pacing.* Armonk, N.Y., Futura; 1993:55.
48. Lau CP, Rushby J, Leigh-Jones M, et al. Symptomatology and quality of life in patient with rate responsive pacemaker: a double blind crossover study. *Clon Cardiol.* 1999;12:505–512.
49. Mabo P, Pouillot C, Kermarrec A, et al. Lack of physiological adaptation of the atrioventricular interval to heart rate in patients chronically paced in the AAIR mode. *PACE.* 1991;14:2133–2142.
50. Lau CP, Tai YT, Leung WH, et al. Rate adaptive pacing in sick sinus syndrome: effects of pacing modes and intrinsic conduction on physiological responses, arrhythmias, symptomatology and quality of life. *Eur Heart J.* 1994;15:1445–1455.
51. Passman R, Banthia S, Garbrez D, et al. The effects of rate-adaptive atrial pacing versus ventricular backup pacing on exercise capacity in patients with left ventricular dysfunction. *PACE.* 2009;32:1–6.
52. Lamas GA, Knight JD, Sweeney MO, et al. Impact of rate-modulated pacing on quality of life and exercise capacity-evidence form the advanced elements of pacing randomized controlled trial (ADEPT). *Heart Rhythm.* 2007;4:1125–1132.
53. van Hemel NM, Holwerda KJ, Slegers PC, et al. The contribution of rate adaptive pacing with single or dual sensors to health-related quality of life. *Europace.* 2007;9:233–238.
54. Wilfkoff BL, Cook JR, Epstein AE, et al. Dual-chamber pacing or ventricular backup-pacing in patients with an implantable defibrillator: The Dual Chamber and VVI Implantable Defibrillator (DAVID) Trial. *JAMA.* 2002;288:3115–3123.
55. Siu CW, Wang M, Zhang XH, et al. Analysis of ventricular performance as a function a pacing site and mode. *Prog Cardiovasc Dis.* 2008;51:171–182.
56. Tse HF, Wong KK, Siu CW, et al. Upgrading pacemaker patients with right ventricular apical pacing to right ventricular septal pacing improves left ventricular performance and functional capacity. *J Cardiovasc Electrophysiol.* 2009 April:1–5.

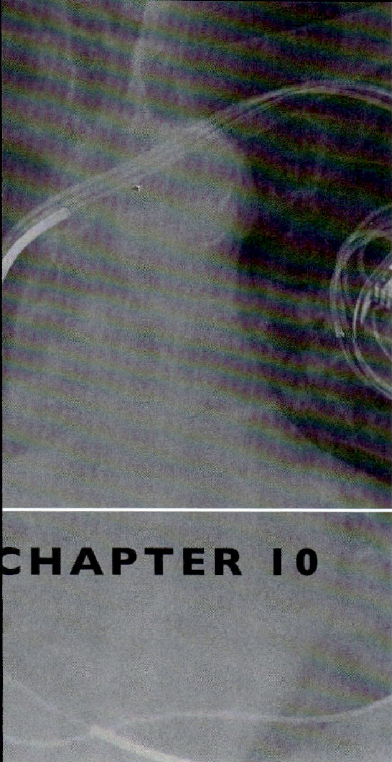

Interpretation of Device Diagnostics

CHAPTER 10

Jordan M. Prutkin and Robert W. Rho

Introduction

Over the last decade, the amount of diagnostic information available in modern pacemakers and implantable cardioverter defibrillators (ICDs) has rapidly increased. At the same time, evaluation of these devices has become increasingly challenging even to the most experienced clinician. A thorough evaluation of modern devices includes an evaluation of the power supply, lead parameters, the capacitor (in ICDs), programmed parameters, arrhythmia logs, pacing and sensing data, sensors, automatic algorithms, and, in some devices, information about the patient's activity and hemodynamics. Differences in the available diagnostics and how the information is displayed vary significantly among device models and manufacturers. An in-depth understanding of all the diagnostic information available in devices is an essential part of routine device follow-up and may greatly enhance the clinician's ability to evaluate acute issues. In order to interpret accurately the diagnostic information, it is important to understand how the device collects the information and what the limitations are. The purpose of this chapter is to provide an overview of the diagnostic information available in modern pacemakers, ICDs, and cardiac resynchronization therapy (CRT) devices from the five major manufacturers.

Programmed Parameters

Programmed parameters in modern pacemakers, ICDs, and cardiac resynchronization devices have become more complicated, in part, because of the many diagnostic and therapeutic features available within these devices. On initial evaluation, it is important to understand the programmed parameters in order to accurately

Pacemakers and Implantable Cardioverter Defibrillators: An Expert's Manual. © 2010 Amin Al-Ahmad, Kenneth A. Ellenbogen, Andrea Natale, and Paul J. Wang, eds. Cardiotext Publishing, ISBN: 978-0-9790164-6-2.

determine the expected behavior of the device in various clinical situations (Fig 10.1). In the event of a significant clinical event, an understanding of the programmed parameters allows the clinician to assess whether the device performed appropriately, whether modifications in programming need to occur, and whether there is evidence of abnormal device behavior. For pacemakers, the basic programmed parameters include pacing mode, lead outputs, and sensitivities. Additional features include whether arrhythmia intervention algorithms are active (eg, interventions for terminating pacemaker mediated tachycardia, mode switching for atrial arrhythmias, algorithms to prevent ventricular pacing) and how diagnostics are set up in the device. For ICDs, programmed parameters are usually divided into bradyarrhythmic and tachyarrhythmic parameters. The basic bradyarrhythmic parameters within an ICD are similar to pacemakers but their expanded parameters are usually more limited in scope. The tachyarrhythmic parameters in ICDs define how many ventricular tachycardia zones are programmed as well as the parameters for meeting detection. The clinician should pay attention to detection criteria, detection cycle lengths, therapies programmed for each zone, supraventricular tachycardia discrimination algorithms, and criteria for detection of atrial fibrillation.

Device Information

Power Supply

The power supply of pacemakers and ICDs are different because their energy demands are significantly different. A pacemaker must be able to deliver low energy pacing impulses using a small current over the course of several years. While pacemaker batteries typically deliver 10 to 15 μJ, an ICD battery must be able to deliver a shock output of up to 40 J while also performing low energy operations. This means an ICD battery must have a high energy density, high current delivery capability, and low rate of internal current leakage.[1]

Pacemaker Batteries

Interpretation of pacemaker battery diagnostic information requires an understanding of basic battery chemistry. Current pacemaker generators are powered with a lithium-iodine battery. Lithium-based batteries have a predictable voltage and intrinsic resistance curve from the beginning to the end of its life. Battery voltage in a lithium-iodine battery decreases slowly throughout most of the life of the battery and then sharply declines toward the end of its life (Fig 10.2).

Diagnostic information relevant to the battery status of a pacemaker includes battery voltage, internal resistance, current, and magnet rate.

Voltage

Because pacemaker batteries follow a predictable voltage curve throughout the life of the battery, when the voltage drops below a determined threshold voltage, replacement is recommended. To provide clinicians with information about the remaining longevity of the battery, descriptions have been created to simplify battery assessment (Table 10.1). Initially, batteries are at beginning of life (BOL) and as time passes, the device enters middle of life (MOL). With normal device function battery depletion will lead to a time when the battery nears the end of its usable life. Manufacturers have selected a voltage threshold triggering a notification that conservatively estimates approximately 3 months of remaining longevity (6 months for Biotronik devices). This notification is called elective replacement indicator (ERI), elective replacement time (ERT), or recommended replacement time (RRT), depending on the manufacturer of the device. This notification occurs at the "knee" of the battery voltage curve at a threshold voltage unique to each pacemaker model. Planning of a generator change should begin at this point depending on the current drain on the battery and whether the patient is pacemaker dependent. It is important to note that the device will automatically reprogram certain features when

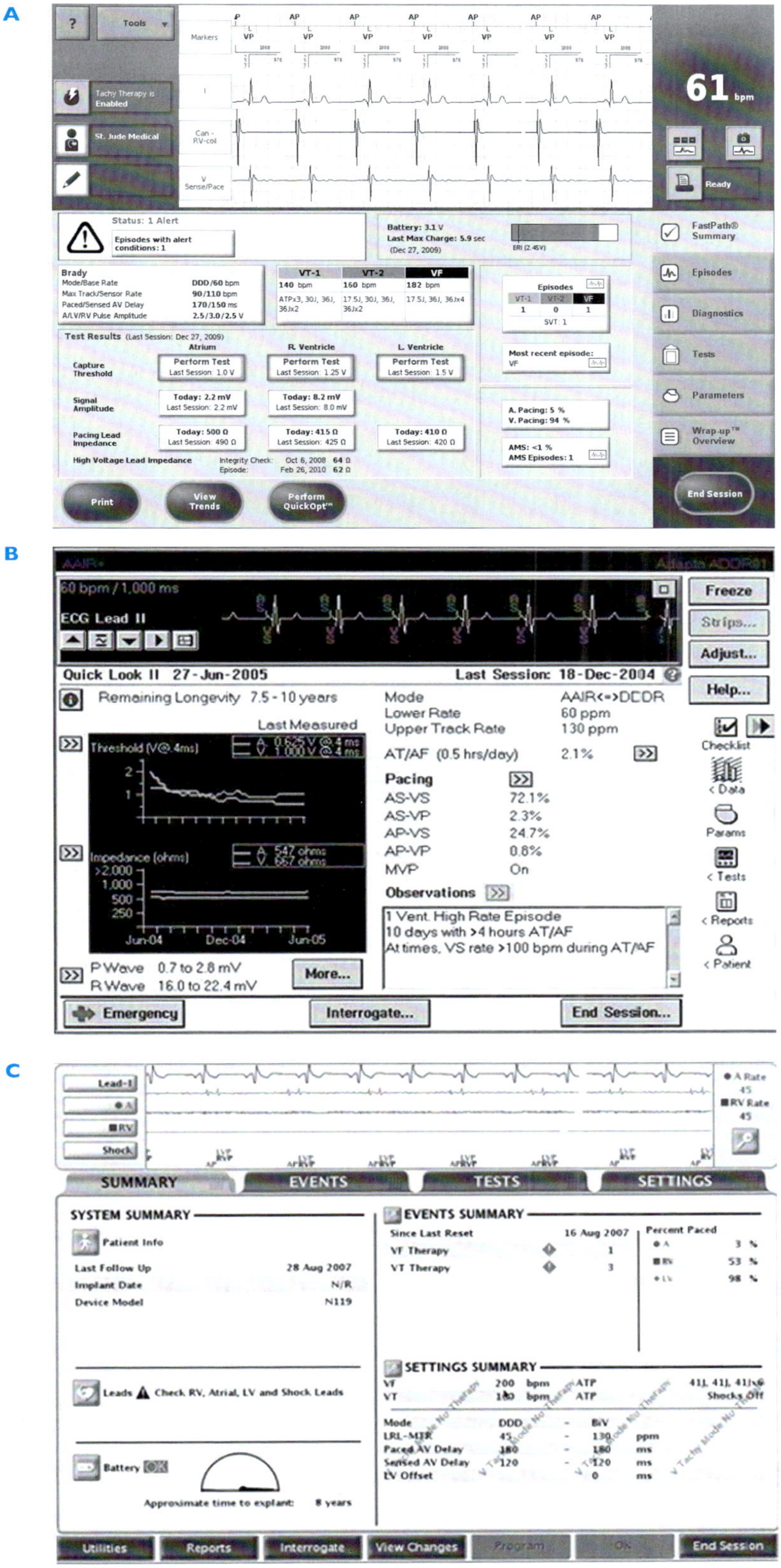

Fig 10.1 Initial opening screens from **A**: St. Jude Medical Atlas II HF ICD, **B**: Medtronic Adapta pacemaker, and **C**: Boston Scientific Teligen ICD.

Abbreviation	Full Name
BOL	Beginning of Life
BOS	Beginning of Service
MOL (MOL1, MOL2)	Middle of Life
ERI	Elective Replacement Indicator/Indication
ERN	Elective Replacement Near
ERT	Elective Replacement Time
RRT	Recommended Replacement Time
EOL	End of Life
EOS	End of Service

Table 10.1 Abbreviations Used to Describe Battery Longevity. Specific abbreviation used varies by manufacturer and model.

it reaches ERI (Table 10.2). When the battery voltage falls further, the device will declare end of life (EOL) or end of service (EOS).

Internal resistance

Another method of measuring battery longevity in pacemakers is by measuring the internal resistance. The internal resistance of a battery has a predictable curve throughout the battery life (Fig 10.2). As a pacemaker battery is gradually depleted, a layer of lithium-iodide is formed which acts a barrier to electron transfer, increasing the internal resistance.[2] In the beginning, the layer is very small and the internal resistance is low. By the time the battery reaches EOL, the layer is very thick and internal resistance is very high.

Note that although most companies' devices will display both voltage and impedance, ELA Medical pacemakers only report an impedance value.

Manufacturer	Nearing Depletion (ie, ERI)	Battery Depleted (ie, EOL)
Biotronik	Rate responsiveness turned Off. Mode is switched to VDD or VVI. Lower rate limit is decreased by 11%. If the device is programmed DDI, DDT, DVI, or DVT, there is no change to the pacing mode but the VA time is extended by 11%.	No change from ERI initially, but features such as autosensing are turned Off as power depletes further.
Boston Scientific	Rate responsiveness turned Off. Features such as sensors, trending, beat-to-beat AutoCapture, and stored electrograms are disabled.	Dual chamber devices revert to VVI mode, lower rate limit is set at 50 ppm, and more features such as hysteresis, histograms, autosensing, and impedance measurements are disabled.
ELA Medical	Rate responsiveness turned Off. Reverts to VVI at 70 ppm with an output of 5 V in a unipolar configuration. Device diagnostics are turned Off.	No change from ERI
Medtronic	Reverts to VVI at 65 ppm. Device diagnostics are turned Off.	No change from ERI
St. Jude Medical	Rate responsiveness turned Off. Pacing interval increases by 100 ms over base rate. AutoCapture features programmed Off. Diagnostic data no longer collected.	No change from ERI

Table 10.2 Pacemaker Changes When the Battery Is Nearing Depletion and Depleted

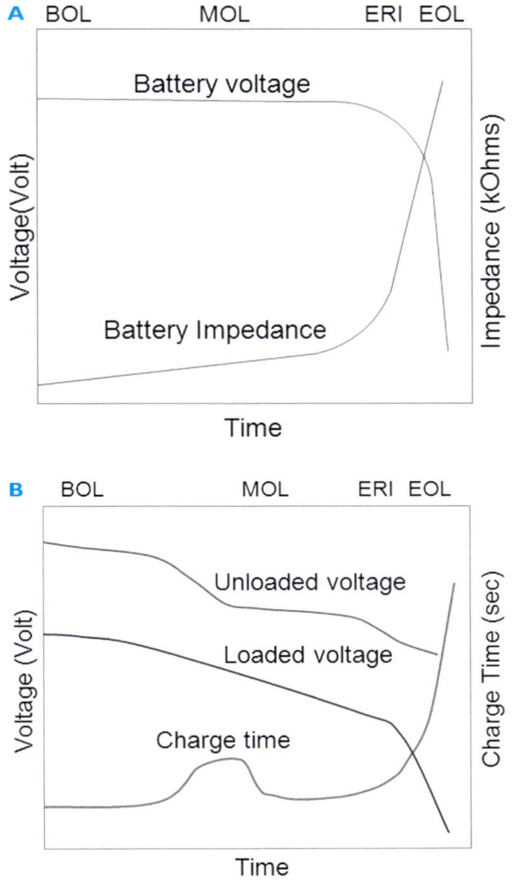

Fig 10.2 A: Pacemaker battery voltage and impedance over time. **B**: ICD battery unloaded voltage, loaded voltage, and charge time over time. BOL, beginning of life; MOL, middle of life; ERI, elective replacement indicator; EOL, end of life.

Magnet rate

When a magnet is applied over a pacemaker, the reed switch or equivalent is closed and, in most devices, will switch to an asynchronous pacing mode with a set pacing rate. The magnet rate is a helpful marker of device longevity because the magnet pacing rate for many pacemakers decreases as the battery is depleted (Table 10.3).

A development among modern pacemakers is the ability to program what the device does in the presence of a magnet. Some St. Jude Medical and Boston Scientific pacemakers allow for programming off of the magnet mode. Biotronik pacemakers have three magnet mode options, called the Magnet Effect. When programmed to *Automatic*, the device paces at 90 ppm for 10 cycles, then returns to the base rate. When programmed *Asynchronous*, the rate remains at 90 ppm until the magnet is removed. Lastly, if the Magnet Effect is programmed *Synchronous*, the magnet does not affect the pacing function. The programmable magnet effect in some pacemakers is important because using magnets for interventions (ie, electrocautery during a surgical procedure) may not have the anticipated effect in some devices.

Estimated longevity

Many modern pacemakers provide estimated longevity based on historical current drain. This involves examining various features including pacing output, mode, current draw, lead impedance, historical pacing percentage, presence of rate responsiveness, and battery impedance to give an estimation of longevity. In addition, a range may be reported using best and worst case scenarios depending on the amount of recent pacing. The estimated longevity reported in devices is usually accurate to within 6 months, assuming no significant changes in pacing parameters.

ICD Batteries

Because of the difference in energy needs of an ICD, different battery chemistries are utilized. Most ICDs have a lithium anode and a silver vanadium oxide (SVO) cathode. In SVO batteries, unloaded battery voltage begins at a plateau phase of about 3.2 V where there is a reduction of the vanadium ($V^{+5} + e^{-} \rightarrow V^{+4}$) and silver ($Ag^{+1} + e^{-} \rightarrow Ag^{+0}$) ions. As the battery is depleted, there is little initial change in voltage (Fig 10.2). After approximately 30% of battery depletion, the voltage drops rapidly, where it again plateaus. At this point the internal battery chemical reaction changes, with the vanadium ion now reduced from V^{+4} to V^{+3}. When there is further battery depletion, the ICD battery reaches ERI.

The addition of silver in the battery cathode improves the conductivity early in battery life. Therefore, unlike a lithium-iodide battery in pacemakers, there is an initial decrease in resistance in the early stages of ICD battery use due to the silver and resistance only increases later after the device has reached MOL.[1] Due to the difference in battery chemistry, ICD battery impedance is not as predictive of battery longevity as in pacemakers.

Medtronic ICDs contain a *charge time-optimized* battery, which uses a different composition of SVO. These batteries have a lower internal resistance buildup, and, therefore, shorter charge times during MOL.[3]

The ELA Medical ICD power supply differs from other manufacturers in that there are two SVO batteries. ELA Medical is also the only company that has a magnet pacing rate in an ICD. The mode is DDD and the rate decreases from 96 ppm to 80 ppm as battery voltage is depleted.

Manufacturer	Programmable Magnet Response? (See text)	Magnet Rate
Biotronik	Yes	Varies depending on Magnet Effect: *Automatic*: 90 ppm for 10 cycles with AV delay shortened to 100 ms, then synchronous with base rate. At ERI, paces at 80 ppm for 10 cycles, then synchronous with base rate. *Asynchronous*: Paces at 90 ppm with AV delay shortened to 100 ms. At ERI, paces at 80 ppm. *Synchronous*: Magnet has no effect.
Boston Scientific	Yes	A rate of 100 ppm is "good," 90 ppm is elective replacement within 1 year, 85 ppm is ERT, < 85 ppm is EOL.
ELA Medical	No	BOL is 96 ppm and gradually reduces to 80 ppm by ERI.
Medtronic	No	The device paces at 100 ppm for three beats, then decreases to 85 ppm, and lowers to 65 ppm at EOL.
St. Jude Medical	Yes	BOL is 98.6 ppm and gradually reduces to 86.3 ppm at ERI, then 66 ppm at EOL.

Table 10.3 Magnet Rate for Each Pacemaker Manufacturer.

Manufacturer	Nearing Depletion (ie, ERI)	Battery Depleted (ie, EOL)
Biotronik	No changes	Tachyarrhythmic detection and therapies unavailable. Pacing parameters are unchanged.
Boston Scientific	No changes	Device reverts to a single VF zone at 165 bpm. No antitachycardia pacing. Pacing becomes VVI at 50 ppm.
ELA Medical	No changes	No changes
Medtronic	No changes	No changes
St. Jude Medical	No changes	No changes

Table 10.4 ICD/CRT-D Changes When the Battery Is Nearing Depletion and Depleted.

Older Boston Scientific ICD and CRT batteries contain SVO and carbon monofluoride (CF_x) as two separate cathodes. Current generation Boston Scientific ICDs and CRT devices use lithium manganese dioxide (Li/MnO_2) batteries, which do not have the MOL impedance buildup of traditional SVO batteries.

Charge times

In addition to battery voltage, the other parameter that provides information about the battery status of ICDs is the capacitor charge time. There is usually a slow increase in charge time, with some devices having a bump during MOL, which then increases more sharply at ERI (Figure 10.2B). A long charge time may be a reflection of either leakage of current across the capacitor (also called deformation) or increased battery internal resistance. Therefore, a second charge 24 hours later is often completed before an excessively long charge time will trigger ERI.

Estimation of longevity throughout the life of the ICD

In ICDs, battery voltage and charge times provide information that the device is nearing the end of its life. It is difficult during the middle of battery life to estimate remaining longevity based on these two parameters. Multiple ICD shocks or other sudden changes in current drain will truncate the remaining longevity of the device. Bearing this limitation in mind, the most recent generation of Boston Scientific ICDs give estimated longevity throughout the life of the battery, derived from a coulomb counter and battery voltage. Power consumption over the previous 2 weeks is then used to project longevity.

Elective replacement indicator/end of life

No programming changes are made in ICDs at ERI, but some manufacturers change settings at EOL to reduce current drain and prolong battery longevity (Table 10.4). Other manufacturers will continue with normal operations until the battery is completely depleted.

Lead Measurements

Another essential component of device diagnostics involves the measurement of lead performance and integrity. This includes three primary measures: sensing, threshold, and impedance.

Sensing

Adequate sensing is of paramount importance for the appropriate function of the device. It is the device's ability to recognize the presence and timing of intracardiac electrograms. The device uses this data to determine the rate within each chamber and then acts in a predetermined manner, such as pacing or delivering antitachyarrhythmic therapies. Factors influencing sensing include lead location, conduction characteristics of the tissue surrounding the lead, the tissue-electrode interface, fixation mechanism, programming in unipolar versus bipolar configuration, the characteristics of the electrogram after signal processing (eg, analog to digital conversion, amplification, rectification, filtering), and the programmed sensitivity threshold. Due to the range of arrhythmias that an ICD must accurately interpret, it is equipped with unique sensing algorithms. Sensing in an ICD is significantly more complicated than in pacemakers. See Chapter 5 for further information regarding automatic sensing.

To allow the clinician to interpret "what the device is thinking," marker channels are provided that designate how the device interpreted the signal and how it responded (Table 10.5 [see pages 210–11]). Marker channels are helpful, but must be interpreted with careful assessment of electrograms and coupling intervals. For instance, a VP designates the device paced in the ventricle but does not mean the pacing output captured. A marker channel may show ventricular tachycardia in a patient in sinus rhythm who is oversensing T waves or double counting a complex ventricular signal.

Ideally, P waves are > 1.5 mV and R waves during sinus rhythm are > 5 to 7 mV. In addition to the amplitude of the signal, trends in ampli-

Table 10.5 Marker Channel Abbreviations by Manufacturer.

Biotronik	
Afib	Atrial fibrillation sensed
Aflut	Atrial flutter sensed
AS	Atrial sensed
AP	Atrial paced
ARS	Atrial refractory sensed
LVp	Left ventricular paced
LVs	Left ventricular sensed
P	Paced event
RVs	Right ventricular sensed
RVp	Right ventricular paced
S	Sensed event
SVT	Supraventricular tachycardia sensed
VES	Ventricular extrasystole (PVC)
VS	Ventricular sensed
VP	Ventricular paced
VRS	Ventricular refractory sensed
VT1	Ventricular event sensed in VT1 zone
VT2	Ventricular event sensed in VT2 zone
VF	Ventricular event sensed in VF zone
1:1	One-to-one arrhythmia sensed
Boston Scientific	
AF	Atrial fibrillation sense
AFib	Atrial fibrillation criteria met
AP	Atrial paced
AS	Atrial sensed
ATR	Atrial tachycardia sense
ATR-Dur	ATR duration started
ATR-FB	ATR fallback started
ATR-End	ATR fallback ended
Chrg	Start/End charge
Detct	Detection met
Dvrt	Therapy diverted
Epsd	Start/End episode
FB	Fallback during A-Tachy Response
FL	Atrial Flutter response
Gradl	Gradual onset
Hy	Hysteresis rate
MT	Atrial tracked at maximum tracking rate
Ns	Sense amplifier noise
P	Paced (single chamber)
PMT-B	PMT termination
PP	Atrial preference pacing
PVC	PVC after refractory
PVP→	PVARP after PVC/PAC
REFR	Refractory interval
S	Sensed (single chamber)
SBR	Sudden brady response
Shock	Shock delivered
Sr	Sensor rate
SRD	Sustained rate duration expired
Stb	Stable
Suddn	Sudden onset
TN	Telemetry noise
Tr	Trigger mode
Unstb	Unstable
VF	VF zone sense
VP	Ventricular paced
VRR	Ventricular rate regulation
VS	Ventricular sensed
VT	VT zone sense
VT-1	VT-1 zone sense
V>A	Ventricular rate faster than atrial rate
()	During refractory
[]	During blanking
↑	Rate smoothing up
↓	Rate smoothing down
—	Unclassified event
ELA Medical	
AMC	Automatic mode conversion
AN	Atrial sense in noise period
AP	Atrial paced

ELA Medical *continues on next page*

Table 10.5 (cont.) Marker Channel Abbreviations by Manufacturer.

Ar	Atrial sense in refractory period
AS	Atrial sense
VN	Ventricular pacing in noise or refractory period
VP	Ventricular paced
Vr	Ventricular sensed in refractory period
VS	Ventricular sensed
Medtronic	
Ab	Atrial sense in PVAB
AP	Atrial pace
AR	Atrial refractory sense
AS	Atrial sense
BV	Biventricular pace
CD	Cardioversion/defibrillation pulse
CE	Charging end
ER	Marker buffer full
FD	Ventricular fibrillation detected
FS	Ventricular fibrillation sensed
HT	High rate timeout period expired
MS	Mode switch
PP	Proactive pace
TD	Ventricular tachycardia detected
TF	Fast ventricular tachycardia detection
TF (with dot next to T)	Fast ventricular tachycardia sensed via VT
TF (with dot next to F)	Fast ventricular tachycardia sensed via VF
TP	Antitachycardia pacing
TS	Ventricular tachycardia sensed
VP	Ventricular pace
VR	Ventricular refractory sense
VS	Ventricular sense
VS (with two lines on marker channel)	Ventricular safety pace
VT	Ventricular tachycardia monitor detected
St. Jude Medical	
AFx	Atrial fibrillation suppression algorithm operation
AMS	Atrial mode switch ongoing
A-noise	Noise reversion mode
AP	Atrial paced
AR	Atrial paced-ventricular sensed
AS	Atrial sensed
ASt	Atrial triggered
AT/AF	Atrial tachycardia/fibrillation detection
(ATP---)	Antitachycardia pacing
AV	Atrial paced-ventricular paced
BP	Biventricular paced
F	Ventricular event sensed in VF zone
(HV)	High voltage therapy
Hys	Rate hysteresis
Magnet	Magnet reversion
(Monitor)	VT or VT-1 diagnosis in monitor only zone
(No more therapies)	No additional therapies available
(nn) J	Programmed energy in Joules
PMT	Pacemaker mediated tachycardia detection
PR	Atrial sensed-ventricular sensed
PV	Atrial sensed-ventricular paced
SIR	Activity sensor indicated rate
SVT	Supraventricular tachycardia diagnosis
T	Ventricular event sensed in VT zone
T1	Ventricular event sensed in VT1 zone
T2	Ventricular event sensed in VT2 zone
VIP	VIP search started
V-noise	Noise reversion mode
VP	Ventricular paced
VS	Ventricular sensed
VSP	Ventricular safety standby
VSt	Ventricular triggered event
VT	Ventricular tachycardia diagnosis
VF	Ventricular fibrillation diagnosis
X	Binned interval reconfirmed
*	Charging for shock delivery
-	Unbinned interval
<	AF/AFL rate zone classification appended to diagnosis
=	Sinus tach rate zone classification appended to diagnosis
>	VT/VF rate zone classification appended to diagnosis

tudes during follow-up are also important. A significant drop in intrinsic amplitude requires close investigation into the sensing properties of the lead. Several factors may affect P- or R-wave amplitude, including antiarrhythmic drug use, fibrosis at the lead/myocardial interface, myocardial infarction, scarring, development of new conduction abnormalities such as right bundle branch block, and lead dislodgement.

If the measured amplitude is low, the consequence is undersensing. In ICDs, low amplitude R waves place the patient at greater risk of undersensing ventricular fibrillation and oversensing of T waves or other undesirable signals. The slew rate of the signal, which is the steepest portion of the intrinsicoid deflection, is measured in addition to the amplitude to increase the likelihood of sensing the desired intracardiac signal.

Medtronic ICDs have an additional feature known as the sensing integrity counter that can help determine whether there might be a breach in the ventricular lead circuit. This counts the number of V-V intervals within 20 ms of the ventricular blanking after a ventricular sensed interval, usually < 130 ms, which are non-physiologic and highly suggestive of a problem with the circuit (Fig 10.3). Other sensing phenomenon that may be binned in this counter include oversensed T wave followed by a premature beat, loose set screws, lead dislodgement, and myopotential oversensing. Therefore, this data should not be taken alone as an indicator of a lead fracture but may be a useful addition to other parameters used to evaluate the lead.[4]

Sensing considerations in CRT devices

Ventricular sensing in a CRT device for tachycardia detection occurs via the right ventricular lead only. Although many devices allow

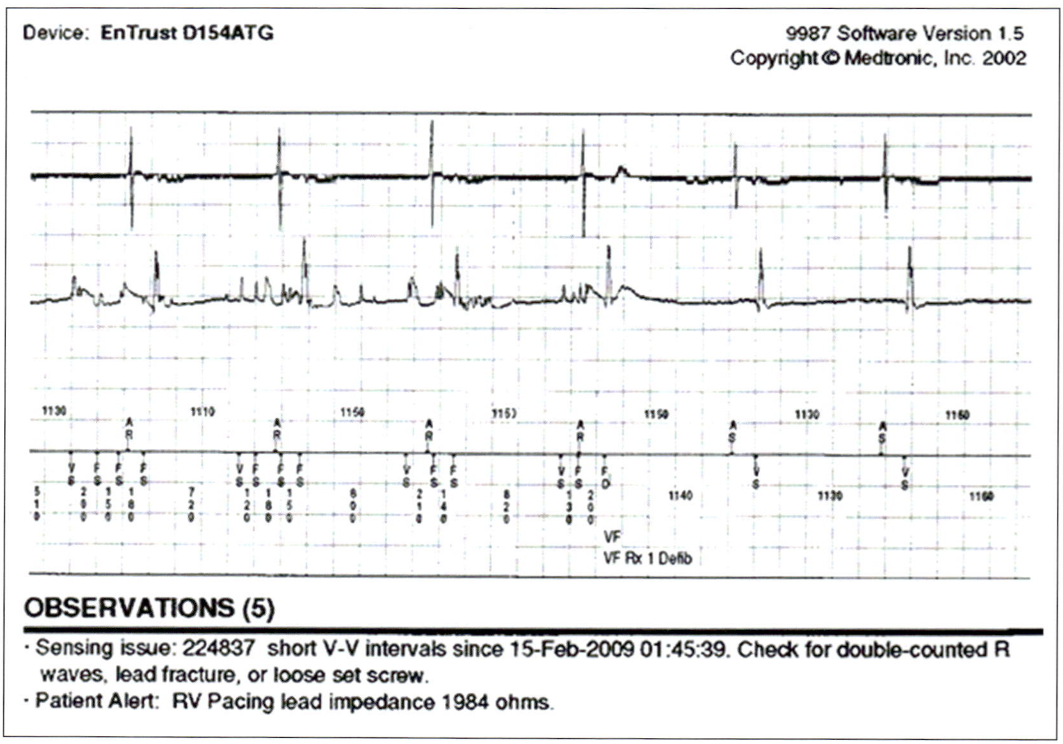

Fig 10.3 Lead fracture which triggers ventricular fibrillation detection in a patient with a Medtronic Sprint Fidelis ICD lead. Noise is evident on the electrogram prior to VF detection. Note the sensing issue demonstrating 224,837 short V-V intervals and elevated pacing impedance. Top line is the atrial channel, middle line is the ventricular channel, and bottom line is the marker channel.

for sensing through the left ventricular lead to check circuit integrity and scanning for PVCs, this is usually not used for sensing and timing of ventricular signals. It prevents double counting of sensed ventricular events, which may cause the device to deliver tachyarrhythmic therapies.

Threshold

The threshold is the minimum energy needed to capture the myocardium with a pacing impulse. In general, the device should be programmed at either twice the threshold voltage or three times the threshold pulse width.

Several lead factors may influence the pacing threshold, including the size of the stimulating electrode, anode surface area, properties of the electrode-tissue interface, inter-electrode spacing, conduction properties of the inter-electrode tissue, and leading edge resistance at the cathode. Changes in the physiological status of the patient, including ischemia or infarction, hyperkalemia, hyperglycemia, acidosis, alkalosis, and hypothyroidism may also transiently or permanently alter pacing thresholds.[5,6]

Some pacemakers and ICDs have automatic threshold testing algorithms that allow the device to pace just above the threshold, which should theoretically allow prolonged battery longevity. See the related discussion in Chapter 8.

Lead Impedance

Impedance is a measure of the resistance of flow within the pacemaker circuit, as demonstrated by the equation, V = IR, where V equals voltage, I equals current, and R equal resistance. Although clinical usage equates resistance and impedance, this is not technically true. Impedance changes as a function of time throughout a pacing impulse, due to the changes in resistance at three locations within the pacing circuit. The first is the conducting element of the lead which, by necessity, provides little resistance. The second location is at the lead-tissue interference. At this part of the circuit there is a higher resistance which, if not too high, is a desirable characteristic as higher resistance allows less current to flow and therefore, less current drain on the battery. The final factor that contributes to the resistance of the circuit is polarization resistance.[7] During the delivery of a pacing pulse, there is the accumulation of positively charged ions (ie, Na^+) in the extracellular space that are attracted to the negatively charged cathode. A short distance away, a layer of negatively charged ions (i.e., Cl^-) is also created, forming an artificial capacitor and increasing the local resistance. This resistance peaks at the end of the pacing impulse, and then decays in an exponential fashion. Therefore, polarization resistance is less important at shorter pulse widths.

Measuring pacing impedance

Measurement of the pacing impedance is an important marker of lead integrity. Each lead has a specified normal impedance and results obtained that are out of this range should be of concern. A relative change in impedance > 300 Ω is also a concern, which may be best seen in trending curves. In general, pacing impedances that are abnormally high may reflect an interruption in the conduction pathway of the lead, such as with a lead fracture. Pacing impedances that are low often reflect an outer insulation breach.

There are differences in the method in which impedance is measured (eg, at the leading edge or mid-pulse), among device manufacturers and among models within the same vendor. These differences in measurement technique can result in different impedance values for the same lead in the same location and may be relevant to decisions made about the lead at the time of implant or during a generator change. Within the same device, however, impedance measurements are an important parameter to measure in assessing the integrity of the conductor and insulation of a lead. When interpreting impedance trends in a device, it is important to realize that impedances are captured intermittently (usually once a day) and intermittent interruptions in the insulation or conducting element of the lead may not be detected. In addition, pacing must be active in a chamber to determine impedance. Ventricular impedance will not be reported if the device is in AAI mode or atrial impedance if in VVI or VDD modes.

High Voltage Impedance

The high-voltage impedance measures the resistance through the shock circuit of the ICD as determined by a high energy shock. This can be performed electively using appropriate sedation, but this parameter may also be recorded if the patient has had a recent clinical shock delivered by the ICD.

In most devices, the high-voltage circuit is checked using a painless subthreshold test pulse, which measures impedance with a paced impulse from the generator to the coils. Although there has been some concern that this does not accurately reflect the clinically relevant impedance during a shock due to nonlinear changes in impedance relative to the paced voltage, clinically, this concern does not seem to be important.[8]

Medtronic, Boston Scientific, and St. Jude Medical ICDs have the capability of checking impedances separately in the SVC and RV coils using different configurations, which may be helpful in identifying the specific component of the lead in which a fracture may exist. Biotronik ICDs measure a combined impedance of the SVC and RV coils. ELA Medical ICDs measure impedance using a pacing impulse, not with the generator but rather from the RV tip to the RV coil and SVC coil, separately. Because of the small size of the RV tip, impedance values are higher. Therefore, ELA Medical ICDs only report the HV impedance as *Normal* or *Open* (> 2000 Ω).

Some St. Jude Medical devices deliver a low energy shock (12 V) to assess the impedance in the high-voltage component of the lead. This test can be uncomfortable and surprising to the patient and, therefore, it is advisable to warn the patient when performing this test. Low energy shocks are not available in the most current generation of St. Jude Medical ICDs. Biotronik ICDs also provide the ability to deliver a 1 J shock through the device to assess impedance in addition to a subthreshold pulse.

Lead performance trends
A very helpful feature in most devices is the availability of graphical lead performance trends (Fig 10.4). This can show stored long-term data on a lead parameter, including sensing, threshold, and impedance. This can demonstrate the time at which an acute change may have occurred, or can show a slower trend that may not be seen if only the last interrogation is examined. It is important to understand that intermittent changes may escape detection in the trended data because they are automatically assessed at various intervals.

Patient Diagnostics

Pacemakers

Underlying rhythm
Assessing whether a patient is pacemaker dependent from sinus node dysfunction or complete heart block is an important clinical fact to know. Pacemaker dependency may be permanent or temporary and may be influenced by medications the patient is taking. The underlying rhythm is checked by temporary suppressing or slowing pacing in the atrium for sinus node dysfunction and in the ventricle for AV block. Care should be taken to have patients lay down flat so that they do not become injured if symptoms develop.

Percent pacing/counters
Many devices will display counters as A-V combinations, atrial-only events, and ventricular-only events. This gives not only the percentage of each paced or sensed events, but also the raw total count of each event.

Several dual chamber pacemakers provide data on how many paced and sensed events occurred in the atrium and ventricle. The data is categorized as atrial-sensed/ventricular-sensed (AS-VS), atrial-sensed/ventricular-paced (AS-

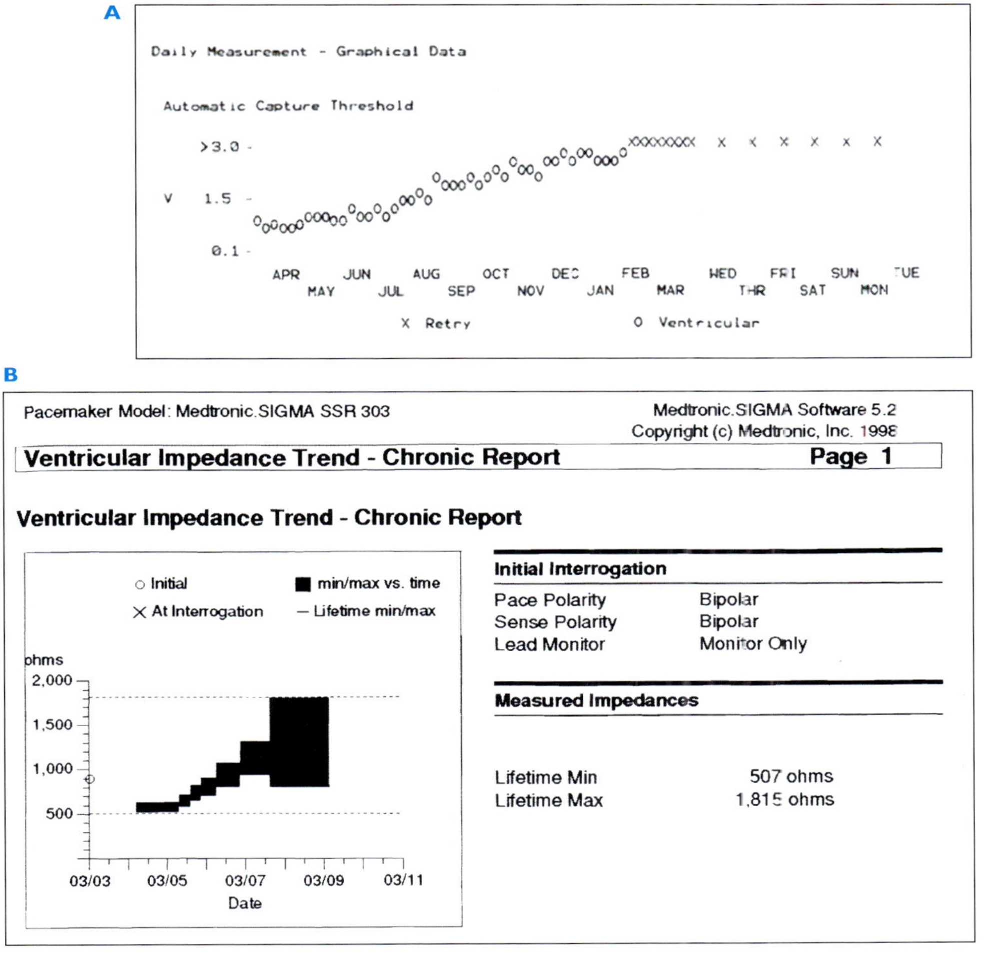

Fig 10.4 Trending feature. **A**: Automatic: capture threshold demonstrating a gradual increase in pacing threshold in a Boston Scientific pacemaker. **B**: Ventricular impedance test demonstrating a slowly increasing pacing impedance in a Medtronic pacemaker.

VP), atrial-paced/ventricular-sensed (AP-VS), or atrial-paced/ventricular-paced (AP-VP). For instance, in Boston Scientific pacemakers, the total combination of events will always equal the number of ventricular events, because the combination events are derived from the underlying ventricular events. The atrial counter, however, may not equal the combination events if there is underlying atrial or ventricular arrhythmias or if the patient is programmed in AAI or VVI modes.

Most devices have separate premature ventricular contraction (PVC) counters. These are defined as two ventricular events with no intervening atrial event. Biotronik pacemakers have more in-depth analysis of PVCs, if this is desired. This includes histograms displaying the number of PVCs at each ventricular rate, percent prematurity, and coupling interval.

One newer feature in devices is the ability of the device to count atrial refractory events as sensed. Therefore, atrial events falling in the postventricular atrial refractory period (PVARP) may be counted, though not all device companies have this feature. Atrial blanked events, which are displayed in current generation Medtronic devices, are not placed in the counter bin but are used for other features like mode switching and given a channel marker (Ab) to aid the clinician in the interpretation of the event.

Boston Scientific uses a pacemaker Wenckebach counter when the device reaches the upper rate limit. If there are 16 atrial-sensed and ventricular-paced events at the maximum tracking rate, the device determines whether the rhythm is pacemaker-mediated tachycardia or pacemaker Wenckebach. If any of the subsequent V-A intervals is > or < 32 ms of the first V-A interval, then the device will bin the episode as a pacemaker Wenckebach event. This is a helpful feature to determine whether the upper rate limit should be programmed higher.

The percentage of pacing can be altered by patient factors and programming. For example, the presence of many ventricular-paced events does not mean that the patient requires ventricular pacing. It may simply indicate that the programmed AV delay is too aggressive. Programming a longer AV delay or activating an algorithm that reduces ventricular pacing, if this feature is available, will prevent ventricular pacing, increase battery longevity, and decrease the likelihood of developing pacing-induced myocardial dysfunction.

Note that these counters are what the device thinks is happening, but may not be what is occurring if these events are analyzed on a 12-lead electrocardiogram (ECG). For instance, the counter will count fusion beats as paced beats. This may be especially important in CRT devices. If the native AV delay is close to the paced AV delay, the counter may report a high percentage of ventricular-paced beats, but may in actuality have a low number of functional paced beats due to fusion.[9] In addition, the counters will not be accurate in the setting of inappropriate sensing or loss of pacing capture.

Counters can be used in some patients to track the amount of atrial tachyarrhythmias in those with tachy-brady syndrome. If the patient is always atrial paced while in sinus rhythm but sensed when in an atrial tachyarrhythmia, the counter can give an approximation of the amount of time in sinus rhythm versus the tachyarrhythmia. This, however, can only give a summation of all tachyarrhythmia beats and does not give a sense of the frequency or duration of episodes.[10]

It is important to understand the clinical characteristics of the patient and whether the counters are represented by the patient's clinical status. Pacemaker system dysfunction may be diagnosed by an abrupt change in the amount of pacing. For instance, if there is a problem with undersensing, there will be more paced beats in that cardiac chamber. Likewise, oversensing of myopotentials or T waves may be reflected by a decrease in pacing. If there is a question, a 24-hour Holter or event monitor may provide additional information (Fig 10.5).

Rate histograms

Although percent pacing gives an overall amount of pacing, a rate histogram can demonstrate the amount of pacing or sensing at each heart rate. This information may be useful in determining whether rate responsiveness is needed or programmed correctly, whether upper and lower rate limits need to be changed, what the underlying rhythm is, or whether the AV delay needs altering. Histograms in dual chamber devices may demonstrate a change in AV nodal conduction in a patient with a device implanted for sinus node dysfunction by showing more ventricular pacing. This may lead to a change in programming to prevent pacing in the ventricle, if possible, by lengthening the AV delay.

Most companies use percent pacing as the percent of total *beats* paced or sensed. St. Jude Medical devices, however, includes information on the amount of *time* paced and sensed as well as the number of beats. The event counter is the percentage of atrial-paced or ventricular-paced beats out of the number of total beats. The histogram, however, is based on the amount of time paced or sensed. This may explain why the two numbers give slightly discrepant results (Fig 10.6A). Note that the event histogram does not include counts while the patient has mode switched.

Elevated heart rates on histograms may have several etiologies, including sinus tachycardia, supraventricular tachycardia, or ventricular tachycardia. Oversensing may result in erroneous numbers of sensed episodes. Furthermore, the rate histogram can be used as a guide to program the appropriate level of sensitivity in the rate response sensor.

Heart rate histograms can also be a marker of autonomic tone. Those with heart failure and higher heart rates are known to have a higher mortality, likely due to increased sympathetic tone.[11] If a patient has a higher heart rate, this may indicate worsening heart failure status, indicating need for closer follow-up or intensification of medical therapy, or may be a marker of patient non-adherence.

Some St. Jude Medical and Medtronic devices also have AV interval histograms, which graphically display the AV intervals. This can be helpful to determine whether the AV interval has been programmed appropriately, especially in those with cardiac resynchronization devices to maximize the amount of pacing (Fig 10.6B). Medtronic devices display rate adaptive AV delays in those with rate responsive-

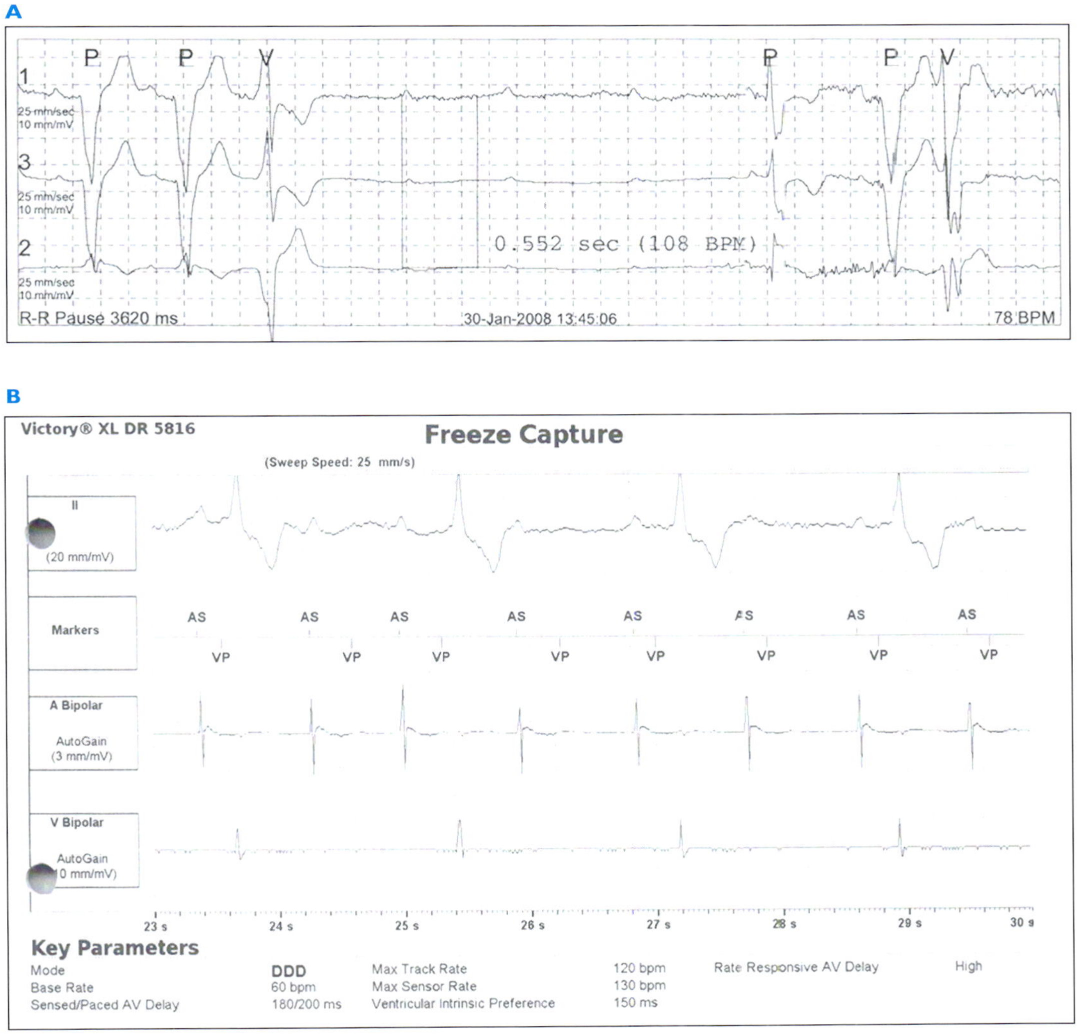

Fig 10.5 **A**: Event monitor showing P waves with no QRS complexes. **B**: Evaluation of the pacemaker demonstrated undersensing and noncapture of ventricular pacing due to a lead fracture.

A

Events

AP Counts	**52%**
VP Counts	**47%**
AV Conduction Counts	**53%**

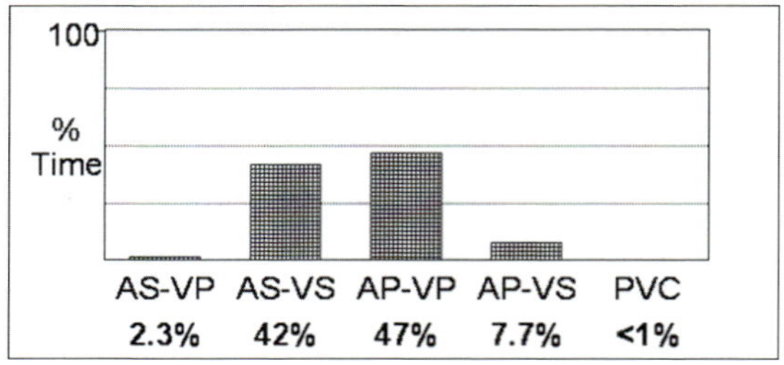

B

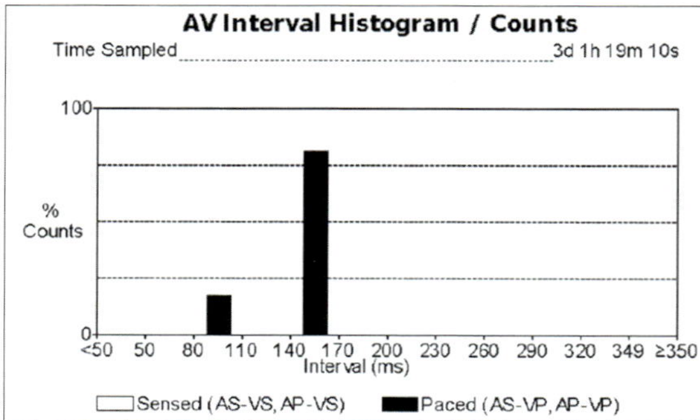

Range (ms)	AS-VP	AS-VS	AP-VP	AP-VS
< 50	0	97	0	0
50 - 79	0	52	0	13
80 - 109	47,419	22	0	5
110 - 139	95	6	4	5
140 - 169	97	7	216,066	2
170 - 199	70	1	0	0
200 - 229	33	1	0	0
230 - 259	0	0	0	0
260 - 289	0	0	0	0
290 - 319	0	0	0	0
320 - 349	0	0	0	0
>= 350	0	0	0	0
Total:	47,714	186	216,070	25

Fig 10.6 A: Event counter and histogram on a St. Jude Medical ICD. The event counter is based on the number of events whereas the histogram is based on the percentage of time. Therefore, the percent of paced beats are not equal.
B: A St. Jude Medical CRT with AV interval histogram. The table on the right demonstrates that most counts in the histogram are AS-VP events with an AV delay of 100 ms and AP-VP events with an AV interval of 150 ms. There are very few ventricular sensed events, indicating appropriate biventricular pacing.

ness programmed, which graphs the amount of atrial sensing/pacing and ventricular sensing/pacing at each heart rate. This can demonstrate whether the patient is experiencing more pacing at higher rates, which may indicate a narrower adaptive AV delay should be programmed.

Atrial arrhythmia trend/AT-AF histograms

Atrial arrhythmia trends and AT-AF histograms may provide helpful data in determining the clinical burden of atrial arrhythmias. It is important to realize that the accuracy of the data provided depends largely in the sensing characteristics of the atrial lead. Low P-wave amplitudes and undersensing during atrial fibrillation may result in underestimation of the number of episodes. Artifact and far-field sensing of the ventricular electrogram may cause an overestimation of the number of episodes. With these limitations in mind, this data may be useful to the clinician in identifying the presence of atrial arrhythmias and in estimating the clinical burden of the arrhythmia.

Medtronic pacemakers display the number of hours each day that atrial arrhythmias are present over a 6-month rolling window. A counter also breaks down the number of episodes by duration into one of eight different time durations, ranging from < 1 min to > 72 hr. This allows the clinician to estimate the frequency and duration of AT/AF episodes.

Biotronik pacemakers also have a histogram that monitors how atrial fibrillation, flutter, or tachycardia initiated. Each episode is divided into whether the rhythm prior to the atrial tachyarrhythmia was normal sinus, sinus tachycardia, or another atrial arrhythmia.

St. Jude Medical devices also report an atrial arrhythmia duration histogram as well as a peak filtered atrial rate histogram. With St.

Jude Medical devices, however, the terminology will vary based on whether mode switch is programmed On. If it is On, the event is called automatic mode switch (AMS), but if mode switch is off and is monitored only, then it is called atrial tachycardia/atrial fibrillation (AT/AF).

For more information regarding automatic mode switching, see Chapter 6.

Ventricular rate during AF/AT

On Medtronic and St. Jude Medical devices, counters can provide the ventricular rate during atrial fibrillation or atrial tachycardia. Both the average and maximum heart rates during atrial tachyarrhythmias are displayed. This can be useful to correlate patient symptoms with episodes of atrial fibrillation. It can also be used to assess whether rate control strategies are providing adequate rate control. Lastly, it may help identify patients at risk for inappropriate shocks from atrial fibrillation associated with a rapid ventricular rate, if the patient has an ICD. Tachyarrhythmic settings may need to be adjusted to prevent inappropriate therapies.

Night heart rate/mean heart rate at rest

Medtronic devices have a feature reporting night heart rate recorded between 12 and 4 AM. Night heart rate has been shown to correlate with various parameters of heart rate variability (HRV), such as the standard deviation of the averaged normal RR intervals (SDANN) and is higher in those with worsening NYHA classification.[12] The absence of a decrease in night heart rate may be a marker of dysregulation of sympathetic tone.

Devices from Biotronik report the mean ventricular heart rate, including all sensed, paced, and premature ventricular beats, over a 24-hr period. The clinician can then set a *resting* period, with the rest period start time and duration being programmable, and the mean heart rate is then calculated specifically during that period. Rolling values over the last 240 days are then displayed.

Sensor indicated rate/sensor replay/sensor rate

St. Jude Medical, Medtronic, and Biotronik pacemakers have the ability to display what the paced heart rate would have been if rate responsiveness were activated, based on data from the sensor. This can serve two functions. It can be used to assess chronotropic incompetence and whether the patient would benefit from rate adaptive pacing or whether the settings need to be changed. In addition, in those with heart failure, it can be used loosely as a marker of sympathetic tone. If the sensor rate demonstrates a greater percentage of the time at lower heart rates, this suggests the heart rate is greater than expected for activity, and the patient may have a worse prognosis due to elevated sympathetic tone, non-adherence of medical therapy such as beta-blockers, or changes in volume status.

ICD Diagnostics

Most diagnostics available in pacemakers are also present in ICDs. However, ICDs have more sophisticated arrhythmia diagnostics as well as diagnostics that may provide insights into the status of a patient's heart failure.

Patient Activity Monitoring

ICDs from each manufacturer except ELA Medical can estimate patient activity using the built-in accelerometer, regardless of whether rate responsiveness is programmed actively. This feature is given different names such as Activity Log, Average Daily Exercise, and Total Daily Activity depending on the manufacturer. Although older devices only reported whether the patient was sedentary or not, newer devices can measure the intensity of exercise. This feature may be useful to determine patient activity level as a surrogate of heart failure status. In particular, this can be an objective marker to help determine whether patients who receive a CRT are responding to therapy.

Additional data provided for heart failure monitoring

Many ICDs and CRT devices provide additional data that may be of interest in the management of patients with heart failure. Medtronic devices have a transthoracic impedance monitor that is a reflection of the amount of fluid that has accumulated in the lung tissue between the distal right ventricular coil and the can of the device. The impedance is converted into an OptiVol fluid index, which may be useful in predicting an impending heart failure decompensation.[13] Other pulmonary processes will affect OptiVol measurement, include pneumonia and pleural effusion, so it cannot be used alone to determine the cause of dyspnea.[14] Likewise, chronic obstructive pulmonary disease may lead to variable amounts of air trapping and differences in the functional residual volume in the lungs. As air has very poor conductance, any change in the amount of air will affect impedance measures. Medtronic collects many of its diagnostics, including OptiVol, into a Cardiac Compass report. This information is only available in a printout and not available on the programmer screen (Fig 10.7).

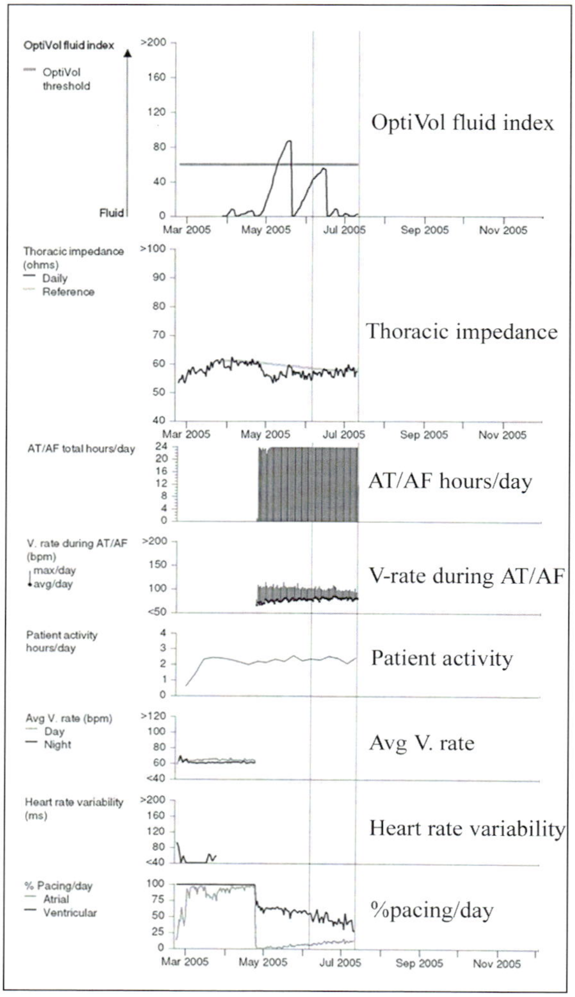

Fig 10.7 A Cardiac Compass report for a patient with a Medtronic CRT. This patient was in sinus rhythm until April 2005, when she developed atrial fibrillation. This led to an increase in the native ventricular rate with a significant decrease in percent biventricular pacing. The thoracic impedance decreased and OptiVol fluid index increased, though the patient activity hours per day was stable. Note that heart rate variability is no longer measured after she went into atrial fibrillation. (Courtesy of Medtronic, used with permission.)

Another parameter available in Medtronic, Boston Scientific, and Biotronik devices is heart rate variability, which is a reflection of autonomic tone. It is has been studied clinically as a predictor of sudden death or arrhythmic events after a myocardial infarction, though the incremental benefit is poor and has been used mostly in research settings.[15] There is evidence that changes in HRV precede a heart failure hospitalization by several days.[16] Although patients with decreased HRV are at higher risk of sudden death, there is insufficient evidence that would support empiric programming of therapies, upgrading of devices to CRT devices, or initiation of antiarrhythmic agents based on HRV alone.

Data for HRV is collected by assessing cycle length variations in sinus rhythm, so the device must be in a dual chamber mode to measure HRV. Different information may be reported depending on the manufacturer. For example, Boston Scientific devices display a HRV footprint plot with heart rate on the X-axis and variability on the Y-axis (Fig 10.8). HRV footprint is then calculated as the area of the graph covered by the HRV plot.

Because of the expanding indication of

ICDs and CRT devices in heart failure patients, a significant effort to provide clinicians with information that will aid in the management of heart failure is being made by most manufacturers. Many of these features require further clinical investigations to clarify their role in the management of patients with heart failure.

Stored Event Evaluation

Many different types of events may be stored in the device, and these may differ depending on whether the device is a pacemaker, ICD, or CRT. Stored arrhythmias may include atrial tachyarrhythmias, sustained or nonsustained ventricular tachyarrhythmias, sudden bradycardiac response events, and mode switch episodes. These data may be displayed in chronologic order or by episode type. Data from stored events can be displayed in a variety of ways varying from device to device. This may involve a description of the episode, marker channels with cycle lengths, and electrograms in most devices. In addition, interval plots may be available in certain devices, which demonstrate the cycle length throughout the duration of the episode. The sensing configuration of the stored electrogram can also be programmed in several devices.

A

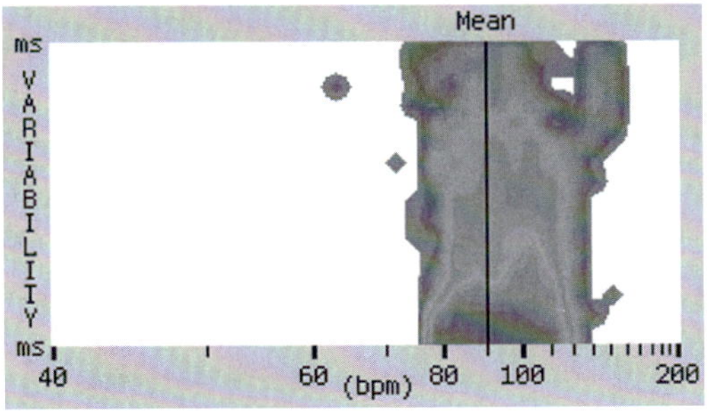

B

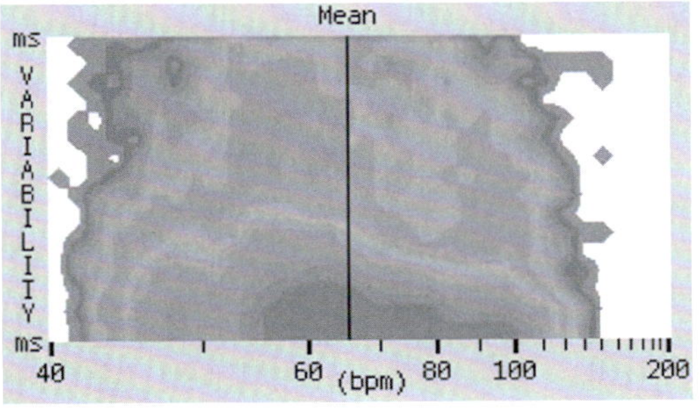

Fig 10.8 Heart rate variability using a HRV footprint plot from a Boston Scientific CRT. **A**: Soon after initial implant, the patient has a mean heart rate of 90 bpm over a narrow range of heart rates and low variability (HRV footprint 24%). **B**: After CRT insertion, the heart rate variability measures have improved significantly. The mean heart rate is 65 bpm with a wide range of heart rates and large variability (HRV footprint 76%). (Courtesy of Boston Scientific. Used with permission.)

Electrogram Evaluation

The optimal stored electrogram should include information on the baseline rhythm, onset, duration, detection, therapies, and outcome of the event, with electrograms from all leads, including marker channels. This allows the operator to determine the mechanism of the arrhythmia and whether the device appropriately classified and treated it.

Examining the real-time electrogram along with its marker channels is useful in evaluating any stored events. This should begin with examination of the amplitude of the signals, the relationship of the atrium and ventricle, and the presence of artifact. The rhythm should be assessed along with the marker channels that demonstrate how the device has interpreted and responded to the signal. This is helpful in determining the mechanism of the arrhythmia, whether the device has the correct interpretation of the arrhythmia, and whether therapies (ie, mode switching, ATP, or shocks) are appropriately executed

To optimize device performance in correctly interpreting the information delivered to the device from the leads, electrograms are processed electronically. This involves a sequence of signal processing including amplification, filtering, and rectification that differs among manufacturers. An important factor to note is that the electrogram available to the clinician examining a paper printout is often taken from a different part of the signal processing chain than the signal that the device stamps marker channels on and "makes decisions" by. This fact is evident in the significant discrepancy between measured R-wave amplitudes on paper and the R waves that the device measures.

Pacemaker Events

Devices may store information on atrial or ventricular high rate episodes, depending on programming. This may include how high the rate must be and how many consecutive beats to trigger storage of the episode, how many beats prior to the onset and at the termination of the arrhythmia are included, and the percent of episodes stored as atrial versus ventricular high rate. There are several options of programming event storage. Event details include a description of the event (ie, atrial rate, ventricular rate, and duration), marker channels, electrograms, and interval plots (in Medtronic devices). Because electrogram storage consumes a significant amount of memory, the tradeoff for more detailed electrogram storage is that fewer or shorter events may be stored. Depending on the event category and memory capacity of the device, storage of electrograms during the event may be a programmable feature, which allows the clinician to confirm the rhythm.

If the electrogram is not available, markers channels may be displayed, which will give a sense of what the device thinks is occurring, but does not allow the clinician to confirm the arrhythmia. Marker channels are present during real-time interrogation or during stored events. Table 10.5 lists some of the markers used by the different device companies. Undersensing or oversensing will limit the sensitivity and specificity of the device in categorizing an arrhythmia. The timing of the marker channel may be helpful in diagnosing some of these episodes. Consistent ventricular sensing at a fixed interval following a ventricular event, for instance, raises the concern for T-wave oversensing.

Most companies have a feature to determine how to handle electrograms once the storage memory is full. This usually involves keeping the earliest events and once the memory is full it will stop storage, or a continuous rolling of events such that a new event overwrites the first stored event. The way the device handles events that occur when maximum storage of events has been exceeded varies between manufacturers and can often be programmed.

Mode switch episodes are stored separately from high rate episodes, and, similarly, the amount of data stored for the episode can be modified. Intermittent undersensing during an atrial arrhythmia may lead to mode switching multiple times during the episode. This may appear that multiple arrhythmias have occurred instead of one continuous arrhythmia. The time that each episode occurred will provide a clue suggesting a continuous rapid atrial arrhythmia associated with intermittent undersensing. Conversely, oversensing may also occur and lead to mode switching. Inspection of the electrograms will determine the cause of frequent mode switching and whether a programming change, such as altering the mode switch rate or atrial sensitivity, is necessary (Fig 10.9).

In some devices, the criteria for triggering a mode switch and whether that episode is stored can be programmed. For instance, the device may be programmed such that mode switch occurs after eight beats, but the event will only be stored if 20 atrial beats meet detection criteria.

ELA Medical pacemakers incorporate an algorithm to minimize ventricular pacing, named AAIsafeR. This enables the device to switch between AAI and DDD depending on intrinsic AV nodal conduction. Mode switching events are stored and can be analyzed to see when and why the device switched modes. In addition, the device stores information on the number of beats while in DDD mode and the amount of time spent in AAI mode.

Boston Scientific, Biotronik, and St. Jude Medical will also store pacemaker mediated tachycardia (PMT) episodes. PMT episodes are defined differently by the various manufacturers but the definitions all share in common an atrial-sensed event following a ventricular-paced event. This relatively nonspecific criterion results in many inappropriate categorization of PMT and requires validation from the clinician.

Medtronic, Boston Scientific, Biotronik, and St. Jude Medical enable patient-activated memory storage in a similar manner as an event monitor. Whereas Medtronic uses a small activator similar to that used for an implantable

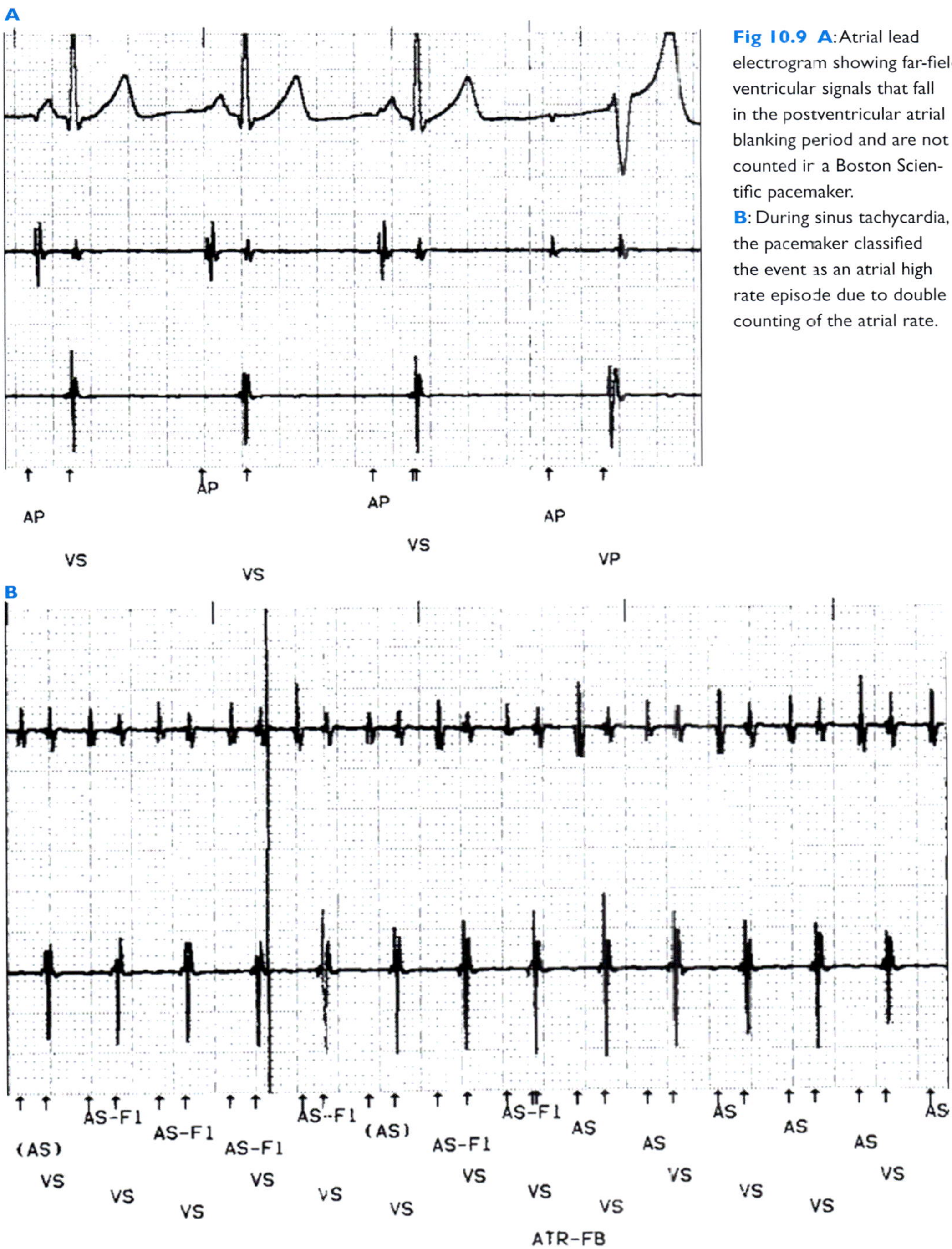

Fig 10.9 **A**: Atrial lead electrogram showing far-field ventricular signals that fall in the postventricular atrial blanking period and are not counted in a Boston Scientific pacemaker.
B: During sinus tachycardia, the pacemaker classified the event as an atrial high rate episode due to double counting of the atrial rate.

loop recorder, the other manufacturers use magnet application to trigger the episode. When this feature is turned On, asynchronous pacing that usually occurs during magnet mode is deactivated. This feature is often underutilized and can be a helpful feature to obtain a rhythm correlation in patients with symptoms concerning for an arrhythmia.

Pacemaker memory

The amount of memory for storing electrograms has significant variability among manufacturers (Table 10.6). This can include how much of the episode is stored pre- and post-trigger, how many channels are selected, and how many episodes can be stored.

Battery longevity may be affected independently of memory storage of pacemaker events. The writing to memory of an event does not require a significant amount of current, as opposed to the continuous monitoring and buffering. Some pacemakers may continue to monitor electrograms, even though the information does not get stored, such that the battery longevity is not impacted by turning electrogram monitoring Off.

Implantable Cardioverter Defibrillation/ Cardiac Resynchronization Therapy Events

Similar to pacemakers, ICDs and CRT devices can store atrial high rate and mode switch episodes. Ventricular high rate episodes are handled differently, because it includes more sophisticated algorithms to determine whether the event is ventricular fibrillation, ventricular tachycardia, or an atrial arrhythmia with rapid ventricular conduction and whether therapies were delivered.

Initial evaluation of ICD events include a list or diagram of recent events that fell into a monitor or therapy zone. Depending on the manufacturer, ICDs will display what it determined the rhythm to be (supraventricular tachycardia, nonsustained ventricular tachycardia, ventricular tachycardia, or ventricular fibrillation) based on rate cutoffs and discrimination algorithms. For therapies the device treated, it can then list whether the therapy was successful.

As in pacemakers, another feature that can be altered is the amount of storage time of the event. This can allow for inspection of the initiation, therapies, and termination of the event.

Current model ELA Medical ICDs store up to 15 episodes with electrograms and interval plots of up to 32 s in length with atrial and ventricular near field electrograms only. Biotronik ICDs and CRT devices, on the other hand, can store up to 32 min of total recording with up to three channels. Each episode can have up to 30 s pretrigger and 15 s post-trigger.

Boston Scientific ICDs have up to 17 min of stored electrogram time, though only 13 min if the Patient Triggered Monitor is enabled. There is a priority to the episodes stored, in the order of ventricular fibrillation, Patient Triggered Monitor (if On), ventricular tachycardia, commanded ventricular therapy, nonsustained ventricular tachycardia, atrial-tachy response,

Manufacturer	Longest Episode Storage	Shortest Episode Storage
Biotronik Cylos	10 s	10 s
Boston Scientific Altrua	28 s pretrigger and 14 s post-trigger	2 s pretrigger and 2 s post-trigger
ELA Medical Reply	16 s	8 s
Medtronic Adapta	24 s pretrigger and post-trigger	2 s pretrigger and post-trigger
St. Jude Medical Zephyr	120 s	4 s

Table 10.6 Shortest and Longest Electrogram Storage Durations in a Representative Pacemaker of Each Manufacturer. Durations vary by model and number of episodes and channels stored and should only used as a rough estimate.

and pacemaker-mediated tachycardia. A maximum of 30 ventricular fibrillation episodes and 25 ventricular tachycardia episodes may be stored.

Medtronic ICDs and CRT devices can hold up to 100 treated episodes of ventricular fibrillation/tachycardia, lasting up to 13.75 min, depending on the specific device. In addition, up to 15 min of monitored VT episodes lasting 2.5 min can be stored. A programmable option of storing 20 s of the electrogram prior to the onset of the arrhythmia is available, but keeping this On continuously can reduce battery longevity by 10% to 15%, which is why there is an option to program this On for only 1 or 3 months.

As with other manufacturers, St. Jude Medical ICDs and CRT devices allow for variability in how episodes are stored, including the duration of storage prior to the detection trigger, the number of channels stored, and which channels are recorded. Up to 45 min total may be stored, depending on settings.

Note that some companies will allow for *stitching* of important parts of events, such as the onset of detection or transitions between zones, to maximize the amount of clinically useful information and to save storage space.

CRT ventricular sensing episodes

Biventricular devices are intended to pace as much as possible to provide the optimal clinical benefit. Medtronic CRT devices display the marker channels of episodes when the device is not pacing due to intrinsic sensed events, which are stored as Ventricular Sensing Episodes. This function reports the duration of the episode, atrial and ventricular rates, and whether the reason for loss of biventricular pacing was due to atrial or ventricular arrhythmias.

Conclusion

Modern pacemakers, ICDs, and CRT devices are capable of storing a significant amount of diagnostic information. In addition to providing information about the software (programmed parameters) and the hardware (battery and leads), modern devices are also ambulatory ECG and physiologic monitors.

Further information on device diagnostics is available in device manuals and from local or telephone technical support from each respective manufacturer.

An in-depth understanding of the diagnostic features available in modern devices can provide a significant amount of information to the clinician and aid in the optimal care of patients during routine follow-up and acute presentations.

References

1. Stroobandt RX, Barrold SS, Sinnaeve AF. *Implantable Cardioverter-Defibrillators Step by Step*. West Sussex, UK: Wiley-Blackwell; 2009.
2. Mallela VS, Ilankumaran V, Rao NS. Trends in cardiac pacemaker batteries. *Indian Pacing Electrophysiol J*. 2004;4(4):201–212.
3. Untereker DF, Cresp AM, Rorvick A, Schmidt CL, Skarstad PM. Power systems for implantable pacemakers, cardioverters, and defibrillators. In: Ellenbogen KA, Kay GN, Lau CP, Wilkoff BL, eds. *Clinical Cardiac Pacing, Defibrillation, and Resynchronization Therapy*. 3rd ed. Philadelphia: Saunders Elsevier; 2007:235–259.
4. Swerdlow CD, Gunderson BD, Ousdigian KT, et al. Downloadable algorithm to reduce inappropriate shocks caused by fractures of implantable cardioverter-defibrillator leads. *Circulation*. 2008;118(21):2122–2129.
5. Patton KK, Levy M, Viswanathan M. Atrial lead dysfunction: an unusual feature of hypothyroidism. *Pacing Clin Electrophysiol*. 2008;31(12):1650–1652.
6. Valettas N, Rho R, Beshai J, et al. Alcohol septal ablation complicated by complete heart block and permanent pacemaker failure. *Catheter Cardiovasc Interv*. 2003;58(2):189–193.
7. Kay GN. Basic concepts of pacing. In: Ellenbogen KA, Wood MA, eds. *Cardiac Pacing and ICDs*. 4th ed. Malden, MA: Blackwell Publishing; 2005:47–121.
8. Vollmann D, Luethje L, Zenker D, Domhof S, Unterberg C. Subthreshold test pulses versus

low energy shock delivery to estimate high energy lead impedance in implanted cardioverter defibrillator patients. *Pacing Clin Electrophysiol.* 2003;26(1 Pt 2):457–460.

9. Kamath GS, Cotiga D, Koneru JN, et al. The utility of 12-lead Holter monitoring in patients with permanent atrial fibrillation for the identification of nonresponders after cardiac resynchronization therapy. *J Am Coll Cardiol.* 2009;53(12):1050–1055.
10. Pollak WM, Simmons JD, Interian A, Jr., Castellanos A, Myerburg RJ, Mitrani RD. Pacemaker diagnostics: a critical appraisal of current technology. *Pacing Clin Electrophysiol.* 2003;26(1 Pt 1):76–98.
11. Gullestad L, Wikstrand J, Deedwania P, et al. What resting heart rate should one aim for when treating patients with heart failure with a beta-blocker? Experiences from the Metoprolol Controlled Release/Extended Release Randomized Intervention Trial in Chronic Heart Failure (MERIT-HF). *J Am Coll Cardiol.* 2005;45(2):252–259.
12. Casolo GC, Stroder P, Sulla A, Chelucci A, Freni A, Zerauschek M. Heart rate variability and functional severity of congestive heart failure secondary to coronary artery disease. *Eur Heart J.* 1995;16(3):360–367.
13. Yu CM, Wang L, Chau E, et al. Intrathoracic impedance monitoring in patients with heart failure: correlation with fluid status and feasibility of early warning preceding hospitalization. *Circulation.* 2005;112(6):841–848.
14. Wang L. Fundamentals of intrathoracic impedance monitoring in heart failure. *Am J Cardiol.* 2007;99(10A):3G–10G.
15. Heart rate variability: standards of measurement, physiological interpretation and clinical use. Task Force of the European Society of Cardiology and the North American Society of Pacing and Electrophysiology. *Circulation.* 1996;93(5):1043–1065.
16. Adamson PB, Smith AL, Abraham WT, et al. Continuous autonomic assessment in patients with symptomatic heart failure: prognostic value of heart rate variability measured by an implanted cardiac resynchronization device. *Circulation.* 2004;110(16):2389–2394.

PART 2
IMPLANTABLE CARDIOVERTER DEFIBRILLATORS

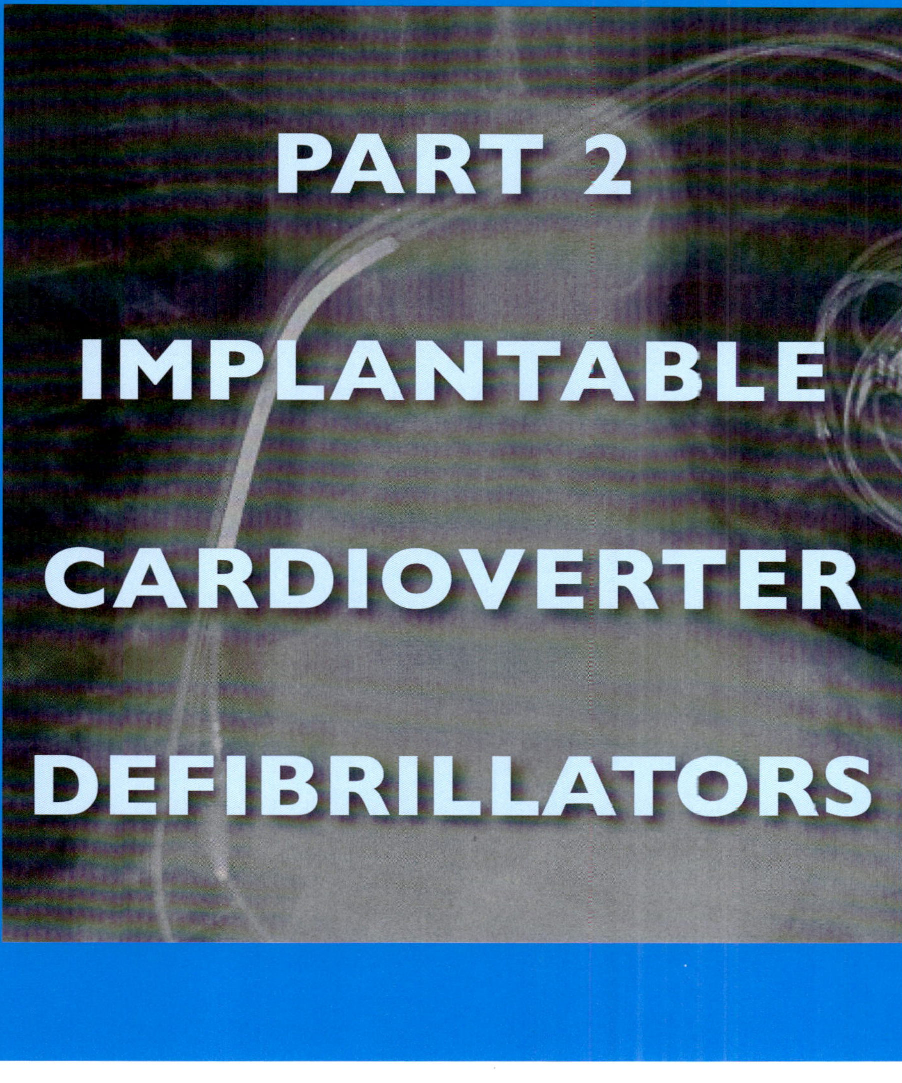

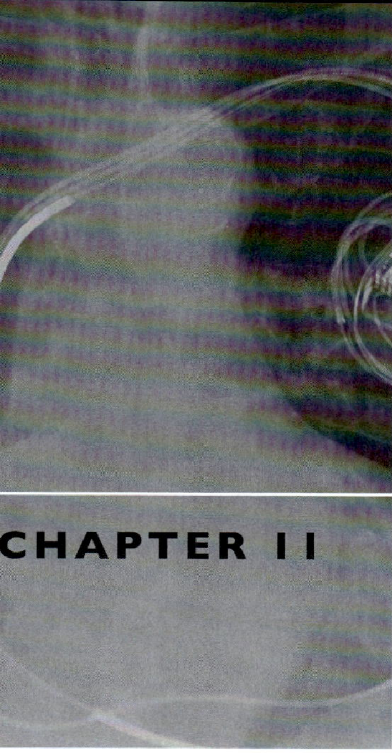

Basic ICD Systems

CHAPTER 11

Jane Chen

Introduction

Each year in the United States, sudden cardiac death (SCD) strikes over 300,000 people, and accounts for > 50% of all cardiovascular deaths.[1–3] Survivors of an initial cardiac arrest have a recurrence rate of 30% within 1 year and 45% in 2 years, with the majority of these events due to ventricular arrhythmias.[4–5] Historically, strategies to reduce the incidence of SCD and prevent its recurrence centered primarily on various medical therapies such as beta-blockers and antiarrhythmic drugs. With the development of the implantable cardioverter defibrillator (ICD), an alternative therapy for the prevention of SCD became available. Various clinical trials have subsequently demonstrated the mortality benefit of ICD over medical management among survivors of SCD (secondary prevention)[6–8] and in patients deemed at high risk for cardiac arrest (primary prevention).[9–11] The initial studies of ICDs as primary prevention therapy of SCD focused on patients with coronary artery disease. The Sudden Cardiac Death in Heart Failure Trial[12] demonstrated that ICDs improve mortality in patients with dilated cardiomyopathy as well. Given the increasing number of ICD implantations, a working knowledge of ICD function is essential for all physicians.

In 1980, the first defibrillator was implanted into a human, and an ICD first received approval by the U.S. Food and Drug Administration in 1985.[13] The original devices were large (~ 205 cc), therefore necessitating placement in the abdomen, and a thoracotomy was required to place epicardial patch electrodes directly onto the heart. With the advent of transvenously inserted defibrillation leads and with improvements in technology, the ICD has become much smaller (< 40 cc), allowing for its placement in the pectoral region. Current-generation ICDs allow programmable multi-tiered algorithms

Pacemakers and Implantable Cardioverter Defibrillators: An Expert's Manual. © 2010 Amin Al-Ahmad, Kenneth A. Ellenbogen, Andrea Natale, and Paul J. Wang, eds. Cardiotext Publishing, ISBN: 978-0-9790164-6-2.

at various heart rates, are able to treat ventricular arrhythmias with high-energy defibrillation shocks and with antitachycardia pacing, and possess the ability to discriminate between rhythm disturbances that may be of supraventricular versus ventricular origin. They can also function as single, dual, or biventricular pacemakers. Finally, almost all ICDs in the present era can be interrogated remotely using radiofrequency or Bluetooth wireless technology. The wide range of functions demanded of an ICD requires a unique power system which will be reviewed in this chapter.

Overview of Defibrillator Components

The basic ICD consists of a pulse generator and a transvenously placed lead in the right ventricle. The pulse generator houses a battery, which serves as the energy source; a capacitor, which allows rapid delivery of current necessary for defibrillation across the myocardium; low power circuits, amplifiers, and microprocessors for sensing, pacing, and other routine operations; and high-output circuits for charging and delivering high energy. The pulse generator is encased in titanium, which is 10 times stronger than steel but weighs much less. The entire casing is welded shut with laser beams for a hermetic seal. This chapter focuses on current battery and capacitor technologies as well as workings of the high-output circuit.

Battery

The battery is the principal energy storage unit for the device. The major components of a battery are the anode, the cathode, and the electrolyte (Fig 11.1). The anode and the cathode must be physically separated from each other, and each must always be in contact with the electrolyte. The anode, which is usually metal, furnishes electrons, and is where oxidation occurs. Therefore, it is the negatively charged electrode. The cathode is the positively charged electrode in a battery, and is where reduction occurs. The electrolyte, a crucial component of the battery, separates the anode and the cathode. The electrolyte can conduct only ions, not electrons, and allows for the buildup of charges at the anode and the cathode to neutralize each other. When an electrolyte is a liquid, a "separator" is required to physically separate the anode and the cathode.

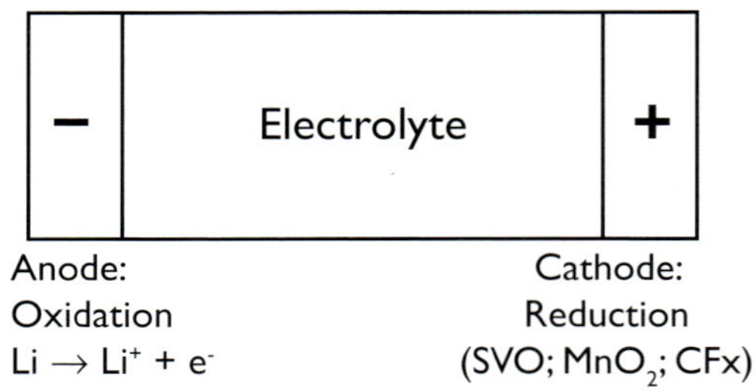

Figure 11.1 Major components of an ICD battery.

The most important feature of a battery that powers an implantable device is reliability. Unlike batteries used for consumer products, batteries for implantable devices cannot be recharged or replaced. Implantable device batteries are expected to power the entire system from the time the generator is sealed at the factory through shelf life, and determine the service life of the generator. The battery must have predictable end-of-life behavior, high-quality performance under various conditions, and be small and lightweight. Materials for implantable device batteries are chosen for their biocompatibility, stability, and ability to perform to the aforementioned specifications.

In pacemakers and ICDs, the most commonly used anodal metal is lithium. Wilson Greatbatch invented the lithium iodide (Li/I_2) battery in 1972,[14] and this battery continues to power all current implantable pacemakers. Lithium is the anode of choice in implantable devices because of its stability and high-energy density (energy stored per volume), which makes small size possible. Although water is an excellent solvent for salts and forms solutions with exceptional ionic conductivity, aqueous electrolytes cannot be used with lithium batteries because lithium reacts violently with water. The Li/I_2 battery is a solid electrolyte system formed from the product of lithium and iodine, which acts as an electronic insulator. The Li/I_2 battery has a low self-discharge rate that makes for a long shelf life.[15] Its internal impedance, which is the resistance of a cell to an alternating current, is high. The higher the internal impedance of a cell, the more difficult it is to pass a current. This is ideal for pacemakers, which has peak power demands of only 100 to 200 μW. Implantable defibrillators, however, are required to deliver peak powers 10,000 times greater than pacemakers, which cannot be achieved using the Li/I_2 battery. The battery for an ICD needs to have low internal resistance to allow passage of high current when defibrillation is required. Electrolytes used in ICDs are nonaqueous, and are commonly mixtures of organic ethers and esters.

One method of decreasing internal resistance is to increase the surface areas of the anode and the cathode, which is one reason ICDs are larger than pacemakers. Another method is to use silver vanadium oxide ($Ag_2V_4O_{11}$) as the cathode. The lithium silver vanadium oxide (Li/SVO) battery is most commonly used in ICDs today. The internal resistance of this battery is very low, allowing the battery to sustain a high current during capacitor charging while maintaining a high voltage. Using SVO as the cathode has resulted in a good balance between the ability to achieve high power rapidly and a gradual decrease in voltage as the cathode is depleted, to give a reasonable battery behavior over time. The Li/SVO cell has a distinctive discharge curve and is independent of models or manufacturers (Fig 11.2).[16] The "background" voltage curve is the voltage during routine operations, including sensing and pacing, and is the voltage reported during interrogations. Typical of SVO cathode behavior, there is a region of nearly constant voltage at beginning of life (3.2 V), followed by an initial drop in voltage, then another plateau phase at 2.6 V which can last a significant period of time, and finally a sharp decline in voltage near end of life. The temporary increases in its internal resistance during use, a behavior inherent to the SVO cathode, can lead to periodically longer charge times. At the 2.6-V plateau, the charge time increases rapidly due to higher internal resistance and lower voltage. The "load" voltage represents the battery voltage at the time the capacitor is being charged, and is much lower than the background voltage. Similar to the background voltage, the load voltage declines over time. Unlike the background voltage, which is the same for all SVO batteries regardless of manufacturers, the slope of the curve of the load voltage can vary widely among models and manufacturers. Elective replacement indicator (ERI) can be triggered by either a drop in background voltage or an increase in charge time.

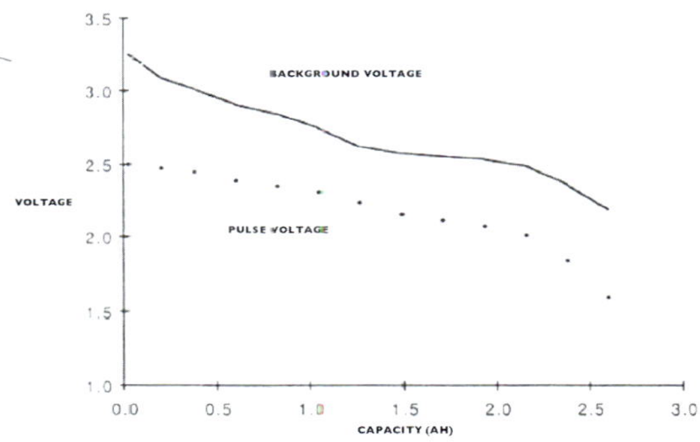

Fig 11.2 Behavior of a typical Li/SVO battery. From: Takeuchi ES, Quattrini PJ, Greatbach W Lithium/silver vanadium oxide batteries for implantable defibrillators. PACE 1988;11:2035-2039. (Courtesy of Wiley and Sons, used with permission.)

The beginning-of-life battery voltage for a typical Li/SVO battery is 3.2 V. Occasionally, two cells may be used in series (6.4 V battery at beginning of life) to reduce charge time. The reduction of charge time with two cells in series compared with a single cell is minimal, on the order of 2 to 3 s, and is generally not worth the increase in generator size required to house two batteries. A typical Li/SVO battery can store 1800 J/cc. Therefore, a 10-cc battery can store 18,000 J/cc, allowing for about 500 shocks at 34 J each during its lifetime.[17] The battery is depleted every time it charges a capacitor, regardless of whether the energy is actually discharged, because the energy used to charge the capacitor cannot be recovered.

Variations of the Li/SVO Battery

Currently two types of SVO are used in ICDs. The decomposition SVO (or DSVO), is an older compound manufactured at low temperature using decomposable starting materials. A newer compound, the combination SVO (CSVO), is manufactured at high temperature using silver and vanadium oxide. The DSVO has an internal resistance that is two to three times higher than CSVO. As a result, the DSVO battery has a longevity approximately 50% less than the CSVO battery.[18] The longevities of DSVO and CSVO batteries are illustrated in Fig 11.3.

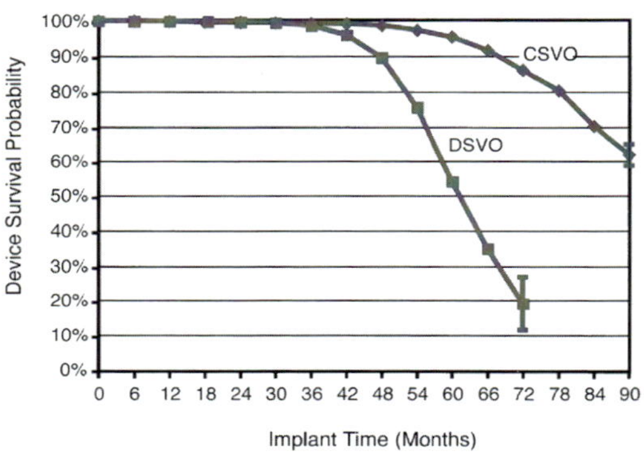

Fig 11.3 Survival curves for CSVO and DSVO batteries. (From *Clinical cardiac pacing, defibrillation, and resynchronization therapy*, 3rd Ed. Ellenbogen, Kay, Lau, & Wilkoff, eds., 249. Copyright Elsevier, used with permission.)

The balance of Li to SVO can be altered to affect charge time. Conventional Li/SVO batteries are cathode limited, meaning they have slightly more capacity at the Li anode than at the SVO cathode, to ensure all cathode can be discharged. The advantage of this design is that it is efficient in packing the maximum capacity into a minimum volume. However, because there is an abundance of lithium to ensure reduction of the SVO occurs well after reaching the 2.6-V plateau, the charge time can rise steeply as the battery approaches ERI. Cathode-limited batteries almost always require frequent capacitor re-formations toward the end of life to reduce charge time (see section on Capacitors). A solution is to rebalance the anode and cathode capacities. The new anode-limited, "charge time optimized" Li/SVO battery has decreased lithium and increased SVO capacities. There is just enough lithium to discharge a short distance into the 2.6-V plateau phase. Thus, the charge time remains low and constant through ERI. Because the battery always remains at higher voltage, it powers the circuit more efficiently and with less energy. The differences in voltage and charge times of conventional cathode-limited DSVO, CSVO, and anode-limited, charge time optimized CSVO (CT CSVO) batteries are illustrated in Fig 11.4.

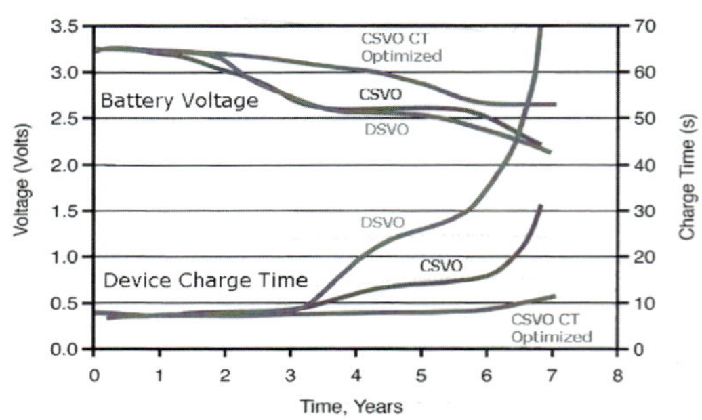

Figure 11.4 Comparison of charge times for different varieties of SVO batteries. (Reproduced with permission of Medtronic, Inc.)

Other Lithium Ion Batteries

Replacing SVO with manganese oxide (Li/MnO_2) solves the problem of temporary increases in internal resistance that is characteristic of SVO batteries. Li/MnO_2 has capabilities for low-power device operations and high-power defibrillation therapy, as well as a predictable voltage behavior. Due to constant low internal resistance, charge times with Li/MnO_2 batteries are more stable over time when compared with LiSVO batteries (Fig 11.5).[19] The lithium carbon monofluoride (Li/CF_x) has a long shelf life and provides medium levels of power, which are ideal for devices that require constant pacing, such as biventricular pacemakers.[20] By itself, Li/CF_x batteries are not capable of providing the high voltage needed for defibrillation. However, a hybrid battery using both carbon monofluoride and SVO (Li/CF_x-SVO) is of interest by many manufacturers for future ICDs. This hybrid battery combines the low- to medium-power capabilities of CF_x for longevity with the high-power capability of SVO for defibrillation.

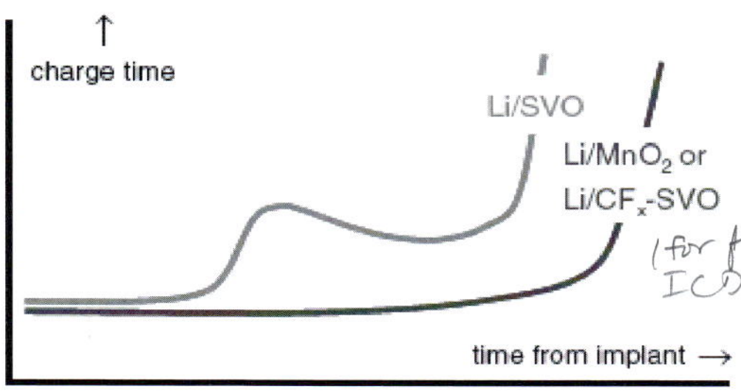

Figure 11.5 Internal resistance behavior and charge times of lithium batteries Used for ICDs. (From *J. of Cardiovasc. Trans. Res.* 2008; 1:254-257. Reprinted with kind permission from Springer Science+Business Media.)

Service Life of ICD Batteries

The lifetime of an ICD battery depends on the requirement of pacing, the number of shocks delivered, and the sophistication of diagnostics and storage data programmed for the device. Most manufacturers continue to rely on battery voltage to determine ERI status. In general, ICD batteries last approximately 5 to 8 years. The generator should be replaced when elective replacement indicator (ERI) is reached. Once ERI is reached, there is sufficient reserve for all ICD operations for several months, although the time available for backup pacing and the number of shocks are limited. When the ERI reserve capacity is used, the generator is at end of life (EOL). At EOL, the device will automatically shut off more sophisticated algorithms, such as antitachycardia pacing, cardioversion, and dual chamber pacing, to conserve battery for high-energy defibrillation. The battery voltages at which ERI and ECL occur vary with individual models of ICDs. The time from ERI to EOL is usually about 3 months, although it depends on the same variables that determine battery depletion. For example, the time from ERI to EOL may be shorter for a biventricular ICD device than a single chamber ICD, because nearly total biventricular pacing is required for the former and likely none for the latter.

Safety

Because the ICD battery contains a large amount of energy and delivers it quickly, if an internal short circuit occurs, the current traveling through the short can heat the cell contents and may cause violent chemical reactions. To avoid catastrophic events, batteries are designed to terminate these potential violent chemical reactions if they occur. The separators, which are used to physically separate the anode and cathode, are made of porous material and are designed to melt at low temperatures. If a short develops and the cell heats up, the separator melts, the porous structure disappears, preventing passage of ions, and the reaction is terminated.[21]

Batteries in Current ICD Systems

Medtronic currently uses Li/CSVO (charge time optimized, anode-limited) batteries in all ICDs, including biventricular ICDs. Boston Scientific has recently switched from Li/SVO to Li/MnO_2 technology for all their high-voltage devices. Biotronik also uses Li/MnO_2 in their ICDs, but their biventricular ICDs have Li/CSVO batteries. St. Jude Medical currently employs the Li/DSVO battery (conventional cathode-limited design).

Capacitors

ICD batteries are designed to function as large energy reservoirs; they are not capable of delivering a current fast enough, or a voltage high enough, when defibrillation is required. Therefore, capacitors are necessary to act as the delivery system. Capacitors contain high-voltage circuitry, which draws large amounts of energy from the battery that can then be discharged across the myocardium. The capacitor itself is unable to store this energy as it leaks voltage over time, and therefore must be charged immediately before defibrillation. High-voltage capacitors largely determine the size of the ICD generator, because they are the bulkiest component in the ICD. A capacitor consists of two plates, or conductors, of opposite charge, separated by a distance (d). The amount of charge (Q) on each conductor is proportional to the difference in voltage between the two conductors. Capacitance (C) is defined as the ability to store charge as a function of voltage, which in turn is dependent on the surface area of the conductors and the distance separating them. The total energy available (in Volts) for discharge is proportional to the product of the capacitance (C) and the voltage (V) stored in the capacitor ($E_{stored} = 1/2C \times V^2$). Inserting insulating materials between the conductors can increase the capacitance. These insulating materials are called dielectrics, and their characteristics determine the properties of the capacitors. Both plates of a capacitor are connected to a transformer, which draws energy from the battery and converts it into high-voltage energy stored in the capacitor (Fig 11.6). Capacitors are passive; the process of storing energy before delivery is called charging. The time for the capacitor to charge is called charge time, and is dependent on the programmed output energy level (ie, higher energy output requires longer charge time).

Electrolytic capacitors are the only type of capacitors used in ICDs, and they are based mostly on aluminum or tantalum materials. These materials are processed to have a high surface area to achieve high capacitance. The anode of aluminum plates are etched with over one million microscopic tunnels. Tantalum anodes are made from a powder that is pressed into a porous pellet, and then heated to make the metal particles bond to one another while remaining porous.[21] The oxide surface for both aluminum and tantalum are formed on the exposed surfaces of the metal and serve as the dielectric. When a voltage is applied to the electrode, the oxide layer forms to a thickness that is proportional to the voltage. Newly formed oxides are fairly free of defects. Defects over time are healed by re-forming the oxide layer when the capacitor is next charged. The oxide that coats the anode surface maintains contact with opposing cathode via the electrolyte, which is usually a conductive organic solvent. Multiple capacitors are usually linked together in series in ICDs to provide sufficient voltage for defibrillation.

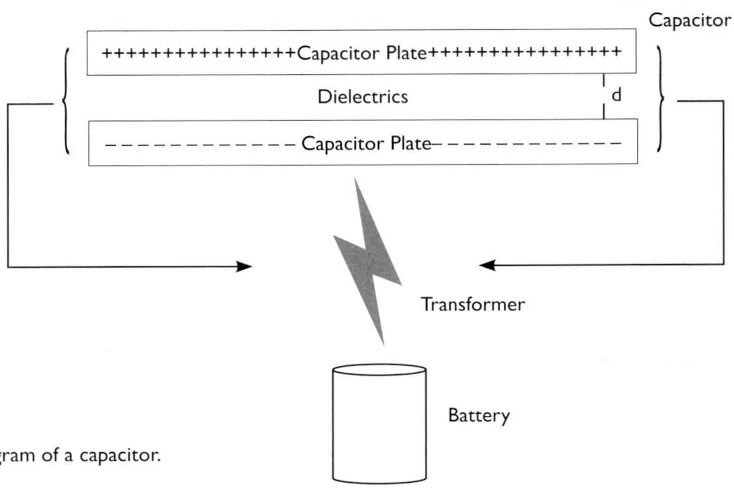

Fig 11.6 Diagram of a capacitor.

In an ideal capacitor system, the energy used to charge the capacitor would be exactly equal to the energy delivered. In reality, however, the energy discharged by the capacitor is usually less than the stored energy. One reason for the reduced delivery of charge is that the waveform during defibrillation is truncated before the voltage on the capacitor reaches zero,[21] which is a more effective way of defibrillating the heart than a waveform that is allowed to decay to zero. Another reason is the deformation of the dielectric material with use. As mentioned before, the oxide layer that forms the dielectric material develops imperfections over time. Additional energy is required to re-form the oxide to heal these defects in a process called re-formation.[22] The additional energy needed to re-form the dielectric is not recovered. A capacitor that has not been used for some time takes longer to charge than a newly re-formed one. Current ICDs have programmable maintenance re-formation, usually at intervals of 1, 3, or 6 months, to routinely charge the capacitors to high voltage to heal the capacitors to avoid excessively prolonged charge times if defibrillation should become necessary. Capacitor re-formation can also be performed manually. In some devices toward end of service, prolonged charge times can be shortened somewhat by performing more frequent capacitor re-formations (eg, devices using conventional cathode-limited Li/SVO batteries). Other factors contributing to non-ideal behavior of capacitors are leakage of current after charging and the presence of internal resistance, which leads to energy loss when the capacitor is discharged.

High-Output Charging Circuit

In ICDs, the low voltage supplied by the battery (3.2 V) must be converted into high-energy voltage (750–800 V) within the capacitors to be discharged across the myocardium. This process takes about 3 to 10 s, and is accomplished through DC-DC converters. DC-DC converters are also called inverters or charging circuits.

The basic components of a charging circuit are the battery (B), the high-current low-voltage switch (S), the fly-back transformer (T), the diode (D), a battery bypass capacitor (C1), and a storage capacitor (C2) (Fig 11.7). The role of the battery bypass capacitor (C1) is to keep the battery voltage above a level at which the rest of the circuit can function. When the switch is open, the battery recharges C1. When the switch is closed, C1 provides the primary current from the battery to the transformer, with the energy stored in the transformer equal to the current squared.[21] When a maximum amount of energy is stored in the transformer (usually takes 5–10 µsec), the switch opens. The energy stored in the transformer cannot cross the open switch, and is therefore transferred to the secondary storage capacitor (C2). Diodes prevent the current from flowing back to the transformer. As soon as the energy is transferred to C2, the switch closes again, and the cycle continues. In this manner, a small amount of energy is stored in the capacitor with each cycle until the desired energy is achieved. Because the energy stored is proportional to the voltage squared ($E_{stored} = 1/2C \times V^2$), the capacitor voltage increases as a function of the square root of elapsed time (Fig 11.8).[23] When the energy stored is not being delivered, an electronic switch diverts the leakage current away from the patient.

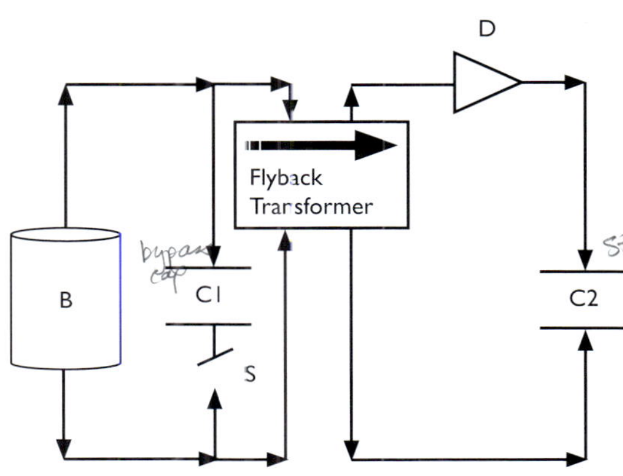

Figure 11.7 Diagram of a basic high-output circuit.

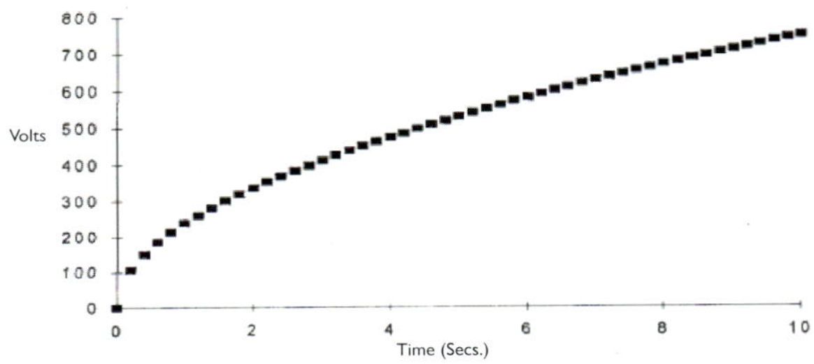

Fig 11.8 Capacitor voltage increase as a function of time. (From Warren JA, Dreher RD, Jaworski RV, Putzke JJ, Russie RJ. *Proceedings of the IEEE* 1996;84:468–479. ©1996 IEEE, used with permission.)

Conclusion

Implantable devices, especially defibrillators, have evolved dramatically in the last 20 years. The battery, capacitors, and high-output circuitry are the basic power systems of the ICD, and constitute the bulk of the ICD generator. Reduction in the size of ICD generators has been limited due to current battery and capacitor technology. The challenges of the future will include exploration of new or combination cathode materials for the battery and development of new capacitors that can store high charges without requirement for increased surface area and dielectrics. The pursuit of these challenges will eventually lead to the increase in longevity, shortened and consistent charge times, and reduction in size of ICD generators sought after by clinicians.

References

1. Myerburg RJ, Kessler KM, Castellanos A. Sudden cardiac death: Epidemiology, transient risk, and intervention assessment. *Ann Int Med.* 1993;119:1187–1197.
2. Gillum RF. Sudden coronary death in the United States: 1980–1985. *Circulation.* 1989;79: 756–765.
3. Zipes DP, Wellens HJ. Sudden cardiac death. *Circulation.* 1998;98:2334–2351.
4. Liberthson RR, Nagel EL, Hirschman JC, and Nussenfeld SR. Prehospital ventricular fibrillation: Prognosis and follow-up course. *N Engl. J Med.* 1974;291:317–321.
5. Baum RS, Alvarez H, Cobb LA. Survival after resuscitation from out-of-hospital ventricular fibrillation. *Circulation.* 1974;50:1231–1235.
6. The Antiarrhythmics versus Implantable Defibrillators (AVID) Investigators. A comparison of antiarrhythmic drug therapy with implantable defibrillators in patients resuscitated from near-fatal ventricular arrhythmias. *N Engl J Med.* 1997;337:1576–1583.
7. Connolly SJ, Gent M, Roberts RS, Dorian P, Roy D, Sheldon RS, Mitchell LB, Green MS, Klein GJ, O'Brien B. Canadian Implantable Defibrillator Study (CIDS): a randomized study of the implantable cardioverter defibrillator against amiodarone. *Circulation.* 2000;101:1297–1302.
8. Kuck KH, Cappato R, Siebels J, Rüppel R. Randomized comparison of antiarrhythmic drug therapy with implantable defibrillator in patients resuscitated from cardiac arrest: the Cardiac Arrest Study Hamburg (CASH). *Circulation.* 2000;102:748–754.
9. Moss AJ, Hall WJ, Cannom DS, and the Multicenter Automatic Defibrillator Implantation Trial Investigators. Improved survival with an implanted defibrillator in patients with coronary disease at high risk for ventricular arrhythmia. *N Engl J Med.* 1996; 335: 1933–1940.
10. Buxton AE, Lee KL, Fisher JD, Josephson ME, Prystowsky EN, Hafley G. A randomized study of the prevention of sudden cardiac death in patients with coronary artery disease. *N Engl J Med.* 1999; 341:1882–1890.
11. Moss AJ, Zareba W, Hall WJ, and the Multicenter Automatic Defibrillator Implantation Trial II Investigators. Prophylactic implantation of a defibrillator in patients with myocardial infarction and reduced ejection fraction. *N Engl J Med.* 2002;346:877–883.
12. Bardy GH, Lee KL, Mark DB, et al. for the Sudden Cardiac Death in Heart Failure Trial Investigators. Amiodarone or an implantable cardioverter-defibrillator for congestive heart failure. *N Engl J Med.* 2005;352:225–237.
13. Mirowski M, Mower MM, Reid RR. The au-

tomatic implantable defibrillator. *Am Heart J* 1980; 100: 1089–1092.

14. Greatbach W, Holmes CF. The lithium/iodine battery: A historical perspective. *Pacing Clin Electrophyiol.* 1992;15:2034–2036.
15. Mallela VA, Ilankumaran V, Rao NS. Trends in cardiac pacemaker batteries. *Indian Pacing Electrophysiol J.* 2004;4:201–212.
16. Takeuchi ES, Quattrini PJ, Greatbach W. Lithium/silver vanadium oxide batteries for implantable defibrillators. *Pacing Clin Electrophyiol.* 1988;11:2035–2039.
17. Eckart RE, Chen J, Epstein LM. Defibrillator function and implantation. In: *Cardiac Pacing for the Clinician*, 2nd ed. Kusumoto FM, Goldschlager NF, eds. Springer 2008.
18. Tachyarrhythmia products. In *Medtronic Product Performance Report*, 2nd ed., vol 14. Minneapolis, Minn., Medtronic, Inc., 2003, p 11.
19. Root MJ. Implantable cardiac rhythm device batteries. *J Cardiovasc Trans Res.* 2008;1:254–257.
20. Greatbach W, Holmes CF, Takeuchi ES, Ebel SJ. Lithium/Carbon monofluoride (Li/CFx): a new pacemaker battery. *Pacing Clin Electrophyiol.* 1996:19:1836–1840.
21. Untereker DF, Crespi AM, Rorvick A, Schmidt CL, Skarstad PM. Chapter 6: Power systems for implantable pacemakers, cardioverters, and defibrillators. In: *Clinical cardiac pacing, defibrillation, and resynchronization therapy*, 3rd ed. Ellenbogen, Kay, Lau, & Wilkoff, eds.
22. Norton J, Anderson C: Proceedings of the 23rd capacitor and resistor technology symposium CARTS 2003, Scottsdale, AZ. 2003, pp 269–277.
23. Warren JA, Dreher RD, Jaworski RV, Putzke JJ, Russie RJ. *Proceedings of the IEEE.* 1996;84: 468–479.

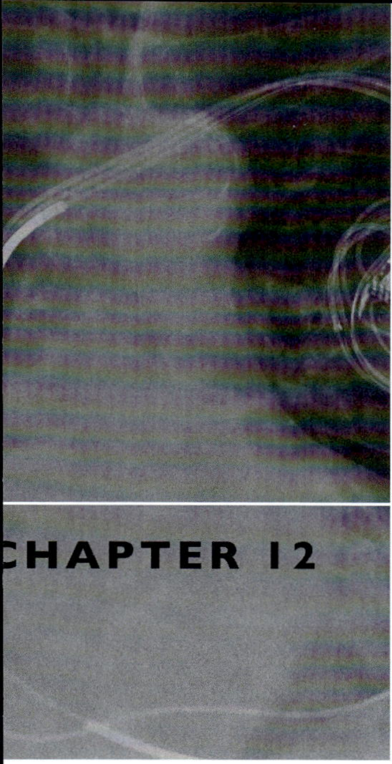

ICD Lead Design

CHAPTER 12

Gautham Kalahasty
and Kenneth A. Ellenbogen

Introduction

The implantable cardioverter defibrillator (ICD) lead is a remarkable medical device that is as critical to the function of the ICD system as the ICD itself. High-voltage leads are required to withstand multiple chronic stresses: mechanical, thermal, electrical, chemical, and oxidative. The purpose of this chapter is not to provide an exhaustive review of ICD lead design principles, suitable for biomedical engineers. Rather, the goal is to explain the design concepts and characteristics of ICD leads and to highlight the relevant differences among current designs in order to provide the implanting physician with the knowledge needed to obtain the safest and most reliable outcomes for their patients. As is true for the ICD itself, it can be argued that any of the current generation of ICD leads is a suitable choice for most patients. However, some lead designs may be a more optimal choice for a specific patient.

The mortality reduction associated with ICDs implanted for primary prevention indications has been made possible by the development of effective and reliable transvenous ICD leads. Mortality rates for implantation of transvenous ICD lead systems is currently < 0.5%. By comparison, mortality rates for epicardial systems requiring thoracotomy were up to 5 times higher.[1]

Since their introduction in 1993, transvenous leads have undergone rapid evolution (Box 12.1). In addition to improvements in reliability, the next generations of leads may offer the ability to monitor hemodynamics and to detect ischemia. Despite advances in design, the high-voltage lead remains the "weakest" component of the ICD system. Long-term data from a prospective registry, published in 2007, showed an overall lead survival rate of 85% at 5 years and as low as 60% at 8 years.[2] Although

Pacemakers and Implantable Cardioverter Defibrillators: An Expert's Manual. © 2010 Amin Al-Ahmad, Kenneth A. Ellenbogen, Andrea Natale, and Paul J. Wang, eds. Cardiotext Publishing, ISBN: 978-0-9790164-6-2.

this study included older leads that are no longer in use (eg, Medtronic 6936), it highlights the importance and limitations of ICD lead design.

1. 1993 First transvenous lead (Guidant ENDOTAK)
2. 1993 First active fixation ICD lead (Medtronic Transvene)
3. 1995 First steroid eluting ICD lead (Guidant ENDOTAK DSP)
4. 1997 First dedicated bipolar lead (Medtronic Sprint)
5. 1997 First dual coil, integrated bipolar lead (Medtronic Sprint)
6. 1997 First silicone backfill of shock coil (Ventritex SPL)
7. 1997 First use of cable conductors (Medtronic Sprint)
8. 2000 First dual coil, dedicated bipolar lead (Medtronic Sprint Quattro)
9. 2002 First 8 Fr ICD lead (St. Jude Medical Riata)
10. 2004 First 7 Fr ICD lead (Medtronic Sprint Fidelis)

Box 12.1 Important Developments in ICD Lead Design

Despite extensive bench, preclinical, and clinical testing, the true reliability and functional characteristics of a lead are often not known until it has been in widespread use. Lead recalls are an unfortunate reality of clinical practice and an understanding of the mechanism of lead failure is essential to proper patient management. Critical appraisal of the literature requires an understanding of lead design.

Basic Concepts

The components of a transvenous ICD lead include the conductors, insulation materials, defibrillation coils, lead electrodes, the fixation mechanism, the yoke, and lead connectors. An example of a dual coil, true bipolar lead is shown in Fig 12.1. The conductor is a composite metal that connects the pin (beyond the yoke) to each of the pace/sense electrodes and to each of the coils. A bipolar ICD lead is similar to a bipolar pacing lead in that there is a tip (cathode) electrode and a ring (anode) electrode. Conductors also connect the DF-1 pin to defibrillation coil or coils. All conductors are arranged in parallel within the lead body until they reach the yoke where the pace/sense conductors and high-voltage conductors separate and terminate in the IS-1 pin or DF-1 pin(s). The yoke is trifurcated in the case of a dual coil lead and is bifurcated in a single coil lead. The length of the distal (right ventricular [RV]) coil is limited by the size of the RV. The proximal coil (superior vena cava [SVC]), if present, is generally longer. Before the development of dual coil leads, a second coil electrode was placed in the SVC in patients with high defibrillation thresholds. Defibrillation efficiency is in part related to the total surface area of the coils. Equal length coils on a smaller diameter lead have less active electrical surface area than ones on a larger diameter lead. Like pacing leads, ICD leads are made in passive fixation and active fixation versions.

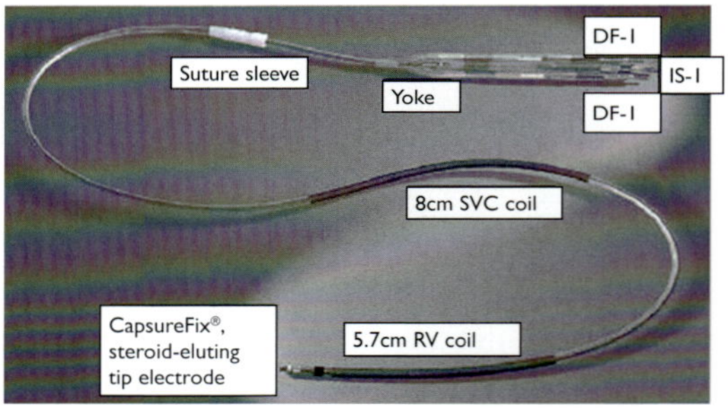

Fig 12.1 Medtronic Sprint Quattro Secure ICD lead. (Reproduced with permission of Medtronic, Inc.)

Active epicardial ICD/patch systems are rarely encountered in clinical practice today. Fig 12.2 shows a schematic of an epicardial patch. Two patches were directly applied to the epicardial surface of the heart with the ICD functioning as an inactive "can." There are two types of patches: titanium mesh patch and a multicoil, platinum-iridium patch. Patch systems have usually been abandoned and replaced with transvenous, nonthoracotomy systems. The patch leads can cover much of the heart surface and may unavoidably reduce the effectiveness of transthoracic defibrillation. Patch lead systems have a high failure rate and the merits of abandoning functioning epicardial patch system (in favor of a new transvenous system), at the time of ICD generator replacement should be weighed.[3] Lead fracture and fluid accumulation in the insulation are among the mechanisms of failure. Constrictive pericarditis due to bacterial infection has also has been reported.[4,5]

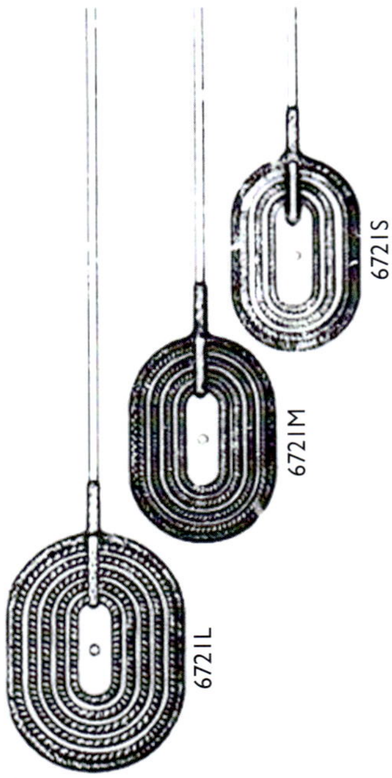

Fig 12.2 Drawings of small, medium, and large unipolar, epicardial patch leads. (Models 6721S, 6721M, and 6721L, Courtesy of Medtronic, Inc.) The lead is made of platinum alloy electrode coils and a low-resistance conductor combined with a polyester outer mesh. The lead is connected to the ICD by a 3.2-mm pin.

Of historical interest is the combination of a nonthoracotomy electrode in the form of a right ventricular catheter (cathode) and a chest wall subcutaneous patch (anode). With a monophasic shock waveform, the epicardial patch system resulted in lower defibrillation thresholds (DFTs) than a nonthoracotomy electrode system. The opposite is true when biphasic waveforms are used.[6,7] The subcutaneous patch was sometimes used in patients with transvenous ICD systems when high thresholds were encountered. The subcutaneous array has an equivalent effect on DFTs and offers greater ease of implant and reliability.[8] Subcutaneous patches are also known to fracture.[9]

Although there are many similarities, each manufacturer has offered a variety of leads with unique specifications and features. Data about older leads that are not currently being marketed, but that may still be in active service, can be found in lead "encyclopedias" published by each manufacturer or other textbooks. Tables 12.1, 12.2, and 12.3 (see pages 242–44) summarize key features and specifications for the most current lead models from each major U.S. manufacturer. Some recent, but not the most current, leads may still be offered by a manufacturer to address specific patient needs or physician preference. For example, the Durata series of leads is the newest ICD lead offered by St. Jude Medical, Inc. The preceding generation (Riata series) of leads is still available for implant.

Materials

The materials used in the construction of ICD leads and lead components are manufactured to very high standards. Although the materials used by each of the major lead manufacturers are similar, there are some differences in how these materials are applied. Some materials, such as copolymer insulation, are unique to a manufacturer. The materials used in the conductor, insulation, shock coil, pace/sense electrode, and connector pin are discussed later. The application of these materials for the construction of leads is also discussed.

Conductors

The primary conductor used in most pacing and ICD leads is MP35N and silver. MP35N (Fort Wayne Metals, Fort Wayne, Indiana) is a superalloy that is double melted to remove

	ENDOTAK RELIANCE G		ENDOTAK RELIANCE SG	
Model/length (cm)	0184/59	0174/59	0180/59	0170/59
	0185/64	0175/64	0181/64	0171/64
	0186/70	0176/70	0182/70	0172/70
	0187/90	0177/90		
Fixation	Active	Passive	Active	Passive
Coils	Dual	Dual	Single	Single
Terminals	IS-1	IS-1	IS-1	IS-1
	DF-1 (2)	DF-1 (2)	DF-1	DF-1
Tip to proximal coil (cm)	18	18	N/A	N/A
Proximal coil Active electrode surface area (mm^2)	660	660	N/A	N/A
Tip electrode surface area (mm^2)	5.7	2.0	5.7	2.0
Isodiametric lead diameter (mm)/(Fr)	2.7/8.1			
Coil electrode diameter (mm)/(Fr)	2.7/8.1			
Distal coil active electrode surface area (mm^2)	450			
Tip-RV coil (mm)	12			
Insulation/external overlay	Silicone rubber/proprietary lubricious coating			
DF-1 pin	Titanium			
IS-1 pin	Stainless steel			
Pace/sense conductor	MP35N, PTFE coated			
Coil material	Platinum clad tantalum with titanium core			
Coil conductor	Drawn brazed stand (DBS) 316L bifilar cable, PTFE coated			
Tip electrode cover	Platinum iridium			
Coil electrode cover	Gore ePTFE			
Multilumen design	Asymmetric			
Sensing	Integrated bipolar			

Table 12.1 Current Boston Scientific (Guidant) ICD Leads

	SPRINT QUATTRO	SPRINT QUATTRO SECURE	SPRINT QUATTRO SECURE S
Model/Length (cm)	6944/58 6944/65 6944/75 6944/100	6947/58 6947/65 6947/75 6947/100	6935—52 6935—58 6935—65 6935—75 6935—100
Fixation	Passive	Active	Active
Coils	Dual	Dual	Single
Terminals	IS-1 DF-1 (2)	IS-1 DF-1 (2)	IS-1 DF-
Tip to proximal coil (cm)	18	18	N/A
Proximal coil active electrode surface area (mm^2)	819	860	N/A
Tip electrode surface area (mm^2)	1.6	5.7	5.7
Isodiametric lead diameter (mm)/(Fr)	2.7/8.1	2.9/8.7	2.8/8.4
Coil electrode diameter (mm)/(Fr)	2.7/8.1	2.9/8.7	2.8/8.4
Distal coil active electrode surface area (mm^2)	584	614	614
Tip-RV coil (mm)	8	8	8
Insulation/external overlay		Silicone rubber/polyurethane	
DF-1 pin		Stainless steel	
IS-1 pin		Stainless steel	
Pace/sense conductor		MP35N, PFTE coated	
Coil material		Platinum clad tantalum	
Coil conductor		MP35N	
Tip electrode cover		Platinized platinum alloy	
Coil electrode cover		Silicone backfill	
Design		Asymmetric	
Sensing		Dedicated bipolar	

Table 12.2 Current Medtronic ICD Leads

	DURATA						
Model/length (cm)	7120/60 7120/65	7121/60 7121/65 7121/75	7122/60 7122/65	7130/60 7130/65	7131/60 7131/65	7170/60 7170/65	7171/60 7171/65
Fixation	Active	Active	Active	Active	Active	Passive	Passive
Coils	Dual	Dual	Single	Dual	Dual	Dual	Dual
Terminals	IS-1 DF-1 (2)	IS-1 DF-1 (2)	IS-1 DF-1	IS-1 DF-1 (2)	IS-1 DF-1 (2)	IS-1 DF-1 (2)	IS-1 DF-1 (2)
Tip to proximal coil (cm)	17	21	N/A	17	21	17	21
Proximal coil active electrode surface area (mm^2)	588	588	N/A	588	588	588	588
Tip electrode surface area (mm^2)	8	8	8	8	8	3.5	3.5
Isodiametric lead diameter (mm)/(Fr)	2.3/6.8						
Coil electrode diameter (mm)/(Fr)	2.3/6.8						
Distal coil active electrode surface area (mm^2)	367						
Tip-RV coil or anode (mm)	11						
Insulation/external overlay	Silicone/Optim overlay with Fast-Pass coating						
DF-1 pin	MP35N and stainless steel						
IS-1 pin	MP35N and stainless steel						
Pace/sense conductor	MP35N and MP35N DFT						
Coil material	Platinum iridium alloy						
Coil conductor	MP35N						
Helix/cover	Platinum iridium alloy/titanium nitride					N/A	N/A
Coil electrode cover							
Multilumen design	Symmetric			Symmetric		Symmetric	
Sensing	Dedicated bipolar			Integrated bipolar		Dedicated bipolar	

Table 12.3 St. Jude Medical ICD Leads

impurities. It is primarily composed of cobalt, nickel, chromium, and molybdenum. It has high tensile strength and is corrosion resistant. Because of its relatively high electrical resistivity (1033 μΩ) MP35N is combined with efficient conductors such as silver. Single conducting filaments (wires) are made in two designs: a drawn brazed strand (DBS) and a drawn filled tube. Figs 12.3 and 12.4 show examples of each. The DBS design consists of the MP5N alloy stranded around the core of softer, highly conductive silver. It is brazed and drawn in the normal wire drawing process (dies). The core size is adjusted to make the silver content between 20% to 25%. The resulting wire combines increased fatigue life, high conductivity, and great solderability with the ability to withstand greater mechanical stresses. The drawn filled tube design has a central core of silver, totally surrounded by MP35N and then coated with platinum or platinum-iridium. Extreme compressive forces are required during the processing of these dissimilar materials in order to form a sound mechanical bond between surfaces. This feature allows the drawn filled tube wire to exist as a round single wire or to be shaped into a ribbon. The tensile strength and electrical resistivity of this wire depends on the amount of silver in the core, which can be manufactured to the needs of the lead engineers. Both drawn filled tube wires and DSB wires can be formed into coils or twisted into cables.

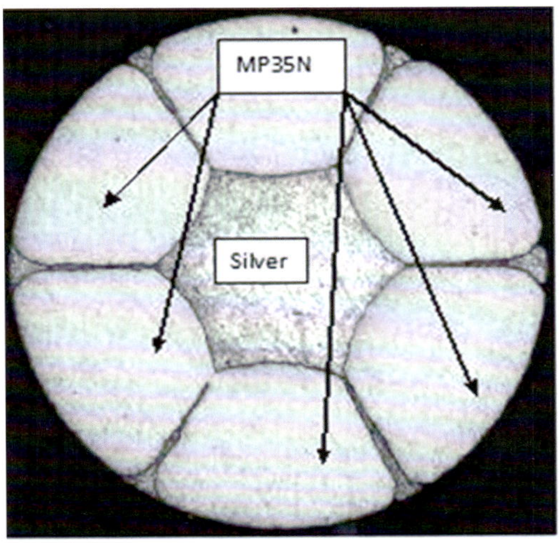

Fig 12.3 Single conducting filaments (wires) are made into a drawn brazed strand (DBS). (Courtesy of Fort Wayne Metals.)

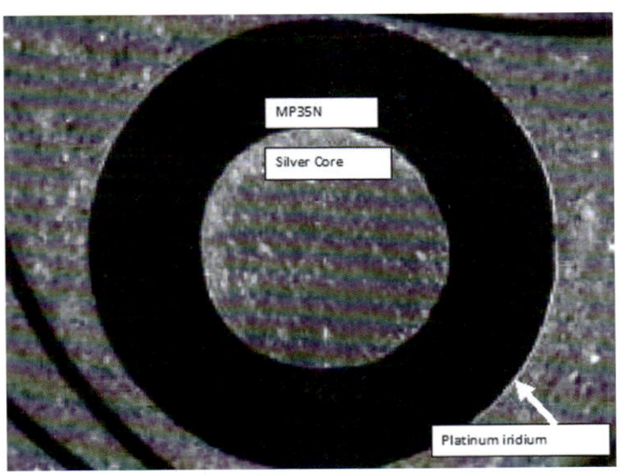

Fig 12.4 Single conducting filaments (wires) are made into a drawn filled tube (DFT). (Courtesy of Fort Wayne Metals, Inc.)

MP35N is not the universal conductor for ICD leads amongst all manufacturers. The Guidant ENDOTAK Reliance series of leads uses a DBS wire composed of silver and a version of 316LMV (Fort Wayne Metals, Fort Wayne, Indiana) as the conductor for the high-voltage coil. This is an austenitic stainless steel composed primarily of chromium, nickel, iron, and molybdenum that is initially electric-arc melted and then vacuum arc remelted (VAR). This process yields a more uniform chemistry with minimal voids and contaminants. 316LMV has good corrosion resistance and many metallurgical studies use it as a reference when evaluating new alloys.

Despite the sophisticated manufacturing process, MP35N can contain foreign inclusions of nitride, oxide, or carbide bodies that can negatively influence the metal fatigue life. Titanium (Ti), which is found in minute quantities in MP35N, can form titanium-carbide or titanium-nitride inclusions that are thought to promote fatigue cracking. A lead containing a modified, low titanium MP35N alloy (US Patent #7138582 assigned to Medtronic, Inc.) may have improved flex life. Low titanium MP35N is not used by all manufacturers and is not yet used clinically in ICD leads.

Insulation

The materials used in ICD leads for insulation play a critical role in the longevity and reliability of the lead as well as handling and implant characteristics. The ideal insulation material should be inert, show no surface erosions, no molecular chain disruptions, no uptake of low-molecular-weight biological materials, no local chemical imbalances, and no tendency to calcification or negative changes of mechanical properties. There is no insulation that can claim all of these properties and there are no ICD leads currently that contain only one insulation material. Silicone rubber, polyurethanes, and fluoropolymers are all used in different combinations within a given lead for various purposes.

Fluoropolymers are fluorocarbon-based polymers with multiple strong carbon-fluorine bonds. They are characterized by a high resistance to solvents, acids, and bases. Therefore, they have maximum biocompatibility and tensile strength but their stiffness limits their use to thin coating (< 0.076 mm) applications. Conductors are coated with a fluoropolymer layer to prevent adverse interactions with silicone tubing. Fluoropolymers will decrease the incidence of metal ion oxidation in polyurethanes, but because ICD leads use silicone tubing, this is not the intended purpose. Examples of fluoropolymers are PTFE (polytetrafluoroethylene, ie, Teflon, DuPont) and ETFE (polyethylene-tetrafluoroethylene).

Silicone rubber is a polymer that has a "backbone" of silicon-oxygen linkages; the same bond that is found in quartz, glass, and sand. It is both biocompatible and biostable. It also has high resistance to extreme temperatures and therefore, less susceptible to damage from electrocautery. Its main disadvantage is its low tensile strength, making it prone to tearing and abrasion wear. Abrasion wear comes from lead-to-lead, can-to-lead, and yoke-to-lead mechanical contact. Silicone rubber is also susceptible to cold flow (also known as creep), defined as increasing deformation under constant or cyclic compression (Fig 12.5). It also has a high coefficient of friction making it difficult to pass alongside other leads. Therefore, when silicone rubber is used as the primary insulation, relatively thick layers are used and covered with a lubricious coating or polyurethane.

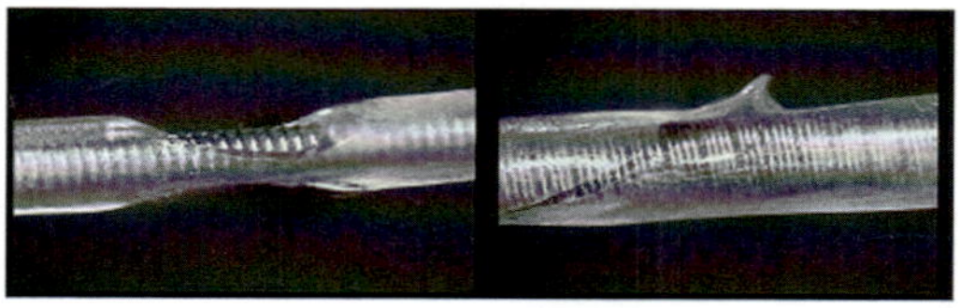

Fig 12.5 Examples of lead abrasion (**left**) and cold flow and abrasion (**right**). (Courtesy of St. Jude Medical, Inc.)

Of the current insulation materials in use today, *polyurethanes* have the least biostability (relatively). They are also characterized by high tear strength, high elasticity, and a low coefficient of friction. They result in limited scar formation and allow for smaller lead diameters. The observed interactions of polyurethane chemistry and body chemistry can lead to significant degradation of lead function resulting from calcification (rare), environmental stress cracking (ESC) and chain scission. ESC occurs, in part, as a result of polyurethane oxidation caused by macrophages that induce hydrogen peroxide formation to the polymer structure. Hydrogen peroxide is also produced by inflammatory cells as they make contact with the conductor. This results in oxidation-induced molecular chain breaks in the polyurethane and metal ion oxidation (MIO). Thermal instability and mechanical stresses also play a role in ESC. Polyurethane is not stable at high temperatures and is prone to melting when electrocautery is applied. Pretreating the polyurethane in an inert gas protects it against ESC. The two most common polyurethanes in clinical use today are Pellethane 80A (Upjohn Co., CPR Division, Torrance, California) and Pellethane 55D. Pellethane 80A has been associated with increased long-term failure rates. Pellethane 55D may be more biostable but it is relatively stiffer and is now the dominant polyurethane.

Elast-Eon (AorTech Biomaterials, Clayton, Victoria, Australia) is a copolymer composed of silicone rubber, polyhexamethylene oxide

(PHMO), and polyurethane. The polyurethane is composed of methylene diisocyanate (MDI) and Butanediol (BDO). Elast-Eon has been specifically designed to be used in biomedical applications because it retains the strengths of each of its primary components (tear and abrasion resistance, lubricity, flexibility, and biostability). Elast-Eon is currently exclusively used by St. Jude Medical in their Durata series of ICD leads and is referred to as Optim Insulation. It is applied as a layer over standard silicone rubber. Although there are in-vitro and in-vivo animal studies, there are as yet no large, long-term human studies that have been completed.[10] At least one study has demonstrated that the co-polymer used in these leads is not protective against thermal injury from cautery.[11] Other co-polymers are being developed.

Although technically not an insulation material, *expanded polytetrafluoroethylene* (ePTFE) or Gore-Tex (WL Gore and Associates, Flagstaff, Arizona) is applied to ICD coils to prevent tissue in-growth. It has a porous structure that allows fluid ingress and therefore is not an electrical insulator and allows efficient defibrillation. In fact, ePTFE can prevent lead chatter from metal-metal interactions when multiple leads are present.[12] The pores are too small to allow cell penetration and help minimize fibrous tissue formation. ePTFE has been shown to improve extractability without compromising electrical performance.[13,14] Most of the data is from animal studies with very limited data from long-term human studies. This material is currently only used in the Guidant Reliance G series of leads. The safety and biostability has been well established through its extensive use in other applications including vascular and plastic surgery.

Defibrillation Coils, Pacing Electrodes, and Connector Pins

The metals used in defibrillation coils include platinum, iridium, tantalum, and titanium. Platinum, in particular, is known for its oxidation-corrosion resistance and biocompatibility. When combined by a process called cladding, these metal alloys offer high-strength, superior conductive properties, stable thermal properties, and enhanced corrosion resistance and biocompatibility. Cladding is the metallurgical process by which dissimilar layers of metals are bonded together with no adhesives or filler materials. It is accomplished through the use of extreme pressure and, in some cases, heat. Combinations include platinum clad-tantalum and platinum clad-tantalum with a titanium core. Neither material has been proven to be superior to the other in clinical applications. Titanium is not used by itself because it produces metallic oxides during high-voltage shocks.

The cathode and anode (of a true bipolar lead) of ICD leads are made of a platinum-iridium alloy. Although a carbon-tipped cathode has been shown to have good mechanical strength and lower chronic stimulation thresholds, most manufacturers are not yet using this in their current lead designs. The electrodes themselves may be coated with a substance to create a microporous, fractal surface that increases the "electrical" surface area. These coatings include titanium nitride, platinum black, and iridium oxide. Electrode efficiency is related to the degree of polarization that takes place at the surface.[15] Titanium nitride has the lowest polarization effect. Connector pins are made with stainless steel or titanium.

Design and Construction

The individual material elements used in each component have specific assembly based on the design goal. The conductors, pace/sense coil, shock coil, and yoke can be thought of as subassemblies that are then combined into an ICD lead. As will be evident later, there is very significant variability to the engineering approaches taken for each component of an ICD lead. The detailed discussion that follows is meant to provide the background to critically appraise clinical and industry literature. Unfortunately, a clinical comparison of design philosophies for each component is not possible. The clinical comparison of leads is really a comparison of the specific combination of design compromises that are represented in a given lead.

Conductors

Single filament drawn filled tubes can be combined into strands and cables (Fig 12.6). Filaments are wound into cables to serve as conductors in ICD leads and pacing leads. Cable conductors offer greater strength, fracture resistance, and redundancy than coiled conductors. Cable conductors are also not compressible. Cable conductors are coated with a fluoropolymer to prevent insulation damage. Multipolar leads that employ cables can be made to smaller diameters than those that use coaxial coiled conductors. The number of filaments and their arrangement within a given cable is variable from manufacturer to manufacturer. Two examples are shown in Fig 12.7. Compared individually, a A 7×7 (49 wire) cable has relatively greater flexibility but relatively lower torquability than a 1×19 (19 wire) design. Neither design has been proven to be clinically superior.

The structure of the pace-sense coil conductor of the cathode is highly variable among manufacturers. Figure 12.8 shows the structure of the coil and the characteristics considered by engineers. These characteristics are important because they affect the flexibility of the coil as well as its resistance to fracture. Wire diameter, number of filars (wires), and pitch are all factors that vary among manufacturers and among lead families of a single manufacturer. Multifilar coils offer lower electrical resistance (optimal) but may have lower fatigue life when compared to bifilar designs. There is no consensus as to the optimal combination of these factors.

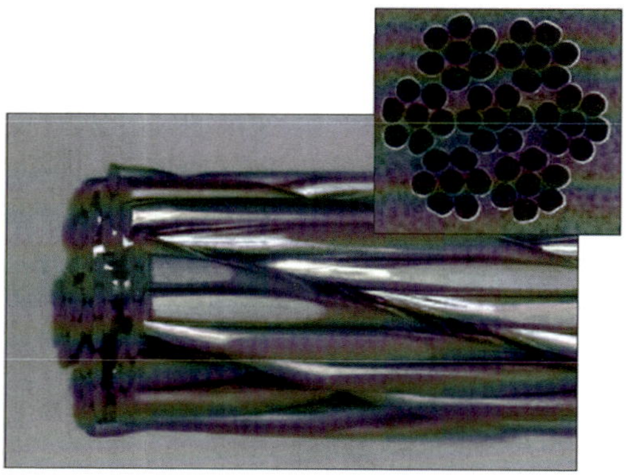

Fig 12.6 Individual wires are combined into strands and then wound into a cable. (Courtesy of Fort Wayne Metals, Inc.)

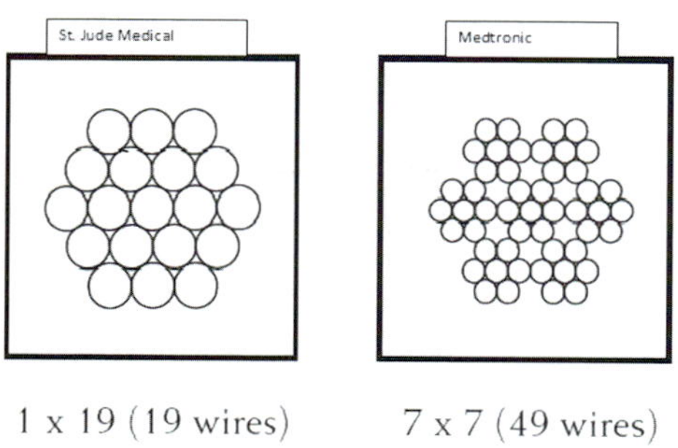

Fig 12.7 Examples of conductor cable structures. (Courtesy of Fort Wayne Metals, Inc.)

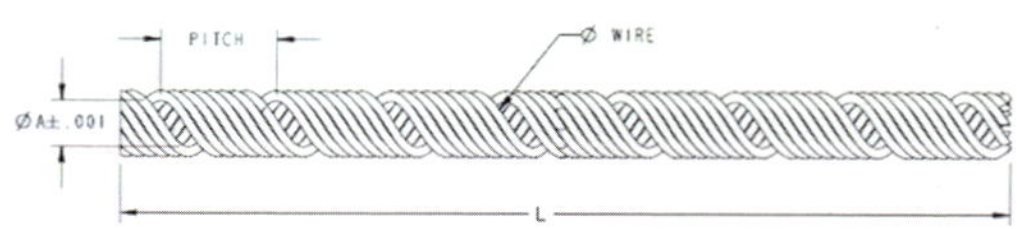

Fig 12.8 Schematic of the coil conductor for the cathode. Each filar has a diameter. Coil filarity is the number of separate wires with the coil. Pitch is a function of the filar diameter *x* the number of filar in the set + the space between filar sets. (Courtesy of St. Jude Medical, Inc.)

Defibrillation Coil

Defibrillation coils on current ICD leads are made with round wires (Medtronic and Boston Scientific) or flat wire (St. Jude Medical Durata and Biotronik). Both designs can be backfilled with silicone or covered with ePTFE. No current designs have bare coils. Wire shape affects surface area and the amount of electrically active surface area which is important to efficient defibrillation. The surface areas of various leads can be found in Tables 12.1 through 12.3. One potential advantage of flat wire coils is the more even and complete distribution of the silicone backfill. This may result in less tissue in-growth. There are no human clinical studies demonstrating the superiority of flat coils versus round coils with respect to tissue in-growth.

ICD Lead Connectors and Yoke Design

All manufactures now follow the Internal Organization for Standards (ISO) guidelines for terminal pin design. Current ICD leads have a bifurcated or trifurcated yoke with terminal pins that connect into the ICD header block. The pace/sense portion of the lead is terminated with an IS-1 pin and the shock coils are terminated with their respective DF-1 (ISO-11318) pins. This design has obvious consequences in terms of pocket bulk. More importantly, the yoke greatly increases the potential for lead-to-lead and lead-to-can interactions resulting in insulation defects. The presence of two DF-1 pins in dual coil leads allows for connection errors in the header block.

The next generation of ICD leads may incorporate a new, in-line design to form a single connector pin, the proposed DF-4 (or IS-4) connector (Fig 12.9). Pocket bulk, as well as the potential for lead-to-lead interactions will be considerably decreased. ICD leads with this design will likely be available by the time this book goes into print. A potential disadvantage is the possibility of multiple component fracture from one critically located stress in the pocket. The DF-4 design will require a compatible header blocker design.

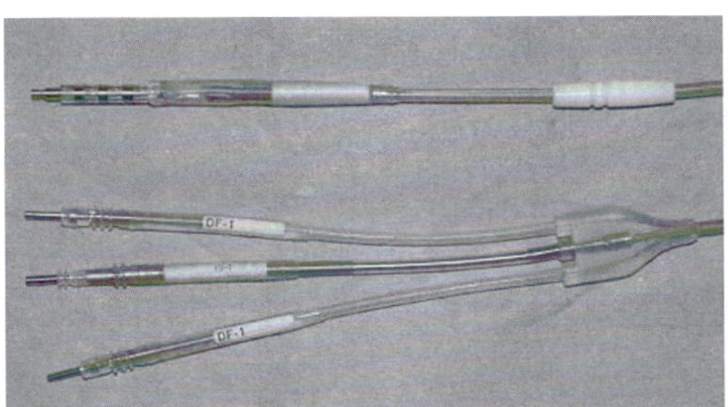

Fig 12.9 Comparison of the current DF-1 connector (**bottom**) and the proposed DF-4 connector (**top**).

The ICD Lead

Early transvenous ICD leads were based on the *coaxial* design of pacemaker leads. In a coaxial lead design, each conductors is coiled around the central (cathode) coil conductor and separated by insulation tubing (Fig 12.10). Examples of these leads include the Medtronic Transvene 6936, St. Jude Medical/Ventritex TVL RV 01, and the Guidant ENDOTAK 0073/75. The central coil allows stylet insertion and helix deployment. Due to the coaxial design and the need for multiple conductors, these leads have large diameters, ranging in size from 9.7 Fr to 12 Fr. This design is more prone to conductor fracture and insulation breach and has been replaced by the multilumen design. Although no longer manufactured, many leads with this design are still in active use. For example, the Medtronic 6936 was released to the U.S. market in 1993 and 23,700 lead were implanted. It is estimated that 3,200 leads are still in active use.

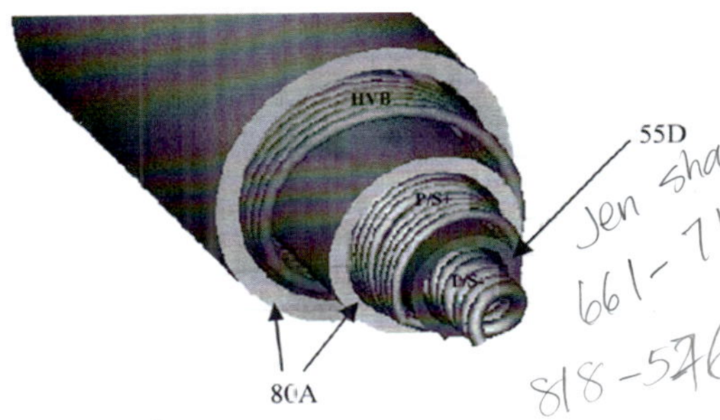

Fig 12.10 Schematic showing the Medtronic Transvene 6936 single coil ICD lead. Coaxial design. Abbreviations: P/S, pace/sense; HVB, high-voltage distal coil; 80A, polyurethane 80A; 55D, polyurethane 55D.

The coaxial design has been replaced by the *multilumen* design. Similar to the coaxial design, a central coil conductor is used as the cathode allowing for stylet insertion and provides the extendable/retractable function of active fixation leads. Conductors for the anode and high-voltage coil(s) are arranged as parallel cables and are distributed around the central coil. The distribution of cables can be *symmetric*, as is the case for current St. Jude Medical

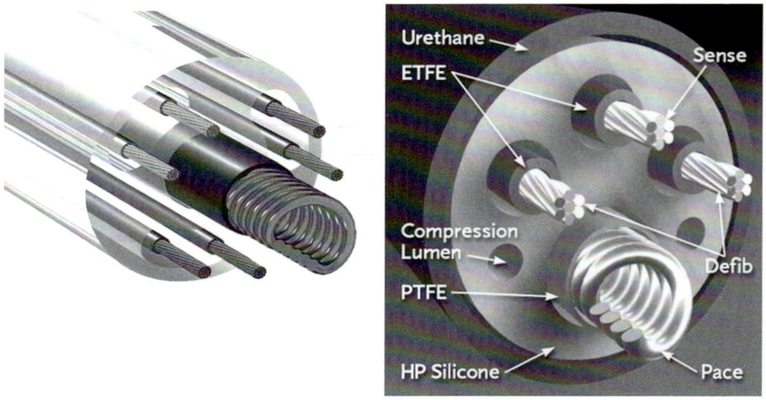

Fig 12.11 Two examples of multilumen lead design. The St. Jude Medical Riata ST (left) has a symmetric structure whereas the Medtronic Sprint 6947 (right) has an asymmetric structure. The cable conductors of the Riata ST are paired and arranged in a common oversized lumen. (Courtesy of St. Jude Medical, Inc., and Medtronic, Inc.)

leads, or *asymmetric* as is the case for current Medtronic and Boston Scientific leads (Fig 12.11). Neither approach has been proven to be superior, but each have theoretical advantages and disadvantages. The symmetric lead design may be more prone to "stacking" of conductors when pressure is applied in any given vector across the lead diameter. Also, because cables are noncompressible, a symmetric design may be less flexible in any given direction than an asymmetrical design. An asymmetric lead is likely to preferentially flex away from the cables, in the direction of the relatively compressible coil. Therefore, the coil and conductor may experience a variable degree of bending and binding stress, depending on the direction that the lead is flexed. Most leads are designed with one conductor for each element. The St. Jude Medical Riata ST series and Durata series of leads are designed with redundant conductors paired into a common oversized lumen. These redundant conductors terminate at a common junction at the coil, electrode, and yoke. There is no proven advantage to this redundancy. The cables and coils are covered by fluoropolymers such as PTFE which protects the cable and improves its dielectric strength.

Figure 12.12 shows a schematic of dedicated bipolar and integrated bipolar leads. A true bipolar lead has one additional conductor that is carried the entire length of the lead, extending from the anode ring to the yoke. Conductor cables are connected to the coils and ring by a variety of methods. Connections are made at the proximal end of the SVC coil and the distal and/or proximal ends of the RV coil (proximal connections are represented in Fig 12.13). Connections at both the distal and proximal ends of the RV coil result in the most uniform distribution of current.[16] Current density is highest at the connection points. Uniform current delivery is thought to improve defibrillation efficiency and delivery of current to the apex is better than delivery to annular region of the septum. All manufacturers connect the SVC coil at the proximal end. Medtronic leads are connected at both the distal and proximal ends of the RV coil. St. Jude Medical (Durata) leads are connected at the distal end of the RV coil and the Boston Scientific ENDOTAK series of leads utilizes a proximal connection. The methods used for connection include spot welding, crimp coupling, and stake joints (or a combination of these methods). Crimp coupling involves crimping the conductor coil to a platinum coupler (jacket). This jacket is then welded to the platinum defibrillation coil. Figure 12.13 shows a schematic illustration of crimp coupling and stake joints. Crimp coupling can increase the rigidity of the lead at the site of cou-

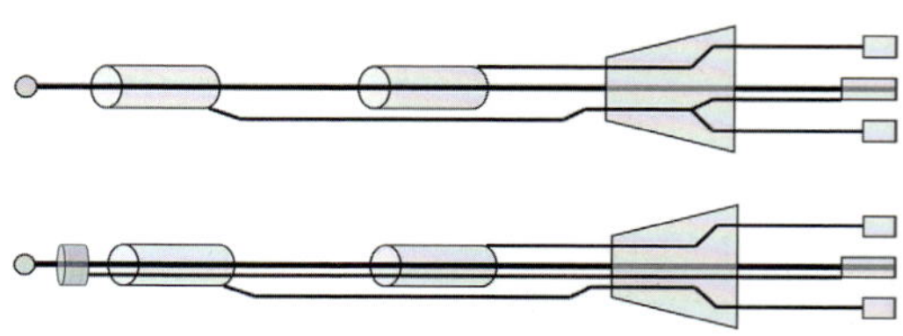

Fig 12.12 Schematic of a dual coil integrated bipolar lead (**top**) and true bipolar lead (**bottom**). Note that in the integrated bipolar lead, the conductor from the distal coil bifurcates in the yoke to connect to the IS-1 and DF-1 pins. (Courtesy of St. Jude Medical, Inc.)

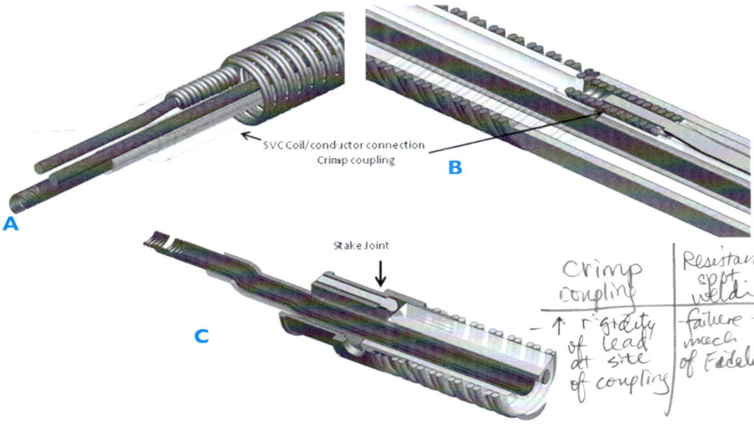

Fig 12.13 Examples of crimp coupling and stake joints. Panel **A** shows the cable conductor connecting to the SVC coil. Panel **B** is a cutaway showing the crimping of the cable conductor to small diameter coil that expands to become the defibrillation coil. Panel **C** shows a stake joint as the means of connection of the cable conductor to the proximal part of the RV coil. (Courtesy of Boston Scientific, Inc.)

pling. The technique of resistance spot welding has been implicated as one of the failure mechanisms for the Medtronic Sprint Fidelis lead. However, this assertion remains controversial and is not substantiated by the manufacturers returned product analysis (see later). Welding of dissimilar metals (platinum and MP35N) is a complicated materials topic and it is an oversimplification to state that two dissimilar metals cannot be welded. The metals must have similar melting points and be metallurgically compatible. Metallurgical incompatibility may lead to uncontrollable weld metal cracking or a weld metal microstructure that cannot provide adequate mechanical or corrosion performance. Adjacent to the fusion boundary there will be a band, typically very narrow, over which there may be a steep composition and melting point gradient due to heat propagation. This fusion boundary region may contain microstructures that are unacceptable for service. It is also known that the technique of welding (ie, resistance spot welding or laser welding) and the use of filler metals can affect the results. The site of welding and the associated structures may be more clinically relevant than the technique. Welding is widely used in pacing and ICD leads.

Another design innovation is the use of compression lumens that may protect against fracture by absorbing crush stress. As shown in Fig 12.11, some leads (Medtronic Sprint Quattro) are designed with separate compression lumens. St. Jude Medical integrates a common lumen around each pair of conductors in its current ICD leads. This approach was also used in the Medtronic Sprint Fidelis lead which was withdrawn from the market. The Guidant (Boston Scientific, Inc.) ENDOTAK Reliance series of leads do not have either separate or integrated crush lumens. There is no clinical data to suggest that the presence of compression lumens or their configuration prevents conductor fracture or affects lead reliability.

The need to place multiple leads into a single patient has highlighted the importance of lead diameter. Pacing leads range in size from 4 to 9 Fr. Current ICD leads range from 6.3 to 8.6 Fr (Fig 12.14). Multiple leads inserted through the subclavian and axillary veins may result in venous obstruction. In an effort to downsize the lead diameter, engineers have had to weigh various design compromises against their potential impact on lead function and reliability. Smaller diameter leads have less insulation material. However, an asymmetric small diameter lead has more insulation than a symmetric small diameter lead. Tip pressure of smaller diameter leads may be greater, increasing the risk

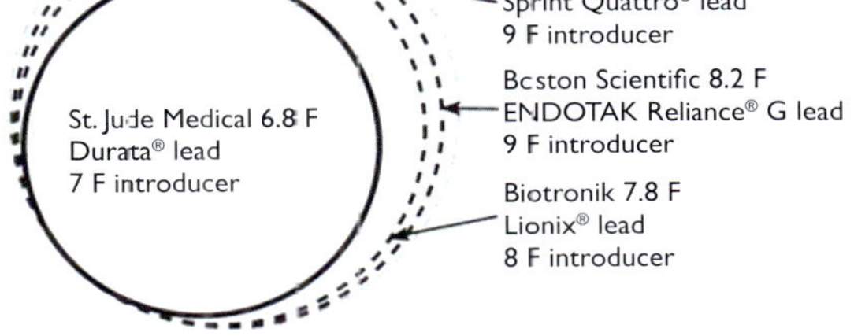

Figure 12.14 Comparison of diameters of current ICD leads. (Courtesy of St. Jude Medical, Inc.)

of perforation. At least one independent study suggests that smaller diameter leads are more prone to early lead failure than larger leads.[17]

Functional Concepts

Integrated Bipolar versus Dedicated Bipolar Leads

From a sensing perspective, there are two types of endocardial ICD leads: true (dedicated) bipolar and integrated bipolar. The true bipolar leads have separate tip and ring electrodes, similar to a standard bipolar pacing lead. Because of the presence of the ring electrode (anode), the defibrillation coil is displaced more proximally and therefore may be farther from the RV apex. The gap between the tip and RV defibrillation coil is referred to as the pullback distance. An integrated bipolar lead uses the RV defibrillation coil as the anode. The primary design difference, therefore, is the need for another conductor in the lead body of the true bipolar lead. Without the intervening ring electrode, the defibrillation coil can be positioned closer to the apex. Other design factors to consider are the size of the anode (ring) and the distance between the tip and ring.

These design differences have important clinical implications. Sensing characteristics are the most obvious consequences of these differences. An integrated bipolar lead may not be suitable for a patient with a small RV or if the defibrillation lead cannot be completely positioned across the tricuspid valve. Far-field oversensing of atrial signals may occur. Because of their similarities to standard pacing leads, true bipolar leads are expected to have the best pacing performance with the fewest sensing errors. Some studies have cast doubt on this generalization. Data gathered at the time of implantation by Frain et al. showed no difference in R-wave amplitude and slew rate between the two lead types. Sensing latency was longer with the true bipolar lead compared to the integrated bipolar lead. The clinical correlate is that a longer programmed AV delay may be needed in patients with true bipolar leads.[18] When used with an automatic gain control ICD, integrated bipolar leads have been shown to yield more oversensing of high-frequency, low-amplitude, respirophasic noise transients (myopotentials).[19] This can be investigated at the time of implant by studying electrograms (EGMs) with the pacing system analyzer (PSA) set to the most sensitive values. This type of oversensing is important to recognize because it could lead to inappropriate tachyarrhythmia detection and therapies and/or pacing inhibition. Inadvertent reversal of the DF-1 terminal pins of an integrated bipolar lead in the header block can lead to inappropriate ICD shocks due to oversensing of myopotentials.[20] T-wave oversensing has been associated with both true bipolar and integrated bipolar lead designs. The mechanism of gain control (fixed or automatic) within the ICD itself[21] as well as patient factors (eg, hypertrophic cardiomyopathy, hyperkalemia, and Brugada Syndrome) can lead to T-wave oversensing.[22–24] Occasionally, the ICD itself needs to be replaced to manage T-wave oversensing.[25,26] In patients with cardiac resynchronization therapy (CRT) devices, it has been shown that true bipolar leads are more likely to manifest anodal stimulation and therefore can affect clinical response to CRT. Contrary to conventional thinking, Freedman and colleagues showed that the rates of oversensing or undersensing did not differ between the two lead designs.[27] However, one study demonstrated that P-wave oversensing was more common with integrated bipolar leads than with true bipolar leads.[28] The sample size in this study was small. The shorter pullback distance may give the integrated bipolar lead better defibrillation performance in selected patients. This has not been proven by clinical trials and may not be an important difference with current high-energy devices. Some newer ICDs will offer the ability to electronically reconfigure a true bipolar lead into a functional integrated bipolar lead.

Single versus Dual Coil Defibrillation Leads

All major manufacturers produce a single and dual coil version of their ICD leads. Dual coil systems are associated with reduced impedance and may lower defibrillation thresholds in select patients. Except in right-sided or abdominal implants, it is rare to use the ICD as an inactive ("cold" can) component. Although controversial, one study showed placement of the proximal coil at the innominate vein-SVC junction yields lower DFTs than when the coil is at the SVC-RA junction. This same study showed the coil separation (17 vs. 21 cm) had no significant effect on defibrillation energy requirements.[29] Frequently, the final position of the proximal coil is dictated by the chamber sizes such that the proximal coil may reside in the right atrium entirely. Some ICD leads have widely spaced coils to maintain an SVC position for the proximal coil even in patients with severe chamber enlargement. It is important to note that coil separation on the lead may not translate into true spatial separation within the heart due to the need to place the appropriate amount of redundancy. Although factors affecting defibrillation thresholds are complex and controversial, a meta-analysis suggested that the optimal defibrillation polarity is with the distal coil functioning as an anode.[30]

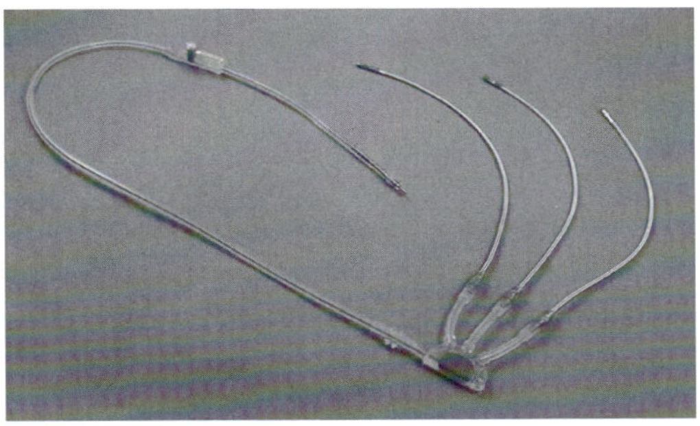

Fig 12.15 A three element subcutaneous array. (Courtesy of Boston Scientific, Inc.)

Hybrid and Subcutaneous Lead Systems and Subcutaneous Arrays

Inadequate defibrillation safety margins are rarely encountered in practice today. Most cases can be managed with reversal of shock polarity or repositioning of the RV lead.[31] Occasionally, an adequate defibrillation safety margin cannot be achieved without the addition of more hardware. An additional defibrillation element that reduces shock impedance or improves the shock vector can be used to achieve successful defibrillation. Subcutaneous patches have also been used for this purpose but have now been replaced by *subcutaneous arrays* (Fig 12.15). Single and multi-coil arrays are more easily implanted and more reliable than patches. These arrays are tunneled into the left posterolateral position (Fig 12.16). The DF-I pin of the array connects to the SVC port of the ICD.

Although epicardial patch systems via thoracotomy are not actively being implanted anymore, epicardial hybrid systems or com-

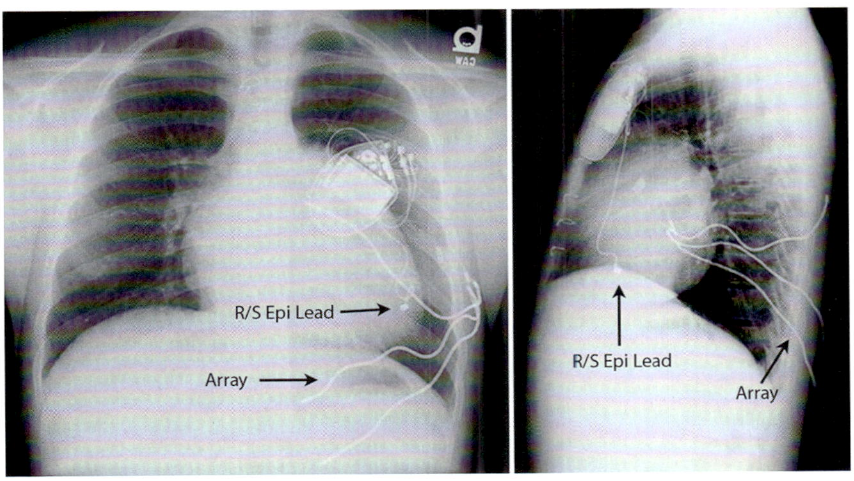

Fig 12.16. A complete epicardial and subcutaneous ICD system implanted in a patient with limited vascular access. The rate sense lead (R/S Epi) is sewn to the epicardial surface. The subcutaneous array is tunneled outside of the thoracic cavity as shown and the shock vector is between the array and the "can."

plete nontransvenous systems via limited thoracotomy are being used in both pediatric and adult patients.[32] Patients with limited or no thoracic vascular access can receive an epicardial pace/sense lead combined with extra-thoracic, tunneled subcutaneous arrays. A pre-existing rate-sense lead in the right ventricle can be combined with subcutaneous arrays to create a hybrid system.

Defibrillation Efficiency

Defibrillation thresholds are affected by multiple interrelated variables. These include ICD, patient, and lead factors. Defibrillation testing and efficiency are discussed more completely in another chapter. In terms of lead design, defibrillation efficiency is affected by high-voltage coil surface area, lead position, location of proximal coil, pullback distance, and the connection site of the conductor to RV coil.

Lead Extraction

Lead extraction has become an increasingly important clinical issue and several aspects of lead design are directly relevant. Lead extraction is a technically demanding practice requiring extensive operator experience. Passive fixation leads may be more difficult to extract due to excessive tissue growth around the tines. Excessive lead length in the heart increases the difficulty of extraction.

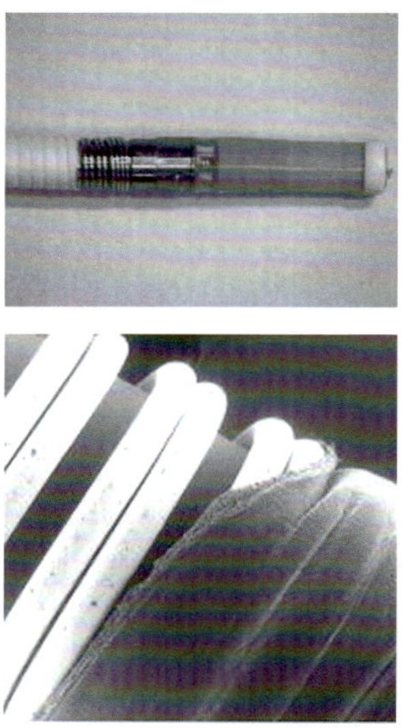

Fig 12.17 Exposed bare coil as the Gore coating "slides off" on a Boston Scientific ENDOTAK lead. (Courtesy of St. Jude Medical.)

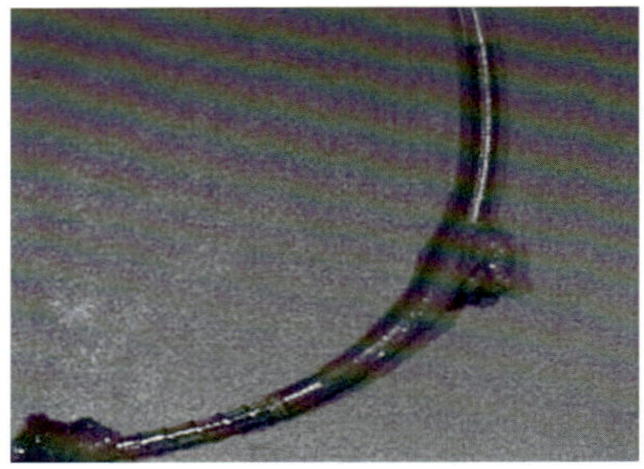

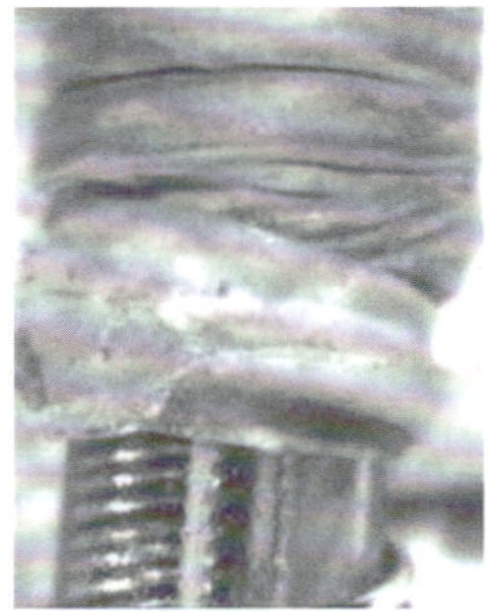

Fig 12.18 Examples of the ePTFE coating "bunching-up" during extraction of a Boston Scientific ENDOTAK lead. (Courtesy of St. Jude Medical.)

Dual coil leads are associated with more fibrosis and tissue in-growth, increasing the difficulty of extraction. Virtually all modern ICD leads have addressed this with backfilling of the coils with medical adhesive (silicone) or covering the coils with ePTFE. Although there is limited human clinical data, it is likely that the backfill method or ePTFE coating method will result in easier extractions compared to bare coils. No clinical data exists comparing ePTFE to silicone backfill. There is also no human clinical data suggesting silicone backfilling of flat coil leads is superior to silicone backfilling of round leads with respect to extraction. Manufacturer reports regarding expected performance of any of these techniques is based on limited animal studies. ePTFE coating of the coils of the current generation of leads is passive with no mechanism to fix the coating to the leads. If not implanted according to manufacturer recommendations, the ePTFE coating may "bunch up" or "slide off," exposing bare coil (Fig 12.17). ePTFE has also been known to bunch up during extraction, potentially making it more difficult to remove these leads (Fig 12.18).

Leads have been known to uncoil during extraction, resulting in failed extraction or retained components. A locking stylet is used to pull the lead from the tip during extraction. Some manufacturers have connected the cable conductors to the body of the lead at the tip and yoke, effectively creating a built-in locking stylet (Tensi-Lock technology, Medtronic, Inc.). This is meant as a redundancy and does not obviate the need for a true locking stylet during extraction. Finally, ineffective sealing of the lead tip can result in blood getting into the lumen of the coil, preventing complete passage of any stylet.

Implantation Technique

Implantation technique can affect lead performance and long-term reliability. Even a well-designed lead can malfunction if it is not implanted with proper care. Implant technique can vary as much among electrophysiologists, cardiologists, and thoracic surgeons as among electrophysiologists themselves. A report showed that the rates of implant-related complications are higher among nonelectrophysiologists compared to electrophyiologists.[33] Despite these differences, there is clearly more than one "right" method of device implantation. However, there are some factors to consider that can help prevent lead-related complications.

Medial subclavian access increases the risk of crush injury and should be avoided when possible.[34] This is due to passage through the costoclavicular ligament and can be recognized by when one encounters difficulty advancing and maneuvering the lead after sheath removal. A more lateral access of the axillary vein is feasible and safe.[35] The technique of "single access with double guidewires" increases the risk of lead-to-lead interaction and is particularly problematic with ICD leads. Leads that have poor lubricity are not good choices for this technique.

When securing the lead in the pocket, the suture sleeve should be kept coaxial with the portion of the lead that penetrates the muscle

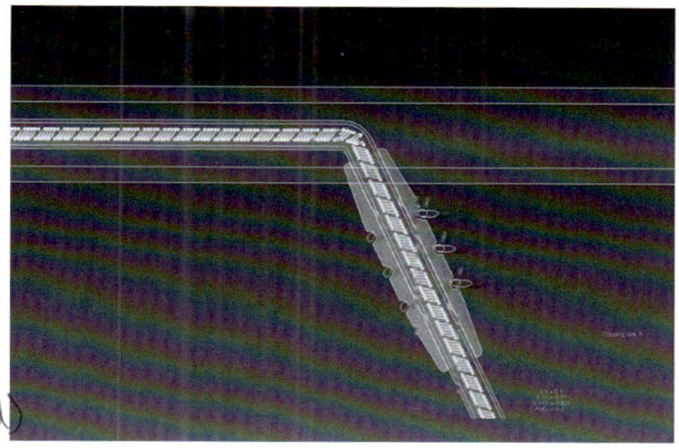

Fig 12.19 A tight bend radius or angle can cause sheet stress and flex fatigue leading to conductor fracture. (Courtesy of St. Jude Medical.)

to avoid a flex point. A sharp bending angle can cause high sheer stress to the conductors and coils, increasing the risk of fracture (Fig 12.19). The best technique for anchoring the lead in the pocket is to not directly tie the lead to the muscle. This can result in tissue compression and bending of the lead. Securing the sleeve to the lead and then tying it to the muscle or fascia is preferred (Fig 12.20). The leads should be coiled under the ICD in such a way as to minimize lead-to-lead interaction. Lead length should be carefully selected to minimize pocket bulk and lead-to-lead interaction.[36]

Abnormally high pacing impedance may suggest poor tissue contact, inadequate deployment of the fixation screw, or coil fracture. The absence of an injury current may suggest inadequate fixation.[37] Abnormally low pacing impedance may suggest an insulation break or cardiac perforation. The fluoroscopic appearance of the lead tip with the helix extended can vary

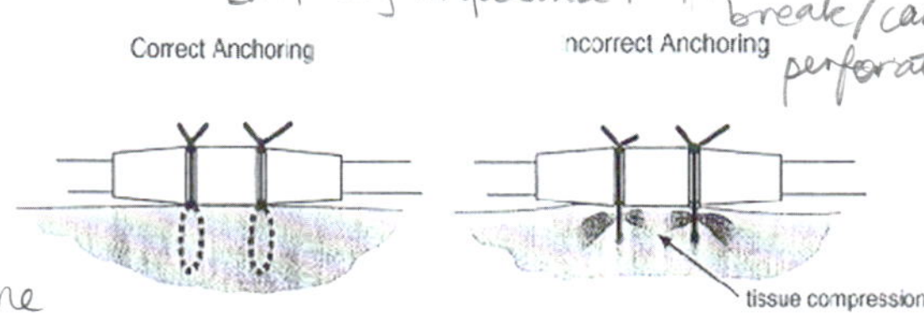

Fig 12.20 Correct technique of anchoring leads in the pocket. (Courtesy of St. Jude Medical.)

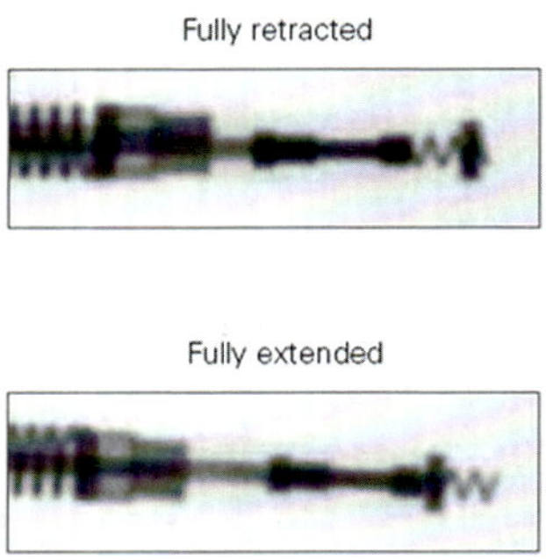

Fig 12.21 Fluoroscopic appearance of an active fixation ICD lead with the helix retracted and extended. Guidant ENDOTAK Reliance G, (Courtesy of Boston Scientific.)

significantly among manufacturers (Fig 12.21). Although the number of turns to fully extend the helix is variable from lead to lead, more turns are generally needed for leads of longer length. In addition to unstable lead fixation and the potential for dislodgment, failure to deploy the helix properly can result in oversensing.[38] The practice of overtorquing the lead to assure adequate fixation has recently been called into question. Overtorquing the lead can cause tissue distortion and therefore worsen electrical parameters.[39] The implanter should be aware of the acceptable ranges for the 5 Volt pacing impedance and shock impedance for a given lead.

Lead Failure Mechanisms and Lead Recalls

Lead failure can have more serious and immediate consequences than failure of the pulse generator. The manifestations of lead failure include high pacing or shock impedance, oversensing, undersensing, nonphysiologic V-V intervals, failure to capture and, less commonly, failure to defibrillate. Inappropriate shocks are the most serious expression of lead failure and can lead to morbidity and mortality.[40] Pulse generator malfunction can be managed by replacement but, in the case of lead failure, the management issues are more complex. In most cases, a new high-voltage lead needs to be implanted and in some cases extraction of the existing lead is indicated. Implantation of an additional pace/sense (P/S) lead is common practice but, as much as 28% of these patients experience lead-related problems during long-term follow-up, including subsequent problems with the retained high-voltage lead in 14% of cases.[41] The addition of a second high-voltage lead can cause lead-to-lead (distal coil-to-coil) interactions and can be particularly problematic if an integrated bipolar lead is used. Lead-to-lead interactions have also been implicated in lead fractures in areas that are otherwise mechanically stress-free.[42] Although some advocate lead extraction for all patients with failed ICD leads, individual patient circumstances should be considered.[43]

When considering lead materials and construction, multiple mechanisms of failure are conceivable. Lead failure can be caused by design features, implantation technique, and patient factors, in isolation or in combination. Patient-induced, repetitive or episodic mechanical trauma to the lead can result in insulation damage and conductor fracture. Twiddler's syndrome has been reported to cause both.[44] Box 2 categorizes the locations of failure. Each of these mechanisms will be considered with clinical examples.

Insulation defects
- Internal
- Outer

Conductor fractures

Conductor-to-coil connection defect

Conductor-to-electrode connection defect

Conductor-to-terminal ring connection defect

Fixation mechanism defect

Box 12.2 Sites and Mechanisms of Lead Failure

Failure of the fixation mechanism has been described for both pacing and high-voltage leads. Individual cases of fixation problems have occurred especially with repeated extensions (and retractions). There have been no widespread problems involving this failure mechanism among ICD leads resulting in a recall.

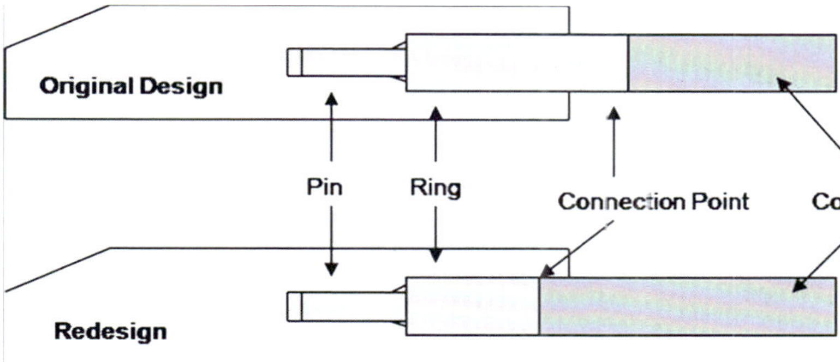

Fig 12.22 Schematic showing the IS-1 terminal inserting into the header of the original (**top**) ENDOTAK DSP 0125 lead (Guidant/Cardiac Pacemakers, Inc.) and the redesigned version (**bottom**).

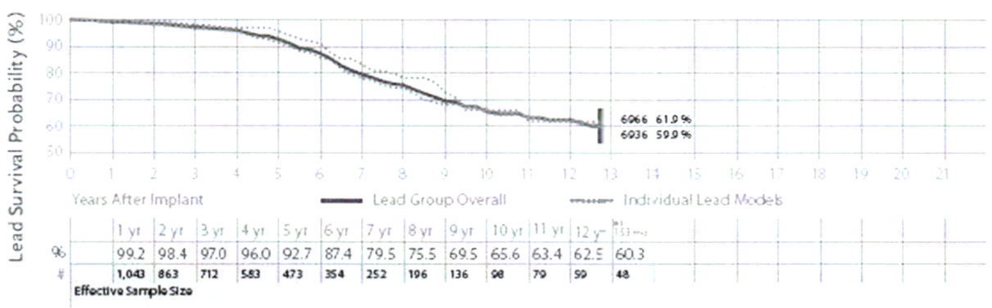

Fig 12.23 Data from the product performance report showing the probability of lead survival for the Transvene 6936 ICD lead. (Courtesy of Medtronic, Inc.)

The initial design of the conductor-to-terminal ring interface of the ENDOTAK DSP Model 0125 lead (Guidant/CPI) had a flexion point that resulted in damage to the conductor and insulation. In one series, this design characteristic resulted in a 3.5% incidence of lead fracture over a 31-month follow-up period and manifested as nonphysiologic V-V intervals.[45] The high fracture rate necessitated a redesign that allowed the connection point to be contained inside the header, thus protecting a vulnerable flexion point (Fig 12.22).

The Medtronic Transvene (Model 6936) is an example of an ICD lead with multiple failure mechanisms. This lead had a coaxial design that is no longer in use. According to the manufacturer approximately 23,700 leads were implanted and an estimated 3200 are in active clinical use. Dorwarth et al reported a 62% lead survival at 8 years with no relationship between lead survival and patient factors or implant technique. Interestingly, conductor fracture due to subclavian crush syndrome is a rare mechanism of failure for this lead.[46] Lead failure rates are not linear over time with a near 90% survival at 4 to 5 years and a 60% to 80% survival at 8 to 9 years (Fig 12.23). There is a higher rate of lead failure following pulse generator replacement suggesting that lead manipulation at the time of the procedure increases the risk of subsequent lead failure. In contrast to studies that showed insulation defects to be the most common mode of failure, one study from the Food and Drug Administration (FDA) database reported that fracture of the high-voltage coil accounted for the majority of failures (38%). This study also reported that the failure of the middle layer of polyurethane 80A (28%) was more likely than failure of the outer layer (13%).[47] Metal ion oxidation is thought to be responsible for the damage to the middle layer. A unique expression of failure of this lead is oversensing after an appropriate or inappropriate shock resulting in additional inappropriate shocks. This may be specific to the failure of the middle insulation layer in a coaxial lead.[48] To test lead integrity at the time of generator replacement, a 1-V pacing pulse can be given between the ring and coil. A value of > 4.4 mA suggests that the middle insulation is intact. In this case, the manufacturer does not recommend replacement. However, given that the rate of lead failure seems

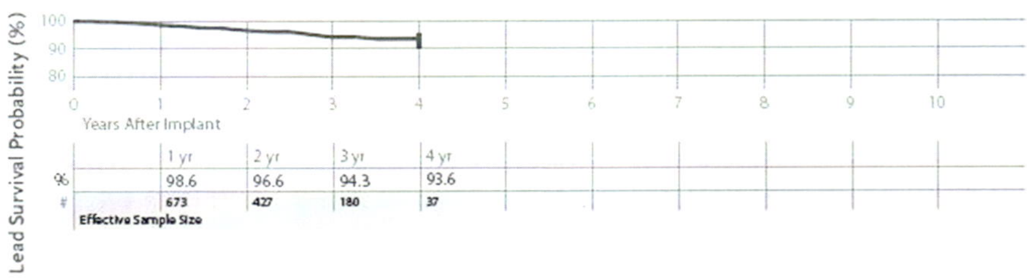

Fig 12.24 Data from the product performance report showing the probability of lead survival for the Sprint Fidelis 6949 ICD lead. (Courtesy of Medtronic, Inc.)

to be higher after generator replacement, lead replacement should also be considered at that time.

Despite the complex mechanisms of failure, the clinic impact of the Transvene 6936 is limited because of the relatively small numbers of leads implanted and still in use today. The Medtronic Sprint Fidelis ICD lead, however, represents a larger clinical problem. An estimated 205,600 leads (Models 6930, 6931, 6948, and 6949) were implanted in the United States and an estimated 150,100 leads are in active clinical use. The vast majority of implanted leads were the dual coil, active fixation model 6949 lead; 186,700 initial U.S. implants with 135,900 remaining in active use. Figure 12.24 shows the estimated lead survival rate at 48 months. This estimate is based primarily on the Medtronic System Longevity Study (SLS). Some attempts at citing design and construction features to explain the mechanism of failure are speculative and based on analysis of a limited number of leads. These theories include an inadequate welding technique, an asymmetric arrangement of conductors leading to stacking and fracture,[49] and a coil filar arrangement with suboptimal sheer stress tolerances. An analysis of a large number of leads is needed to arrive at reliable conclusions and to associate (if appropriate) design characteristics with failure mechanisms. The manufacturer's returned product analysis (RPA) is the best means to understand the mechanism of lead failure. This analysis, to date, reveals that conductor fracture is the primary (90%) mechanism of failure. About 10% of chronic fractures have occurred at the DF-1 connector segment or the proximal portion of the RV coil. Therefore, the inability to deliver high-voltage therapy is an uncommon expression of failure of this lead. Oversensing, loss of pacing, and inappropriate shocks are more likely presentations. The two sites of conductor fracture have been localized to the distal portion of the lead (conductor cable), near the anode (see Figs 12.25 and 12.26), and at the

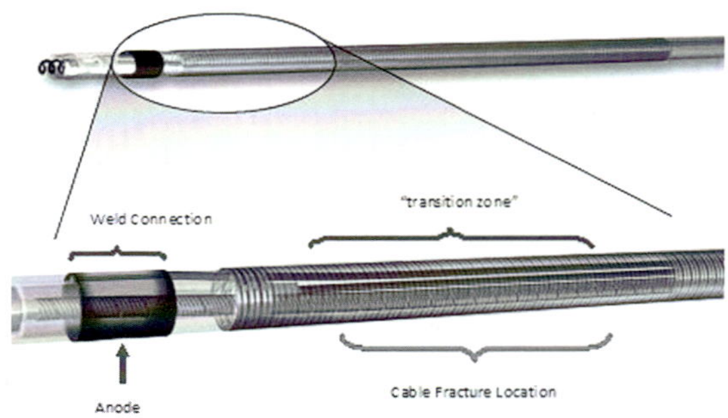

Fig 12.25 The "stiffness transition and seal zone" (see text) and distal fracture site of the Sprint Fidelis ICD lead. (Reproduced with permission of Medtronic, Inc.)

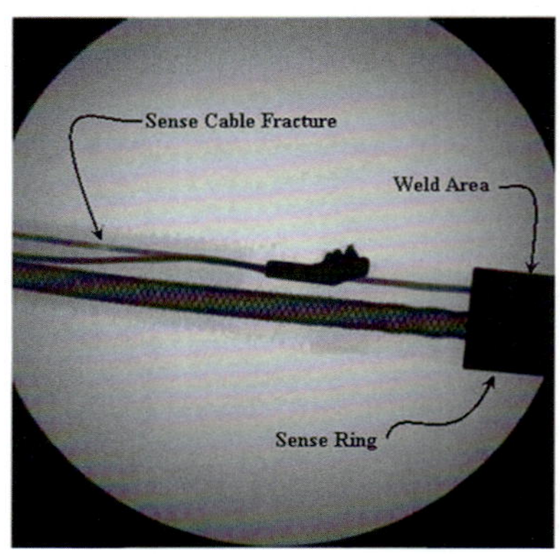

Fig 12.26 Radiograph of Sprint Fidelis demonstrating distal fracture site. (The defibrillation coil has been removed for illustration purposes.) Note: the site of fracture is remote from the weld site of the conductor and anode ring. (Reproduced with permission of Medtronic, Inc.)

proximal portion of the lead (conductor coil) near the anchoring sleeve. The "stiffness transition and seal zone" is the area of the lead where the transition of the relatively flexible lead body to the rigid sleeve head is made (to improve implant handling) and the lead is sealed from body fluid leakage. This is an area of transitioning stiffness of the lead body as a whole and may contribute to the fracture mechanism. It is proximal to the weld site of the conductor and anode. Propagation of heat from the weld site to the fracture sites is an unlikely contributor to the fracture mechanism due to the distance. Of the proximal coil fractures, 60% have occurred immediately past the anchoring sleeve (potentially within the muscle) and 30% have occurred between the sleeve and yoke. Although the locations of these fractures have been well defined, the relationship to design and construction is yet to be defined. Furthermore, the incidence of lead fracture seems to be increasing[50] and the impact of upcoming generator replacements on the failure rate is unknown. In an effort to identify impending lead fractures and reduce the risk of inappropriate shocks, Medtronic has made several recommendations. These including enabling lead impedance alerts and extending tachycardia detection intervals. The lead-integrity algorithm (LIA) is a downloadable RAMware that should be added to all ICDs with a Fidelis lead. The LIA algorithm is effective in identifying impending fractures, but cannot capture all fractures before they present especially if the change in impedance is less than the recommended alert level.[51,52]

Monitoring, Detecting, and Reporting of Lead Malfunction and Failure

A remarkable amount of research (bench and animal studies) and engineering skill go into the development of every pacing and defibrillation lead, even before premarket testing. As evidenced by the history of lead recalls, these practices alone are inadequate predictors of lead performance and reliability. Sample sizes are too small, in-vivo variables and implant technique are difficult to account for. Manufacturers use a set of standard tests when assessing lead performance on the bench. Each manufacturer also uses unique tests to meet their own internal standards. Lead design is an evolutionary process but there are no accepted definitions of a "new" lead such as to warrant a new series of clinical data.

The true incidence of lead failure is difficult to ascertain because of underreporting. Most failed leads are usually not explanted and returned to the manufacturer for analysis. Leads may be damaged during removal, complicating the analysis of the failure mechanism. Current monitoring of lead performance relies primarily on industry-based postmarket surveillance and voluntary reporting to the FDA. The MedWatch program (www.fda.gov/medwatch) allows physicians to report on any variety of concerns including those related to medical devices. This information is the entered into the Manufacturer and User Device Experience (MAUDE) database. In addition to underreporting and reporting bias, the utility of the MAUDE database is limited by nonvalidated entries. HeartNet is a subnetwork of the FDA's Medical Product Surveillance Network (MedSun) that focuses specifically on medical devices used in the electrophysiology laboratory. Entries are made into a publicly searchable database by specialists from a very large number of preselected medical facilities. Postmarket surveillance is also conducted by industry. This includes prospective registries, RPA, and adverse event reports. RPA has the potential to provide insight into the mechanism of lead failure but is limited by the fact that many failed leads are abandoned and not extracted. In addition, several independent registries now exist that specifically follow ICD leads. These registries include the Danish Pacemaker and ICD registry, the United Kingdom Pacemaker and ICD Registry, the Minneapolis Heart Institute Multicenter Registry and the National Cardiovascular Data Registry (NCDR). The data in the NCDR is derived from the Centers for Medicare and Medicaid Services (CMS) primary prevention implant data and represents over 88% of all ICDs implanted in the United States. This will be the largest database of its kind and has the potential to yield useful information and identify uncommon lead performance issues. Finally, remote monitoring using proprietary Internet-based software and equipment specific to each manufacturer can provide enhanced surveillance and assist in the management of individual patients.[53] The Heart Rhythm Society has published a set of guidelines addressing the monitoring, detecting, and reporting of lead malfunction and failure.[54] In order for these various systems to be effective in identifying potential lead problems, the individual clinician needs to be proactive in reporting suspected malfunctions to the regulatory agencies and to the manufacturer. Once a problematic lead is identified, RPA will likely remain the most effective means of identifying the mechanism of failure.

Summary

The continued expansion of indications for ICD implantation and improved mortality rates for patients receiving ICDs will place greater and greater demand on ICD leads. They will routinely need to withstand two or perhaps three generator replacements during their service lifetime. Clearly, the evolution of lead design is influenced as much by lead failures as it is by successes. The last 15 years of lead design have yielded the following:

1. A multilumen ICD lead is superior to a coaxial design.
2. Conductor fracture and insulation breach are the primary mechanisms of failure.
3. Lead size, reliability, and safety are not mutually exclusive.
4. A combination of silicone and polyurethane or a copolymer is superior to silicone or polyurethane alone.
5. Engineering and design cannot completely protect against improper implant technique or patient factors.
6. A comprehensive approach from all participants and regulatory agencies is needed to identify and remove problematic leads from the market. An objective and transparent analysis of returned products is needed to identify the mechanism of failure.

Acknowledgments

I would like to acknowledge Boston Scientific, Inc., Medtronic, Inc., and St. Jude Medical, Inc. for technical assistance in the preparation of this chapter.

References

1. Kelly PA, Cannom DS, Garan H, et al. The automatic implantable cardioverter-defibrillator: efficacy, compliance and survival in patients with malignant ventricular arrhythmias. *J Am Coll Cardiol.* 1998;11(6):1278–1286.
2. Kleeman T, Becker T, Doenges K, et al. Annual rate of transvenous defibrillation lead defects in implantable cardioverter-defibrillators over a period of >10 years. *Circulation.* 2007;115 (19):2474–2480.
3. Brady PA, Freidman PA, Trusty JM, et al. High failure rate of epicardial implantable cardioverter defibrillator lead: Implications for long-term follow-up of patients with an implantable cardioverter defibrillator. *J Am Coll Cardiol.* 1998;31(3):616–622.
4. Almassi GH, Champan PD, Troup PJ, et al. Constrictive pericarditis associated with patch electrodes of the automatic implantable cardioverter-defibrillator. *Chest.* 1987;92(2):369–371.
5. Kassanoff AH, Levin CB, Wyndham CR, et al. Implantable cardioverter defibrillator infection causing constrictive pericarditis. *Chest.* 1992; 102(3):960–963.
6. Thakur RK, Souza JJ, Troup PJ, et al. A director comparison of epicardial and nonthoracotomy defibrillation using monophasic and biphasic shocks. *Pacing Clin Electrophysiol.* 1995;18(1):70–74.

7. Wellens F, Brugada P, Guiraudon G, et al. The implantable cardioverter defibrillator: the end of the thoracotomy approach. *Eur J Cardiothorac Surg.* 1994;8(12):628–634.
8. Trusty JM, Hayes DL, Stanton MS, et al. Factors affecting the frequency of subcutaneous lead usage in implantable defibrillators. *Pacing Clin Electrophysiol.* 2000;23(5):842–846.
9. Milasinovic G, Jelic V, Savic D, et al. Fracture of the subcutaneous patch electrode in a patient with an implanted cardioverter-defibrillator. *Circ J.* 2005;69(1):116–118.
10. Collier TO, Kao JW. In-vivo biocompatibility and biostability of modified polyurethanes. *J Biomed Res.* 1997;36:246–257.
11. Lim KK, Reddy S, Desai S, et al. Effects of electrocautery on transvenous lead insulation materials. *J Cardiovasc Electrophysiol.* 2009;20(4):429–435.
12. Cooper JM, Sauer WH, Garcia FC, et al. Covering sleeves can shield the high-voltage coils from lead chatter in an integrated bipolar ICD lead. *Europace.* 2007;9(2):137–142.
13. Koplan BA, Weiner S, Gilligan D, et al. Clinical and electrical performance of expanded polytetrafluoroethylene-covered defibrillator leads in comparison to traditional leads. *Pacing Clin Electrophysiol.* 2008;31(1):47–55.
14. Wilkoff BL, Belot PH, Love CJ, et al. Improved extraction of ePFTE and medical adhesive modified defibrillation leads from the coronary sinus and great cardiac vein. *Pacing Clin Electrophysiol.* 2005;28:205–211.
15. Neibauer MJ, Wilkoff B, Yamanouchi Y, et al. Iridium oxide-coated defibrillation electrode: reduced shock polarization and improved defibrillation efficacy. *Circulation.* 1997;96:3732–3736.
16. Lang DJ, Heil JE, Hahn SJ, et al. Implantable cardioverter-defibrillator lead technology: improved performance and lower defibrillation thresholds. *Pacing Clin Electrophysiol.*;18(3 Pt2):548–559.
17. Borleffs CW, van Erven L, van Bommel RJ, et al. Abstract 4695: Risk of failure of implantable cardioverter defibrillator leads. *Circulation.* 2008;118:S926.
18. Frain BH, Ellison KE, Michaud GF, et al. True bipolar leads have increased sensing latency and thresholds compared with integrated bipolar configurations. *J Cardiovasc Electrophysiol.* 2007;18(2):192–195.
19. Sweeney MO, Ellison KE, Shea JB, et al. Provoked and spontaneous high-frequency, low-amplitude, respirophasic noise transients in patient with implantable cardioverter defibrillators. *J Cardiovasc Electrophysiol.* 2001;12(4):402–410.
20. Issa ZF. Inadvertent transposition of defibrillator coil terminal pins causing inappropriate ICD therapies. *J Interv Cardiol Electrophysiol.* 2008;22(1):63-8.
21. Thibault B, Roy D, Guerra PG, et al. Anodal right ventricular capture during left ventricular stimulation in CRT-implantable cardioverter defibrillators. *Pacing Clin Electrophysiol.* 2005;28(7):613–619.
22. Sperry RE, Ellenbogen KA, Wood MA, et al. Failure of a second and third generation implantable cardiovertor defibrillator to sense ventricular tachycardia: Implications for fixed-gain sensing devices. *Pacing Clin Electrophysiol.* 1992;15:749–755.
23. Kapa S, Curwin JH, Coyne RF, et al. Inappropriate defibrillator shocks from depolarization-repolarization mismatch in a patient with hypertrophic cardiomyopathy. *Pacing Clin Electrophysiol.* 2007;30(11):1408–1411.
24. Otmani A, Rey JL, Leborgne L. T-wave oversensing during exercise one year after cardioverter defibrillator implantation for Brugada syndrome. *Arc Cardiovasc Dis.* 2008;101(4):292–294.
25. Tuzcu V. Resolution of T-wave oversensing with implantable cardioverter defibrillator generator replacement in an adolescent. *Pacing Clin Electrophysiol.* 2007;30(7):929–932.
26. Srivasthan K Scott LR, Altemose G. T-wave oversensing and inappropriate shocks: a case report. *Europace.* 2008;10(5):552–555.
27. Freedman RA, Petrakian A, Boyce K, et al. Performance of dedicated versus integrated bipolar defibrillator leads with CRT-defibrillators: results from a Prospective Multicenter Study. *Pacing Clin Electrophysiol.* 2009;32(2):157–165.
28. Weretka S, Michaelsen J, Becker R, et al. Ventricular oversensing: A study of 101 patients

implanted with dual chamber defibrillators and two different lead systems. *Pacing Clin Electrophysiol.* 2003;26(1 Pt 1):65–70.

29. Gold M, Val-Mejias J, Leman RB, et al. Optimization of superior vena cava coil position and usage for transvenous defibrillation. *Heart Rhythm.* 2008;5(3):394–399.
30. Kroll MW, Efimov IR, Tchou PJ. Present understanding of shock polarity for internal defibrillation: the obvious and non-obvious clinical implications. *Pacing Clin Electrophysiol.* 2006;29(8):885–891.
31. Day JD, Olshansky B, Moore S, et al. High defibrillation energy requirement are encountered rarely with modern dual-chamber implantable cardioverter-defibrillator systems. *Europace.* 2008;10(3):347–350.
32. Kaltman JR, Gaynor JW, Rhodes LA, et al. Subcutaneous array with active can implantable cardioverter defibrillator configuration: a follow-up study. *Congenital Heart Dis.* 2007;2(2):125–129.
33. Curtis JP, Luebbert JJ, Wang Y, et al. Association of physician certification and outcomes among patients receiving and implantable cardioverter-defibrillator. *JAMA.* 2009;301(16):1661–1670.
34. Ramza BM, Rosenthal L, Hui R, et al. Safety and effectiveness of placement of pacemaker and defibrillator leads in the axillary vein guided by contrast venography. *Am J Cardiol.* 1997;80(7):892–896.
35. Roelke M, O'Nunian SS, Oswald SS, et al. Subclavian crush syndrome complicating transvenous cardioverter defibrillator systems. *Pacing Clin Electrophysiol.* 1995;18(10):1968–1970.
36. Mehta D, Nayak HM, Singson M, et al. Late complications in patients with pectoral defibrillator implants with transvenous defibrillator lead systems: high incidence of insulation breakdown. *Pacing Clin Electrophysiol.* 1998;21(10):1893–1900.
37. Saxonhouse SJ, Conti JB, Curtis AB. Current of injury predicts adequate active lead fixation in permanent pacemaker/defibrillation leads. *J Am Coll Cardiol.* 2005;1;45(3):412–417.
38. Laske TG, Vieau SA, Skadsberg ND, et al. High pacing impedances: are you overtorquing your leads? *Pacing Clin Electrophysiol.* 2005;28(9):883–891.
39. Mela T, Ngarmukos T, Rosenthal L, et al. Inappropriate ICD therapy due to lead-related noise in an active fixation ICD lead. *J Invasive Cardiol.* 2001;13(5):406–408.
40. Messali A, Thomas O, Chauvin M, et al. Death due to an implantable cardioverter defibrillator. *J Cardiovasc Electrophysiol.* 2004;15(8):953–956.
41. Wollman CG, Bocker D, Loher A, et al. Incidence of complications in patients with implantable cardioverter/defibrillator who received additional transvenous pace/sense leads. *Pacing Clin Electrophysiol.* 2005;28(8):795–800.
42. Noma M, Kuga K, Matsushita S, et al. Intracardiac lead fracture in an implantable cardioverter-defibrillator. *Int Heart J.* 2005;46(5):903–907.
43. Bracke FA, Meijer A, Van Gelder LM. Malfunction of endocardial defibrillator leads and lead extraction: where do they meet? *Europace.* 2002;4(1):25–26.
44. Budzikowski AS, Uyguanco E, Gunsburg MY, et al. Twisting until it breaks: a rare cause of ICD lead failure. *Cardiol J.* 2008;15(6):558–560.
45. Mera F, DeLurgio DB, Langberg JJ, et al. Transvenous cardioverter defibrillator lead malfunction due to terminal connector damage in pectoral implants. *Pacing Clin Electrophysiol.* 1999;22(12):1797–1801.
46. Dorwarth U, Frey B, Dugas M, et al. Transvenous defibrillation leads: high incidence of failure during long-term follow-up. *J Cardiovasc Electrophysiol.* 2003;14:38–43.
47. Hauser RG, Cannom D, Hayes DL, et al. Long-term structural failure of co-axial polyurethane implantable cardiovascular defibrillator leads. *Pacing Clin Electrophysiol.* 2002;25(6):879–882.
48. Ellenbogen KA, Wood MA, Shepard RK, et al. Detection and management of an implantable cardioverter lead failure: incidence and clinical implications. *J Am Coll Cardiol.* 2003;41:73–80.
49. Nilsson KRJ, Hranitzky P. Early failure of a small diameter high-voltage implantable cardioverter lead. *Heart Rhythm.* 2008;5:168–169;author reply 169.
50. Farwell D, Green MS, Lemery R, et al. Accelerating risk of Fidelis lead fracture. *Heart Rhythm.* 2008;5:1375–1379.

51. Swerdlow CD, Gunderson BD, Ousdigian KT, et al. Downloadable algorithm to reduce inappropriate shocks caused by fractures of implantable cardioverter-defibrillator leads. *Circulation.* 2008;118:2122–2129.
52. Vlay SC. Limitation of programmed alerts to predict ICD lead failures. *Pacing Clin Electrophysiol.* 2009;32(4):554–555.
53. Spencker S, Coban N, Koch L, et al. Potential role of home monitoring to reduce inappropriate shocks in implantable cardioverter-defibrillator patients due to lead failure. *Europace.* 2009;11(4):483–488. Epub 2008 Dec 22.
54. Maisel WH, Hauser RG, Hammill SC, et al. Recommendations from the Heart Rhythm Society Task Force on Lead Performance Policies and Guidelines. *Heart Rhythm.* 2009. http://www.hrsonline.org/News/Media/press-releases/upload/lead_performance_recommendations.pdf.

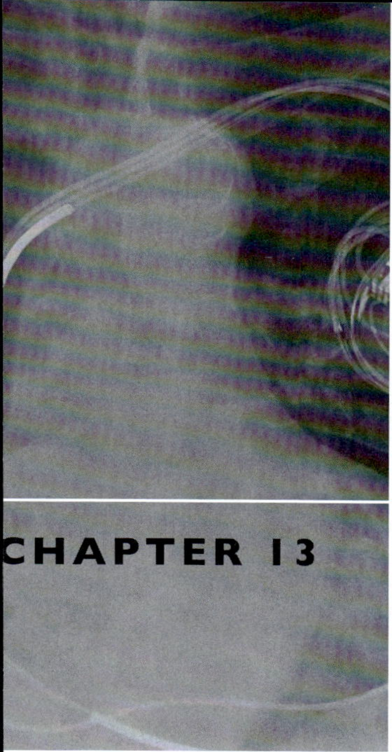

Sensing in ICDs

CHAPTER 13

Sergio L. Pinski

Introduction

Sensing is the process by which an implantable cardioverter defibrillator (ICD) determines the timing of each ventricular depolarization (and also atrial if dual chamber) from electrogram signals. A basic requirement of ICDs is reliable sensing of low amplitude and oftentimes highly variable ventricular depolarization signals during ventricular fibrillation (VF), while simultaneously avoiding sensing of T waves and extracardiac noise. Oversensing can lead to spurious ICD discharges (with associated psychological morbidity,[1] battery consumption, and occasional proarrhythmia[2]) and to inhibition of pacing, which can defeat the therapeutic objective (ie, resynchronization) or be potentially catastrophic in the pacemaker-dependent patient. In contrast to traditional antibradycardia pacemakers with fixed sensitivity, this technically challenging process is accomplished by an automatic adjustment of the sensitivity.[3,4,5] Generally, these autoadjusting algorithms function adequately. Life-threatening tachyarrhythmias are correctly detected (Fig 13.1), while spurious device activations due to oversensing are infrequent. In 518 patients with ICDs followed for 1.6 years, ventricular oversensing was documented in 38 patients (7.3%) and resulted in inappropriate therapies in 10 (2.3 %).[6] In another study of 336 patients followed for a mean of 3 years, inappropriate shocks due to ventricular oversensing occurred in 3.9% of the patients.[7] In the MADIT II study, 6.1% of total shock episodes (20% of inappropriate shock episodes) were due to oversensing.[8] Improvement in sensing circuits and algorithms together with better awareness of sources of electromagnetic interference (EMI) that can induce oversensing are likely to further reduce this incidence in the future. Only the incidence of shocks due to oversensing of "make-and-break" signals of lead fracture appears on the rise.[9]

Pacemakers and Implantable Cardioverter Defibrillators: An Expert's Manual. © 2010 Amin Al-Ahmad, Kenneth A. Ellenbogen, Andrea Natale, and Paul J. Wang, eds. Cardiotext Publishing, ISBN: 978-0-9790164-6-2.

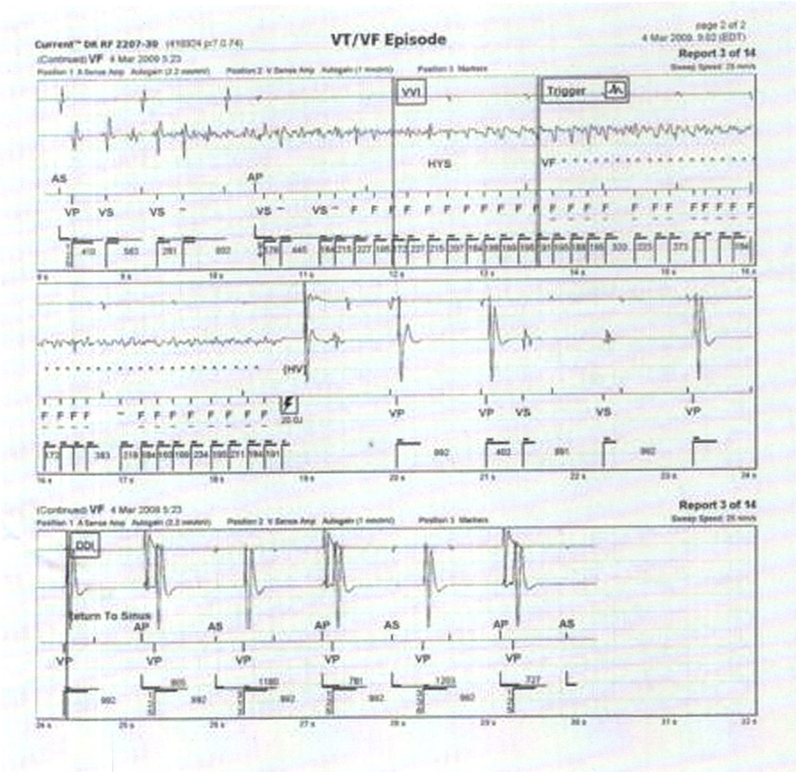

Fig 13.1 Rapid detection of spontaneous VF. Stored electrogram from an episode of *de novo* VF in a woman with cardiomyopathy and 1st degree AV block. After an initial atrial sensed/ventricular paced beat, a large amplitude ventricular premature beat triggers VF. There is initial intermittent undersensing of the low-amplitude VF signals and an atrial pacing artifact is delivered. The automatic sensitivity algorithm then allows sensing of the next depolarization before the ventricular pacing pulse is delivered. From there, sensing is accurate, with only an occasional "dropped" beat. A high-energy shock terminates VF. Postshock pacing is seen in the bottom strip.

Standard bradycardia pacemakers do not "need" to detect VF. On the other hand, an ICD faces a dilemma in the absence of sensed complexes. Two potentially life-threatening diagnoses must be considered: asystole (requiring pacing) and fine VF (requiring an increase in sensitivity for proper detection). To ensure VF detection, pacing onset triggers a rapid increase in ventricular channel sensitivity in most ICDs (Table 13.1; Figs 13.2 and 13.3). These very high sensitivity levels can promote oversensing of intracardiac or extracardiac signals. If the patient is pacemaker-dependent, oversensing perpetuates because the absence of spontaneous large amplitude escape beats maintains the high operating sensitivity.

Ventricular sensing in all ICDs (even biventricular ones) occurs from the RV lead. Although a large number of scenarios could exist,[10] current ICDs capable of biventricular pacing sense and trigger timing cycles from the RV electrogram alone. Devices from Boston Scientific and Biotronik incorporate LV sensing, but this information is only used to set a "left ventricular protection window" to avoid pacing in the vulnerable period of the left ventricle.

There are two basic bipolar designs for ICD lead sensing functions.[11] The first is the *integrated* bipolar configuration with sensing between the tip electrode and the RV distal shock coil, set about 1–1.5 cm back from the tip. The second is the *dedicated* or *true* bipolar configuration that is identical to a conventional pacing lead with sensing between the tip electrode and a ring electrode also located about 1–1.5 cm proximal to the tip. The major differences, therefore, between the two lead configurations are the need for a separate anode ring, the size of the anode, and the need for an extra conductor. Although early integrated bipolar leads (with the distal coil very close to the tip) could undersense VF after a failed shock,[12]

Device	Ventricular Sensitivity after Sensing or Pacing at Nominal Settings	Programmability
Biotronik Lumax	After a sensed event, the sensitivity is set at 50% of measured R wave at the end of the 100-ms refractory (upper threshold). The threshold then decays 0.125 ms every 250 ms through the T-wave discrimination period (hold of. upper threshold, nominally 360 ms since R-wave detection). The threshold is then decreased to 25% of the measured R wave (lower threshold) and then decreases 0.125 ms every 500 ms until the maximum sensitivity (0.8 mV) is reached or the next paced or sensed event. After a paced event, the threshold is immediately placed at the maximum sensitivity at the end of the paced refractory period.	P: Maximum sensitivity: 0.5; 0.6; … 2.5 mV (**0.8 mV**) P: Upper threshold: **50**; 75; 87.5% of R wave P: Lower threshold: 12.5; **25**; 50% of R wave P: Hold of upper threshold: 100; 120;…600 ms (**360 ms**) P: **Standard**, Enhanced T-Wave Suppression, Enhanced VF Sensitivity
Boston Scientific COGNIS Teligen	After a sensed or paced event the device calculates a search area for the next event with MAX and MIN boundaries that are based on a weighted average of the peak amplitude of all previous beats and the peak amplitude of the last beat. See following calculations. After a sensed beat, once the peak is found (up to 32 mV), sensitivity is held at the peak level for 65 ms, and then drops to 75% of the sensed peak. Afterwards, it decreases to $^7/_8$ of the previous value every 35 ms until either the MIN or the AGC floor is reached, whichever is first. After a paced event, the sensitivity is held to 4.8 mV for absolute refractory + 15 ms, and then drops to 75% of the peak average. After this, it will decrease to $^7/_8$ of the previous value in a series of steps. The duration of each step is automatically calculated based on the LRL to reach MIN or the AGC floor 150 ms prior to the next scheduled pace.	P: maximum sensitivity of the AGC algorithm 0.15, 0.2, 0.25, 0.3, 0.4, … 1.0, 1.5 mV (**0.6 mV**)
Medtronic Concerto Consulta Secura Virtuoso	After a ventricular sensed event, the ventricular sensitivity threshold increases to 75% of the peak measured R wave (maximum at nominal sensitivity 3 mV: 10 times the programmed value). After a ventricular paced event, sensitivity is set at 4.5 times maximum at the end of the post-pace blanking (nominal 1.35 mV; maximum 1.8 mV) Sensitivity then decays toward 0.3 mV with a 450 ms constant.	Maximum sensitivity: 0.15; **0.3**; 0.45; 0.6; 0.9; 1.2 mV
St. Jude Current Promote	After a ventricular sensed event, the ventricular sensitivity threshold is set at 62.5% of the peak R wave (but not > 3.75 mV or < 1.875 mV) at the end of the 125-ms refractory and holds there for 60 ms. The threshold then decays at a rate of 3 mV/sec toward 0.3 mV. After a paced event, the threshold start and decay delay automatically adjusted at the end of the post-pace refractory according to a "look-up table" to provide increased sensitivity at faster rates (eg, at a rate of 70 bpm, the threshold start is set at 1.6 mV and the decay delay at 187 ms; at a rate of 103 bpm, the threshold start is set at 1.5 mV and the decay delay at 62 ms).	Maximum sensitivity: Defibrillator: 0.2 **0.3**; … to 1 mV Pacemaker: **same as defib**; 0.2; 0.3; … to 2 mV Decay delay: 0; 30; 60; 95; 125; 160; 190; 220 ms Post sense: **60 ms** Post pace: **auto** Threshold start: Post sense: 50; **62.5**; 75; 100% of maximum peak amplitude Post pace: **auto**, 0.2; 0.3; … 3.0 mV

Table 13.1 Ventricular Sensing Algorithms of Some Current Dual- and Triple-Chamber ICDs

bold, nominal; LRL, lower rate limit; MAX, maximum; MIN, minimum; NP, non-programmable; P, programmable.

CRT-Ds from Biotronik and Boston Scientific allow programming of sensitivity settings in the LV. Sensing in the LV triggers a "LV protection period" but does not otherwise affect timing cycles or tachyarrhythmia detection. Calculations of sensing algorithm in Boston Scientific ICDs. Postventricular sense: Peak $Average_n = {}^3/_4 \times$ Peak $Average_{n-1} + {}^1/_4 \times Peak_{n-1}$; $MAX_n = {}^3/_2 \times$ Peak $Average_n$; $MIN_n = {}^1/_8 \times$ Peak $Average_n$. Postventricular pace: Same calculations as postventricular sense, except the peak value for paced event = Greater of (8 × programmed AGC floor) and 4.8 mV.

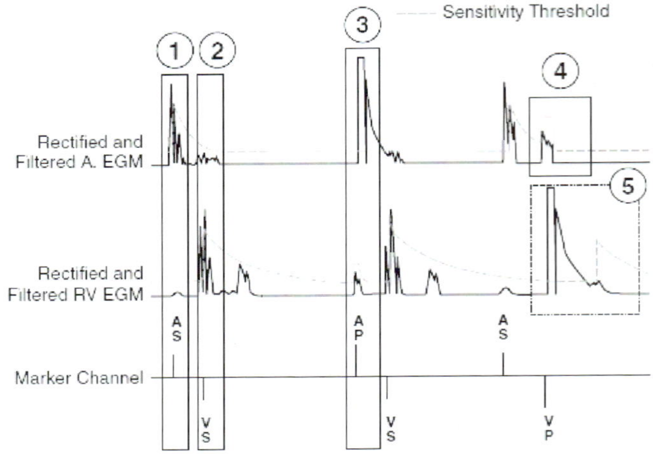

Fig 13.2 Autoadjusting sensitivity thresholds in Medtronic Concerto CRT-D.

1 After an atrial sensed event, the atrial sensitivity threshold increases to 75% of the EGM peak (maximum: 8x the programmed value).
2 After a ventricular sensed event, the ventricular sensitivity threshold increases to 75% of the EGM peak (maximum: 10x the programmed value).
3 After an atrial paced event, the device does not adjust the atrial sensitivity threshold. The ventricular sensitivity threshold increases to 0.45 mV.[2]
4 After a ventricular paced event, the atrial sensitivity threshold increases to 4x the programmed value[3] (maximum: 2.0 mV).
5 After the ventricular pace blanking period is finished, the ventricular threshold increases to 4.5x the programmed value (maximum: 1.8 mV).

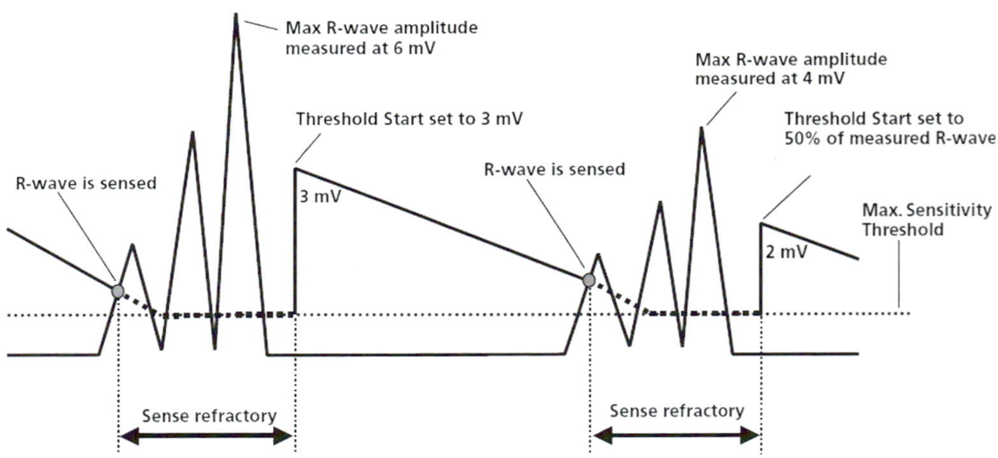

Fig 13.3 Automatic sensitivity control in the right ventricle in St. Jude Medical devices. Nominal settings have been reprogrammed. The R wave is sensed when its amplitude crosses the autoadjusting sensitivity threshold, starting the sense refractory. The signal is then tracked to its peak (in this case 6 mV). Sense channel begins to measure R waves at the Post-Sensed Decay Delay setting (in this example, 50% of maximum measured signal or approximately 3 mV). It maintains this gain level for the duration of the Decay Delay setting (in this example, 0 ms) and then linearly increases the grain (reduces the mV setting) until the next sensed beat or until it reaches the Max Sensitivity setting (1 mV in this example). The cycle restarts when the next R wave is sensed.

more recent studies have not shown sensing advantages for dedicated bipolar leads versus current integrated bipolar leads.[13,14] Dedicated bipolar designs may have a lower rate of detection of far-field signals.[15] The larger length and surface area of the RV coil electrode compared to a ring could increase the opportunity for oversensing with integrated bipolar leads. This is particularly so in patients with small right ventricles in whom a portion of the shock coil may extend back across the tricuspid valve into the right atrium, where it becomes susceptible to sensing atrial signals.[16] Dedicated bipolar leads may also be less susceptible to oversensing of EMI. Thus, they may be preferable in patients who will have workplace or recreational exposure to known sources of EMI, such as arc welding. Except in these circumstances, there is no clear reason to prefer dedicated bipolar leads, in view of their need for an extra conductor with its attendant complications. Newer Medtronic ICDs allow the programming of the sensing vector (true bipolar or integrated bipolar) when using a dedicated bipolar lead (Fig 13.4). Switching to integrated bipolar sensing could be useful (at least as a temporary maneuver), when there is oversensing due to conductor fracture to the distal ring electrode (which, for example, is the most common failure mode in the Sprint Fidelis lead). The specificity of the "sensing integrity counter," an algorithm in Medtronic devices aimed at providing an early warning of lead failure, may be less when used in combination with an integrated bipolar lead due to transient, otherwise undetected oversensing.[17]

Blanking periods, during which the ICD does not sense electrical signals, are necessary to avoid sensing the same event more than once, pacing pulses, postpacing polarization, and T waves. However, the need to detect rapid rhythms in both chambers precludes the relatively long blanking periods used in standard pacemakers. Most devices implement longer blanking periods following paced events (to avoid sensing the depolarization signal on the electrodes), whereas the blanking periods after sensed events are short. Some devices also present different blanking periods for antibradycardia pacing and antitachycardia function[18] (Table 13.2). The way the terminology is used differs among manufacturers. Strictly speaking, a blanking period occurs when the sensing amplifier is completely disabled (ie, shut off) and sensing cannot occur. During a refractory period a signal can still be sensed but cannot start certain pacing timing intervals. For practical purposes, however, if a signal sensed during a refractory period is ignored by *all* timing cycles in the device, the refractory period

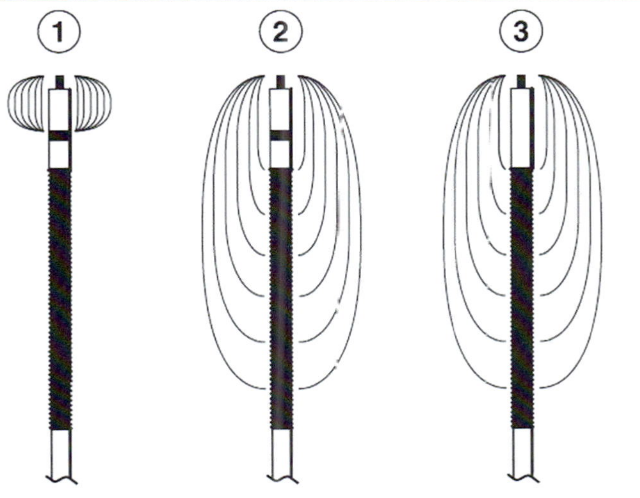

Fig 13.4 Programmability of the sensing vector in current Medtronic devices. (1) Sensing with a true bipolar lead and RV Sense Polarity programmed to Bipolar. (2) Sensing with a true bipolar lead and RV Sense Polarity programmed to Tip to Coil. (3) Sensing with an integrated bipolar lead and RV Sense Polarity programmed to either Bipolar or Tip to Coil.

operates as a blanking period. Devices from several manufacturers incorporate short retriggerable "noise windows" within refractory periods. The window is initiated by either a sensed or paced event. Recurrent high-frequency noise activity will retrigger the noise window and possibly the effective refractory period or blanking period beyond the programmed pacing escape interval. Depending on the programming, this could result in asynchronous pacing. This function is useful to prevent asystole in response to EMI in pacemaker-dependent patients.

T-Wave Oversensing

Avoidance of oversensing of the T wave is easy in conventional pacemakers and is achieved by a fixed low sensitivity (typically 2.5 mV) and a relatively long (> 200 ms) and fixed blanking or refractory period, which is similar after a paced or sensed ventricular event. In contrast, the need to detect rapid rhythms precludes a long and fixed ventricular blanking in ICDs. Most devices implement longer blanking periods following paced events (to avoid sensing the depolarizations signal on the electrodes), whereas

Model	Postatrial Paced Blanking	Postventricular Paced Refractory	Postventricular Sense Refractory
Biotronik Lumax	P: **50**; 60;... 100 ms NP VSP	P: **auto**; 100; 110; ... 350 ms	Fixed at 100 ms
Boston Scientific COGNIS, Teligen	P :"**smart**"*, 45; 65; 85 ms) No VSP	P: **fixed** (150; 160; ... 500 ms) (**250 ms**) or dynamic (Min: 150; 160; ... 500 ms) **(230 ms)** (fixed absolute refractory, last 40-ms noise detection window)	Fixed at 135 ms (50 ms absolute refractory + 40-ms noise detection window + 45 tachy refractory)
Medtronic Concerto, Consulta, Virtuoso	Fixed at 30 ms P VSP: **ON**, OFF	P: 170; 180; ... 450 ms (**200 ms**)	P: **120**; 130; ... 170 ms
Sorin Ovatio, Paradym	Fixed at 16 ms NP VSP	Fixed at 220 ms	Fixed at 95 ms
St. Jude Current, Promote	NP: 44 or 52 ms.** P VSP: **ON**, OFF	P: 125; 160; 190; ... 400; 440; 470 ms (**250 ms**) P: Rate-responsive: OFF, **Low**, Medium, High Shortest: 125; 150; ... 475 ms (**225 ms**) P: "Arrhythmia Unhiding": OFF, 2; **3**;... 15 intervals	P: **125** or 157 ms

Table 13.2 Ventricular Blanking and Refractory Periods in Some Current Dual- and Triple-Chamber ICDs.
bold: nominal; max: maximum; min: minimum; NP: non-programmable; P: programmable VSP: ventricular safety pacing.
CRT-Ds from Biotronik and Boston Scientific allow programming of separate ventricular refractory periods in the LV. These periods are used to set up a "LV protection period" and do not otherwise affect timing cycles or tachyarrhythmia detection.
*SMART—37.5-ms absolute refractory with no noise window. If the Automatic Gain Control setting is < $^3/_8$ of the current peak average, SMART blanking will increase it to $^3/_8$ of the current peak average to avoid far-field oversensing.
**When pulse amplitude and pulse width settings or capture test results are high, the device automatically selects 52 ms.

the blanking periods after sensed events are kept very short, not much longer than the true minimal myocardial refractory period of around 100 to 140 ms.

Oversensing of T Waves after Sensed Beats

Oversensing of the spontaneous T wave manifests clinically as spurious ICD interventions (antitachycardia pacing or shocks) during a supraventricular rhythm. This requires a relatively elevated base rate, so "double-counting" of each complex fulfills the ventricular tachycardia/fibrillation detection rate. Thus, a common scenario is the occurrence of multiple spurious shocks during exercise. If a ventricular tachycardia (VT) zone with antitachycardia pacing is programmed, pacing can be proarrhythmic and induce true ventricular tachyarrhythmia (Fig 13.5). Oversensing of T waves followed by close-coupled VPDs can increase the "sensing integrity counter" in Medtronic ICDs and falsely suggest a lead problem.[19]

Despite a short post-sense refractory period, oversensing of T waves after spontaneous beats is rare as long as the R wave is of adequate voltage. The autoadjusting algorithms adjust the sensing threshold according to the R-wave voltage, which then decreases over time (in steps, linearly, or exponentially with variable constants, according to how the algorithm is implemented). Thus, the sensitivity is still relatively low by the time of the T wave, which is then "hopped over." In the presence of an adequate R-wave voltage, oversensing of spontaneous T waves is likely to happen only in patients with long QT syndrome, in whom repolarization can be sufficiently delayed so that the local T-wave deflection is inscribed at a time when sensitivity is already high.

T-wave oversensing is more likely to occur when the R wave is of a lower voltage (ie, < 3 mV), as sensing will start from a relatively high sensitivity at the end of the blanking period. A low R-wave voltage is uncommon in patients with ischemic cardiomyopathy. In contrast, it is more common in conditions that affect the right ventricle, such as cardiac sarcoidosis,[20] arrhythmogenic RV cardiomyopathy or dysplasia,[21] some forms of dilated cardiomyopathy, or Brugada syndrome.[22,23] In Brugada syndrome, transient changes in RV depolarization/repolarization can make T-wave oversensing evanescent and difficult to circumvent.[24] A marked reduction in the amplitude of the R wave that

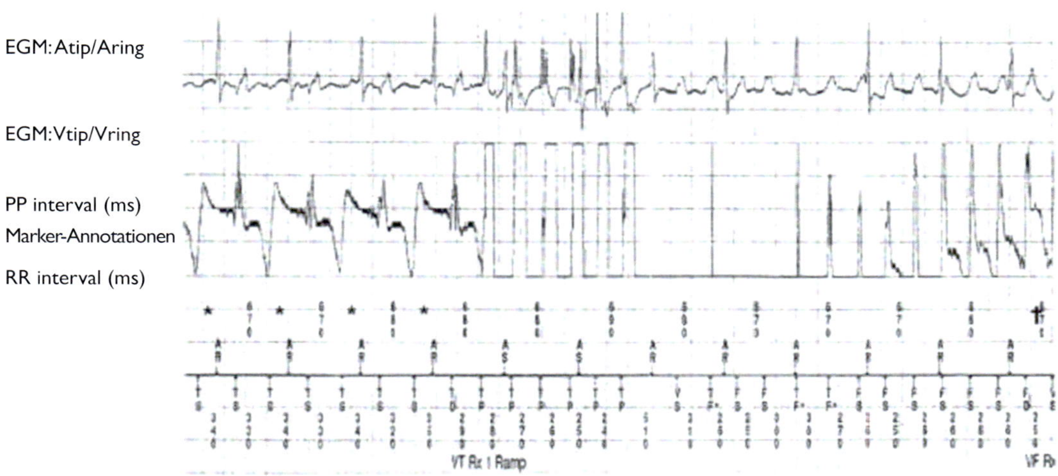

Fig 13.5 Proarrhythmic inappropriate therapy due to T-wave oversensing. T-wave oversensing (*) during sinus rhythm at 95 bpm resulted in detection of VT for which inappropriate antitachycardia pacing was delivered. The inappropriate therapy induced a rapid VT which was detected as VF (†) and then terminated by a shock (not shown). (From Watanabe et al.[26] with permission.)

occurs soon after implant is often a manifestation of lead microdisplacement, which may not be diagnosed from chest X-rays.[25] Prompt lead revision is indicated when lead displacement is present. In patients with diseases that affect the right ventricle, deterioration in the amplitude of the R wave due to disease progression is common despite adequate amplitude at implant and often results in spurious shocks due to T-wave oversensing.[26] In one case, T-wave oversensing only occurred after successful ablation of ventricular ectopy from the Purkinje system close to the RV lead. Ablation caused a reduction in R-wave amplitude and an unfavorable R-to-T wave ratio.[27] "Unexplained," nonreproducible transient reduction in R-wave amplitude leading to T-wave oversensing has been described.[28] Lead microdislodgment should be suspected in those instances.

Less commonly, T-wave oversensing is due to high amplitude T waves, such as those described in hypertrophic cardiomyopathy,[29] the short QT syndrome,[30,31] and the long QT syndrome. Hyperkalemia is a well-known cause of an increase in the amplitude of the surface ECG T wave. A high-amplitude surface T wave correlates with a high-amplitude T wave in the endocardial electrogram.[32] Hyperkalemia can thus result in transient T-wave oversensing that is corrected when the plasma potassium level normalizes.[33,34] In one case double-counting, due to T-wave oversensing in the setting of hyperkalemia, triggered an "inappropriate appropriate" ICD shock for VT below the detection cutoff rate.[35] Hyperglycemia has also been described as a rare cause of transient T-wave oversensing.[36]

A minor decrease in sensitivity is often the first step considered to circumvent oversensing spontaneous T waves and is generally effective in the presence of R waves of good amplitude. St. Jude Medical devices allow programming of separate maximum sensitivity for the pacemaker and defibrillator function of the ICD (nominally the same). Reducing the bradycardia sensitivity may be useful to eliminate T-wave oversensing (especially after paced beats) without compromising detection of VF. Devices from St. Jude and Biotronik allow additional fine programming of the decay in sensitivity after a sensed QRS (Fig 13.6). These features can be particularly useful in patients with long QT syndrome.[37] For example, the Enhanced T-wave Suppression setting in Biotronik Lumax ICDs introduces several changes in sensing aimed at avoiding double-counting of T waves: (1) high pass filtering is increased to reduce low-frequency signal components such as T waves and respiratory artifacts; (2) the upper threshold is increased to 75%; and (3) the upper threshold is no longer retriggered with each sensed event, but only when the new R wave crosses the previous 50% threshold. The new R-wave amplitude is only used to recalculate the thresholds if its amplitude exceeds that of the previous R wave. Although in some

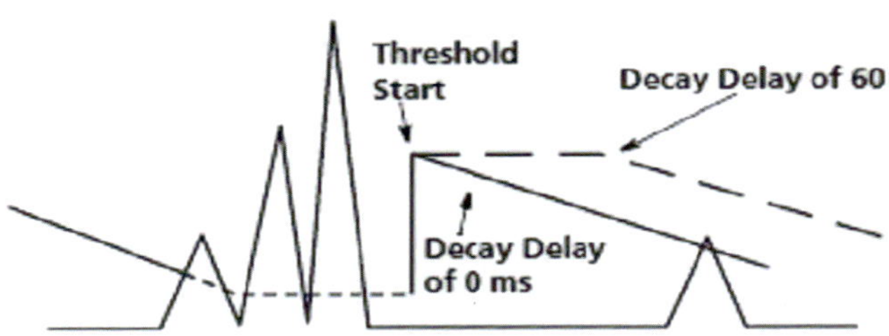

Fig 13.6 Programmability of the sensing decay delay in St. Jude Medical ICDs. The Decay Delay parameter determines the amount of time after the sensed or paced refractory period that the threshold remains at the programmed Threshold Start setting before beginning its decay. Increasing the Decay Delay (in this case from the nominal of 0 to 60 ms) may prevent oversensing of T waves.

cases T-wave oversensing can be eliminated by forced pacing[38] (mostly because the postventricular paced refractory period allows greater programmability, see later), this strategy is not recommended because of the possible detrimental hemodynamic effects of unnecessary RV pacing and because oversensing could still occur during sinus tachycardia above the upper tracking limit or during mode switch for atrial fibrillation. The addition of morphology enhancement criteria (such as the electrogram width) to the detection algorithm could also prevent the delivery of spurious shocks for T-wave oversensing, without abolishing oversensing *per se*.[39] Other maneuvers destined to prevent tachyarrhythmia detection and therapy delivery without eliminating T-wave oversensing, such as changing the tachycardia detection rate, prolonging detection time, or attempting to blunt the sinus rate with beta blockers are generally ineffective.

Any change in the sensitivity settings aimed at eliminating T-wave oversensing can compromise reliable detection of VF, especially in the common scenario of a low-amplitude R wave.[40] T-wave oversensing in the setting of a low-amplitude R wave is a warning that detection of VF may be unreliable and should be assessed with the intended programming changes at noninvasive electrophysiological study with induction of VF. Repeat testing should be performed even when appropriate detection of VF with "worst-case scenario" (ie, lowest sensitivity) has been demonstrated during implant. The ventricular lead should be revised if the safety margin for sensing VF is insufficient.

Oversensing of T Waves after Paced Beats

A high operating sensitivity makes T-wave oversensing much more common after ventricular-paced beats, despite the longer blanking/refractory period present after pace than after sensed ventricular events.[41] For example, in Medtronic ICDs, ventricular sensitivity is set at 4.5 times the maximum sensitivity (but only up to 1.8 mV; 1.35 mV at the nominal maximum sensitivity of 0.3 mV) at the end of pace blanking, and then decays toward the maximum-programmed sensitivity with a 450-ms constant. These very high-sensitivity levels can promote oversensing of intracardiac or extracardiac signals. Oversensing of paced T waves is therefore not uncommon.

In patients with continuous ventricular or AV sequential pacing, T-wave oversensing will result in inhibition of the next pacing stimulus, consequently lengthening the effective pacing escape interval (Fig 13.7). Most instances are of little clinical consequence, but the resulting bradycardia may become symptomatic. In patients with long QT syndrome, the slower paced rate further prolongs the QT interval, may perpetuate oversensing,[42,43] and lead to development of torsade de pointes. During atrial tracking, T-wave oversensing can be clinically unapparent (except for a spurious increase in PVC counts). However, loss of tracking of sinus rhythm can also occur when the oversensed T wave is interpreted as a PVC. Depending on the device, this can trigger an extended postventricular atrial refractory period (PVARP) and result in functional undersensing of the following P wave. If there is spontaneous conduction, a typical pattern of pacing alternans with tracking of every other P wave is seen.[44,45] If there is no spontaneous conduction, ventricular pacing could maintain nonreentrant AV synchrony.[46] Oversensing of paced T waves can also invoke "rate-stabilization" algorithms and perpetuate pacing in patients without bradycardia (Fig 13.8).[47] Paced T-wave oversensing can inhibit the delivery of antitachycardia pacing.[48] Oversensing of paced T waves will not result in spurious tachyarrhythmia detection, except in the rare patient with a St. Jude Medical device and concomitant ventricular bigeminy (Fig 13.9).

A small decrease in the maximum sensitivity, an extension of the postventricular pace blanking period, or both are in general useful to eliminate oversensing of T waves that occur after pacing,[49] but these maneuvers can entail a trade-off with sensing and detection of ventricular tachyarrhythmias. St. Jude Medical devices

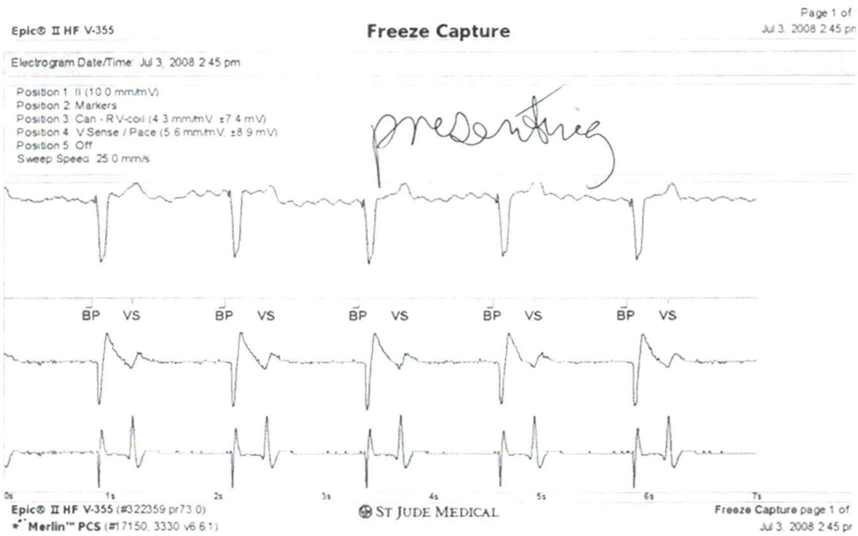

Fig 13.7 Oversensing of paced T waves resulting in bradycardia below the lower rate limit. Patient with chronic renal failure on ambulatory peritoneal dialysis, permanent atrial fibrillation, and complete heart block with a St. Jude Medical CRT-D. Pacing was programmed VVIRV 60 to 120 bpm, with nominal sensing and refractory periods. He presented with increased fatigue and the ECG showed biventricular pacing at 45 bpm. ICD interrogation disclosed continuous resetting of the timing cycle by oversensing of high-amplitude sharp T waves. Plasma potassium was 5.6 mEq/L. Oversensing was circumvented by fine-tuning of the postpace threshold and decay settings without extending the refractory period or reducing maximum sensitivity.

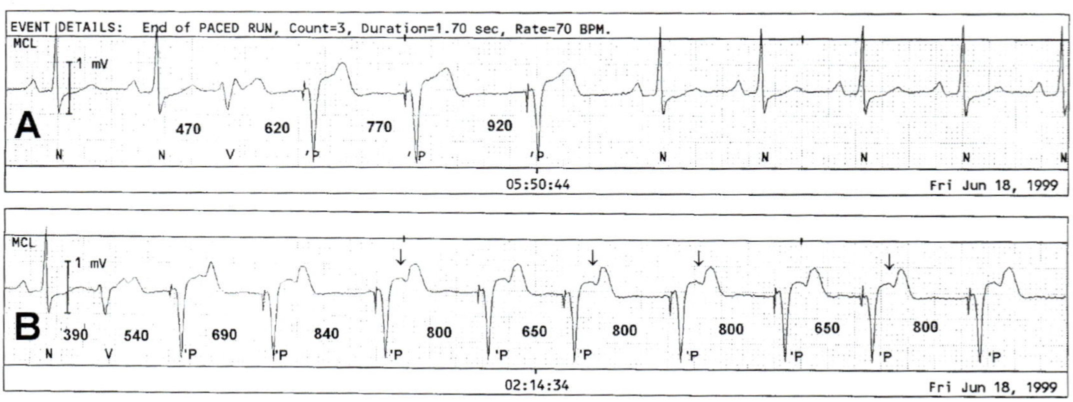

Fig 13.8 Oversensing of paced T waves resulting in unnecessary pacing due to autoperpetuation of the ventricular stabilization algorithm in a single chamber Medtronic ICD. Single lead monitor ECG recordings with numbers indicating intervals in ms. **A**: Normal functioning of the algorithm after a VPD sensed 470 ms after the sinus beat. Three ventricular pulses at progressively longer cycles are delivered before resumption of sinus rhythm. **B**: Autoperpetuation of ventricular pacing. Intermittent T-wave oversensing (arrows) 300 ms after the previous pulse repetitively invokes the ventricular stabilization algorithm. (From Pinski,[47] courtesy of Wiley-Blackwell. Used by permission.)

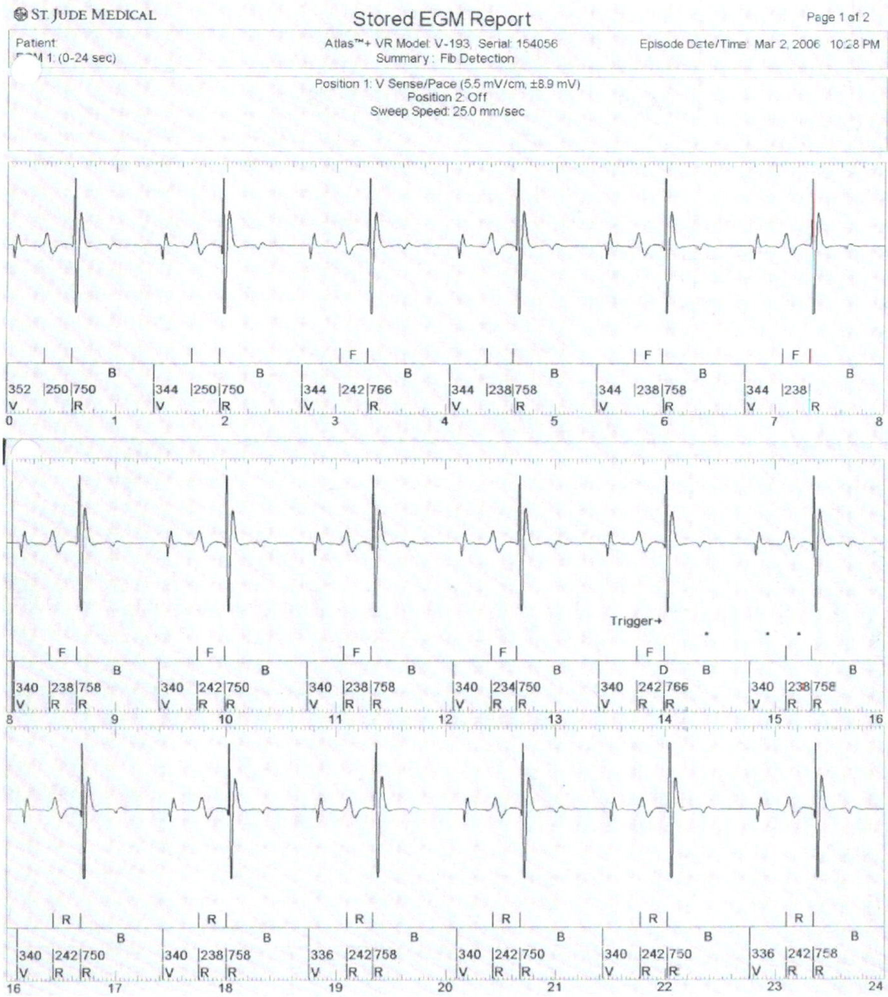

Fig 13.9 Spurious shock due to oversensing of paced T waves during ventricular bigeminy. A woman with hypertrophic cardiomyopathy, permanent atrial fibrillation, and complete heart block and VT presented with multiple shocks from a single chamber Atlas St. Jude Medical ICD with a chronic bipolar pacing/sensing lead in the RV outflow tract. Pacing was programmed at 70 bpm, VT detection at 152 bpm (395 ms), and VF detection at 200 bpm (300 ms). All other parameters were at nominal settings. Stored electrogram from one of the episodes shows demand pacing with escape interval of 750 ms, with consistent oversensing of the paced T wave 344 ms afterwards. There is ventricular bigeminy with coupling interval to the paced beat of 580 ms, (but occurring 242 ms after the T wave and sensed in the VF zone). Detection and therapy occurred because St. Jude Medical ICDs classify detected events based on both the current interval and a running interval average (an average of the current interval and the previous three intervals). To satisfy the detection criteria and be counted toward detection, both the current interval and the running interval average must be shorter than or equal to the longest tachyarrhythmia detection interval (in this case 395 ms). The interval is classified as the shorter of either (1) the interval or (2) the interval average. Detection occurs when a detection zone classifies its required number of intervals (in this case 12 intervals at 300 ms). Bigeminy without T-wave oversensing will not trigger therapy because the device must detect more tachyarrhythmia intervals than sinus intervals before it delivers therapy. Pacing threshold was 0.75 V at 0.5 ms. Paced T-wave oversensing was eliminated by prolonging the baseline ventricular blanking (while maintaining dynamic shortening during rate-responsive pacing) and reducing the maximum pacer sensitivity to 2 mV. The defibrillator sensitivity was left unchanged at 0.3 mV. Appropriate detection of induced VF with the new settings was confirmed. Spurious shocks did not recur in 3.5 years of follow-up.

allow additional fine programming of sensing after a paced beat (Fig 13.10). Ventricular tachyarrhythmias that emerge during relatively rapid pacing due to tracking or sensor activation may be temporarily masked by a lengthy blanking period thereby delaying detection.[50] During AV sequential pacing, the postatrial paced ventricular blanking further shortens the detection window. A similar phenomenon can occur when the initial tachycardia beats trigger rate-smoothing pacing at or close to the upper rate limit in devices from Guidant/Boston Scientific, in which atrial pacing in the detection zone can occur. Underdetection of VT can occur if the VT rate is not very fast and the programmed AV delay is long, as this demands delivery of the atrial pulses shortly after the tachycardia-sensed beats.[51,52] In general, the Boston Scientific programmer screen displays Parameter Interaction Attentions and advisory messages to inform about programming combinations that could interact to cause these scenarios; the interactions can be resolved by reprogramming the pacing rate, AV Delay, and/or refractory/blanking periods.

When the postventricular paced blanking is fixed, the upper rate limit(s) may need to be lowered to ensure maintenance of a tachycardia detection window during ventricular pacing. This is critical in patients with slow VT. Sequential biventricular pacing with a long V-V time can further extend blanking and reduce

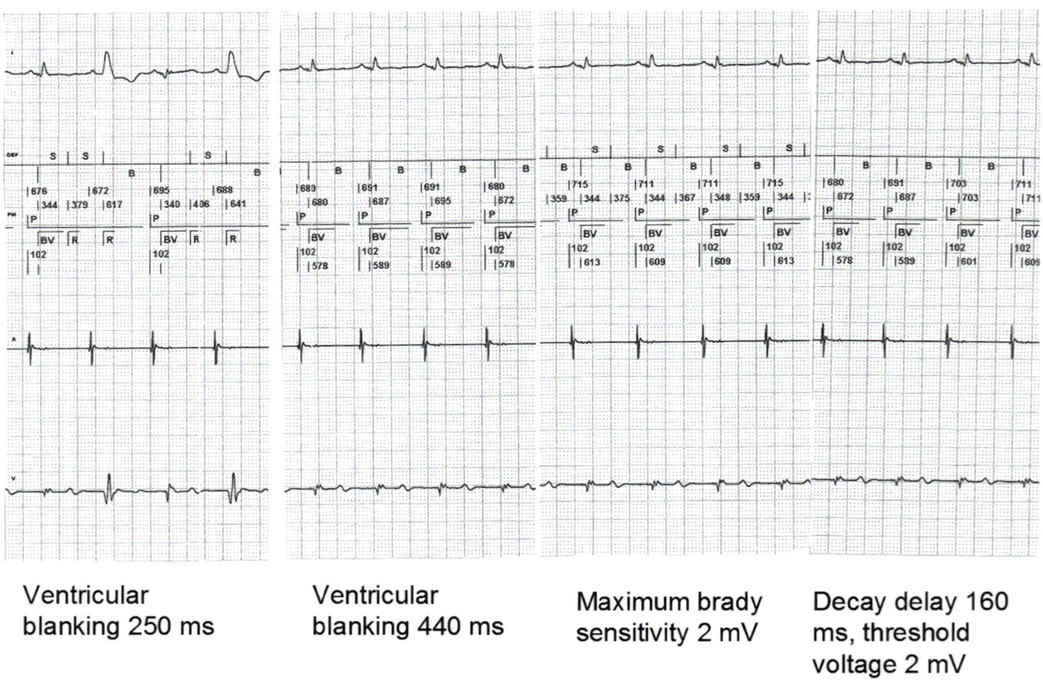

Fig 13.10 Troubleshooting of paced T-wave oversensing in a St. Jude Medical CRT-D. From top to bottom, surface ECG, markers for defibrillation (DEF) and pacing (PM) function, atrial (A) and right ventricular (V) electrograms. The first panel, with nominal parameters, shows paced T-wave oversensing, with the classical pattern of 2:1 tracking. The P wave after the sensed T waves falls in the extended PVARP and it is not tracked. The second panel shows elimination of T-wave oversensing by extending the postpace blanking to 440 ms. This is not recommended as it leaves a very narrow alert window for arrhythmia detection. The third panel shows the ventricular blanking again at 250 ms. Oversensing is eliminated by programming the minimum sensitivity in the bradycardia channel at 2 mV. Note that the T waves are still oversensed by the defibrillator (marked as S) but do not affect pacing timing. In the last panel, the brady sensitivity is again nominal, but the sensing decay after pacing has been changed to "hop" over the T wave.

the alert window. Although current ICDs allow maximum tracking rates and maximum sensor-driven rates >140 bpm, the maximum achievable pacing rate is limited by a series of parameter interlocks. In Medtronic devices, parameter interlocks prevent pacing in the detection zone (Fig 13.11). ELA/Sorin devices provide a detection algorithm (PARAD) that allows overlap between the pacing rate and the slow VT detection rate.[53]

Shorter ventricular blanking periods can maintain a wider alert window during rapid pacing. The cross-chamber ventricular blanking after atrial pace shows in general little programmability among different models. The post-ventricular paced blanking is more extensively programmable (Table 13.2). The QT interval shortens at faster paced rates. Guidant/Boston Scientific and St. Jude Medical devices take advantage of this phenomenon via programmable dynamic ventricular paced blanking periods. When this feature is enabled in Guidant/Boston Scientific devices, the ventricular blanking period shortens automatically and in a linear fashion from the programmed baseline value at the lower rate limit down to the minimum "dynamic" value at the upper rate limit. In St. Jude Medical ICDs, the rate-responsive ventricular pace refractory starts to shorten when the filtered atrial rate, the sensor-indicated rate, or the AF suppression algorithm rate exceeds 90 bpm. The slope of the decrease is programmable Low (shortening of 1 ms for each bpm), Medium (2 ms for each bpm), or High (3 ms for each bpm). Shortening continues until the maximum sensor rate, the maximum tracking rate, or the shortest refractory (also programmable) is reached. In St. Jude Medical devices, the rate-responsive PVARP and ventricular refractory periods are programmed simultaneously. St. Jude Medical devices provide additional functions to promote detection during rapid paced rates. When the ventricular Post-Paced Decay Delay is set nominally to Auto, the device automatically adjusts the Decay Delay used after a ventricular paced pulse to compensate for QT-interval shortening associated with fast pacing rates. Similarly, with Ventricular Post-Paced Threshold Start set to Auto, the device automatically adjusts the Threshold Start used after a ventricular paced pulse to provide increased sensitivity at fast pacing rates. In Biotronik Lumax devices the nominal postpace ventricular refractory is automatically adjusted according

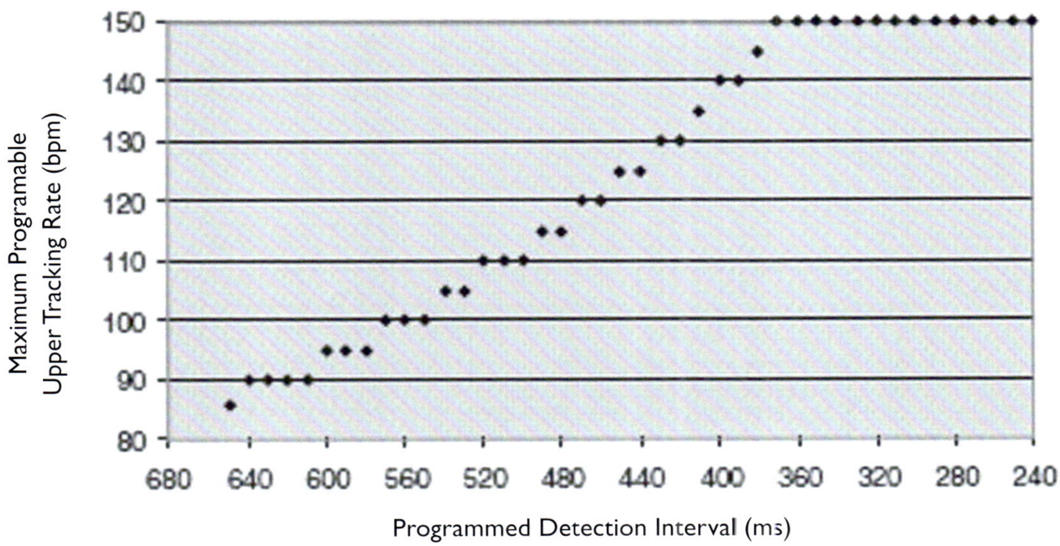

Fig 13.11 Maximum programmable upper tracking rate in Medtronic devices according to the programmed detection intervals.

to the maximum programmed pacing rate and (when applicable) the V-V interval.

St. Jude Medical devices also provide an additional "arrhythmia unhiding" function that increases the alert period (through an adaptive relative refractory period) to unmask arrhythmias hidden by pacing (Fig 13.12). An adaptive relative refractory period is enabled when the ventricular pacing cycle length is < 2 times the longest tachycardia detection interval or 2 times the pacing refractory, whichever is shorter. If a sensed event occurs during the adaptive relative refractory and the next event is paced, the adaptive relative refractory period is enabled again. If no sense event occurs during the adaptive relative refractory period or the next event is not paced, the pace refractory period returns to normal. Once the number of intervals with a sensed event during the adaptive relative refractory period specified by the arrhythmia unhiding function have occurred consecutively, the pacing cycle length is extended for six cycles in an attempt to reveal the arrhythmia. If no arrhythmia is revealed during the extended pacing interval, the adaptive relative refractory period will not be reenabled for 10 cycles to prevent unnecessary extension of the pacing interval.

The Guidant/Boston Scientific algorithm has been tested clinically. Worst-case scenario testing (maximum pacing output and ventricular sensitivity, shortest blanking period of 150 ms, maximum rate of 120 bpm) suggests that this feature prevents oversensing of paced T waves while maintaining a wide tachyarrhythmia detection window.[54] Another study confirmed safe and rapid detection of VF occurring in the setting of rapid paced rates (DDD pacing at 150 bpm and DDDR pacing at 175 bpm) in Guidant devices with programmed minimum dynamic postpace ventricular blanking at 150 ms.[55] There is little safety information on tachyarrhythmia detection during rapid pacing by ICDs with fixed postpace ventricular blanking.

In a patient with a Medtronic CRT-D, oversensing of paced T waves was eliminated

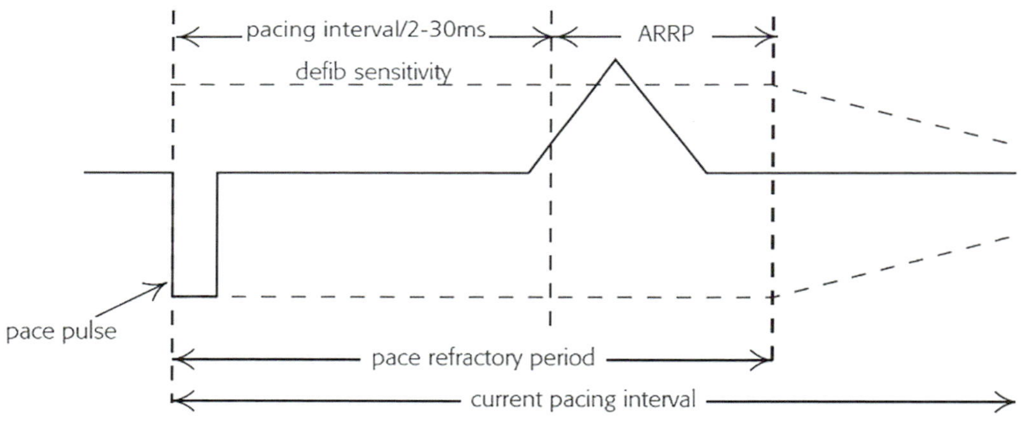

Fig 13.12 Arrhythmia "unhiding" function during high-rate ventricular pacing in St. Jude Medical devices. Arrhythmia Unhiding increases the alert period (through an adaptive relative refractory period or ARRP) to unmask arrhythmias hidden by pacing. An ARRP is enabled when the ventricular pacing cycle length is < 2 times the longest tachycardia Detection Interval/Rate or 2 times the Atrial Pace Refractory, whichever is shorter. If a sensed event occurs during the ARRP and the next event is paced, then the ARRP is enabled again. If no sensed event occurs during the ARRP or the next event is not paced, then the pace refractory period returns to normal. Once the number of intervals specified by Arrhythmia Unhiding have occurred consecutively with a sensed event during the ARRP, the pacing cycle length is extended for six cycles in an attempt to reveal the arrhythmia. If no arrhythmia is revealed during the extended pacing interval, the ARRP is not reenabled for 10 cycles in order to prevent unnecessary extension of the pacing interval.

by switching from simultaneous to sequential (LV first 30 to 50 ms) biventricular pacing.[56] This is equivalent to extending the blanking. In Medtronic CRT-Ds, blanking duration is measured from the end of the second ventricular pace.

Operative Intervention for T-Wave Oversensing

Operative intervention is required if T-wave oversensing cannot be eliminated without compromising reliable detection of VF. Review of published cases and anecdotal evidence[57,58] suggest that oversensing of T waves (spontaneous or paced) is much more common with devices from Medtronic or St. Jude Medical than with devices from Guidant/Boston Scientific. In the presence of a high-amplitude R wave, the initial sensing threshold is adjusted much higher in the Boston Scientific ICDs, and the "slow" component of the automatic gain control algorithm tends to prevent achievement of maximum sensitivity.[59]

T-wave oversensing can be site-specific (Fig 13.13). Insertion of a new pace/sense lead is necessary when T-wave oversensing cannot be safely circumvented by reprogramming, especially in the setting of a low-amplitude R wave. When a new lead is implanted in the right ventricle without removing a pre-existent one, it is important to avoid contact between the leads to avoid another source of oversensing. When there is severe RV pathology it may be necessary to institute left ventricular (LV) epicardial pacing, via a bipolar coronary venous lead[60] or epimyocardial leads[61] to ensure adequate R-wave sensing and avoid T-wave oversensing.

P-Wave Oversensing

Oversensing of the far-field atrial activation is uncommon, but can be life-threatening when it results in prolonged inhibition of pacing. It occurs almost exclusively with "integrated" bipolar leads when the distal coil goes through the tricuspid valve.[15] Oversensing of the spontaneous

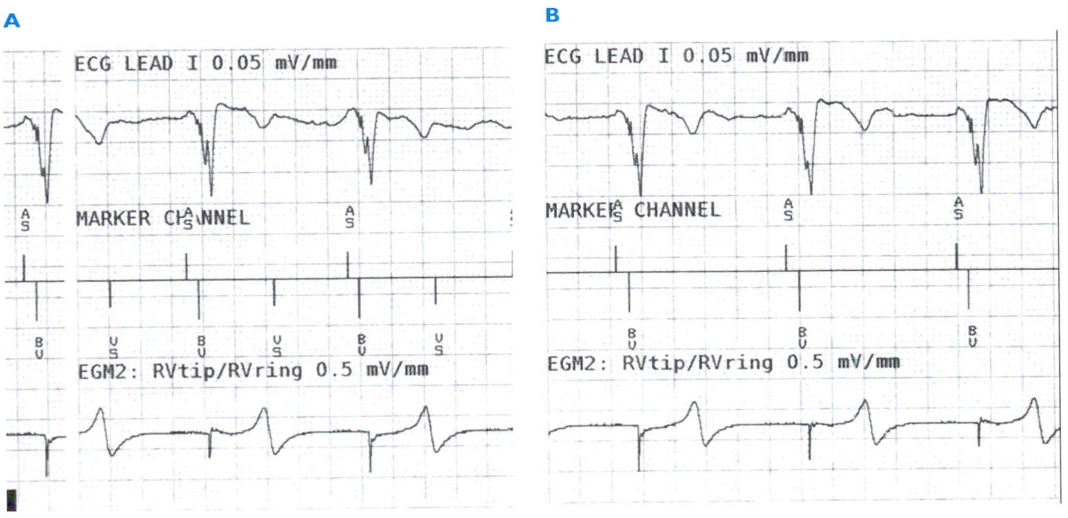

Fig 13.13 Site-dependency of T-wave oversensing. At the time of elective replacement of a Medtronic CRT-D, a Fidelis lead was "prophylactically" switched to the LV port and the bipolar LV lead was inserted in the RV port.[117,118] Panel **A** shows oversensing (VS) of paced T waves with nominal sensitivity of 0.3 mV. The RV tip/RV ring channel is indeed recording the LV electrogram. Because the sinus rate is slow, T-wave oversensing does not affect tracking of the following sinus beat. The patient had not had T-wave oversensing from the RV in 4 years of follow-up. Panel **B** shows that the oversensing was eliminated by reducing sensitivity to 0.45 mV.

sinus P wave can be asymptomatic or result in inappropriate discharges during sinus tachycardia. For double-counting to occur, the sensed PR interval must exceed the ventricular blanking. Oversensing of the paced P wave is unlikely to cause double-counting as it will manifest in most devices as ventricular safety pacing. Oversensing of the paced P wave outside of the ventricular safety-pacing window, followed by a conducted QRS, can result in a "short V-V interval," and increase the sensing integrity counters in Medtronic ICDs (Fig 13.14). On the other hand, oversensing of atrial depolarizations during atrial flutter or atrial tachycardia in the setting of continuous or intermittent ventricular pacing is likely to cause spurious shocks (independent of the ventricular rate) and possible asystole.[62–65] Ensuring that the distal coil lies entirely within the RV chamber minimizes oversensing of atrial signals.

Atrial oversensing in sinus rhythm can occur with lead dislodgment and migration to the tricuspid annulus or coronary sinus. In one case, oversensing of P waves during VT co-

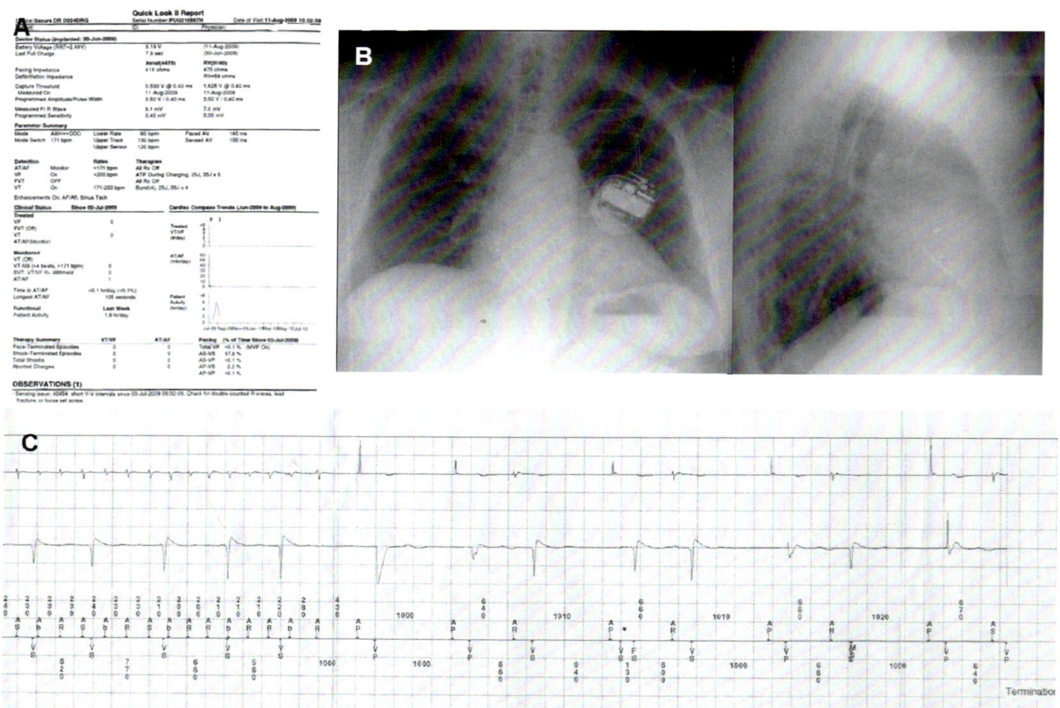

Fig 13.14 Intermittent oversensing of P waves resulting in short RR intervals in a patient with a Medtronic dual chamber ICD. **A**: At the first postoperative visit, more than 40,000 short RR intervals were logged in the sensing integrity counter, suggesting a lead or header problem. Lead impedance was repeatedly normal. Oversensing could not be provoked with deep respiration, Valsalva maneuver, pectoral muscle contraction, or pocket manipulation. **B**: Chest X-ray showed that the lead was relatively "shallow" in the right ventricle, with the distal coil possibly going through the tricuspid valve. It was assumed that the short RR intervals were due to intermittent oversensing of far-field atrial activity, possibly during atrial fibrillation. Sensitivity was empirically decreased from 0.3 to 0.45 mV. **C**: At a follow-up visit the strip stored after termination of an episode of atrial fibrillation showed a single example of oversensing of the paced P wave (*), with the following conducted QRS sensed in the VF zone and accounting for the "short RR" interval of 130 ms. Note that oversensing did not occur during atrial fibrillation, as the relatively rapid conduction maintained the sensitivity low. Oversensing could only occur late in diastole after atrial pacing at the escape interval, when the sensitivity was probably already at its maximum. As pacing has been programmed AAI+ (ie, no rate response), it was concluded that this oversensing was "innocent" and could not result in spurious shocks and did not require further reprogramming or intervention.

incided with an acute decrease in the amplitude of R waves, suggestive of lead dislodgment. A defibrillation shock was synchronized to the P wave (rather than to the R wave) and induced VF from which the patient could not be resuscitated.[66] Oversensing of P waves during sinus tachycardia triggering inappropriate shocks can be the initial manifestation of lead failure. An increase in the sensitivity to compensate for the reduction in R-wave amplitude has been invoked as the causal mechanism.[67]

In older biventricular ICDs that sensed and timed from both ventricular channels (ie, composite electrogram) proximal migration of the LV lead toward the main coronary sinus (where a sizable atrial electrogram is recorded) could lead to triple-counting (in the presence of spontaneous conduction) or asystole due to continuous ventricular inhibition (in case of AV block).[68] In current ICDs from Biotronik and Boston Scientific that sense from the LV lead to prevent pacing in the vulnerable period, such oversensing will result in withholding of the biventricular pulse (Fig 13.15). However, asystole does not occur as pacing will be delivered after the end of the LV protection window.

Double-Counting of R Waves

Double-counting of R waves is rare in current ICDs. (It was common in early CRT-Ds that sensed from the composite RV-LV electrogram[69]). It occurs if the duration of the sensing electrogram exceeds the postsensed ventricular blanking period of around 120 to 140 ms in most devices. Rarely, it can be triggered by hyperkalemia or sodium-channel–blocking drugs, particularly at high heart rates, which increase use-dependent sodium-channel blockade. In a patient with hypertrophic cardiomyopathy, double-counting of the R wave only occurred after transcoronary alcohol septal ablation which resulted in the development of new complete right bundle branch block and widening of the intraventricular electrogram to 200 ms.[70] The most common manifestation of double-counting of R waves is spurious

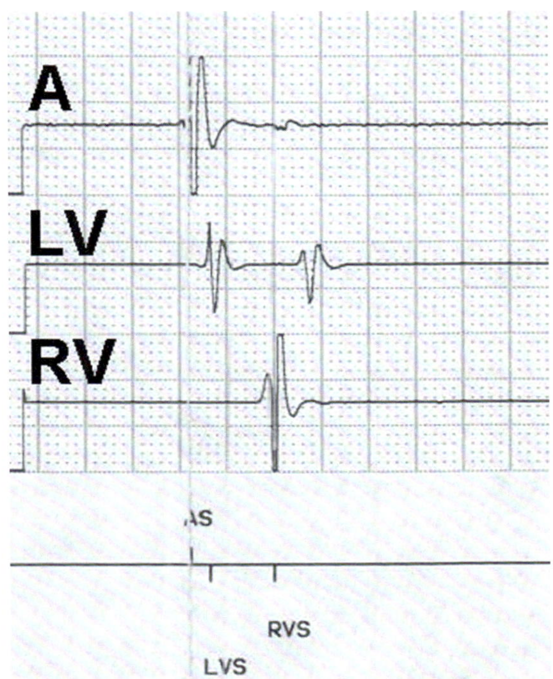

Fig 13.15 Oversensing of the P wave after displacement of the LV lead into the main coronary sinus in a patient with a Boston Scientific COGNIS CRT-D. Real-time electrograms of atrial (A), left ventricle (LV), and right ventricle (RV) activity. Left atrial activation is sensed in the LV lead (LVS), and triggers the "left ventricular protection period." The biventricular pacing pulse is withheld despite a programmed sensed AV delay of 140 ms. There is spontaneous conduction with a long PR, with sensing in the right ventricle first (RVS). In older models, this phenomenon could have resulted in asystole in the presence of AV block. In this case, a pacing pulse would have been delivered at the end of the LVVP (nominal 400 ms) if there had been no conduction.

tachyarrhythmia detection, with a typical pattern of alternation of ventricular cycle lengths with an isoelectric interval between sensed events. A characteristic "railroad track" pattern is seen in interval plots.[59] Double-counting of the R wave during VT can result in detection of VF and the delivery of shocks instead of antitachycardia pacing.

With St. Jude Medical and recent generation Medtronic R-wave double-counting may be overcome by increasing the postsense ventricular refractory period from the nominal value. Otherwise, lead revision is necessary if the cause of the double-counting is not reversible.

Oversensing of Diaphragmatic Myopotentials

Myopotentials are high-frequency, low-amplitude electrical transients recorded from the sensing leads that are generated by skeletal muscles, including intercostal muscles or the diaphragm. Diaphragmatic myopotentials can often be distinguished from other potential sources of noise because they are generally of low amplitude (ie, they do not saturate the amplifier), they are most prominent on the sensing electrogram, they persist for variable fractions of the cardiac cycle, and they are respirophasic. Even when the amplitude of the signal is constant, oversensing usually occurs after long diastolic intervals or after ventricular paced events when sensitivity

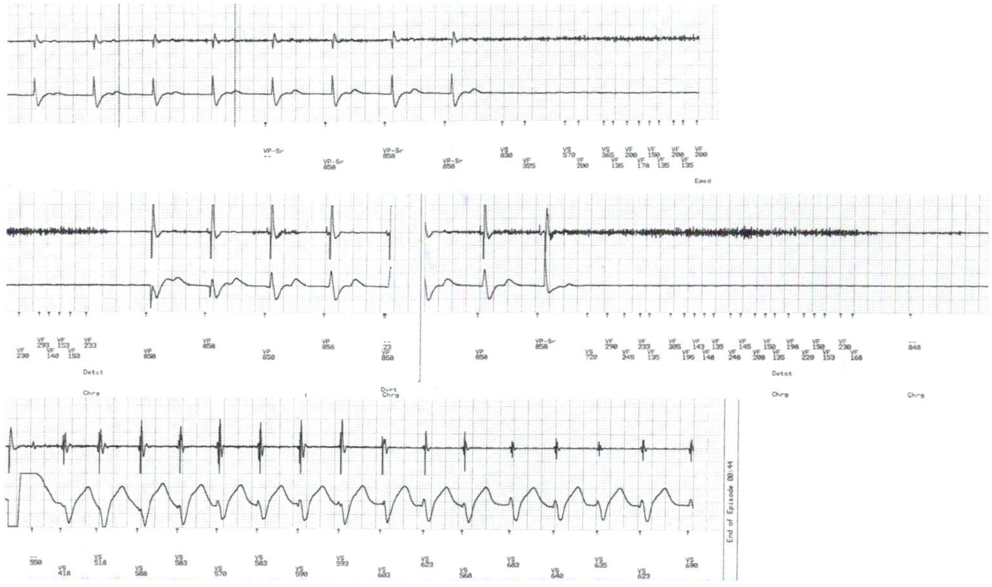

Fig 13.16 Oversensing of myopotentials during Valsalva maneuver during defecation. Patient with ischemic cardiomyopathy, permanent atrial fibrillation, and complete heart block who the day before had received a new Contak Renewal 3 HD CRT-D. An old pacemaker had been removed. He presented with syncope followed by a shock while defecating. Programming was VVIRV 70 to 120 bpm, VF detection at 180 bpm, duration 1 second, nominal sensitivity, reconfirmation On. Continuous recordings showing near-field and far-field electrograms. There is oversensing of myopotentials at the end of the top strip with inhibition of pacing. VF is eventually detected and capacitor charge is initiated. At the same time, Valsalva is released and myopotentials disappear. Charge is diverted and appropriate pacing resumes. A few seconds later, the patient strains again and the sequence repeats. This time charge proceeds. Although myopotentials disappear as the Valsalva is released (possibly coinciding with syncope), a committed shock is nevertheless delivered after a 3-second "confirmation" window with asystole. Guidant/Boston Scientific devices will not divert two shocks in a row for the same episode of arrhythmia. Oversensing was eliminated by reprogramming sensitivity to "least." Appropriate detection of induced VF at "least" sensitivity had been demonstrated during implant. This oversensing of myopotentials is unlikely with current Boston Scientific devices.

is maximal and often ends with a sensed R wave, which abruptly reduces sensitivity.

Oversensing of diaphragmatic myopotentials is a well-described cause of pacing inhibition and spurious shocks[71–74] (Fig 13.16). Prospective provocative testing demonstrated that myopotential oversensing was more likely during ventricular pacing, in men, and with integrated bipolar leads in the RV apex. However, in the absence of hardware problems (eg, lead insulation failure) the particular sensing algorithm appeared to be the main determinant of this occurrence. It was relatively common (10%–20%) with older Guidant/Boston Scientific devices (and also with ELA Defender ICDs), but practically nonexistent with Medtronic devices.[16,75–77] A narrower frequency band pass filter and a new Dynamic Noise Algorithm (DNA) in current Boston Scientific devices make oversensing of diaphragmatic myopotentials much less likely. The algorithm uses the characteristics of a noise signal—frequency and energy—to identify a signal as noise. When noise is present, DNA keeps the automatic gain control floor above the noise. Additionally, the nominal floor sensitivity is now higher than before (0.6 versus 0.18 or 0.24 mV) and the new automatic control algorithm makes achievement of maximum sensitivity after a paced event less rapid.

With previous generation Guidant devices, myopotential oversensing amenable to reprogramming had to be differentiated from structural lead failure or other problems requiring operative revision. Oversensing exclusively during deep breathing or the Valsalva maneuver favors the former, whereas reproduction of oversensing by pocket manipulation or arm movements and measurement of abnormal or changing lead parameters (impedance, pacing threshold, electrogram amplitude) suggest hardware problems. In unclear cases, frequent follow-up could elucidate the cause. Oversensing of diaphragmatic myopotentials without hardware problems could frequently be circumvented by reprogramming the maximum sensitivity to a less-sensitive setting.[78,79] The recommendation to always test VF detection at lowest sensitivity during implant arose when oversensing of diaphragmatic myopotentials was frequent. It was argued that this allowed safe reprogramming of the sensitivity in follow-up without the need to retest VF detection. This recommendation is less relevant today, as most current causes of oversensing (except paced T waves) are not "innocent."

Because oversensing of diaphragmatic myopotentials is much less common with current systems, a hardware problem should be suspected in most instances and the threshold for operative revision should be low.[80,81] For example, with small-caliber leads, inappropriate discharges due to diaphragmatic myopotential oversensing can be the first manifestation of subacute RV perforation.[82,83] Although oversensing of pectoral myopotentials (ie, provoked during isometric pectoral muscle contraction or forceful arm movements) with normal lead function has been reported,[84] this finding is highly likely to be associated with hardware problems. For example, it could be a manifestation of an incipient abrasion in the lead insulation inside the pocket or of chronic damage to the seal plugs that cover the setscrews in the header of the ICD

When using a dual coil integrated bipolar lead with Boston Scientific ICDs, reversal of the DF-1 pins (ie, right ventricular [RV] coil in the receptacle for the superior vena cava [SVC] coil and vice versa) often results in oversensing of pectoral myopotentials (and also high defibrillation thresholds).[85–87] Due to the hardwiring at the lead yoke and at the generator header itself, transposition of the DF-1 terminal pins results in a shocking vector from the proximal coil to the distal coil and the can and in a sensing vector both from the lead tip to the distal RV coil and from lead tip to the generator can (Fig 13.17). The proximal (SVC) coil electrode does not enter the abnormal sensing circuit. This configuration potentiates extracardiac oversensing, particularly of pectoralis muscle myopotentials. The mistake may not be recognized intraoperatively, especially if the implant is performed under general anesthesia and defibrillator threshold testing is not performed.

Pin reversion can be suspected when recording an atrial deflection from the far-field channel (which normally is recorded from the distal coil to the can but in case of transposition from the proximal coil to the can).[88,89] Pin transposition should be strongly suspected when myopotential oversensing occurs shortly after a device replacement[90] or upgrade.[91]

On the other hand, recording of high-frequency myopotentials exclusively from sensing vectors that include the generator can (eg, with St. Jude Medical devices that allow collection of the SVC coil to can electrogram) does not indicate a lead integrity problem.[92] Although this oversensing will not result in pacing inhibition or false detection of tachycardia, it can interfere with algorithms that utilize the morphology of signals recorded between the pulse generator and a proximal or distal coil to discriminate between supraventricular rhythms and VT.[93]

Crosstalk Inhibition

Crosstalk occurs when atrial output signals are sensed by the ventricular channel and result in the inhibition of the ventricular pulse. Crosstalk typically occurs with high atrial pulse amplitude or pulse width settings and high ventricular sensitivity. All dual and triple chamber ICDs incorporate a cross-chamber ventricular blanking to prevent it. This cross-chamber blanking must be kept short to maintain a ventricular alert window. To prevent crosstalk inhibition,

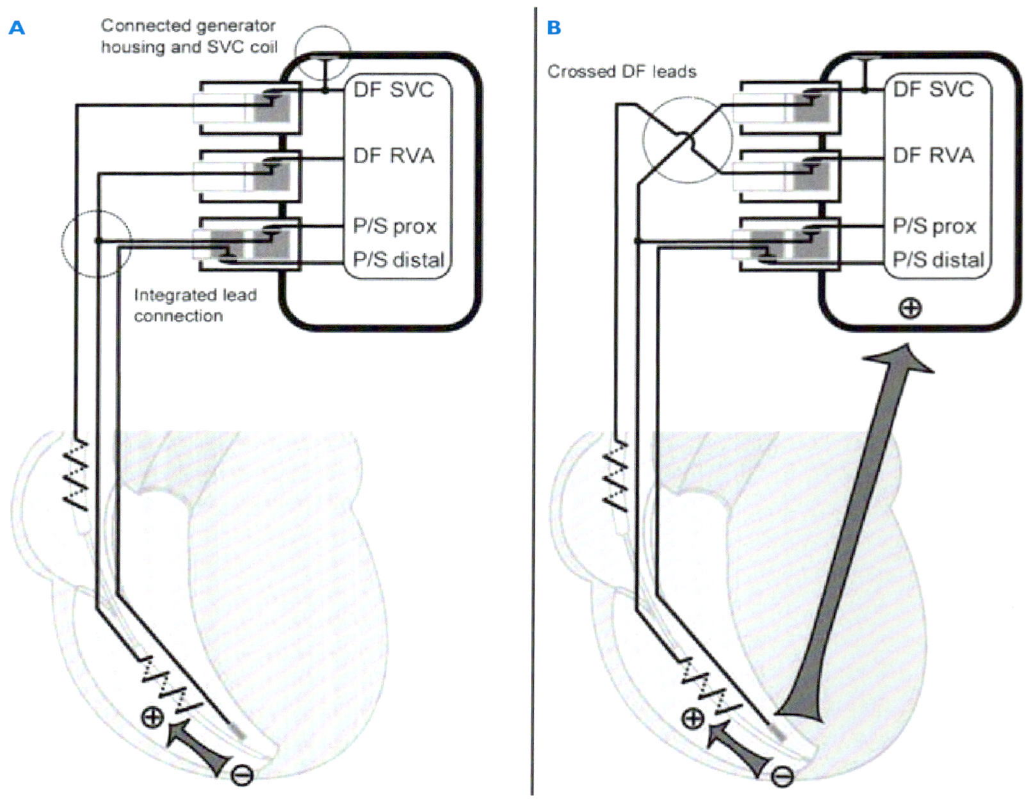

Fig 13.17 A:The intended design of integrated bipolar lead and sensing function. The bipolar ventricular sensing is from the right ventricular apex (RVA) pace/sense (P/S) distal electrode to the RVA defibrillator (DF) coil. The connection between the superior vena cava (SVC) DF coil and generator housing itself allows for an "active-can" configuration for defibrillation purpose. **B**:When DF pins are transposed, the generator housing acts as a second anode, markedly expanding the volume of interest. The SVC DF coil is not involved in the sensing function in either scenario. (Reproduced from Eckart[90] with permission.)

all ICDs (except those from Guidant/Boston Scientific) incorporate an additional ventricular safety pacing algorithm that delivers a backup ventricular pulse when ventricular sensing occurs outside the blanking but in the initial 100 to 110 ms of the AV delay. Thus, crosstalk inhibition is extremely rare in ICDs.

Asystole is the typical manifestation of crosstalk inhibition. Another possible presentation (in patients with preserved conduction) is *pacemaker alternans*. During continuous atrial pacing, an alternation of paced and conducted beats is seen. After a paced beat, high ventricular sensitivity promotes crosstalk and inhibition. The conducted QRS resets the sensitivity higher, and the next atrial pacing pulse is not oversensed. Ventricular pacing ensues, restarting the sequence.[94]

Pacing capture thresholds rise immediately after an ICD shock,[2,95,96] and most ICDs nominally provide for some form of high-output pacing for a brief period after a shock. Crosstalk inhibition causing asystole after an ICD shock has been described in a patient with complete heart block and a Biotronik Tachos DR.[97] The short (23 ms) nonprogrammable ventricular blanking after atrial pacing, absence of "safety pacing," high nominal ventricular sensitivity (0.5 mV), and high-output postshock atrial pacing (7.2 V at 1 ms) in that device promoted this complication. These shortcomings have been corrected in newer Biotronik devices. Devices from Medtronic and St Jude also nominally provide high-output atrial pacing after a shock, but crosstalk inhibition should not occur as long as the default ventricular safety pacing is not turned Off.

To prevent crosstalk inhibition in the absence of safety pacing, older Guidant devices had a relatively long 65-ms nominal postatrial-paced ventricular blanking. If the AV delay was programmed long (ie, ≥ 200 ms), undersensing of a late-coupled ventricular premature depolarization (VPD) falling during ventricular blanking followed by ventricular capture in the vulnerable period could result in arrhythmia induction.[98]

Current Boston Scientific ICDs have a nominal "smart blanking" function during the cross-chamber ventricular blank after atrial pace, that includes a 37.5-ms fixed blanking followed by a transient decrease in sensitivity if already high. Because residual polarization in the integrated bipolar lead after shock delivery can promote crosstalk, the cross-chamber blanking is automatically extended and fixed to 85 ms during the post-therapy period (nominally 30 seconds).[99] In one patient with complete heart block, post-shock crosstalk inhibition and asystole occurred after expiration of this 30-second period.[100] In patients with complete heart block, the cross-chamber blanking should be programmed longer or the post-therapy period extended.

Hardware Problems

Several different hardware problems, including lead conductor fracture, by far the most common, and loose setscrews can result in intermittent connection and transient "make-and-break" signals in the sensing channel that result in oversensing and possibly spurious shocks (Fig 13.18). Oversensing from lead or connector (header, adaptor, or setscrew) problems is intermittent. Usually it occurs only during a small fraction (< 10%) of the cardiac cycle and often saturates the amplifier. It may be limited to the sensing electrogram and may be associated with postural changes. Often, the pacing lead impedance is abnormal, indicating complete or partial interruption of the pace-sense circuit. However, abnormal impedance measurements may be intermittent or not significant, even after oversensing causing multiple shocks occurs.[101,102] At least with the coaxial Medtronic 6936 lead model, oversensing after an appropriate shock (resulting in multiple subsequent spurious shocks) was a common form of presentation.[103] An algorithm in Medtronic devices that looks at changes in lead impedance and early evidence of oversensing (short RR intervals, detection of runs of nonsustained VT), can oftentimes provide advance warning of impending spurious shocks.[104]

A defective connection between the header block and the terminal pin of the sensing lead can induce intermittent electrical noise (Fig 13.19) and result in oversensing and spurious shocks. Interestingly, it often manifests in the first days after implant. The problem can often be diagnosed from a radiograph, as the pin does not extend beyond the header post. Although often assumed to be due to operator error, physical characteristics of the device headers and setscrews can make particular devices more prone to the complication.[105] It is important to follow the manufacturer's recommendations regarding proper lead connection technique.[106]

Seal plugs that cover the setscrews in the header of an ICD allow setscrew wrench insertion while preventing body fluids from entering the header cavities. If minor damage prevents resealing of the preslit passage in the seal after removing the wrench, body fluid from the pocket may enter the header, creating an additional sensing pathway. Minor body fluid infiltration generally does not disrupt sensing. However, if air is trapped in the header during the lead insertion process, it may escape through a damaged seal plug. An escaping air bubble can momentarily displace body fluid in the seal plug and disrupt the conductive accessory pathway. This momentary disruption causes a change in impedance, generating an artificial noise signal. Although this oversensing is generally very transient, it can result in pacing inhibition and spurious tachyarrhythmia detection.[107–109] The noise signals are discrete (one deflection per each bubble that escapes) (Fig 13.20). Lead impedance is normal and oversensing cannot be provoked with pocket manipulation. This form of oversensing disappears once entrapped air is dissipated and pressure equilibrium is achieved (a few hours or a day or two at most). If oversensing is observed while the pocket is still open, relieving trapped air by reopening the seal plug with a setscrew wrench may hasten stabilization, but care should be taken to avoid further damage to the seal plug. Conservative management is recommended if this type of oversensing is observed after pocket closure; in the majority of clinical cases reported, sporadic

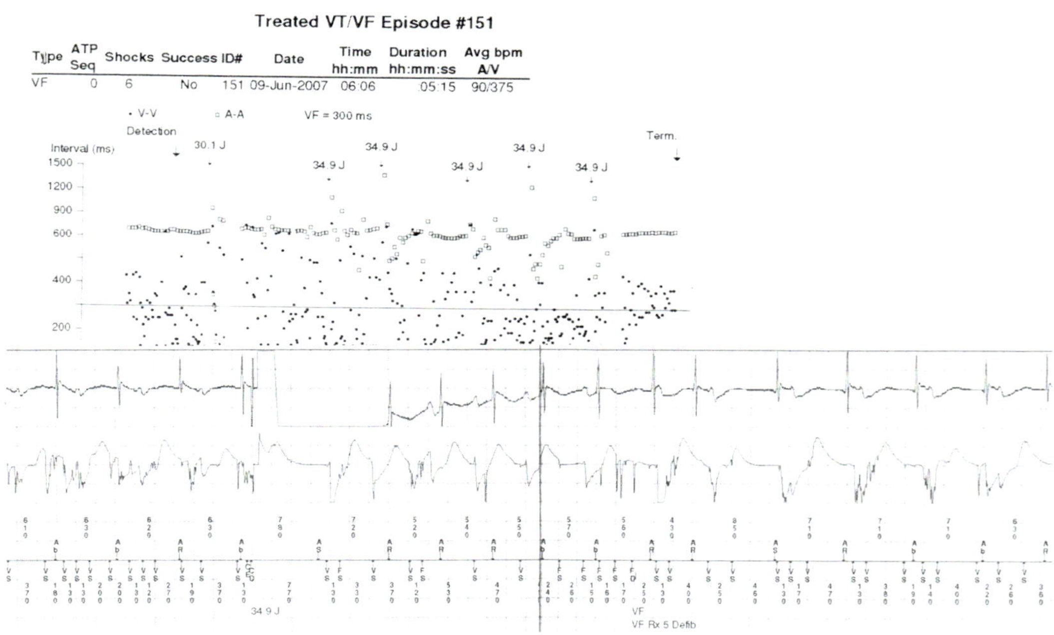

Fig 13.18 Multiple inappropriate shocks in a patient with a fractured Sprint Fidelis lead. High amplitude, intermittent signals are seen in the stored intracardiac electrogram. The interval plot depicts very irregular RR intervals.

oversensing disappeared without intervention within a few hours or at most a few days.[110] Oversensing due to transient seal plug damage could cause an early increase in the sensing integrity counter in Medtronic devices that then recedes.[111] On the other hand, chronic more-severe damage to the seal plugs can create a persistent aberrant sensing pathway that manifests

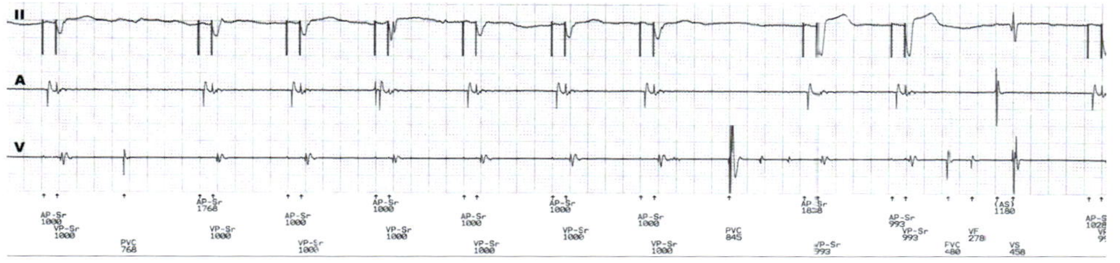

Fig 13.19 Oversensing due to loose setscrew. Pauses during pacing were first noted the day after implant. Real time electrograms (surface ECG, atrium, right ventricular near-field) show intermittent, at times high-amplitude deflections in the RV, which are detected as PVCs, and reset the escape interval. A loose setscrew was confirmed at operative revision.

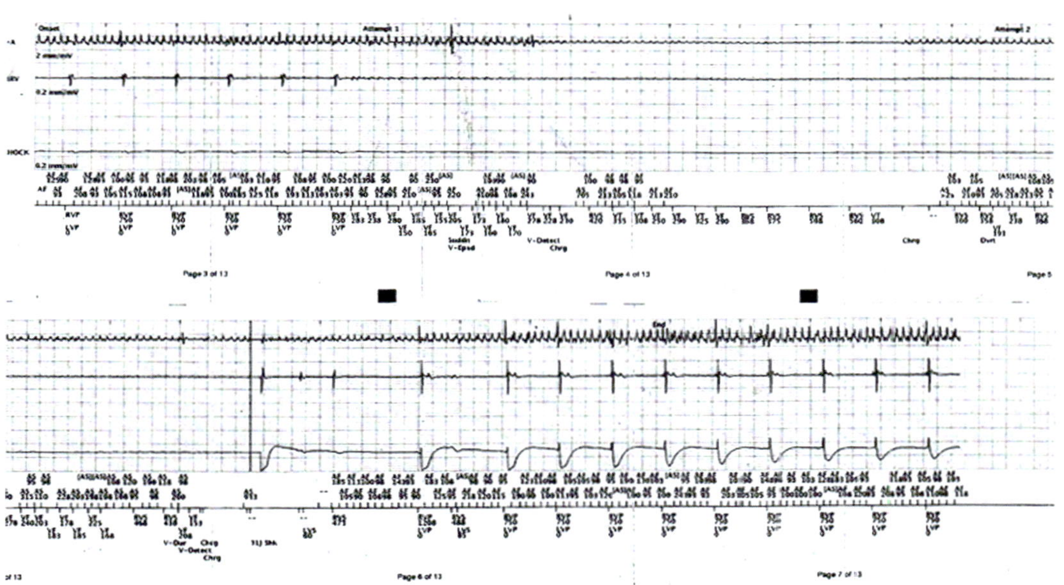

Fig 13.20 Oversensing caused by air bubbles escaping through a seal plug that has not completely resealed following wrench insertion. Stored electrogram of a spurious shock that occurred immediately after closing the pocket in a patient with permanent atrial fibrillation and complete heart block who received a Boston Scientific CRT-D. The atrial port was plugged, but the recommended settings to completely ignore information from the atrial channel were not programmed.[119] The device was programmed VVIRV. There is initial ventricular pacing followed by oversensing of rapid, low-amplitude, discrete signals, seen in the near-field RV channel but not in the shock electrogram. Oversensing results in pacing inhibition and asystole. VF is detected and charge commences. The escape of bubbles "slows" below the tachycardia detection rate and the shock is initially diverted. However, another rapid "bubble salvo" shortly thereafter results in VF redetection and a "committed" shock follows. Bubbles cease after the shock and appropriate postshock pacing ensues. Telemetry and fluoroscopy testing immediately did not disclose any other abnormality. The device was left programmed in "electrocautery-mode" (ie, VOO with therapies Off) while the patient was observed overnight in the intensive care unit. Extensive testing the next day, including defibrillation threshold testing, was normal and detection and therapies reenabled. Oversensing did not recur.

as oversensing of pectoral myopotentials and requires surgical correction.

To avoid damage to the seal plugs during implant, one has to carefully locate the slit and then guide the wrench through the slit to the setscrew cavity beneath. If the slit cannot be located or if wrench insertion damages the seal plug (ie, the slit does not properly reseal following wrench removal), the pulse generator should be discarded and a new one used.[110]

Mechanical contact between two defibrillation leads,[112,113] or even between a defibrillation lead and a retained fragment of a pacemaker lead[114] can result in oversensing. When it is not possible to extract an abandoned lead, it is important to implant the new lead far from the old one. Absence of contact should be confirmed in several different fluoroscopic projections. In saline tank simulation studies, a Guidant Reliance integrated bipolar lead with coils covered by expanded polytetrafluoroethylene was immune to oversensing electrical signals due to contact with other leads.[115] Covered leads thus should be considered in patients with abandoned leads to reduce the risk of oversensing.

Electromagnetic Interference (EMI)

Multiple sources of EMI in daily life, the workplace, and the medical environment can interfere with ICDs and induce oversensing.[116] Discussion of these sources is beyond the scope of this chapter. In stored electrograms, noise is seen in all channels. Signal amplitude is greater on the high-voltage electrogram recorded from widely spaced electrodes than on the sensing electrogram recorded from closely spaced electrodes (Fig 13.21). The interference signal may

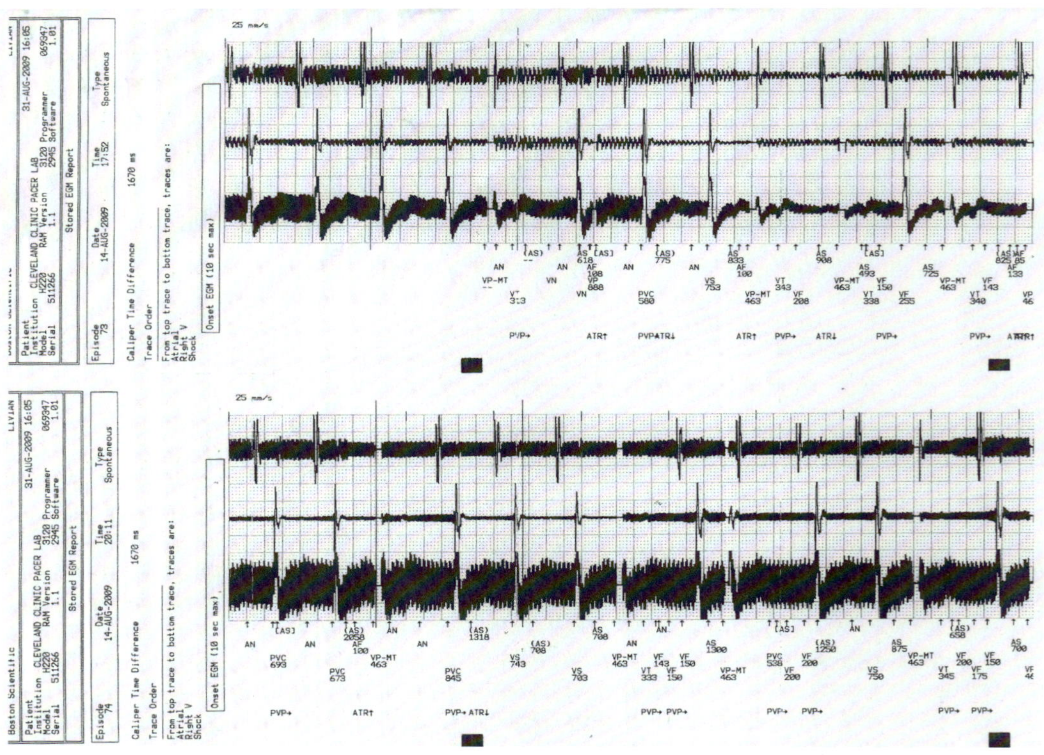

Fig 13.21 Oversensing of EMI. Multiple spurious arrhythmia detections (without shock) recorded in a patient at the time of a routine visit. The day of the episodes the patient had been working with a poorly maintained power drill on top of a wet roof. Noise is first detected in the atrial channel, resulting in mode switch. The amplitude of the noise signals is much larger in the shock electrogram than in the RV electrogram.

be continuous. The source of EMI is often clinically obvious. Avoidance of known sources is the only reliable strategy to prevent EMI. Close-coupled dedicated bipolar leads should be used in patients who are expected to return to a work environment suspected of high-level EMI.

References

1. Jacq F, Foulldrin G, Savouré A, et al. A comparison of anxiety, depression and quality of life between device shock and nonshock groups in implantable cardioverter defibrillator recipients. *Gen Hosp Psychiatry.* 2009;31:266–273.
2. Pinski SL, Fahy G. The proarrhythmic potential of implantable cardioverter-defibrillators. *Circulation.* 1995;92:1651–1664.
3. Jones GK, Bardy GH. Considerations for ventricular fibrillation detection by implantable cardioverter defibrillators. *Am Heart J.* 1994;127:1107–1110.
4. Brumwell DA, Kroll K, Lehmann MH. The amplifier: sensing the depolarization. In: Kroll MW, Lehmann MH, eds. *Implantable cardioverter-defibrillator therapy: the engineering-clinical interface.* Norwell, Massachusetts: Kluwer Academic Publishers; 1996: 275–302.
5. Swerdlow CD, Gillberg JM, Olson WH. Sensing and detection. In: Ellenbogen KA, Kay GN, Lau CP, Wilkoff BL, eds. *Clinical cardiac pacing, defibrillation and resynchronization therapy.* 3rd edition. Philadelphia, PA: Saunders Elsevier; 2007:75–160.
6. Rauwolf T, Guenther M, Hass N, et al. Ventricular oversensing in 518 patients with implanted cardiac defibrillators: incidence, complications, and solutions. *Europace.* 2007;9:1041–1047.
7. Occhetta E, Bortnik M, Magnani A, Francalacci G, Marino P. Inappropriate implantable cardioverter-defibrillator discharges unrelated to supraventricular tachyarrhythmias. *Europace.* 2007;8:863–869.
8. Daubert JP, Zareba W, Cannom DS, et al; MADIT II Investigators. Inappropriate implantable cardioverter-defibrillator shocks in MADIT II: frequency, mechanisms, predictors, and survival impact. *J Am Coll Cardiol.* 2008;51:1357–1365.
9. Hauser RG, Hayes DL. Increasing hazard of Sprint Fidelis implantable cardioverter-defibrillator lead failure. *Heart Rhythm.* 2009;6:605–610.
10. Wang P, Kramer A, Estes III NAM, Hayes DL. Timing cycles for biventricular pacing. *Pacing Clin Electrophysiol.* 2002;25:62–75.
11. Haqqani HM, Mond HG. The implantable cardioverter-defibrillator lead: principles, progress, and promises. *Pacing Clin Electrophysiol.* 2009;32:1336–1353.
12. Cooklin M, Tummala RV, Peters RW, Shorofsky SR, Gold MR. Comparison of bipolar and integrated sensing for redetection of ventricular fibrillation. *Am Heart J.* 1999;138:133–136.
13. Frain BH, Ellison KE, Michaud GF, et al. True bipolar defibrillator leads have increased sensing latency and threshold compared with the integrated bipolar configuration. *J Cardiovasc Electrophysiol.* 2007;18:192–195.
14. Freedman RA, Petrakian A, Boyce K, et al. Performance of dedicated versus integrated bipolar defibrillator leads with CRT defibrillators: results from a prospective multicenter study. *Pacing Clin Electrophysiol.* 2009;32:157–165.
15. Gunderson BD, Pratt T, Johnson WB, et al. Ventricular oversensing in ICD patients: true bipolar versus integrated bipolar sensing. *Pacing Clin Electrophysiol.* 2001;24:560 (Abstract).
16. Weretka S, Michaelsen J, Becker R, et al. Ventricular oversensing: A study of 101 patients implanted with dual chamber defibrillators and two different lead systems. *Pacing Clin Electrophysiol.* 2003;26:65–70.
17. Vollmann D, Erdogan A, Himmrich E, et al. Patient alert to detect ICD lead failure: efficacy, limitations, and implications for future algorithms. *Europace.* 2006;8:371–376.
18. Barold SS, Cantens F. Characterization of the 16 blanking periods of the Medtronic GEM DR dual chamber defibrillators. *J Interv Card Electrophysiol.* 2001;5:319–325.
19. Vollman D, Lüthje L, Zabel M. Unusual cause for an increase of the sensing integrity counter in a patient with inappropriate implantable cardioverter-defibrillator therapy. *Europace.* 2007;9:275–277.
20. Schuller JL, Lowery CM, Weinberger HD, Sauer WH. Fluctuation in ventricular sensing lead-

ing to underdetection of ventricular fibrillation in a patient with cardiac sarcoidosis. *J Interv Card Electrophysiol.* 2009 Jul 23. [Epub ahead of print]

21. Boriani G, Artale P, Biffi M, et al. Outcome of cardioverter-defibrillator implant in patients with arrhythmogenic right ventricular cardiomyopathy. *Heart Vessels.* 2007;22:184–192.
22. Porres JM, Brugada J, Marco P, García F, Azcarate B. T wave oversensing by a cardioverter defibrillator implanted in a patient with the Brugada syndrome. *Pacing Clin Electrophysiol.* 2004;27:1563–1565.
23. Veltmann C, Kuschyk J, Schimpf R, et al. Prevention of inappropriate ICD shocks in patients with Brugada syndrome. *Clin Res Cardiol.* 2009 Sep 16. [Epub ahead of print]
24. Alizadeh A, Haghjoo M, Arya A, et al. Inappropriate ICD discharge due to T-wave oversensing in a patient with the Brugada syndrome. *J Interv Card Electrophysiol.* 2006;15:65–68.
25. Hsu SS, Mohib S, Schroeder A, Deger FT. T wave oversensing in implantable cardioverter defibrillators. *J Interv Card Electrophysiol.* 2004; 11:67–72.
26. Watanabe H, Chinushi M, Izumi D, et al. Decrease in amplitude of intracardiac ventricular electrogram and inappropriate therapy in patients with an implantable cardioverter defibrillator. *Int Heart J.* 2006;47:363–370.
27. Strohmer B, Schernthaner C, Pichler M. T-wave oversensing by an implantable cardioverter defibrillator after successful ablation of idiopathic ventricular fibrillation. *Pacing Clin Electrophysiol.* 2006;29:431–435.
28. Baranchuk A, Ribas S, Divakaramenon S, Morillo CA. An unusual mechanism causing inappropriate implantable cardioverter defibrillator shocks: transient reduction in R-wave amplitude. *Europace.* 2007;9:694–696.
29. Kapa S, Curwin JH, Coyne RF, Winters SL. Inappropriate defibrillator shocks from depolarization—repolarization mismatch in a patient with hypertrophy cardiomyopathy. *Pacing Clin Electrophysiol.* 2007;30:1408–1411.
30. Sun Y, Zhang P, Li X, Guo J. Inappropriate ICD discharge due to T-wave oversensing in a patient with short QT syndrome. *Pacing Clin Electrophysiol.* 2009 Sep 30. [Epub ahead of print]
31. Schimpf R, Wolpert C, Bianchi F, et al. Congenital short QT syndrome and implantable cardioverter defibrillator treatment: inherent risk for inappropriate shock delivery. *J Cardiovasc Electrophysiol.* 2003;14:1273–1277.
32. Hosaka Y, Chinushi M, Iijima K, et al. Correlation between surface and intracardiac electrocardiogram in a patient with inappropriate defibrillation shocks due to hyperkalemia. *Intern Med.* 2009;48:1153–1156.
33. Koul AK, Keller S, Clancy JF, et al. Hyperkalemia induced T wave oversensing leading to loss of biventricular pacing and inappropriate ICD shocks. *Pacing Clin Electrophysiol.* 2004;27:681–683.
34. Khan E, Voudouris A, Shorofsky SR, Peters RW. Inappropriate ICD discharges due to "triple counting" during normal sinus rhythm. *J Interv Card Electrophysiol.* 2006;17:153–155.
35. Oudit GY, Cameron D, Harris L. A case of appropriate inappropriate device therapy: hyperkalemia-induced ventricular oversensing. *Can J Cardiol.* 2008;24:e16–18.
36. Krishen A, Shepard RK, Leffler JA, Wood MA, Ellenbogen KA. Implantable cardioverter defibrillator T wave oversensing caused by hyperglycemia. *Pacing Clin Electrophysiol.* 2001;24:1701–1703.
37. Srivathsan K, Scott LR, Altemose GT. T-wave oversensing and inappropriate shocks: a case report. *Europace.* 2008;10:552–555.
38. Wieczorek M, Hoeltgen R, Djajadisastra I. [Avoidance of intermittent T-wave oversensing with device programming]. *Herzschrittmacherther Elektrophysiol.* 2006;17:106–111. German.
39. Duru F, Bauersfeld U, Candinas R. Avoiding inappropriate ventricular tachycardia detection due to T-wave oversensing in an implantable cardioverter defibrillator: a novel application of the electrogram width criterion. *Europace.* 2001;3:80–84.
40. Lin D, Dixit S, Russo AM, Hsia HH. Total failure to sense ventricular fibrillation with inappropriate defibrillator sensitivity adjustment. *Pacing Clin Electrophysiol.* 2004;27:1321–1323.
41. Reiter MJ, Mann DE. Sensing and tachyarrhythmia detection problems in implantable cardio-

verter defibrillators. *J Cardiovasc Electrophysiol.* 1996;7:542–558.
42. Perry GY, Kosar EM. Problems in managing patients with long QT syndrome and implantable cardioverter-defibrillators: a report of two cases. *Pacing Clin Electrophysiol.* 1996;19:863–867.
43. Böhm A, Pintér A, Préda I. QT dependent T wave sensing. *Pacing Clin Electrophysiol.* 1998;21:1290–1291.
44. Pinski SL. 2:1 tracking of sinus rhythm in a patient with a dual-chamber ICD: what is the mechanism? *J Cardiovasc Electrophysiol.* 2001; 12:503–504.
45. Lezcano AO, Aracama JM, Ayestaran VU, Urra FG. T wave oversensing and low percentage of biventricular pacing in cardiac resynchronization therapy. *Cardiol J.* 2009;16:580–581.
46. Barold SS, Levine PA. Pacemaker repetitive nonreentrant ventriculoatrial synchronous rhythm. A review. *J Interv Card Electrophysiol.* 2001;5:45–58.
47. Pinski SL. Inappropriate pacing due to autoperpetuation of the ventricular rate stabilization algorithm: a manifestation of T-wave oversensing by ICDs. *Pacing Clin Electrophysiol.* 2000;23:1446–1447.
48. Manolis AG, Chatzis DG, Kouvelas K, Kyriakides ZS. Partial inhibition of ongoing antitachycardia pacing sequence due to T-wave oversensing. *Pacing Clin Electrophysiol.* 2008; 31:780–781.
49. Mann DE, Damle RS, Kelly PA, et al. Comparison of oversensing during bradycardia pacing in two types of implantable cardioverter-defibrillator systems. *Am Heart J.* 1998;136:658–663.
50. Shalaby AA. Delayed detection of ventricular tachycardia in a dual chamber rate adaptive pacing implantable cardioverter defibrillator: a case of intradevice interaction. *Pacing Clin Electrophysiol.* 2004;27:1164–1166.
51. Shivkumar K, Feliciano Z, Boyle NG, Wiener I. Intradevice interaction in a dual chamber implantable cardioverter defibrillator preventing ventricular tachyarrhythmia detection. *J Cardiovasc Electrophysiol.* 2000;11:1285–1288.
52. Glikson M, Beeman AL, Luria DM, et al. Impaired detection of ventricular tachyarrhythmias by a rate-smoothing algorithm in dual-chamber implantable defibrillators: intradevice interactions. *J Cardiovasc Electrophysiol.* 2002;13:312–318.
53. Sadoul N, Mletzko R, Anselme F, et al; Slow VT Study Group. Incidence and clinical relevance of slow ventricular tachycardia in implantable cardioverter-defibrillator recipients: an international multicenter prospective study. *Circulation.* 2005;112:946–953.
54. Pinski SL, Haw J, Trohman RG. Usefulness of a dynamic post-pace ventricular blanking period in dual-chamber, rate-responsive implantable defibrillators. *Pacing Clin Electrophysiol.* 1999;22:897 (Abstract).
55. Ellenbogen KA, Edel T, Moore S, et al. A prospective randomized-controlled trial of ventricular fibrillation detection time in a DDDR ventricular defibrillator. *Pacing Clin Electrophysiol.* 2000;23:1268–1272. Erratum in: *Pacing Clin Electrophysiol.* 2000;23(11 Pt 1):viii.
56. Silver JS, Gray ME, John RM. Strategy to eliminate inappropriate shocks secondary to T-wave oversensing in a biventricular ICD. *Pacing Clin Electrophysiol.* 2009;32:134–136.
57. Gilliam FR 3rd. T-wave oversensing in implantable cardiac defibrillators is due to technical failure of device sensing. *J Cardiovasc Electrophysiol.* 2006;17:553–556.
58. Tuzcu V. Resolution of T-wave oversensing with implantable cardioverter defibrillator generator replacement in an adolescent. *Pacing Clin Electrophysiol.* 2007;30:929–932.
59. Swerdlow CD, Friedman P. Advanced ICD troubleshooting: part I. *Pacing Clin Electrophysiol.* 2005;28:1322–1346.
60. Bilchick KC, Judge DP, Calkins H, Marine JE. Use of a coronary sinus lead and biventricular ICD to correct a sensing abnormality in a patient with arrhythmogenic right ventricular dysplasia/cardiomyopathy. *J Cardiovasc Electrophysiol.* 2006;17:317–320.
61. Cohen MI, Anagnostopoulos PV, Papez A. An unusual resolution of T-wave oversensing in an implantable cardioverter defibrillator in a child with long QT syndrome. *J Interv Card Electrophysiol.* 2009;25:235–238.
62. Curwin JH, Roelke M, Ruskin JN. Inhibition of bradycardia pacing caused by far-field atrial

sensing in a third-generation cardioverter defibrillator with an automatic gain feature. *Pacing Clin Electrophysiol.* 1996;19:124–126.

63. Schecter SO, Greenberg SM, Hoch DH, Cesa M, Levine JH. Inappropriate discharges of an implantable cardioverter defibrillator secondary to automatic adjustable gain of atrial tachycardia. *Pacing Clin Electrophysiol.* 1997;20:1721–1722.
64. Peters W, Kowallik P, Wittenberg G, Scholl C, Meesmann M. Inappropriate discharge of an implantable cardioverter-defibrillator during atrial flutter and intermittent ventricular antibradycardia pacing. *J Cardiovasc Electrophysiol.* 1997;8:1167–1174.
65. Scaglione J, Socas AG, De Palma C, Kreutzer E. Inappropriate single chamber ICD discharges due to supraventricular tachycardia with high degree atrioventricular block. *J Interv Card Electrophysiol.* 2004;11:73–76.
66. Dimitri H, John B, Young GD, Sanders P. Fatal outcome from inappropriate defibrillation. *Europace.* 2007;9:1059–1060.
67. Vollmann D, Lüthje L, Zabel M. Far-field oversensing of atrial signals: an unusual cause for very short V-V intervals and inappropriate implantable cardioverter defibrillator therapy. *Europace.* 2008;10:1009–1011.
68. Vollmann D, Luthje L, Gortler G, Unterberg C. Inhibition of bradycardia pacing and detection of ventricular fibrillation due to far-field atrial sensing in a triple chamber implantable cardioverter defibrillator. *Pacing Clin Electrophysiol.* 2002;25:1513–1516.
69. Barold SS, Herweg B, Gallardo I. Double counting of the ventricular electrogram in biventricular pacemakers and ICDs. *Pacing Clin Electrophysiol.* 2003;26:1645–1648.
70. Shah P, Harris L, Hill A, Schwartz L, Cameron D. Inappropriate therapy from a defibrillator complicating transcoronary ablation of septal hypertrophy in a patient with hypertrophic obstructive cardiomyopathy. *Pacing Clin Electrophysiol.* 2004;27:677–680.
71. Kelly PA, Mann DE, Damle RS, et al. Oversensing during ventricular pacing in patients with a third-generation implantable cardioverter-defibrillator. *J Am Coll Cardiol.* 1994;23:1531–1534.
72. Rosenthal ME, Paskman C. Noise detection during bradycardia pacing with a hybrid nonthoracotomy implantable cardioverter-defibrillator system: incidence and clinical significance. *Pacing Clin Electrophysiol.* 1998;21:1380–1386.
73. Deshmukh P, Anderson K. Myopotential sensing by a dual chamber implantable cardioverter-defibrillator: two case reports. *J Cardiovasc Electrophysiol.* 1998;9:767–772.
74. Babuty D, Fauchier L, Cosnay P. Inappropriate shocks delivered by implantable cardioverter-defibrillators during oversensing of activity of diaphragmatic muscle. *Heart.* 1999;81:94–96.
75. Sweeney MO, Ellison KE, Shea JB, et al. Provoked and spontaneous high-frequency, low amplitude respirophasic noise transients in patients with implantable cardioverter-defibrillators. *J Cardiovasc Electrophysiol.* 2001;12:402–410.
76. Kopp DE, Burke MC, Lin AC, et al. Oversensing in dual chamber implantable cardioverter-defibrillators. *Pacing Clin Electrophysiol.* 2000;23:591 (Abstract).
77. Santos KR, Adragão P, Cavaco D, Morgado FB, Candeias R, Lima S, Silva JA. Diaphragmatic myopotential oversensing in pacemaker-dependent patients with CRT-D devices. *Europace.* 2008;10:1381–1386.
78. Niehaus M, Neuzner J, Vogt J, et al. Adjustment of maximum automatic sensitivity (automatic gain control) reduces inappropriate therapies in patients with implantable cardioverter-defibrillators. *Pacing Clin Electrophysiol.* 2002;25:151–155.
79. Schulte B, Sperzel J, Carlsson J, et al. Inappropriate arrhythmia detection in implantable defibrillator therapy due to oversensing of diaphragmatic myopotentials. *J Interv Card Electrophysiol.* 2001;5:487–493.
80. Mortensen PT, Hansen PS, Jensen HK, et al. Oversensing by implantable defibrillators is most often caused by sensing lead failure as verified by surgical exploration. *Pacing Clin Electrophysiol.* 2000;23:630 (Abstract).
81. Salukhe TV, Wright I, Wright M, Kanagaratnam P, O'Neill MD. A fortuitous syncope. The pitfalls of integrated bipolar defibrillator leads. *Indian Pacing Electrophysiol J.* 2008;8:312–316.
82. Wiegand UK, Wilke I, Bonnemeier H, Eberhardt F, Bode F. Inadequate ICD discharges

due to diaphragmatic electromyopotential oversensing as the first sign of right ventricular lead perforation. *Pacing Clin Electrophysiol.* 2006;29:1176–1178.

83. Ueda-Tatsumoto A, Fukamizu S, Nishizaki M, Sakurada H, Hiraoka M. Inappropriate ICD discharges due to noise oversensing as the first sign of repetitive perforations of the right ventricular lead. *Pacing Clin Electrophysiol.* 2009;32:1481–1484.
84. Barakpour H, Emkanjoo Z, Alizadeh A, Sadr-Ameli MA. Inappropriate shock delivered by implantable cardioverter defibrillator-cardiac resynchronization therapy (ICD-CRT) due to myopotential oversensing. *Indian Pacing Electrophysiol J.* 2009;9:71–74.
85. Karanam S, John RM. Inappropriate sensing of pectoral myopotentials by an implantable cardioverter defibrillator system. *Pacing Clin Electrophysiol.* 2004;27:688–689.
86. Maagh P, Trappe HJ, Meissner A. Non-determinable defibrillation threshold and inefficacy of implantable cardioverter/defibrillator shocks due to defective connections of the defibrillator lead terminals in the device header port. *Europace.* 2007;9:1161–1162.
87. Issa ZF. Inadvertent transposition of defibrillator coil terminal pins causing inappropriate ICD therapies. *J Interv Card Electrophysiol.* 2008;22:71–74.
88. Issa ZF. Noninvasive diagnosis of inadvertent transposition of defibrillator coil terminal pins. *Pacing Clin Electrophysiol.* 2009;32:1060–1062.
89. Chawla P, Hanon S, Lam P, Schweitzer P. An uncommon cause of myopotentials leading to inappropriate ICD therapy. *Pacing Clin Electrophysiol.* 2009; Epub ahead of print.
90. Eckart RE, Hruczkowski TW, Stevenson WG, Epstein LM. Myopotentials leading to ventricular fibrillation detection after advisory defibrillator generator replacement. *Pacing Clin Electrophysiol.* 2006;29:1273–1276.
91. Francisco GM, Sharma S, Dougherty AH, Kantharia BK. Multiple shocks after upgrade of an implantable cardioverter-defibrillator to a cardiac resynchronization therapy-defibrillator device. *Cardiol J.* 2009;16:473–476.
92. Kowalski M, Ellenbogen KA, Wood MA, Friedman PL. Implantable cardiac defibrillator lead failure or myopotential oversensing? An approach to the diagnosis of noise on lead electrograms. *Europace.* 2008;10:914–9147.
93. Swerdlow CD, Brown ML, Lurie K, et al. Discrimination of ventricular tachycardia from supraventricular tachycardia by a downloaded wavelet-transform morphology algorithm: a paradigm for development of implantable cardioverter defibrillator detection algorithms. *J Cardiovasc Electrophysiol.* 2002;13:432–441.
94. Shalaby AA. Cross-talk in a dual-chamber defibrillator presenting as pacemaker alternans. *J Cardiovasc Electrophysiol.* 2003;14:325–328.
95. Kudenchuk PJ, Poole JE, Dolack GL, et al. Prospective evaluation of the effect of biphasic waveform defibrillation on ventricular pacing thresholds. *J Cardiovasc Electrophysiol.* 1997;8:485–495.
96. Kessler DJ, Canby RC, Horton RP, et al. Effect of biphasic endocardial countershock on pacing thresholds in humans. *Am J Cardiol.* 1996;77:527–528.
97. Helguera ME, Pinski SL. Cross-talk inhibition and asystole resulting from postshock high-output pacing: a new form of implantable cardioverter-defibrillator proarrhythmia. *Heart Rhythm.* 2005;2:310–312.
98. Pinski SL, Trohman RG. Permanent pacing via implantable defibrillators. *Pacing Clin Electrophysiol.* 2000;23:1667–1682.
99. Cross-chamber blanking periods in ICDs and CRTDs. Accessed on December 25, 2009. http://www.bostonscientific.com/template data/imports/HTML/CRM/A_Closer_Look/pdfs/ACL_CrossChamber_Blanking_121908.pdf
100. Boveda S, Aubert JT, Albenque JP, Marijon E. Report of a pacing-dependent patient implanted with a dual-chamber ICD: Smart, but not always smart enough. *Heart Rhythm.* 2009;6:1674–1676.
101. Kallinen LM, Hauser RG, Lee KW, et al. Failure of impedance monitoring to prevent adverse clinical events caused by fracture of a recalled high-voltage implantable cardioverter-defibrillator lead. *Heart Rhythm.* 2008;5:775–779.

102. Donaldson DM, Singh JP, Heist EK, et al. Multiple ICD discharges associated with lead fracture without triggering of high impedance alert. *Pacing Clin Electrophysiol.* 2009;32:543–546.
103. Ellenbogen KA, Wood MA, Shepard RK, et al. Detection and management of an implantable cardioverter defibrillator lead failure: incidence and clinical implications. *J Am Coll Cardiol.* 2003;41:73–80.
104. Swerdlow CD, Gunderson BD, Ousdigian KT, et al. Downloadable algorithm to reduce inappropriate shocks caused by fractures of implantable cardioverter-defibrillator leads. *Circulation.* 2008;118:2122–2129.
105. Pickett RA 3rd, Saavedra P, Ali MF, Darbar D, Rottman JN. Implantable cardioverter-defibrillator malfunction due to mechanical failure of the header connection. *J Cardiovasc Electrophysiol.* 2004;15:1095–1099.
106. Connecting leads to Boston Scientific ICDs and CRT-Ds with white seal plugs. Accessed on December 25, 2009, http://www.bostonscientific.com/templatedata/imports/HTML/CRM/A_Closer_Look/pdfs/ACL_Connecting_Leads_White_Seal_Plugs_082108.pdf.
107. Cheung JW, Iwai S, Lerman BB, Mittal S. Shock-induced ventricular oversensing due to seal plug damage: A potential mechanism of inappropriate device therapies in implantable cardioverter-defibrillators. *Heart Rhythm.* 2005;2:1371–1375.
108. Lee BP, Wood MA, Ellenbogen KA. Oversensing in a newly implanted dual-chamber implantable cardioverter-defibrillator: What is the mechanism? *Heart Rhythm.* 2005; 2:782–783.
109. McManus DD, Rosenthal LS, Robotis DA. Inappropriate shock from nonphysiologic noise during implantation of a Boston Scientific COGNIS N119 biventricular implantable cardioverter-defibrillator (CRT-D). *Heart Rhythm.* 2009;6:1066–1068.
110. Preventing and detecting oversensing due to damaged, torn or missing seal plugs. Accessed on December 26, 2009, http://www.bostonscientific.com/templatedata/imports/HTML/CRM/A_Closer_Look/pdfs/ACL_Prevent_Detect_Ovsn.pdf.
111. Arias MA, Puchol A, Castellanos E, Pachón M, Rodríguez-Padial L. Ventricular oversensing after replacement of an implantable cardioverter-defibrillator. *Pacing Clin Electrophysiol.* 2009;32:925–927.
112. Pfitzner P, Trappe HJ. Oversensing in a cardioverter defibrillator system caused by interaction between two endocardial defibrillation leads in the right ventricle. *Pacing Clin Electrophysiol.* 1998;21:764–768.
113. Gardas R, Mlynarski R, Staszak K, et al. Lead interaction: rare cause of oversensing during implantation procedure of implantable cardioverter-defibrillator system. *Pacing Clin Electrophysiol.* 2006;29:1174–1175.
114. Lickfett L, Wolpert C, Jung W, et al. Inappropriate implantable defibrillator discharge caused by a retained pacemaker lead fragment. *J Interv Card Electrophysiol.* 1999;3:163–167.
115. Cooper JM, Sauer WH, Garcia FC, et al. Covering sleeves can shield the high-voltage coils from lead chatter in an integrated bipolar ICD lead. *Europace.* 2007;9:137–142.
116. Pinski SL. Electromagnetic interference and implantable devices. In: Ellenbogen KA, Kay GN, Lau CP, Wilkoff BL, eds. *Clinical cardiac pacing, defibrillation and resynchronization therapy.* 3rd ed. Philadelphia, PA: Saunders Elsevier; 2007:1149–1176.
117. Otten RF, Foreman LD, Groh WJ. Pacemaker/implantable cardioverter-defibrillator problem: right ventricular lead missensing in a biventricular implantable cardioverter-defibrillator. *Heart Rhythm.* 2008;5:158–159.
118. Venkataraman G, Moore H, Karasik P, Singh S, Fletcher R. Biventricular implantable cardioverter defibrillator right ventricle pace-sense ring electrode failure: lead switch fix. *Pacing Clin Electrophysiol.* 2008;31:899–903.
119. Appropriately programming a dual-chamber ICD or multi-chamber CRT-D when atrial information is not needed. Accessed on December 25, 2009. http://www.bostonscientific.com/templatedata/imports/HTML/CRM/A_Closer_Look/pdfs/ACL_ICD_CRTD_Atrial_Not_Needed.pdf

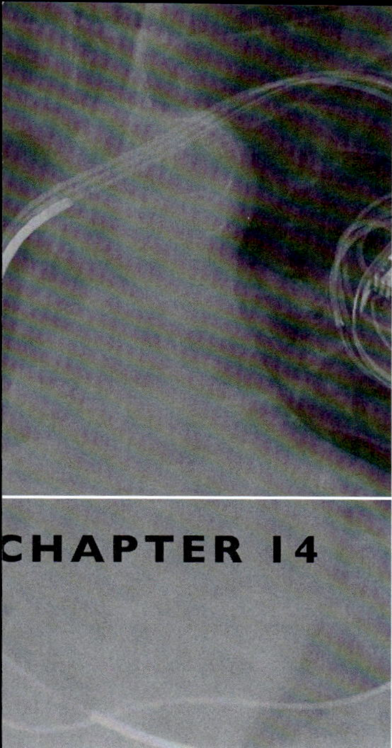

ICD Therapy—ATP

CHAPTER 14

Karin K. M. Chia, Luigi Di Biase, Paolo Pieragnoli, Giuseppe Ricciardi, Laura Perrotta, Robert Canby, Amin Al-Ahmad, Mark S. Wathen, Andrea Natale, and Luigi Padeletti

Introduction

Implantable cardioverter defibrillator (ICD) therapy has been shown to be effective in reducing mortality in both secondary prevention and primary prevention of sudden cardiac death.[1,2] This reduction of mortality by defibrillator shock therapy does, however, come at a cost. Defibrillator shocks can have detrimental effects on the mental and physical well-being of patients leading to a decreased quality of life.[3] ICD shocks may trigger maladaptive psychocognitive responses that can increase the incidence of depression and anxiety.[4,5] In addition, the pain associated with a shock can be significant.[6,7] Rarely, some shocks may also be proarrhythmic.[8–10] Appropriate and inappropriate shocks as compared to no shock at all was associated with a significant increase in subsequent risk of death from all causes in both the Multicenter Automatic Defibrillator Implantation Trial II (MADIT II) and Sudden Cardiac Death in Heart Failure Trial (SCD-HeFT) populations,[11,12] although a causal relationship has not yet been proven. These factors, along with the significant cost of shocks to battery drain and device longevity, would indicate that the reduction of shocks, both appropriate and inappropriate is an important goal.

The current overall shock reduction strategies are antitachycardia pacing (ATP), prolonged time to detection, and the avoidance of inappropriate shocks with reduced oversensing from T wave or electronic noise and improved supraventricular tachycardia discrimination, which is discussed in depth in chapter 16. In this chapter, the evidence for the safety of ATP in general and its mechanisms of action are reviewed along with the success of ATP as a therapy for ventricular tachycardia. The clinical factors that affect the efficacy of ATP are discussed as well as the evidence supporting

Pacemakers and Implantable Cardioverter Defibrillators: An Expert's Manual. © 2010 Amin Al-Ahmad, Kenneth A. Ellenbogen, Andrea Natale, and Paul J. Wang, eds. Cardiotext Publishing, ISBN: 978-0-9790164-6-2.

increased time to detection for shock reduction. Finally the two commonest ATP pacing schemes are reviewed with a brief primer on the programmable ATP variables in modern ICDs.

Safety of ATP

In the past, there have been concerns that complicating the ICD with the therapeutic option of ATP and replacing shock as the first therapy with ATP may increase the failure rate by acceleration of the tachycardia (Fig 14.1) and also increasing delay to successful therapy. If true, this effect should be detected by measuring the rate of sudden death, syncope, or near syncope.

Prior to the Pacing Fast Ventricular Tachycardia Reduces Shock Therapies (PainFREE Rx) trials,[13,14] the data on ATP safety was limited. The data came largely from the Bilitch Registry, a voluntary registry of implanted ICDs and pacemakers. The Bilitch Registry measured the effect on mortality by comparing 1553 shock-only ICDs to 550 ATP-capable ICDs. At 2 years' follow-up, the total mortality in the shock group was 89% but was improved in the ATP group to 94%, $p<0.05$.[15] Although the two groups differed in the ATP capability of their ICDs, improved survival in the ATP-capable ICD group may have been secondary to other factors such as broadly improved cardiovascular and other health care. Nonetheless, at the very least, it did

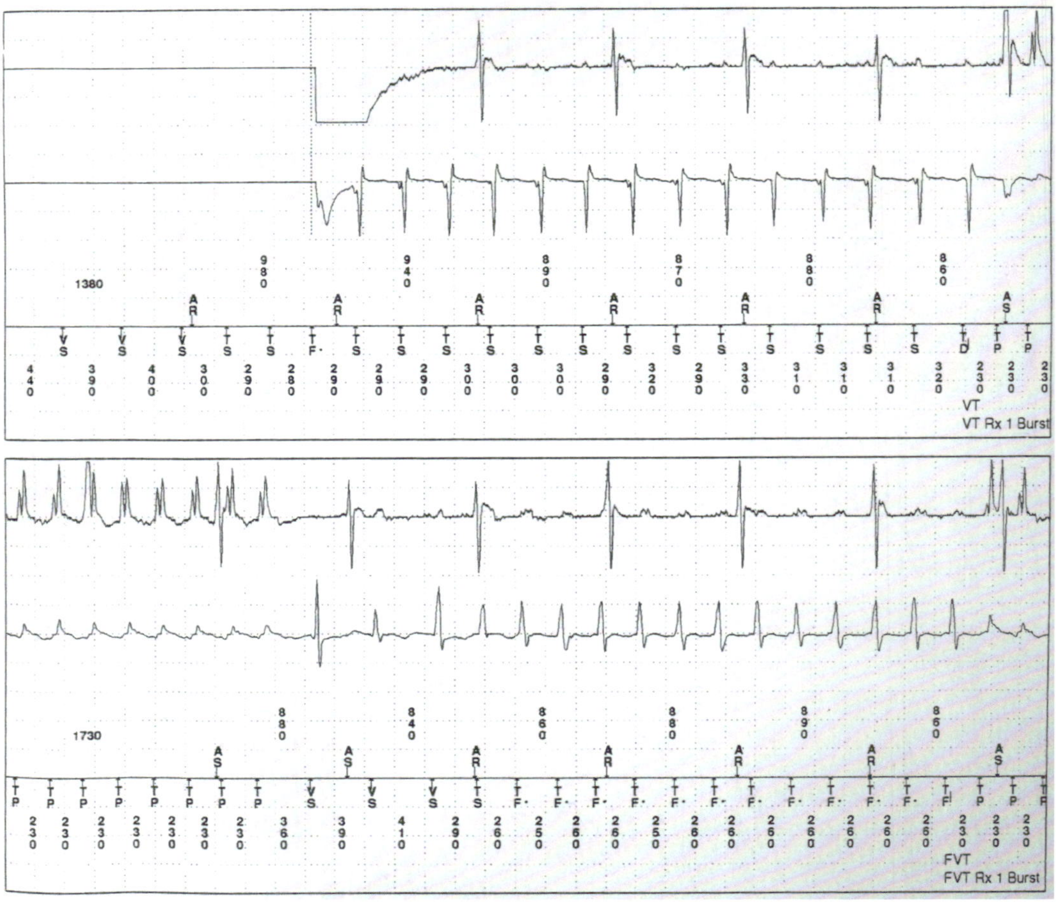

Fig 14.1 Example of burst ATP (annotated by TP on the EGM marker channel) accelerating a VT from a cycle length of 290 to 330 ms to 230 to 260 ms.

not appear that ATP-capable ICDs worsened mortality.

Subsequent nonrandomized studies in the 1990s that assessed the outcomes of ICD patients in ATP therapy trials showed mortality rates in patients with ATP as first therapy to be consistent with prior ICD trials, thus not implicating failed ATP therapy as a contributor to death. The PainFREE Rx II study randomized ICD patients to ATP versus shock. This trial carefully captured and adjudicated all causes of death. There were 2 sudden deaths in each of the shock and ATP arms among the 634 enrolled patients who were followed for a year, again showing that ATP ICDs did not appear to worsen mortality.[14]

In addition, a composite analysis of the Pain FREE Rx, Pain FREE Rx II, and Proven Shock Reduction for Primary Prevention Patients (PREPARE) trials found that in comparison to patients without ventricular tachycardia (VT) or ventricular fibrillation (VF) events, patients with episodes treated successfully with ATP had no reduced survival whereas patients treated with shock had reduced survival (relative risk 1.2, $p<0.001$).[16]

In summary, there is no trial evidence of worsened mortality with ATP. More data will be necessary to fully answer this question.

Mechanism of ATP Efficacy

Most VTs appear to originate within relatively small areas of diseased myocardium and are thought to be largely due to reentry. Although single capture tachycardia termination using critically timed premature extrasystoles falling in the "termination zone" of the tachycardia cycle length can be effective, particularly with slower tachycardias, multiple captures using burst pacing has proven to be more effective.[17–19] Burst pacing from a site not necessarily in the circuit requires distant capture and conduction into the circuit. Essentially, the success of ATP depends on the pacing stimulus penetrating an "excitable gap" in the circuit, and colliding both antidromically with the "head" of the VT wavefront and orthodromically with the VT "tail" at a point of absolute refractoriness, thus extinguishing the tachycardia[20,21] It stands to reason that the faster the reentry circuit, the shorter the time period the critical tissue is available for capture from extraneous pacing. Thus, it has been observed that slower tachycardias are more amenable to pace termination, as supported by evidence from the electrophysiology laboratory.[19,22,23] Not surprisingly there has been an initial reticence to apply ATP to faster VTs and the initial studies to demonstrate clinical efficacy were in slower, presumably hemodynamically tolerated VTs.

ATP Success

Prior studies have demonstrated that ATP was able to successfully treat spontaneous "slow" VTs with success rates of 89% to 94%.[24–28] These studies were limited in that they did not utilize a specific ATP regimen and ATP therapies involving both burst and ramp pacing were evaluated. In addition, the slow VT was variably defined by the investigators from 188 bpm (and even less in some devices) up to 220 bpm. Despite this variation in programmed parameters, ATP seemed to work for slow VT with a low failure rate of 6% to 11%. The rates of VT acceleration by ATP were between 2.0% to 3.7%[29] (Fig 14.2).

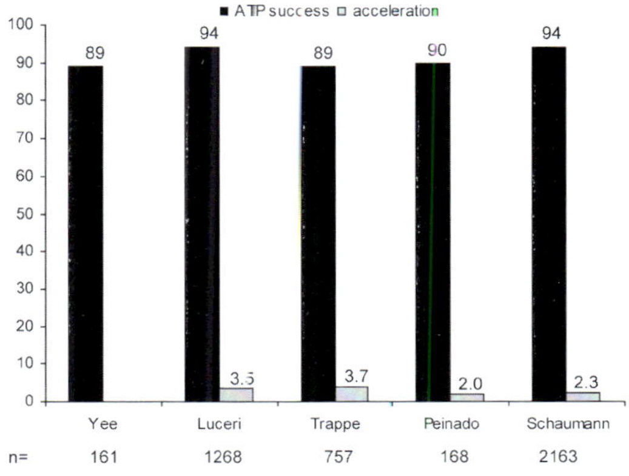

Fig 14.2 Antitachycardia pacing success for "slow" VT < 220 bpm. Abbreviation: n, number "slow" VT episodes. (Modified from Fig 1, Wathen M.[29] Reproduced with permission from Elsevier.)

Supportive evidence of the safety of ATP in fast ventricular tachycardia (FVT) was gained from the German Ventritex MD-Register[30] where the success rate of ATP-induced termination of the episodes was 63.9% for FVT (> 200 bpm). The PainFREE Rx I trial,[13] published in 2001, was a prospective multicenter study that examined the question of whether ATP could reliably and safely terminate FVT in patients with coronary artery disease (CAD). Two hundred twenty patients with indications for ICD therapy were enrolled. They underwent implantation of a Medtronic system capable of delivering ATP for FVT within the VF detection zone. FVT detection and initial therapy programming were standardized across all patients such that FVT zone was defined as 240 to 320 ms (188 to 250 bpm), with detection in FVT zone requiring 12 of the previous 16 RR intervals to have CL = 320 ms and the first therapy in the FVT zone to be 2 ATP sequences (8 pulses at 88% the FVT cycle length minus 10 ms between bursts) with sequences delivered at maximum voltage and pulse duration. During a mean follow-up period of 6.0 ± 3.6 months, 1100 episodes of ventricular arrhythmias occurred of which 624 (57%) were slow VT and 446 episodes (40%) were FVT with only 3% of episodes being VF (Fig 14.3). Eighty-five percent (85%) of the 446 FVT events were successfully treated with the first ATP attempt. There were no episodes where shock therapy was not successful after failed ATP therapy. Analyzing the results on a per-patient basis, 48 (76%) of the 63 patients who had FVT had every episode of FVT successfully treated with ATP, and 90% of patients had at least 1 episode of successful ATP. Only 2% of patients with FVT treated with ATP experienced syncope and only 4% had acceleration of the arrhythmia.

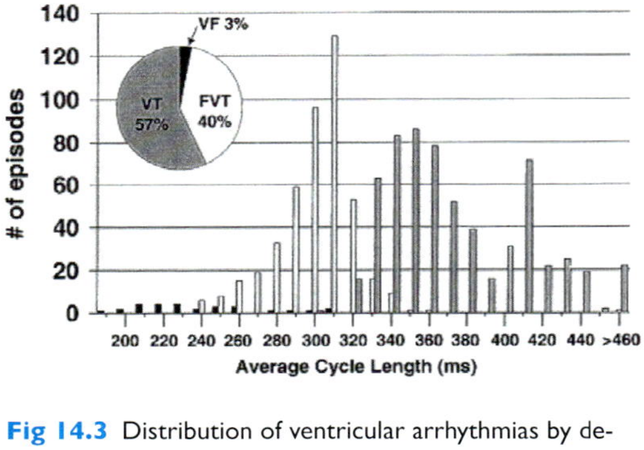

Fig 14.3 Distribution of ventricular arrhythmias by detection zone and median CL during follow-up period of PainFREE Rx I trial. (From Wathen M, et al.[13] Reproduced with permission from Wolters Kluwers Health.)

Some limitations of the study were that it was nonrandomized, studied only CAD patients, and may have deemed ATP to be successful in episodes that may have been nonsustained VT due to a detection interval of only 12 out of 16.

The PainFREE Rx II attempted to resolve some of the limitations that were seen in the PainFREE Rx I trial.[14] This was a prospective randomized, multicenter trial whereby the primary end point was to test whether empiric ATP would be as safe and effective as shocks in a broad ICD population. The inclusion criteria for PainFREE Rx II was broader than in the PainFREE Rx I trial excluding only ICD patients believed unlikely to have substrate for stable monomorphic VT susceptible to ATP (eg, hypertrophic cardiomyopathy, long QT syndrome, or Brugada syndrome). A total of 634 patients were randomized to 2 arms: 313 received standardized empirical ATP therapy while 321 received shock for their initial therapy of spontaneous FVT. Compared to PainFREE Rx I, detection intervals were extended out such that all ICDs were programmed to detect FVT when 18 of 24 intervals were 188 to 250 bpm (320 to 240 ms) and 0 of the last 8 intervals were > 250 bpm (VF rate). In the ATP arm, the first therapy in the FVT zone was a single ATP sequence. Over the 11 ± 3-month follow-up period, 1342 episodes in 159 patients of adjudicated ventricular arrhythmias occurred and were used for analysis. Of these, 32% were FVTs. ATP was effective in 229 of the 284 (72% adjusted, 95% CI 60% to 81%) of FVT episodes (Fig 14.4). When compared to the shock arm, programming ATP as first therapy resulted in a relative shock reduction of 70%. On a per-patient basis, 80% of patients benefited from

ATP. There was no statistically significant difference between the ATP and shock therapy arms in terms of acceleration (2% in ATP arm versus 1% in shock arm), syncope, episode duration (10 seconds for ATP arm versus 9.7 seconds for shock arm), and mortality. In addition, as compared to the shock arm, the ATP arm had statistically significant improvement in quality of life measurements. Hence, PainFREE Rx II provided clear evidence that ATP is highly effective in treating ventricular arrhythmias. More recently, the Comparison of Empiric to Physician-Tailored Programming of Implantable Cardioverter-Defibrillators (EMPIRIC) study,[31] published in 2006, gave further supportive evidence of the safety of ATP in FVT. While not designed specifically to look at ATP safety, patients in the empiric arm had ATP programmed for VTs > 200 bpm and showed no increase in mortality or the rate of syncope when compared to the patients who received physician-tailored therapies.

Factors Influencing the Success of ATP

Determinants of ATP success have been repeatedly evaluated. Although there is conflicting evidence, two factors have more consistently predicted lower ATP success: faster VT rates and reduced left ventricular ejection fraction (LVEF).

VT cycle length: Success rates for ATP treating spontaneous VTs < 200 to 220 bpm are between 89% and 94% in multiple trials.[24,27,28] This is in contrast to published success rates of 63.9 % to 89% for FVT. In addition, the incidence of acceleration of monomorphic VT increases with VT CL.[32,33]

LVEF: In the PainFREE Rx II trial, individuals with an EF < 30% had ATP efficacy of 52% versus EF > 30% having ATP efficacy of 72%, p=0.01.[21]

Site of pacing: Interestingly, with the advent of biventricular pacing, the site of ATP

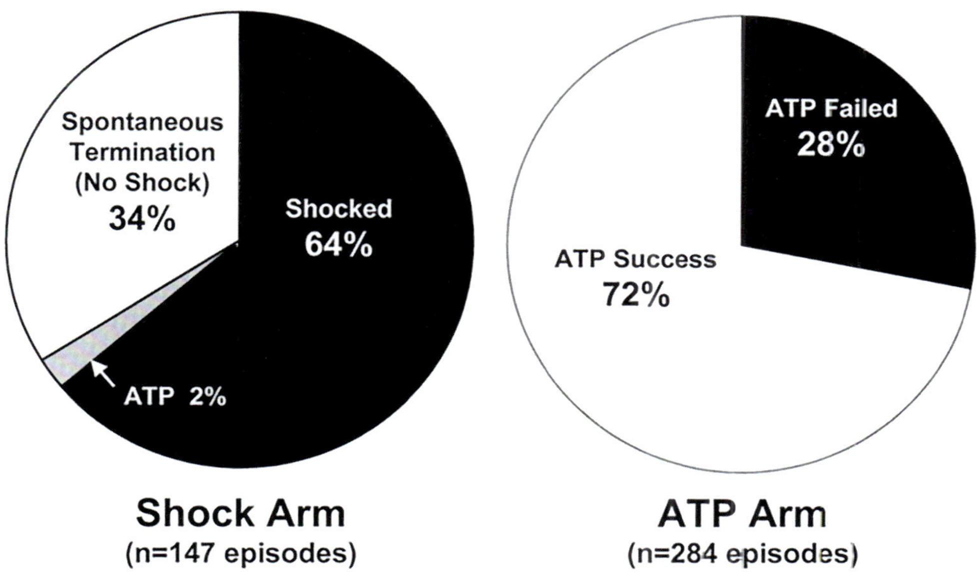

Fig 14.4 Terminating therapy for FVT episodes in each arm of the PainFREE Rx II trial. (From Wathen M et al.[14] Reproduced with permission from Wolters Kluwers Health.)

stimulation has come up as a possible factor influencing ATP success, because the distance and conduction time between the pacing stimulation site and the site of origin of the VT circuit may influence the ability of the pacing stimuli to interact with the circuit. In the InSync ICD OUS (Outside United States) study, biventricular (biV) ATP was 2.4 times more successful than right ventricular (RV) ATP and was associated less with VT acceleration.[34] A study by Yee et al demonstrated that ATP delivered from a left coronary vein lead offers no efficacy advantage over pacing from the right ventricular artery (RVA) in terminating induced VTs in patients undergoing electrophysiology testing.[35] However the applicability of its conclusions to patients with an implanted LV lead with spontaneous VT is unclear. The ADVANCE CRT-D trial, which was a prospective, randomized, multicenter parallel trial comparing RV ATP with biV ATP in terminating VT in patients receiving CRT, demonstrated no significant difference in RV versus biV pacing in their efficacy of terminating VT in all patients. In the subset of patients with ischemic cardiomyopathy, biV ATP was significantly more effective in terminating VT.[36] The current data regarding alternate ATP stimulation sites is insufficient to draw conclusions on.

Increasing Detection Intervals to Reduce Shocks

Ventricular arrhythmias may terminate spontaneously, therefore increasing the intervals for detection of VT/VF would reduce the inappropriate delivery of therapies for nonsustained VT. The safety of such a strategy was seen when comparing outcomes in PainFREE Rx I and PainFREE Rx II. The cohort in PainFREE Rx I[13] had devices programmed such that detection in the FVT zone required 12 of the last 16 beats to fall below the cycle length limit of 320 ms. In comparison, subjects in both arms of the PainFREE Rx II[14] trial had devices programmed such that detection in the FVT zone required that 18 of the last 24 RR intervals had a cycle length of < 320 ms. Extending the number of intervals to detect (NID) between the two studies did not increase the rate of arrhythmic syncopal episodes or sudden cardiac death.

Most recently, the PREPARE study[37] provides additional evidence that increased detection intervals coupled with ATP as strategic ICD programming can safely reduce shocks in patients receiving an ICD for primary prevention. This was a multicenter, prospective, cohort-controlled study that analyzed 700 patients with primary indications for an ICD. They included both biV and non-biV ICDs and patients were followed for 12 months. The control cohort was a historical control group composed of the entire subset of subjects from the MIRACLE ICD and the physician-tailored arm of the EMPIRIC trials. The PREPARE study cohort had tachyarrhythmia detection and therapy settings programmed to only detect fast and sustained tachycardias along with applying ATP as the first therapy for FVTs and employing high-output first shock. The detection interval for FVT and VF were 30 of 40 beats. The primary end point measured was a morbidity index. Strategic programming in the PREPARE study patients resulted in a statistically significant 62% risk reduction in the primary end point compared to the control group. Arrhythmic syncope experienced by the PREPARE study patients was rare, with 12 (1.6%) patients experiencing such, of which 10 were judged to be related to the PREPARE study programming. Unfortunately similar data had not been collected from the historical control cohort for comparison. Nonetheless, PREPARE demonstrated that extension of detection intervals to 30 out of 40 along with the use of fast rate cutoffs and the application of ATP in faster rate zones together with SVT discrimination algorithms can be safely used to reduce the combined morbidity of spontaneous shocks, arrhythmic syncope, and untreated sustained symptomatic VT/VF events. The Avoid Delivering Therapies for Nonsustained Fast Ventricular Tachyarrhythmia in Patients with Implantable Cardioverter/Defibrillator (ADVANCE III) trial is underway to address whether prolonged detection interval for life-threatening VT is able to reduce therapies delivered by an ICD in patients with a Class I–IIa indication for an ICD. This trial is expected to finish in 2011.[38]

Programming Options of ATP Modalities for VT

The two most commonly applied and studied ATP schemes are burst and ramp pacing. Burst pacing is a stimulation pattern whereby a train of pacing pulses is delivered with an equal interstimulus interval. Some manufacturers permit an increased duration of the train with each successive train. Biotronik has a modification of burst pacing whereby an additional programmed extrastimulus is added at the end of the burst pacing drive train (Burst + PES). Ramp pacing is where the train of pacing pulses have an automatically decrementing interstimulus interval (Fig 14.5). There have been conflicting results in studies that have compared the efficacy of burst versus ramp pacing in terminating spontaneous VT. Most recently, this has been addressed by the PITAGORA ICD trial which randomly compared a burst pacing scheme of 8 pulses at 88% coupling interval against a ramp pacing scheme of 8 pulses with a 91% coupling interval ramp in 216 ICD patients followed for a median of 36 months.[39] Burst pacing was significantly more efficacious than ramp pacing in terminating FVT episodes (75.2% versus 54.3%, p=0.015). Older studies have either shown no difference between the two pacing schemes[32,40] or demonstrated ramp pacing to be more successful, though by a small margin only.[28] The difference in risk of acceleration by the two schemes is similarly conflicting. One study has reported increased risk with ramp pacing[41] whereas another has observed no difference in the risk.[42] This lack of consensus amongst studies probably suggests the likelihood that there is no important clinical difference between the various pacing schemes that can be programmed in modern ICDs.

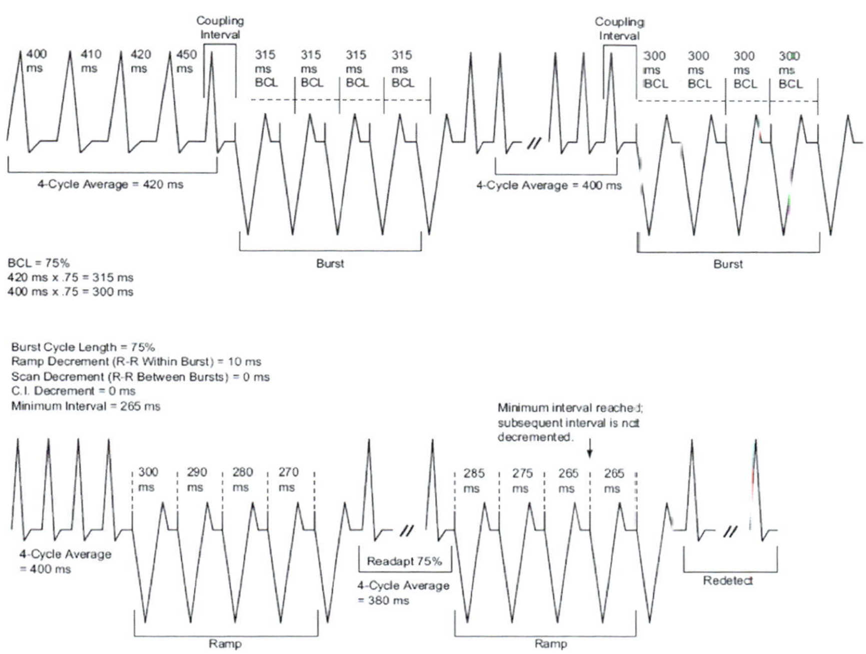

Fig 14.5 Top: Schematic representation of a burst pacing scheme with equal intervals between each stimulus. **Bottom**: Schematic representation of a ramp pacing scheme with the interstimulus interval decreasing by 10 ms (ramp decrement) and no decrement in the coupling interval between each sequence of pacing. Note the last 2 paced stimuli are at the same interval of 265 ms, even though it is a ramp pacing scheme, due to the minimum interval being reached. (Reproduced with permission of Boston Scientific Corporation.)

Table 14.1 Summary of Differences in ATP Features in Current ICD Models.

	St. Jude Medical	Biotronik	ELA/Sorin	Medtronic	Boston Scientific
ATP pulse amplitude	Fixed at 7.5 V	Fixed at 7.5 V	Fixed at 7.0 V	Programmable independent of brady therapies but common to all ATP schemes and postshock pacing. 1–8 V	Programmable independent of brady therapies but common to all ATP schemes and postshock pacing. 0.1–7.5 V
ATP pulse width	1.0, 1.5 ms	Fixed at 1.5 ms	Fixed at 1.5 ms	Programmable independent of brady therapies but common to all ATP schemes and postshock pacing. 0.1–1.5 ms	Programmable independent of brady therapies but common to all ATP schemes and postshock pacing 0.2–2.0 ms
Coupling interval to last sensed ventricular event	Same as the BCL	Programmable independent to BCL, fixed/adaptive	Same as the BCL	Adaptive	Programmable independent to BCL, fixed/adaptive
Ability to add stimuli per burst	Available (up to 1 additional pulse per sequence)	Available (up to 1 additional pulse per sequence)	Available (by programmable number of pulses per sequence)	Unavailable in burst pacing. Automatically adds an additional pulse per ramp pacing sequence.	Available (by programmable number of pulses per sequence)
BCL	Fixed/adaptive	Fixed/adaptive	Fixed/adaptive	Adaptive	Fixed/adaptive
Pacing schemes	Ramp (+/– scan) Burst (+/– scan)	Ramp (+/– scan) Burst (+/– scan) Burst (+/– scan)+PES	Ramp (+/– scan) Burst (+/– scan)	Ramp (+/– scan) Burst (+/– scan)	Ramp (+/– scan) Burst (+/– scan
Pacing site	RV only	RV/biV	RV/LV/biV	RV/LV/biV	RV
ATP associated with charging for fast VTs	None	ATP One Shot: ATP before charging that commences after ATP delivery without redetection with reconfirmation prior to charge delivery	None	ATP During/Before Charging	Quick Convert
ATP time out	VT therapy timeout	Available	Available	Available	Available
Progression of therapy	Default	Requires programming on "Progressive Course of Therapies"	Default	Requires programming on "Progressive Episode Therapies"	Default

Although each defibrillator manufacturer has some unique proprietary features to their devices, many programmable variables in relation to antitachycardia pacing are common to most. We review these programmable variables here and highlight some of the differences between and features unique to certain device manufacturers in their most current defibrillators (see Table 14.1).

Number of sequences/bursts: One can determine the number of sequences of ATP that can be delivered to treat the tachycardia if it remains within the same rate zone. Though this can be programmed up to 15, it is more typically set at 3 to 4 sequences.

Number of stimuli/pulses per sequence: This is also programmable and is seldom set at more than 10 because of concerns with reinduction of the tachycardia. However, it may be necessary at times to increase the number of stimuli in order to penetrate the VT circuit. All sequences have the same number of pulses in Medtronic devices programmed to burst ATP. Medtronic devices programmed to ramp ATP will have an additional pacing pulse per sequence of ATP. St. Jude Medical, Boston Scientific, Biotronik, and ELA/Sorin devices can have an increment in the number of stimuli in successive sequences programmed (burst and ramp).

Burst cycle length (BCL): The pacing interval between pulses within a sequence of ATP. This may be fixed as an interval in ms or adaptive, whereby the cycle length is a percentage of the average tachycardia cycle length.

Coupling interval or R-S1: This is the interval between the last sensed event and the first pulse in the ATP sequence. In Boston Scientific and Biotronik devices, the interval between the sensed event and the first pulse in the sequence can be separately programmable to the BCL as a fixed or adaptive interval with subsequent pulses determined by the previously discussed BCL. A decrement in this interval is determined by the scan decrement in Biotronik devices, whereby the interval between the first and second pulse is equal to the R-S1 interval in all pacing schemes. In contrast, in Boston Scientific devices, the coupling interval can be decremented between sequences independently of the interval between the first and second pulse which itself is determined by the programmed scan decrement. In Medtronic, St. Jude Medical, and ELA/Sorin devices, this R-S1 interval is determined by the BCL.

Scan: Scanning controls the BCL between sequences or bursts of ATP and the decrement in the BCL is determined by the programmed scan step or scan decrement which is a fixed duration and often nominally programmed at 10 ms. In contrast to St. Jude Medical, Boston Scientific, Biotronik, and ELA/Sorin devices, the same feature in Medtronic devices is only available in burst pacing schemes and is referred to as the interval decrement within burst therapy.

Ramp: If programmed On, this feature decreases the interval between successive pulses/stimuli within a sequence by the programmed ramp step. The ramp step is referred to as the interval decrement within ramp therapy in Medtronic devices, the S1 decrement in Biotronik ICDs, and the ramp decrement in Boston Scientific and ELA/Sorin ICDs. In addition, each sequence may add one pacing pulse in Medtronic devices.

Ramp+: This ATP therapy scheme is available in Medtronic devices only. It allows for the interval of the first pulse, the second pulse, and the subsequent pulses to be independently programmed as a percentage of the tachycardia cycle length. This creates a pacing scheme that is a hybrid of ramp pacing for the initial 3 pulses, then burst pacing for the subsequent pulses. In addition, each sequence may add one pacing pulse (Fig 14.6).

Minimum BCL/antitachycardia pacing minimum interval: This is the minimum pacing interval for all ATP therapies and is nominally set at 200 ms for most devices.

ATP pulse amplitude and pulse width: These are fully programmable in Medtronic and Boston Scientific devices but is fixed at maximum output for St. Jude Medical, Biotronik, and ELA/Sorin devices.

ATP timeout: This is a programmable duration of time during which a patient may receive ATP therapies. When this time has expired,

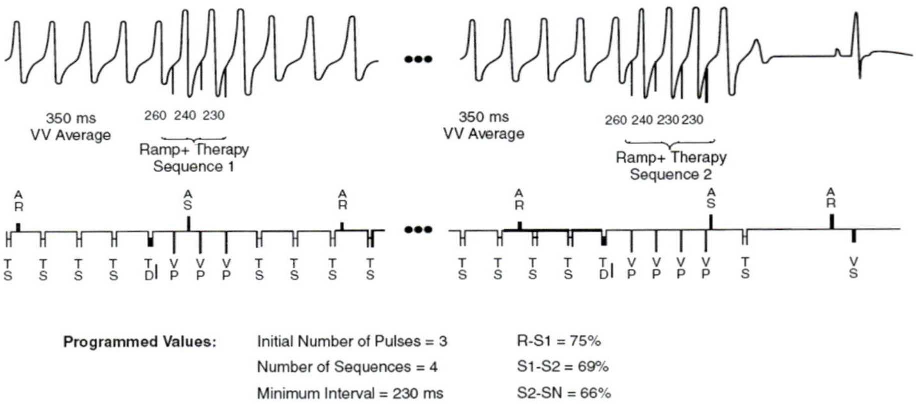

Fig 14.6 Schematic representation of ramp+ pacing scheme. The coupling interval of the first pacing pulse to the sensed ventricular beat, the interval between S1 and S2, and the interval of subsequent beats in the sequence are all independently programmable as a percentage of the BCL, that must still fulfill the criteria of being greater than the minimum interval. (Reproduced with permission of Medtronic, Inc.)

the device will cease delivering ATP for that episode and progress to the first programmed shock therapy for that rate zone. This feature is present in Biotronik, Boston Scientific, and ELA/Sorin devices. A similar feature in St. Jude Medical devices is VT Therapy Timeout, although this limits the duration that therapies (both ATP and shock therapies) programmed for the VT zones are delivered, rather than limiting ATP alone.

Autoswitch of ATP schemes: In case multiple and complex ATP schemes are programmed to increase the success rate of ATP before delivering shocks, a function in ELA/Sorin devices has been implemented to attempt to further improve ATP efficacy and to reduce the time-to-terminate an arrhythmia. The basic principle is that the most effective ATP scheme (within a certain detection zone) is applied in priority at every new VT occurrence within the same detection zone (basing upon "repeatability" of monomorphic VTs). If a first VT (VT1) occurs within the VT zone, and only the second ATP scheme (ATP2) is effective in terminating the VT1, when a second VT (VT2) occurs, the priority is given to the ATP2 scheme. After many VT episodes, ATP2 might be ineffective (maybe another form of VT occurs with similar rate): in this case, the system goes back to the previous priority scheme, to respect the empiric approach given by the original programming (see Fig 14.7). In addition, Medtronic devices have an algorithm that disables ATP when four consecutive episodes are unsuccessful with the programmed block of ATP, this is called "Smart mode." For example, if ATP is programmed to Scan followed by Ramp, the device will disable the Scan ATP is it fails four times. It will not disable the next therapy (Ramp in this case). Of note, Smart mode is programmable for all types of ATP in Medtronic devices.

Fast VT Therapy: The optimal programming of ATP would be to minimize shocks delivered via the treating of FVT with ATP instead. This

Fig 14.7 The principles of ATP Autoswitch (Paradym ICDs). (Reproduced with permission of ELA/Sorin CRM.)

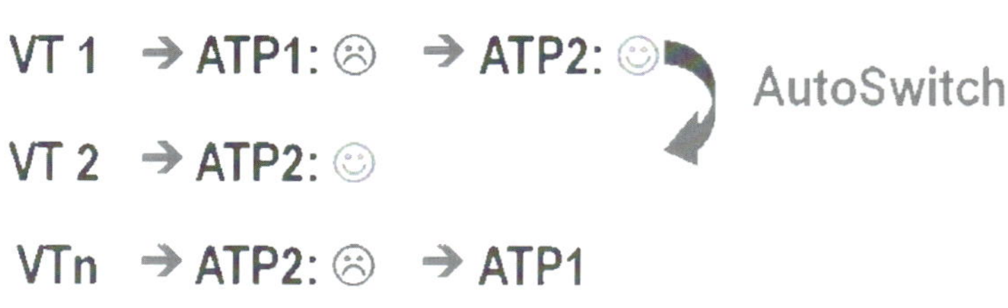

is determined by the programming of the rate zones such that different therapies can be delivered for slower VTs, faster VTs, and VF. In current Medtronic devices, this is achieved by programming a FVT via VF zone whereby it utilizes the detection interval of the VF zone and results in VV intervals falling between the FVT interval and the VF interval being marked as FVT events and being treated by the programmed FVT therapies of ATP sequences followed by shocks. If, however, at least 1 of the last 8 intervals falls in the VF interval, the episode is classified as VF and treated as such with shock as first and subsequent therapy. With ELA/Sorin group devices, a similar analysis of the VT stability occurs. After the device first analyzes the mean ventricular rate, an option is available to analyze the stability of the Fast VT: if it is a stable rhythm, ATPs are delivered (because a monomorphic stable VT is suspected), whereas a shock is delivered if the Fast VT is unstable (eg, polymorphic VT VF onset) or the V rate exceeds the upper limit of the Fast VT zone (it is a true VF) (Fig 14.8). ELA/Sorin devices also allow for separately programmed therapies for FVT and VF episodes though, utilizing the same detection criteria. A similar effect is achieved in Biotronik, Boston Scientific, and St. Jude Medical devices where more than one VT zone can be programmed, allowing for a FVT zone to be programmed separately to a slower VT and VF zone. In addition Boston Scientific's most current devices have a Quick Convert ATP feature, which if programmed

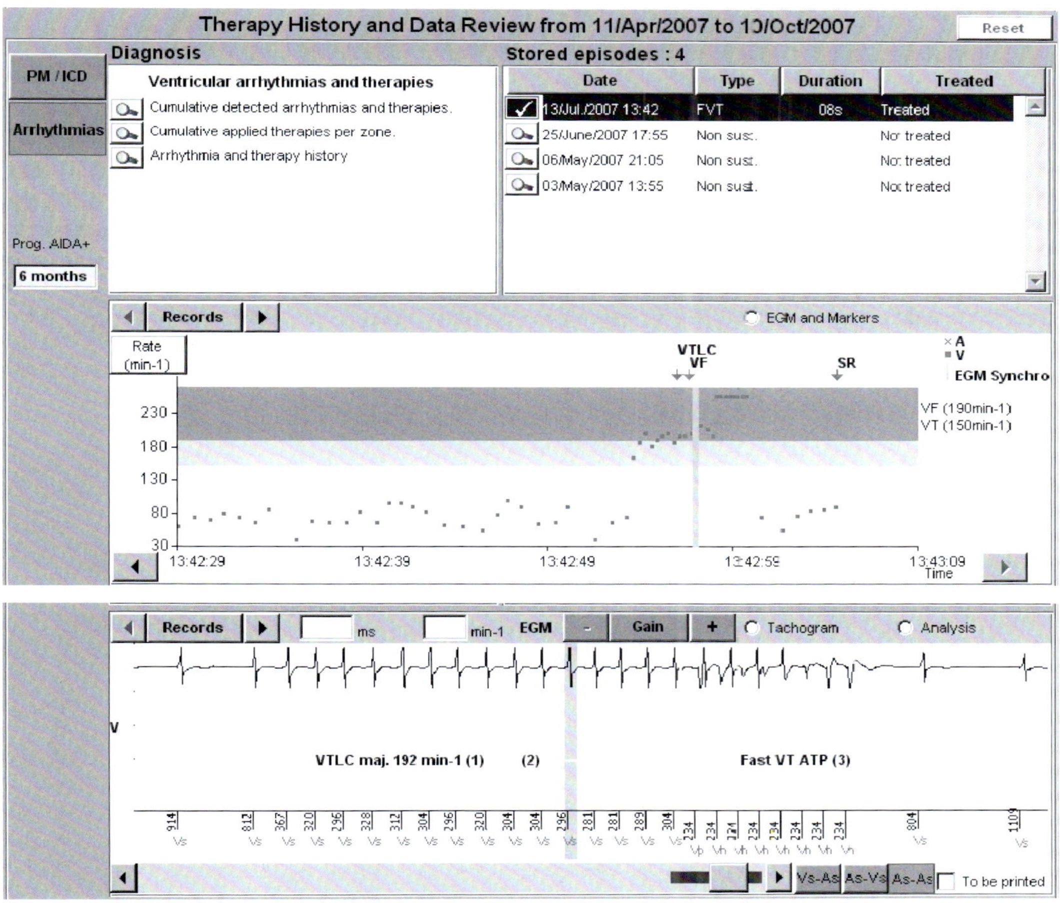

Fig 14.8 The rhythm falls into the VF zone and fulfills the rate criterion to be classified as a Fast VT (FVT). Furthermore, it is stable, and it is then primarily—and successfully—treated with ATP instead of shock.

On, delivers 1 burst of ATP for an episode in the VF zone, provided the rate is < 250 bpm, with no redetection before charging, followed by reconfirmation before proceeding to the shock sequence if required. This allows an attempt at ATP while minimizing the delay to begin charging and is a feature called ATP One Shot in Biotronik devices. The ATP During Charging feature in current Medtronic devices achieves a similar effect with no delay in the shock therapy if needed. However, these features are as efficacious as programming a FVT via VF zone (available in Medtronic and ELA/Sorin only) but comes at the costs of depleting the battery by charging the capacitors unnecessarily if ATP is successful. If one still chooses to program ATP During Charging, the Charge-Saver feature should be programmed On to conserve battery life. This allows the device to switch from ATP During Charging to ATP before charging (where charging only commences after reconfirmation of VF after delivery of one sequence of ATP) if ATP has successfully terminated VT on a programmable number of previous attempts.

Progression of therapies: St. Jude Medical, ELA/Sorin, and Boston Scientific devices default to delivering more aggressive therapies even if the arrhythmia were to be redetected in a slower rate zone. For example, if a patient has received a shock as a second therapy and then slows to a slower VT zone, ATP would not be delivered even if that is the first therapy for the new redetected slower zone. In contrast, in Medtronic and Biotronik devices, the default setting of the ICD is to deliver the zone-specific therapy that the arrhythmia is redetected in, even if this is a less aggressive therapy unless Progressive Episode Therapies and Progressive Course of Therapies are programmed On, respectively.

Conclusion

ATP when appropriately programmed can significantly reduce both ICD shock as well as any reduced quality of life that results from shock therapy. Reduction in shocks has an important role in terms of patient acceptance and potentially the reduction of any deleterious effect of shock therapy. The routine use of ATP for the treatment of VT, including fast VT should be considered in all patients with implantable cardioverter defibrillators. Although there are many ways to program ATP, it is important that the clinician become familiar with the different algorithms and aspects of programming. In addition, recent studies have been important in elucidating the both the safety of ATP as well as the safety of prolonging the NID to reduce the overtreatment of nonsustained VT. Although ATP may occasionally fail to terminate VT or accelerate VT into VF, consideration of a change in the ATP programming may be more useful than eliminating ATP altogether in most patients.

Acknowledgments

The authors would like to thanks all the following engineers for their excellent contribution for the realization of this work: Danilo Contardi (Sorin Group), Lorenzo Zanchetta (Biotronik), Sergio Valsecchi (Medtronic), Paolo Silvestri (St. Jude Medical), Cristina Dondina (Boston Scientific).

References

1. Moss AJ, et al. Improved survival with an implanted defibrillator in patients with coronary disease at high risk for ventricular arrhythmia. *N Engl J Med.* 1996;335(26):1933–1940.
2. The Antiarrhythmics versus Implantable Defibrillators Investigators. A comparison of antiarrhythmic-drug therapy with implantable defibrillators in patients resuscitated from near-fatal ventricular arrhythmias. *N Engl J Med.* 1997;337(22);1576–1584.
3. Passman R, et al. Implantable cardioverter defibrillators and quality of life: results from the Defibrillators in Nonischemic Cardiomyopathy Treatment Evaluation Study. *Arch Intern Med.* 2007;167(20):2226–2232.

4. Mark DB, et al. Quality of life with defibrillator therapy or amiodarone in heart failure. *N Engl J Med.* 2008;359(10):999-1008.
5. Sears S, Matchett M, Conti J. Effective management of ICD patient psychosocial issues and patient critical events. *J Cardiovasc Electrophysiol.* 2009;20(11):1297–1304.
6. Dunbar SB, Warner CD, Purcell JA. Internal cardioverter defibrillator device discharge: experiences of patients and family members. *Heart Lung.* 1993;22(6):8.
7. Ahmad M, Bloomstein L, Roelke M, Bernstein AD, Parsonnet V. Patients' attitudes toward implanted defibrillator shocks. *PACE.* 2000;23(6):3.
8. Germano JJ, et al. Frequency and causes of implantable cardioverter-defibrillator therapies: Is device therapy proarrhythmic? *Am J Cardiol.* 2006;97(8):1255–1261.
9. Pires LA, Hull ML, Nino CL, May LM, Ganji JR. Sudden death in recipients of transvenous implantable cardioverter defibrillator systems: terminal events, predictors, and potential mechanisms. *J Cardiovasc Electrophysiol.* 1999;108.
10. Mitchell LB, Penada EA, Titus JL, Bartosch PM, Benditt DG. Sudden death in patients with implantable cardioverter defibrillators: the importance of post-shock electromechanical dissociation. *J Am Coll Cardiol.* 2002;39:6.
11. Daubert JP, et al. Inappropriate implantable cardioverter-defibrillator shocks in MADIT II: frequency, mechanisms, predictors, and survival impact. *J Am Coll Cardiol.* 2008;51(14):1357–1365.
12. Poole JE, et al. Prognostic importance of defibrillator shocks in patients with heart failure. *N Engl J Med.* 2008;359(10):1009–1017.
13. Wathen MS, et al. Shock reduction using antitachycardia pacing for spontaneous rapid ventricular tachycardia in patients with coronary artery disease. *Circulation.* 2001;104(7):796–801.
14. Wathen MS, et al. Prospective randomized multicenter trial of empirical antitachycardia pacing versus shocks for spontaneous rapid ventricular tachycardia in patients with implantable cardioverter-defibrillators: Pacing Fast Ventricular Tachycardia Reduces Shock Therapies (PainFREE Rx II) trial results. *Circulation.* 2004; 110(17):2591–2596.
15. Gross JR, Sackstein RD, Song SL, et al. The anti-tachycardia pacing ICD: impact on patient selection and outcome. *PACE.* 1993;16(1(Pt 2)):5.
16. Sweeney MO, Wathen MS, Sherfesee L, et al. Differences in effects of electrical therapy type for ventricular arrhythmias on mortality in ICD patients. *Heart Rhythm.* 2009;7 (3)353–360.
17. Fisher JD, Mehra R, Furman S. Termination of ventricular tachycardia with bursts of rapid ventricular pacing. *Am J Cardiol.* 1978;41(1):9.
18. Fisher JD, et al. Role of implantable pacemakers in control of recurrent ventricular tachycardia. *Am J Cardiol.* 1982;49(1): 194–206.
19. Roy D, Waxman HL, Buxton AE, et al. Termination of ventricular tachycardia: role of tachycardia cycle length. *Am J Cardiol.* 1982;50(6):5.
20. Callans DJ, Hook BG, Josephson ME. Comparison of resetting and entrainment of uniform sustained ventricular tachycardia. Further insights into the characteristics of the excitable gap. *Circulation* 1993;87(4):1229–1238.
21. Sweeney MO, Antitachycardia pacing for ven tricular tachycardia using implantable cardioverter defibrillators. *PACE.* 2004;27(9): 1292–1305.
22. Fisher JD, Kim SG, Waspe LE, Matos JA. Mechanisms for the success and failure of pacing for termination of ventricular tachycardia: clinical and hypothetical considerations. *PACE.* 1983;6(5 pt 2):12.
23. Naccarelli GV, Zipes DP, Rahilly GT, Heger JJ, Prystowsky EN. Influence of tachycardia cycle length and antiarrhythmic drugs on pacing termination and acceleration of ventricular tachycardia. *Am Heart J.* 1983;105(1):5.
24. Luceri RM, Salem, MH, David IB, et al. Changing trends in therapy delivery with a third generation noncommitted implantable defibrillator: results of a large single center clinical trial. *PACE.* 1993;16(1 pt 2):6.
25. Leitch JW, Gillis AM, Wyse DG, et al. Reduction in defibrillator shocks with an implantable device combining antitachycardia pacing and shock therapy. *J Am Coll Cardiol.* 1991;18(1):7.
26. Yee R, Klein, GJ, Guiraudon, GM, et al. Initial clinical experience with the pacemaker-cardioverter-defibrillator. *Can J Cardiol.* 1990;6(4):10.

27. Trappe HJ, Klein H, Fieguth HG, et al. Clinical efficacy and safety of the new cardioverter defibrillator systems. *PACE.* 1993;16(1 pt 2):6.
28. Schaumann A, et al. Empirical versus tested antitachycardia pacing in implantable cardioverter defibrillators : aprospective study including 200 patients. *Circulation.* 1998;97(1):66–74.
29. Wathen M. Implantable cardioverter defibrillator shock reduction using new antitachycardia pacing therapies. *Am Heart J.* 2007;153(4, Suppl 1):44–52.
30. Grosse-Meininghaus D, Siebels J, Wolpert CH, et al, for the German Ventritex MD-Investigators. Efficacy of antitachycardia pacing confirmed by stored electrograms. A retrospective analysis of 613 stored electrograms in implantable defibrillators. *Z Kardiol.* 2002;91(5):8.
31. Wilkoff BL, et al. A comparison of empiric to physician-tailored programming of implantable cardioverter-defibrillators: results from the prospective randomized multicenter EMPIRIC trial. *J Am Coll Cardiol.* 2006;48(2):330–339.
32. Gillis AM, et al. A prospective randomized comparison of autodecremental pacing to burst pacing in device therapy for chronic ventricular tachycardia secondary to coronary artery disease. *Am J Cardiol.* 1993;72(15):1146–1151.
33. Fiek M, Hoffmann E, Dorwarth U, et al. Long-term efficacy of antitachycardia pacing for treatment of ventricular tachycardia in patients with implantable cardioverter/defibrillator. *Z Kardiol.* 1999;88(10):8.
34. Krater L, Lamp B, Heintze J, et al. Influence of antitachy pacing location on the efficacy of ventricular tachycardia termination. *J Am Coll Cardiol.* 2002;39:124A.
35. Yee R, Birgersdotter-Green U, Belk P, et al. The relationship between pacing site and induction or termination of sustained monomorphic ventricular tachycardia by antitachycardia pacing. *PACE.* 2009 Nov 18. [Epub ahead of print].
36. Gasparini M, et al., Abstract 5893: Biventricular versus right ventricular delivered anti-tachycardia pacing for the termination of ventricular tachyarrhythmias in heart failure patients receiving a biventricular ICD: results from the ADVANCE CRT-D trial. *Circulation.* 2008;118(18):S1024.
37. Wilkoff BL, et al. Strategic programming of detection and therapy parameters in implantable cardioverter-defibrillators reduces shocks in primary prevention patients: results from the PREPARE (Primary Prevention Parameters Evaluation) study. *J Am Coll Cardiol.* 2008;52(7):541–550.
38. Schwab JO, Gasparini M, Lunati M, et al. Avoid delivering therapies for nonsustained fast ventricular tachyarrhythmia in patients with implantable cardioverter/defibrillator: the ADVANCE III trial. *J Cardiovasc Electrophysiol.* 2009;20(6):663–666.
39. Gulizia MM, et al. A randomized study to compare ramp versus burst antitachycardia pacing therapies to treat fast ventricular tachyarrhythmias in patients with implantable cardioverter defibrillators: the PITAGORA ICD trial. *Circ Arrhythm Electrophysiol.* 2009;2(2):146–153.
40. Newman D, Dorian P, Hardy J. Randomized controlled comparison of antitachycardia pacing algorithms for termination of ventricular tachycardia. *J Am Coll Cardiol.* 1993;21:6.
41. Peters RW, Zhang X, Gold MR. Clinical predictors and efficacy of antitachycardia pacing in patients with implantable cardioverter defibrillators: the importance of the patient's sex. *PACE.* 2001;24(1):5.
42. Nasir N, et al. Spontaneous ventricular tachycardia treated by antitachycardia pacing. *Am J Cardiol.* 1997;79(6):820–822.

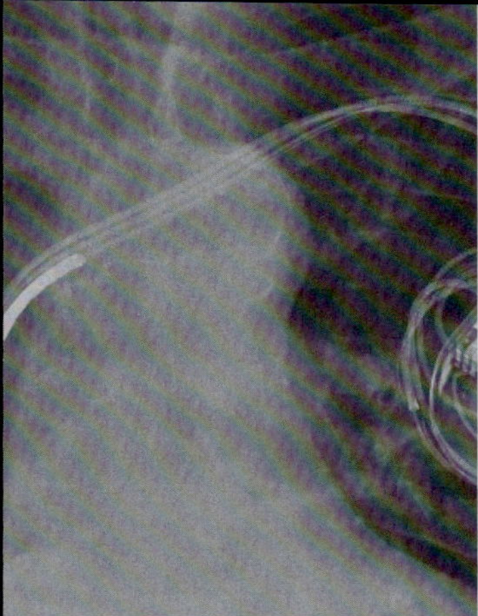

ICD Therapy—Shock

CHAPTER 15

T. Jared Bunch, Jeffrey S. Osborn, and John D. Day

Introduction

Sudden cardiac death (SCD) from ventricular fibrillation (VF) remains a major cause of mortality in the western world. The majority of VF cardiac arrests occur outside of the hospital. Implantation of an ICD is strongly supported by evidence from many randomized trials for the primary (Fig 15.1) and secondary prevention of sudden death.[1–4] In these high-risk patients, coronary artery disease is the most common cause of left ventricular dysfunction and heart failure in industrialized countries.

VF results when an electrical wavebreak induces reentry and results in propagated new wavebreaks. Tissue heterogeneity in patients with underlying cardiomyopathy results in a predisposition to wavebreak, reentry, and ultimately VF.[5] These wandering wavelets of VF are generally self-sustaining once initiated. There have been significant advances in the technology required for defibrillation of VF/tachycardia. However, less is known about the basic underlying mechanisms of defibrillation. Contemporary theories exist that account for how an electric shock terminates VF. These theories

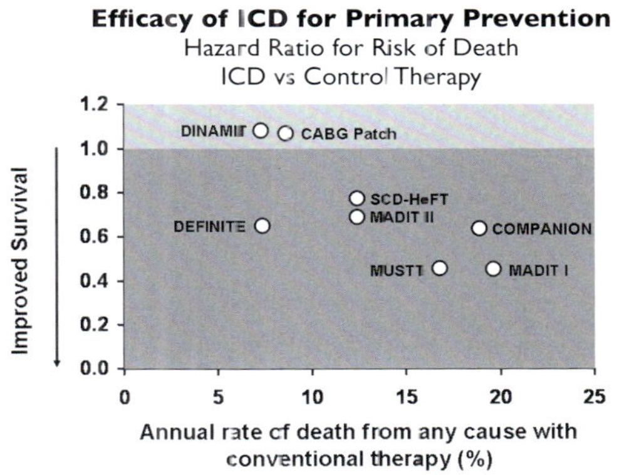

Fig 15.1 Illustrated are hazard ratios for the risk of death after the implantation of an ICD compared with control or conventional therapy in eight primary-prevention trials. All but two trials showed a significant survival benefit with an ICD. (Figure adapted from Sanders et al.[31])

Pacemakers and Implantable Cardioverter Defibrillators: An Expert's Manual. © 2010 Amin Al-Ahmad, Kenneth A. Ellenbogen, Andrea Natale, and Paul J. Wang, eds. Cardiotext Publishing, ISBN: 978-0-9790164-6-2.

are broadly defined as: critical mass, upper limit of vulnerability, progressive depolarization, and virtual electrode depolarization.[6] The theories underscore the two most important components of an ICD shock. First, the shock must successfully terminate the arrhythmias. Second, the ICD shock must not restart the arrhythmia in the process.

Critical Mass

The "critical mass theory," reflects the premise that shocks need to only eliminate fibrillatory wavelets in a critical amount of myocardium to terminate VF. In support of this concept were canine studies in which an injection of potassium chloride was used to depolarize defined regions of the myocardium. In these studies injections into the right coronary artery or the left circumflex artery failed to terminate VF as often as injections made simultaneously into both the left circumflex and the left anterior descending arteries. In a second part of the study, electrical shocks of equal magnitude terminated VF most frequently when the electrodes were positioned at the right ventricular apex and the posterior left ventricle in comparison to two right ventricular electrodes. These observations supported the concept that if a critical mass of myocardium was rendered unavailable for VF either by potassium chloride injection or by high-voltage shocks, the remaining excitable tissue was insufficient to support the wandering wavelets and thereby terminated the arrhythmia.[7]

Upper Limit of Vulnerability

Investigation into unsuccessful shocks led to the upper limit of vulnerability (ULV) theory (Fig 15.2). In these investigations, after the initial shock an isoelectric interval was seen before resumption of VF. In some cases there was a relatively long pause that suggested the VF terminated with the first shock and then regenerated again from the shock.[8] This concept was supported by review on postshock conduction patterns that were distinct from the preshock patterns supportive of the concept that failed shocks are unsuccessful because they gave rise to a new focus of fibrillation rather than failing to terminate the initial rhythm.[9] VF frequently reinitiated in the regions of lowest shock intensity, suggesting that these low-intensity regions were particularly vulnerable. Figure 15.3 shows a failed defibrillation attempt at low power with conversion of coarse VF to fine VF immediately after the shock.

Further investigation into shock intensity demonstrated that shocks with potential gradients less than a minimum critical value or "upper limit of vulnerability," defined as 6 V/cm for monophasic shocks or 4 V/cm for biphasic shocks, could induce fibrillation when applied to vulnerable myocardium. Under this concept low-energy shocks create regions of functional block in vulnerable myocardium that can serve as critical points of reentry and ultimately recurrent fibrillation (Fig 15.2).[10]

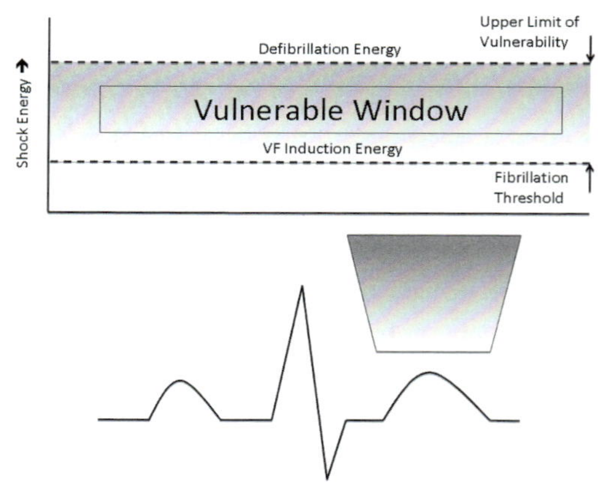

Fig 15.2 The period of vulnerability during sinus rhythm is illustrated. In this vulnerable period the ventricles are susceptible to VF when a shock is delivered in the vulnerable window. However, to induce VF the shock has to be above the fibrillation threshold or below the upper limit of vulnerability. Shocks that fall outside of this range will not induce VF.

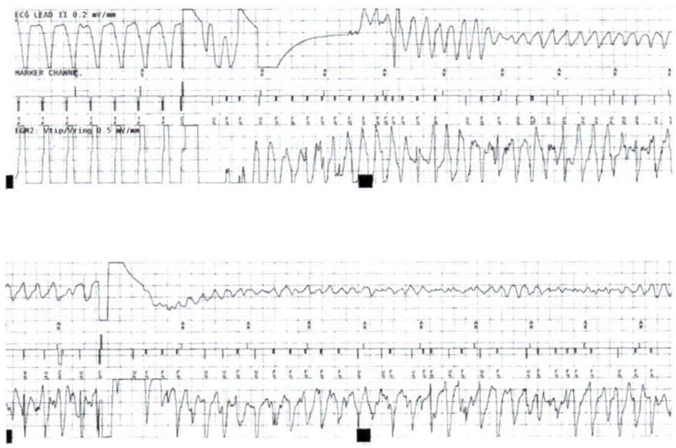

Fig 15.3 Intracardiac electrograms are shown during defibrillation testing shortly after an ICD was implanted. VF was induced with a shock during the vulnerable window on the T wave. VF is initially coarse in nature. VF is rapidly detected, but the initial shock fails to terminate VF. Of interest is that VF immediately changes after the shock to a fine pattern.

In sinus rhythm, low-energy shocks delivered during the T wave induce VF whereas higher energy shocks that are above the ULV do not. During defibrillator testing, low-energy shocks are intentionally delivered in the vulnerable zone to induce fibrillation (Fig 15.2). The observation that the vulnerable zone exists and that the ULV has been correlated with the defibrillation threshold (DFT) support this hypothesis as a mechanism of defibrillation.[11] The use of the ULV in an inductionless strategy at ICD implant remains a viable approach to assess long-term risk as reported in the ASSURE study (Arrhythmia Single Shock Defibrillation Threshold Testing Versus Upper Limit of Vulnerability: Risk Reduction Evaluation With Implantable Cardioverter Defibrillator Implantations).[12]

Progressive Depolarization

On the heels of the two prior theories, the progressive depolarization theory or refractory period extension theory incorporates some elements of both the critical mass and ULV theories. Initial studies demonstrated that shocks of sufficient strength were able to bring out active responses from what was felt to be refractory myocardium.[13] This observation showed that the action potential duration could be prolonged if a sufficiently strong shock is applied.[14] The degree of prolongation in depolarization time is a function of both the shock intensity and timing.[15] By doing such, the high-energy shock that defibrillates extends the overall ventricular refractoriness which limits the excitable tissue available for fibrillation (Fig 15.4). Just as discussed in the critical mass theory, this will limit the amount of tissue vulnerable to reinitiate fibrillation. In contrast, lower-energy shocks may result in a graded lower response that can potentially create transient block and a critical point, thereby reinducing fibrillation.[15]

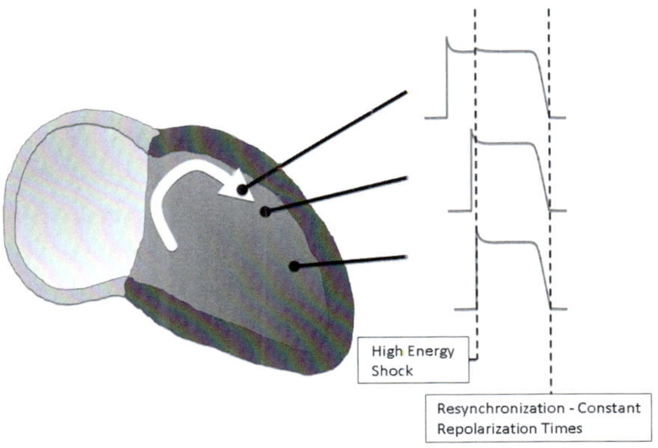

Fig 15.4 Progressive depolarization is illustrated by the figure. The VF wavefront is illustrated by the arrow. A high voltage shock is illustrated. The region in which the wavefront just passed was in its' plateau phase which typically would be refractory. However, the shock was of high enough intensity that a small active response was generated and the action potential prolonged. The next region is at the leading edge of the wavefront and the shock impacts the tissue at phase 0 of the action potential and has little effect on its duration. The final region is in the excitable gap and the shock initiates a new action potential. (Adapted from Figure 1.23, Bunch et al.[6])

Virtual Electrode Depolarization

A relatively new concept centers on the premise that the defibrillation electrode or "virtual electrode" can be made effectively larger than the physical electrode. The regions of depolarization or hyperpolarization near the physical electrode are surrounded by adjacent regions with opposite polarity.[16] During an anodal shock a wavefront initiates a positively charged region boundary that spreads toward the physical anode to other negatively charged areas that ultimately collapse with other wavefronts and becomes neutralized.[16] This produces "collapsing" wavefronts that frequently collide and neutralize one another,[17] whereas cathodal shocks initiate a negatively charged wavefront that expands and propagates away from the physical cathode. The expanded region sensitive to the cathodal shocks increases success and thereby incorporates many aspects of the aforementioned mechanisms.[17]

After review of these basic theories of shock it would seem that the concepts presented would favor using the highest energy shock possible. However, high-energy shocks may have untoward side effects and may also be proarrhythmic. Very high-energy shocks can lead to toxic effects, including disruption of cell membranes by extraporation, postshock block, myocardial and mechanical dysfunction, and new tachyarrhythmias (Fig 15.5).[15]

Monophasic and Biphasic Shock Waveforms

Energy delivery platforms have evolved to improve the shock efficacy at lower energy levels. The advent of the biphasic waveform significantly reduced the energy required to achieve a successful defibrillation. In theory, with biphasic shocks the function of the first phase is to extinguish as many wavefronts as possible or enough critical mass. In a basic sense this is achieved by prolonging the action potential of stimulated cells and activating recovered cells.[18–21] As stated previously, unsuccessful shocks can lead to disruption of cell membranes, initiation of new wavefronts, or inadequate reach in obtaining a critical mass. The second phase of the waveform is to counter all of these possible effects. DFT is directly related to the second phase duration of the biphasic waveform (Fig 15.6). Shock optimization can be performed by modifying the percentage-voltage delivered (tilt-based waveform) or the pulse width (fixed-duration waveform) in each phase of the biphasic shock. The ability to optimize the shock waveform is available in some ICD manufacturers and fixed in others.

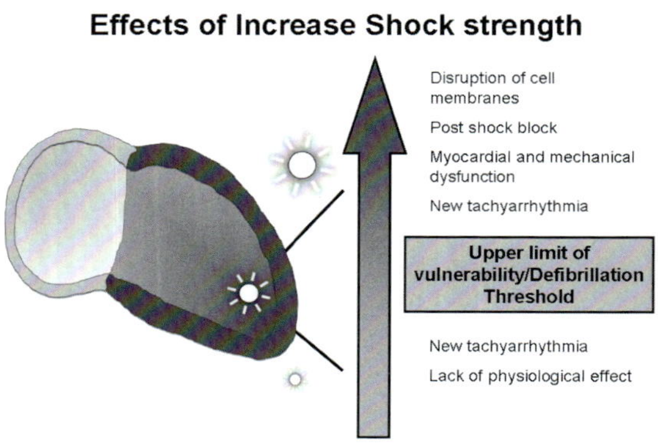

Fig 15.5 The tissue effects of increasing electric field strength are apparent as referenced to the region in which the upper limit of vulnerability and defibrillation threshold are encountered.

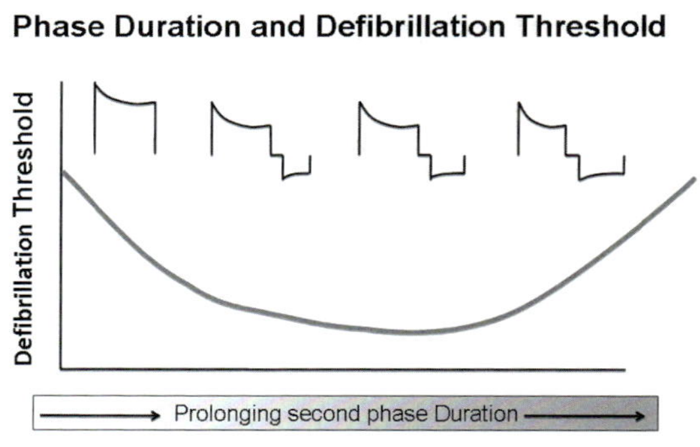

Fig 15.6 Idealized curve that demonstrates the relationship of the second phase of a biphasic waveform and the defibrillation threshold. (Adapted based upon data from Wessale et al.[32])

With shock theories it is important to recognize that successful defibrillation is probabilistic in nature. Variance in outcome is likely due to the spatial and temporal heterogeneities of ventricular myocardium during VF. DFT is commonly defined as the minimum shock energy required to terminate VF and this will be discussed in a subsequent chapter, 18. Although a favorable DFT provides some reassurance of device efficacy, there is no single energy level above which defibrillation is uniformly successful or an energy level below which it uniformly fails.[22]

ICD Shock Efficacy Dependence on Stage and Type of Heart Disease

Current ICDs have multiple features to enhance diagnostics, minimize unnecessary pacing, conserve energy use, and deliver pain-free therapies such as antitachycardia pacing. Of all of these features, the most important remains the ability to recognize a life-threatening ventricular arrhythmia and terminate it with a shock. The benefit and significance of an ICD shock is dependent on the type of heart disease, stage of heart disease, and the presence of structural heart disease. These concepts are illustrated in a brief overview of ICD trials in patients with ischemic and nonischemic heart disease.

For example, the benefit of ICD therapy in patients with ischemic heart disease is directly related to the time from myocardial infarction (MI) to implant. The Defibrillator in Acute Myocardial Infarction Trial (DINAMIT) trial,[23] that randomized patients to receive an ICD or standard medical therapy 4 to 40 days after MI showed no difference in overall mortality between the two treatment groups (62 were in the ICD group versus 58 in the control group). This study was in contrast to the majority of prior ICD trial patients that included patients with a remote MI (average time from myocardial to enrollment for Multicenter Unsustained Tachycardia Trial Investigators [MUSTT] was 39 months and for Multicenter Automatic Defibrillator Implantation Trial [MADIT]-II 81 months), which showed a survival benefit with ICD therapy. The dramatic variance in outcomes with an ICD in these studies likely reflects the underlying significance of ventricular arrhythmias after MI. Early after MI, ventricular arrhythmias are surrogate markers of worsening myocardial function, recurrent ischemia, and infarction. By comparison, late ventricular arrhythmias are often related alterations of the electrophysiologic substrate in the setting of compensated heart failure due to scar and reentry mechanisms.[2] In support of this hypothesis, is a subanalysis of the MADIT-II trial Wilber et al[24] found only those who received an ICD with a remote MI (> 18 months) benefited (hazard ratio 0.55 [0.39–0.78], p = 0.001) versus those with a relatively recent MI (< 18 months, hazard ratio 0.97 [0.51–1.81], p = 0.92).

In comparison, those patients that have nonischemic cardiomyopathy have a distinct temporal benefit to ICD implantation. In the Defibrillators in Nonischemic Cardiomyopathy Treatment Evaluation (DEFINITE) trial,[25] 458 patients with nonischemic dilated cardiomyopathy (ejection fraction ≤ 0.36) were randomized to an ICD versus conventional therapy. In this trial there was a significant reduction in sudden death (hazard ratio, 0.20; 95% confidence interval, 0.06–0.71; p = 0.006) and a trend toward a reduction in total mortality (hazard ratio, 0.65; 95% confidence interval, 0.40–1.06; p = 0.08). In a DEFINITE trial subanalysis, the benefit of ICD therapy was seen predominantly in those who had nonischemic dilated cardiomyopathy of < 3 months (p = 0.049) compared to those with older disease (p = 0.483). The findings of this subsequent study were in drastic contrast to those in ischemic populations in which the benefit of ICD therapy is in patients with remote/chronic disease.

Significance of an ICD Shock for VT/VF

Despite the type and stage of cardiac disease, the presence of an ICD shock signifies a high-risk patient. In a subanalysis of the DINAMIT trial, Dorian et al[26] studied 55 patients who had an appropriate ICD shock. Of these patients who had an ICD shock, 40% died within 1 year, a finding independent of age, ejection fraction, and low-heart-rate variability. In the MADIT-II trial, patients who received appropriate ICD therapies had an increased risk for first (HR 1.90, $p = 0.01$) and recurrent (1.74, $p < 0.001$) congestive heart failure events within a relatively short period after the shock. These heart failure events were independently associated with increased mortality.[27] In a large review of patients who underwent ICD implantation for primary prevention, an appropriate ICD shock compared to no shock was associated with a significant increase in the subsequent risk of death from all causes (hazard ratio, 5.68; 95% confidence interval [CI], 3.97–8.12; $p < 0.001$).[28] As important, the most common cause of death was from progressive cardiac dysfunction and heart failure. It is unknown whether aggressive pharmacologic and nonpharmacologic therapies for heart failure after an ICD shock can mitigate this negative prognostic significance.

Significance of an Inappropriate ICD Shock

Initially, avoidance of inappropriate ICD shocks was heralded to improve quality of life and improve device longevity. However, additional studies have shown that these shocks are also significant for both alterations in morbidity and mortality. In both patients who received an ICD for primary or second prevention, an inappropriate shock was associated with an increase in total mortality.[28,29] In a study by Daubert et al,[29] the most common cause of an inappropriate shock was atrial fibrillation, followed by supraventricular tachycardia, and abnormal sensing. The significance of new onset atrial fibrillation after ICD implantation has been investigated as well.[30] Atrial fibrillation was associated with an increased risk of heart failure hospitalization, appropriate and inappropriate shocks, and total mortality. These data in aggregate suggest that inappropriate shocks, often a marker of atrial arrhythmias, identify a patient at high risk of poor long-term cardiovascular outcomes.[30]

References

1. Bardy GH, Lee KL, Mark DB, et al. Amiodarone or an implantable cardioverter-defibrillator for congestive heart failure. *N Engl J Med.* 2005; 352(3):225–237.
2. Bunch TJ, Hohnloser SH, Gersh BJ. Mechanisms of sudden cardiac death in myocardial infarction survivors: insights from the randomized trials of implantable cardioverter-defibrillators. *Circulation.* 2007;115(18):2451–2457.
3. Buxton AE, Lee KL, DiCarlo L, et al. Electrophysiologic testing to identify patients with coronary artery disease who are at risk for sudden death. Multicenter Unsustained Tachycardia Trial Investigators. *N Engl J Med.* 2000;342(26):1937–1945.
4. Moss AJ, Zareba W, Hall WJ, et al. Prophylactic implantation of a defibrillator in patients with myocardial infarction and reduced ejection fraction. *N Engl J Med.* 2002;346(12):877–883.
5. Weiss JN, Qu Z, Chen PS, et al. The dynamics of cardiac fibrillation. *Circulation.* 2005;112 (8): 1232–1240.
6. Bunch TJ, Hayes DL, Friedman PA. Clinically relevant basics of pacing and defibrillation. In: Hayes DL, Friedman PA, eds. *Cardiac pacing, defibrillation, and resynchronization. A practical approach.* Vol II. West Sussex: Wiley-Blackwell; 2008:1–42.
7. Zipes DP, Fischer J, King RM, Nicoll AD, Jolly WW. Termination of ventricular fibrillation in dogs by depolarizing a critical amount of myocardium. *Am J Cardiol.* 1975;36(1):37–44.
8. Chen PS, Shibata N, Dixon EG, et al. Activation during ventricular defibrillation in open-chest dogs. Evidence of complete cessation and regeneration of ventricular fibrillation after unsuccessful shocks. *J Clin Invest.* 1986;77(3): 810–823.
9. Chen PS, Wolf PD, Melnick SD, Danieley ND, Smith WM, Ideker RE. Comparison of activation during ventricular fibrillation and following

unsuccessful defibrillation shocks in open-chest dogs. *Circ Res.* 1990;66(6):1544–1560.
10. Frazier DW, Wolf PD, Wharton JM, Tang AS, Smith WM, Ideker RE. Stimulus-induced critical point. Mechanism for electrical initiation of reentry in normal canine myocardium. *J Clin Invest.* 1989;83(3):1039–1052.
11. Chen PS, Feld GK, Kriett JM, et al. Relation between upper limit of vulnerability and defibrillation threshold in humans. *Circulation.* 1993;88(1):186–192.
12. Day JD, Doshi RN, Belott P, et al. Inductionless or limited shock testing is possible in most patients with implantable cardioverter- defibrillators/cardiac resynchronization therapy defibrillators: results of the multicenter ASSURE Study (Arrhythmia Single Shock Defibrillation Threshold Testing Versus Upper Limit of Vulnerability: Risk Reduction Evaluation With Implantable Cardioverter-Defibrillator Implantations). *Circulation.* 2007;115(18):2382–2389.
13. Dillon SM, Kwaku KF. Progressive depolarization: a unified hypothesis for defibrillation and fibrillation induction by shocks. *J Cardiovasc Electrophysiol.* 1998;9(5):529–552.
14. Sweeney RJ, Gill RM, Steinberg MI, Reid PR. Ventricular refractory period extension caused by defibrillation shocks. *Circulation.* 1990;82(3):965–972.
15. Dillon SM. The electrophysiological effects of defibrillation shocks. In: Kroll M, Lehmann M, eds. *Implantable Cardioverter Defibrillator Therapy: The Engineering-Clinical Interface.* Norwell, MA: Kluwer Academic Publishers; 1996:31–61.
16. Yamanouchi Y, Cheng Y, Tchou PJ, Efimov IR. The mechanisms of the vulnerable window: the role of virtual electrodes and shock polarity. *Can J Physiol Pharmacol.* 2001;79(1):25–33.
17. Efimov IR, Cheng Y, Yamanouchi Y, Tchou PJ. Direct evidence of the role of virtual electrode-induced phase singularity in success and failure of defibrillation. *J Cardiovasc Electrophysiol.* 2000;11(8):861–868.
18. Efimov IR, Cheng Y, Van Wagoner DR, Mazgalev T, Tchou PJ. Virtual electrode-induced phase singularity: a basic mechanism of defibrillation failure. *Circ Res.* 1998;82(8):918–925.
19. Hillebrenner MG, Eason JC, Campbell CA, Trayanova NA. Postshock arrhythmogenesis in a slice of the canine heart. *J Cardiovasc Electrophysiol.* 2003;14(10 Suppl):S249–256.
20. Seidl K, Denman RA, Moulder JC, et al. Stepped defibrillation waveform is substantially more efficient than the 50/50% tilt biphasic. *Heart Rhythm.* 2006;3(12):1406–1411.
21. Zheng X, Walcott GP, Smith WM, Ideker RE. Evidence that activation following failed defibrillation is not caused by triggered activity. *J Cardiovasc Electrophysiol.* 2005;16(11):1200–1205.
22. Kowalski M, Huizar JF, Kaszala K, Wood MA. Problems with implantable cardiac device therapy. *Cardiol Clin.* 2008;26(3):441–458, vii.
23. Hohnloser SH, Kuck KH, Dorian P, et al. Prophylactic use of an implantable cardioverter-defibrillator after acute myocardial infarction. *N Engl J Med.* 2004;351(24):2481–2488.
24. Wilber DJ, Zareba W, Hall WJ, et al. Time dependence of mortality risk and defibrillator benefit after myocardial infarction. *Circulation.* 2004;109(9):1082–1084.
25. Kadish A, Dyer A, Daubert JP, et al. Prophylactic defibrillator implantation in patients with nonischemic dilated cardiomyopathy. *N Engl J Med.* 2004;350(21):2151–2158.
26. Dorian P, Connolly S, Hohnloser SH, Investigators D. Why don't ICDs decrease all-cause mortality after MI? Insights from the DINAMIT Study. *Circulation.* 2004;502(Supplement S): 2356.
27. Goldenberg I, Moss AJ, Hall WJ, et al, Multicenter Automatic Defibrillator Implantation Trial III. Causes and consequences of heart failure after prophylactic implantation of a defibrillator in the multicenter automatic defibrillator implantation trial II. *Circulation.* 2006;113(24):2810–2817.
28. Poole JE, Johnson GW, Hellkamp AS, et al. Prognostic importance of defibrillator shocks in patients with heart failure. *N Engl J Med.* 2008;359(10):1009–1017.
29. Daubert JP, Zareba W, Cannom DS, et al. Inappropriate implantable cardioverter-defibrillator shocks in MADIT II: frequency, mechanisms, predictors, and survival impact. *J Am Coll Cardiol.* 2008;51(14):1357–1365.
30. Bunch TJ, Day JD, Olshansky B, Stolen KQ, Mullin CM. Newly detected atrial fibrillation

in patients with an implantable cardioverter-defibrillator is a strong risk marker of increased mortality. *Heart Rhythm.* 2009;6(1):2–8.

31. Sanders GD, Hlatky MA, Owens DK. Cost effectiveness of implantable cardioverter-defibrillators. *N Engl J Med.* 2005;353(14):1471–1480.

32. Dixon EG, Tang AS, Wolf PD, Meador JT, Fine MJ, Calfee RV, Ideker RE. Improved defibrillation thresholds with large contoured epicardial electrodes and biphasic waveforms. *Circulation.* 1987;76(5):1176–84.

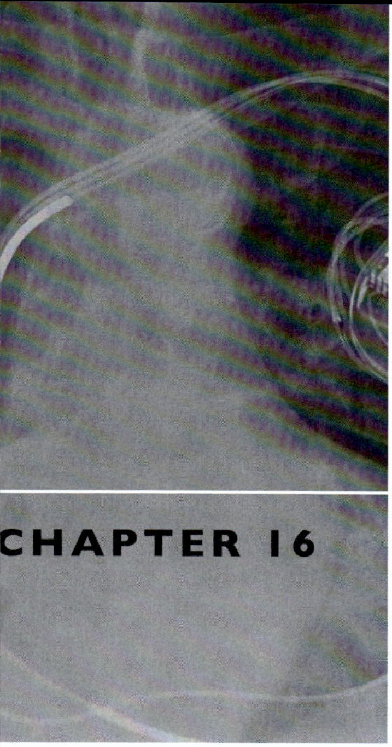

Discrimination Algorithms and Arrhythmia Detection

CHAPTER 16

Irina Suman Horduna and Paul Khairy

Introduction

Since the commercial release of the first generation of implantable cardioverter defibrillators (ICDs), remarkable technologic advances have enhanced their efficacy and safety and improved the accuracy of arrhythmia detection algorithms. The introduction of dual chamber devices was an important milestone that incorporated additional atrial information into discrimination algorithms, while offering dual chamber pacing. Nevertheless, despite these developments, inappropriate therapy for supraventricular tachyarrhythmias (SVT) remains a major limitation of contemporary ICDs, with 7% to 27%[1,2] of implanted patients receiving inadequate therapies.

In this chapter, we review current detection algorithms included in modern single and dual chamber devices developed by the various manufacturers and describe particularities and performance issues. In so doing, the following definitions pertaining to tachycardia detection will be adopted (Table 16.1 on following page): true positive (TP), false positive (FP), true negative (TN), and false negative (FN).

MEDTRONIC DEVICES

Single Chamber ICDs

Single chamber ICDs from Medtronic currently incorporate four elements into detection algorithms: (1) RR interval analysis; (2) RR onset; (3) RR regularity or stability, and (4) Ventricular electrogram (VEGM) morphology.

RR Interval Analysis

The RR interval analysis is the first and simplest criterion used to classify high ventricular

Pacemakers and Implantable Cardioverter Defibrillators: An Expert's Manual. © 2010 Amin Al-Ahmad, Kenneth A. Ellenbogen, Andrea Natale, and Paul J. Wang, eds. Cardiotext Publishing, ISBN: 978-0-9790164-6-2.

Device Classification	Physician Classification	
VT	VT (TP)	SVT (FP)
SVT	VT (FN)	SVT (TN)

Table 16.1 Tachycardia Detection. Abbreviations: FN, false negative; FP, false positive; SVT, supraventricular tachycardia; TN, true negative; TP, true positive; VT, ventricular tachycardia.

rates according to the cycle length of each programmed zone. It provides the highest sensitivity for detecting true VT but does not distinguish VT from SVT with a high ventricular rate that overlaps with VT/VF zones. Counting algorithms based on RR interval analyses are similar in single and dual chamber devices and consist of two counters with three programmable rate detection zones: VF, VT, and fast VT (FVT).

The VF counter nominally requires that 18 of the last 24 intervals be shorter than the fibrillation detection interval (FDI), the latter indicating the "window size." This counter relies on a "sliding window" principle; as long as intervals are binned within this window, an interval that meets the FDI threshold will increment the counter by one whereas a sinus or a VT interval will "freeze" the counter (Fig 16.1).

I

BEAT	1	2	3	4	5	6	7	8	9	10	11	12	13	14	15
INTERVAL	VF	VF	VF	Sinus	VF	VF	VF	Sinus	Sinus	Sinus	Sinus	Sinus	Sinus	VF	Sinus
COUNTER	1	2	3	3	4	5	6	6	6	6	6	6			

VF counter: 6/12

II

BEAT	1	2	3	4	5	6	7	8	9	10	11	12	13	14	15
INTERVAL	VT	VT	VF	Sinus	VF	VT	VF	Sinus	Sinus	Sinus	Sinus	Sinus	Sinus	VT	Sinus
COUNTER	x	1	2	2	3	4	5	5	5	5	5	5	5		

VF counter: 5/12

III

BEAT	1	2	3	4	5	6	7	8	9	10	11	12	13	14	15
INTERVAL	VT	VF	VF	Sinus	VF	VT	VF	Sinus	Sinus	Sinus	Sinus	Sinus	Sinus	VT	Sinus
COUNTER	x	x	1	1	2	3	4	4	4	4	4	4	4	5	

VF counter: 5/12

IV

BEAT	1	2	3	4	5	6	7	8	9	10	11	12	13	14	15
INTERVAL	VF	VF	VF	Sinus	VF	VF	VF	Sinus	Sinus	Sinus	Sinus	Sinus	Sinus	VF	Sinus
COUNTER	x	x	x	0	1	2	3	3	3	3	3	3	3	4	4

VF counter: 4/12

Fig 16.1 The sliding window principle: a window progressively slides beat by beat from I to IV. Shown are the numbered beats, intervals binned, and the VF zone counter (in this example set to 9/12). (Reproduced from Mansour and Khairy.[3])

The VT counter nominally requires 16 *consecutive* RR intervals that fall within the tachycardia detection interval (TDI) but are greater than or equal to the FDI. The emphasis on consecutive intervals may be useful in rejecting variable rates during rapidly conducted AF. Thus, an interval meeting the VT threshold will increment the counter, whereas a slower interval will reset the counter to 0; of note, an interval binned in the VF zone will neither increase nor reset the counter.[3]

To avoid delays in detecting tachyarrhythmias with overlapping rates between VT and VF zones, a combined count feature was added that is automatically enabled when a VT zone is programmed On. This count is triggered when at least 6 RR intervals are in the VF zone. It increments if VF or VT counters increment and decrements if the VT counter is reset or if the VF counter decrements.[3] Detection occurs when the sum of the VT and VF counters reaches a value of 7/6 multiplied by the programmed number of intervals needed to detect VF (rounded down). The nature of subsequent delivered therapy is based on the last 8 intervals: if *all* fall within the VT zone, VT therapy is delivered; if *any* fall within the VF zone,

VF therapy (or FVT therapy, see following) will be triggered.

The third programmable rate zone is the fast VT (FVT) zone, which is intended to allow therapies while avoiding unnecessary shocks.[4] If the fast tachycardia interval (FTI) is less than FDI, the FVT zone becomes a subset of the VF counter (FVT via VF). For FVT via the VF zone, FVT therapy is delivered if *all* of the last 8 intervals are in the FVT zone. If not, VF therapy is delivered. If the FTI is greater than FDI, FVT intervals are considered in the VT counter (FVT via VT). FVT therapy is delivered if *any* of the last 8 intervals are in the VF or FVT zone, otherwise VT therapy is provided.

RR Onset

"RR onset" relies on sudden ventricular rate changes to discriminate VT from sinus tachycardia (ST) of progressive onset. This feature is nonspecific for ventricular arrhythmias, because atrial tachycardia that conducts 1:1 may exhibit a similar pattern, and may miss detection of VT that initiates during ongoing ST. "RR onset" is functional only in single chamber ICDs (until EnTrust) and is exclusively applicable for initial detection. The onset algorithm is based upon a rolling counter that uses the 8 most recent intervals. "Sudden onset" is declared if the average of the 4 most recent intervals is less than the average of the previous 4 intervals, multiplied by the programmed onset percentage (nominally set to 81%). Once this occurs, the VT counter is activated. This criterion only pertains to the VT counter.

RR Stability

This feature is used to discriminate monomorphic, presumably regular, VT from rapidly conducted atrial fibrillation (AF) with an irregular cycle length. It may prevent detection of unstable VT such as polymorphic forms. Conversely, it may misclassify a supraventricular arrhythmia with 2:1 conduction block, such as atrial flutter (Aflutter), or a rapidly conducted AF with a pseudoregular ventricular pattern.

The algorithm operates with a rolling counter, which uses the 4 most recent intervals. When the VT counter reaches 3, if the current interval varies from *any* of the previous 3 by more than the programmed value, the rhythm is considered unstable and the VT counter is reset to zero. The "stability interval" nominal value is set to 50 ms. Of note, the VT counter requires consecutive intervals to fall within the programmed zone, thus providing a complementary feature to the stability criterion. It is the only discriminator that applies to both initial and redetection periods.

Wavelet Dynamic Discrimination Criterion

"Wavelet" (or morphology) criterion is used to classify rapid rhythms as SVT if the arrhythmia template is similar to that recorded during baseline rhythms. SVT with aberrancy is a well-recognized source of misclassification. To minimize this drawback, the morphology is analyzed after the fourth fast beat and withholds detection when at least 3 of the last 8 complexes match the stored template. Morphology analysis continues until insufficient normal beats are recognized (and VT detection occurs) or until the heart rate slows out of the detection zone. This comparison is expressed as a percent-match score that reflects the degree of similarity of sinus and tachycardia electrograms.

Nominally, beats with match scores $< 70\%$ are classified as ventricular in origin. The 70% value (programmable feature) is based on results of a previous, retrospective, postprocessing analysis of electrograms recorded during electrophysiologic study[2] and was subsequently confirmed to be a reasonable cutoff with high specificity, without compromising sensitivity.[5,6]

The morphology algorithm

The morphology algorithm functions as follows:

1. The "wavelet transform" of the composite baseline-rhythm template electrogram is constructed as shown in Fig 16.2 on the following page and stored;

2. Each of the last 8 tachycardia electrograms preceding detection is aligned with the template electrogram in the time domain. Alignment is based on the positive or negative peak with the greatest absolute value (dotted vertical line);

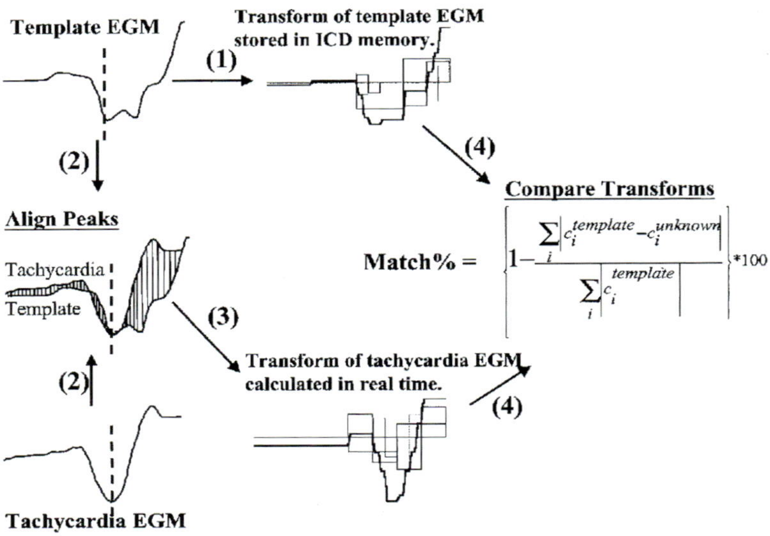

Fig 16.2 Morphology analysis using the wavelet transform. (Adapted from Swerdlow et al.[5])

3. The "wavelet transform" of each tachycardia electrogram is calculated in real time;

4. A match-percent score that describes the degree of similarity of each tachycardia electrogram to the template is calculated.[7]

Performance of this discrimination algorithm was assessed in several studies.[5,6] In 23 patients with single chamber ICDs (model 7277) and a nominally programmed match-percent threshold of 70%,[5] the sensitivity for detecting VT was 100%, with a specificity for SVT rejection of 78%. The Worldwide Application of Marquis VR Enhancements (WAVE)[6] study found that the wavelet morphology discrimination algorithm provided a 58% reduction in inappropriate SVT detection (independent of rate onset and interval stability), with a > 99% sensitivity for sustained VT/VF. These results were comparable to the performance of dual chamber devices from another study.[1] When only episodes with a median cycle length ≥ SVT limit were considered, wavelet-based therapies for SVT were reduced by 78%, with a sensitivity for sustained VT of 98.6%. The very low rate of misclassification of VT as SVT (< 1.5%) may be attributed, in part, to the nominal use of a far-field EGM source (RV coil-can) that more accurately captures cardiac depolarization than a near-field (tip-ring or tip-coil) EGM source. However, SVT was inappropriately classified as VT in 18% of patients, mostly due to subtle or major rate- or ischemia-related aberrancy, signal clipping due to peak-peak amplitudes exceeding the programmed EGM range (7%), postshock signal distortion (3%), and myopotential noise (2%). Wavelet performance was independent of ventricular cycle length and was not influenced by preexisting BBB.

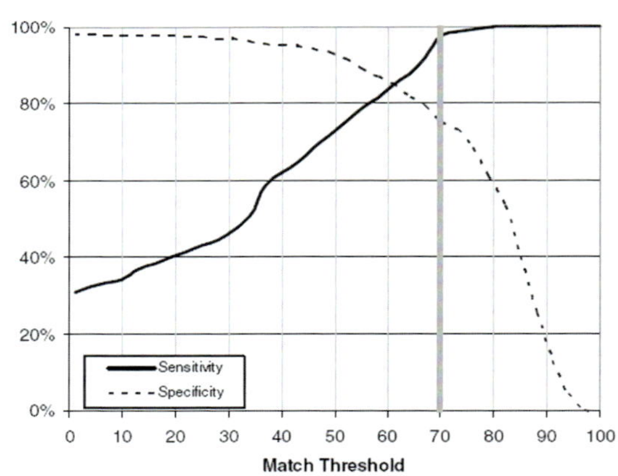

Fig 16.3 Percentage of appropriately classified VT/VF (sensitivity) and SVT (specificity) as a function of match threshold. (Adapted from Klein, Gillberg et al.[6])

The influence of match threshold on wavelet VT/SVT discrimination performance was assessed retrospectively in the same study.[6] The nominal match threshold of 70% appears to provide the best compromise between SVT rejection and high sensitivity for true VT for the overall patient population (Fig 16.3).

High-rate timeout
This feature overrides all SVT discriminators (including onset and stability) if tachycardia persists for a duration that exceeds the programmed value. It is nominally inactivated.

SVT limit
This feature overrides wavelet classification of SVT (as well as the PR Logic algorithm in dual chamber devices) when the median RR interval < SVT limit (nominally 320 ms).

Dual Chamber ICDs

The PR Logic algorithm classifies rhythms within the programmed number of intervals needed for detection (NID) and only during initial detection. Some particular features are noteworthy: RR onset is not included in the algorithm, mainly because of the concern for underdetecting VTs that occur during SVT; Wavelet (morphology criterion) is not yet part of the decision tree in Medtronic dual chamber ICDs; the chamber of origin of the arrhythmia is not used in PR Logic because of the risk of under/oversensing or blanking; the stability of the ventricular rhythm is assessed by using a specific function called "RR modesum" (see later).

Four programmable parameters are currently available,[8] that is, 3 On/Off switches allowing to enable or disable SVT rejection for rapidly conducted AF/Aflutter, ST, and SVTs with nearly simultaneous atrial and ventricular activation (eg, junctional tachycardia and SVT with 1:1 conduction). The fourth programmable parameter is an RR interval-based feature, the "SVT limit," defined as the shortest ventricular cycle length for which PR Logic may withhold therapies for VT.

If the median RR interval is shorter than the SVT limit, the discrimination algorithm is bypassed and detection is forced to the rate-only criterion. The SVT limit is nominally set to the FDI, but it can be programmed independently of the boundaries of the detection zones,[8] between 240 ms and 650 ms with EnTrust devices and thereafter.

PR Logic Detection Elements

Six dual chamber detection elements are incorporated in the PR Logic algorithm: (1) RR intervals, (2) PR patterns, (3) RR regularity, (4) PR dissociation, (5) PP intervals, and (6) PP regularity. SVT rejection algorithms do not apply during redetection when only ventricular-rate detection criterion is used.

RR Intervals

Ventricular cycle length is estimated by the median of the last 12 RR intervals. Median statistics are less sensitive to outliers arising from under- or oversensing than mean values. This value will classify episodes according to the "SVT limit." The counting algorithm consists of 2 counters and 3 rate detection zones, as in single chambered devices.

PR Pattern

PR pattern is analysed for each ventricular event using the two previous RR intervals and intervening P events (Fig 16.4). The number and position of atrial events within two consecutive RR intervals are analyzed to define a particular pattern. A letter is assigned to each couple code and a syntax is built based upon this series of letters. A sustained tachycardia is diagnosed by a unique sequence of codes, which is compared with the predetermined patterns assigned to different types of arrhythmia. Each pattern syntax denotes a given tachyarrhythmia.

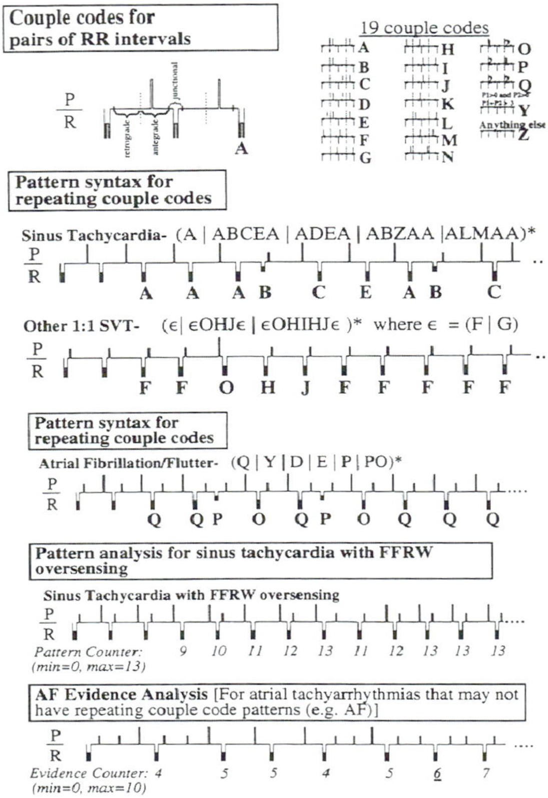

Fig 16.4 Top: PR analysis for 1:1 rhythms. The timing of P waves relative to R waves within a given RR interval is shown series of 19 couple codes is attributed to each sequence of P and R events encompassed within two RR intervals and a pattern syntax series is subsequently created by assembling a specific sequence of letters. Note that some "violations" from the classic pattern attributed to one specific arrhythmia (ie, AAA pattern for ST) are allowed: for example, ABCEA is still recognized as ST if premature ventricular complexes (PVC) occur. **Middle** and **bottom**: Analysis for > 1:1 rhythms. In case of a regular ventricular rhythm, an Aflutter pattern is recognized by using a specific pattern syntax. In the case of an irregular rhythm, no specific pattern can be identified because the PR relationship is highly variable. The AF evidence counter (bottom) is enabled in these situations (see text for more details). In the case of ST with FFRWs, no couples codes are used, but rather a combination of PR pattern and PP regularity (see text for more details). (Adapted from Gillberg and Olson.[8])

<1:1 rhythms

The rhythm is classified as < 1:1 if P events are insufficient to be consistent with SVT. RR intervals frequently do not contain P waves. PR patterns for rhythms in this class have no more than 3 of 5 RRs with a P event. Because this pattern is not compatible with SVT, the detection algorithm reverts to the RR interval-only criterion.

1:1 rhythms

The episode is classified as a 1:1 rhythm if most RR intervals have only 1 P event, and no more than 1 of 5 RR intervals has 0 or 2 P waves. The PR pattern in this branch allows establishing 3 diagnoses: ST/atrial tachycardia, junctional tachycardia (labelled as "Other 1:1 SVT") and VT with 1:1 retrograde conduction (assumed by default when the patterns for ST/atrial tachycardia are not recognized). Each RR interval is divided into 3 segments (Fig 16.4, top). For defining the boundary between antegrade and retrograde conduction, a threshold of 50% of the current RR interval is used.

- If the PR interval is < 50% of the current RR interval but > 80 ms, the atrial event is considered antegrade and supports a diagnosis of ST. Evidence of ST is maintained by a counter. The ST pattern counter has a maximum value of 13 and a recognition threshold of 6 (diagnosis established). Below this threshold, each event that does not match the criterion for ST resets the counter to 0. Above this threshold each event with no PR pattern match decrements the counter by 4, 8, 16, and so on (ie, exponential decay or decrement property). The decrement value is reset to 4 when the counter reaches 6 for the first time after counting up from 0 or when it reaches 13.[8]

- If the P wave is recorded 80 ms before a ventricular event or < 50 ms after a ventricular event, tachycardia is considered "junctional" (ie, "other 1:1 SVT"). Evidence of such PR pattern is also maintained by a counter. The counter has a maximum value of 6 and it resets to 0 for each event outside this range. It does not have an exponential decrement property.

- If the PR interval is ≥ 50% of the current RR interval and the RP interval is > 50 ms, the P event is considered retrograde (evidence for VT with 1:1 retrograde conduction).

In Gem DR and Gem II DR ICDs, the antegrade-retrograde boundary is fixed at 50% of the RR interval. A programmable parameter, the "1:1 VT-ST boundary" has been added to PR Logic in the Gem III DR and Marquis DR ICDs, which allows changing this limit to values that could vary between 35% and 85% of the RR interval. More recent ICDs models do not use this fixed VT-SVT boundary, but rely on an adaptive ST algorithm, as described later.

> 1:1 rhythms
The PR pattern-only cannot discriminate among the following 4 possible diagnoses: rapidly conducted AF, Aflutter with a regular ventricular response, VT/VF arising during ongoing SVT (double tachycardia), or ST with a far-field R wave (FFRW) pattern. PR Logic uses all 6 features mentioned previously to classify the rhythm. To distinguish between *ST with FFRW* or AF/Aflutter, PR Logic combines the PR pattern and PP regularity features described later (Fig 16.4).

Regularly conducted *Aflutter* (2:1, 3:1) is recognized using a particular PR pattern and a specific counter that increments by 1 when a couple code matches the predetermined syntax and resets to 0 in case of no match. It has a maximum value of 6. In the case of irregularly conducted AF/Aflutter, when a consistent PR pattern is not recognized, PR Logic uses a counter to maintain evidence of > 1:1 rhythm. The *AF evidence counter* increments for a given RR interval if there are 2 or more intervening P waves, unless 1 P event is classified a FFRW oversense (see following). In this case, the counter remains unchanged. If there is only one atrial event in a VV interval, the counter holds for one interval and than decrements by 1. The counter also decrements by 1 if there is no atrial event in a given RR interval. This up-down counter has a maximum value of 10 with a recognition threshold of 6 and remains recognized until the count falls below 5 (Fig 16.4).

RR Regularity

This criterion is particularly useful in cases of dual tachycardia detected in the VT zone (VT + SVT). Regularity is determined using a function called modesum. The last 18 ventricular intervals are measured and a frequency histogram is computed. The modesum is determined by comparing the number of intervals in the two largest interval bins to the total number of intervals. A cut-off value of 75% establishes the regularity/irregularity pattern. The lower this ratio, the more irregular is the rhythm.

PR Dissociation

This qualifier helps to improve diagnostic accuracy in the case of VT/VF or double tachycardias (VT + SVT or VF + SVT). PR dissociation is first determined by analyzing each beat and then the entire rhythm. The current AV interval is compared with the average of the last 8 AV intervals. A ventricular event is considered dissociated if this value varies by > 40 ms (not programmable) or if there is no P event recorded within the current VV interval. The rhythm is deemed dissociated if at least 4 of the last 8 beats are dissociated.

PP Intervals

This discriminator is helpful in appropriately detecting rapidly conducted AF. Atrial rate is determined as the median of the last 12 atrial beats, updated with each atrial event on a beat-to-beat basis and then compared against the median ventricular rate. A median atrial rate at least 6% faster than the median ventricular rate provides evidence for AF.

PP Regularity

This element is particularly useful to reject FFRW oversensing. For 2:1 rhythms (FFRW oversensing during sinus rhythm and 2:1 conducted Aflutter) the detection algorithm combines PP regularity and PR pattern elements. Consistent alternations of PP intervals avoid misclassification of the rhythm as 2:1 Aflutter. In the Gem DR and Gem II DR devices, 10 or more of the last 12 RR intervals must contain P waves identified as FFRW oversensed events in order to diagnose ST with FFRW. With Gem III DR models only 4 of the last 12 RR intervals are required to reject P events as FFRWs. The following criteria are required to diagnose ST with FFRW:

- Exactly 2 atrial events for every ventricular event
- A short-long alternating A-A pattern (> 30 ms)
- Low VA interval variability (< 50 ms)
- Consistent AV or VA intervals (< 20 ms from average AV or VA)
- One atrial event labeled as nonphysiologic (A-V < 60 ms or V-A < 160 ms)
- If this pattern consistently recurs

ST with FFRW Pattern Counter

This counter increments by 1 when there are 1 or 2 atrial events within the RR interval with one of them falling in the antegrade region of the RR interval. It does not use couple codes, but relies on criteria described earlier. It has a recognition threshold of 6, a maximum value of 13, and an exponential decrement property. Once the counter reaches 6, each nonmatching event decrements the counter by 2, 4, 8, and so on, in an exponential manner (Fig 16.4). This counter has similar reset behavior to the ST counter: its decrement value resets to 2 when the counter reaches 6 for the first time when counting up from 0 or when reaching 13.

PR Logic Decisional Tree

The PR Logic algorithm is applied only during initial detection and not during redetection of VT/FVT/VF.[8,9] If a VT/FVT/VF is detected, the PR Logic discrimination algorithm is reactivated only after 8 consecutive RR intervals longer than TDI are counted (when episode termination criterion is satisfied). "Transition" is a property of a specified element included in PR Logic and Wavelet algorithms, which allows withholding therapy for 6 (Jewel AF, Gem DR, and Gem II DR) or 10 intervals (Gem III DR and newer models) after this criterion is no longer satisfied. During this period all PR Logic criteria that are at the same level or higher in the decisional tree than the most recent satisfied criterion (see later) are evaluated. If SVT cannot be recognized until the end of the transition period, VT/FVT/VF is detected. As the RR interval criterion is the lowest in this hierarchy, the VT/FVT/VF detection is withheld during the transition period.

The decisional process begins with a PR, RP, PP, RR pattern that is updated with each new ventricular event[8] (Fig 16.5). PR Logic criteria are not assessed until the median RR interval is ≤ TDI (or FDI if tachycardia zone is disabled) or when the sum of VT and VF counters is > 8 in order to reduce computational burden at slower rates and to preserve the device longevity. The next step consists of determining the ventricular rate. If the ventricular rate is faster than the SVT limit (the median RR interval must be less than the SVT limit interval), PR Logic is bypassed and only the RR interval-based detection of VT/FVT/VF is applied. If the median RR interval is ≥ SVT limit, a stepwise approach is enabled by applying and combining different algorithmic criteria, beginning with the double tachycardia criteria, followed by SVT criteria, and eventually, the RR interval-based criterion as follows:

1. Double tachycardia (VT/VF + SVT: therapy delivered)

   PR Logic will identify a double tachycardia using the following set of discriminators:

- Median RR interval ≥ SVT limit
- AF evidence recognized (AF evidence counter)
- PR dissociation

a. For the detection of a double tachycardia (VT + SVT) in the VT zone (or FVT via VT zone), RR regularity (> 75%) is also required (modesum ≥ 14/18)

b. For a double tachycardia in the VF zone (or FVT via VF zone), RR regularity is not part of a detection algorithm because true VF usually has an irregular pattern.

2. AF/Aflutter (SVT: therapy withheld)
PR Logic will define an AF/Aflutter SVT if one of the following 2 sets of elements are simultaneously satisfied:

a. Irregularly conducted (AF)

- Median RR interval ≥ SVT limit
- AF/Aflutter with specific PR pattern or AF evidence (no repeating couple code patterns)
- RR regularity ≤ 50% (modesum ≤ 9/18)
- Median PP interval < 0.94 median RR interval (atrial rate is at least 6% faster than the ventricular rate)
- FFRW not met (< 10/12 FFRW)

b. Regularly conducted (Atrial Flutter)

- Median RR interval ≥ SVT limit
- AF/Aflutter specific PR pattern recognized
- FFRW not met (< 10/12 FFRW)

3. ST (SVT: therapy withheld)
PR Logic will detect a ST for ventricular rates that fall within the range programmed when the following set of criteria are simultaneously met:

- Median RR interval ≥ SVT limit
- PR pattern with 1:1 rhythm detected and the intervening P event falling in the antegrade region of the RR interval (ST pattern)
- or ST with FFRW pattern if ≥10/12 FFRWs (or ≥ 4/12 in Gem III DR)

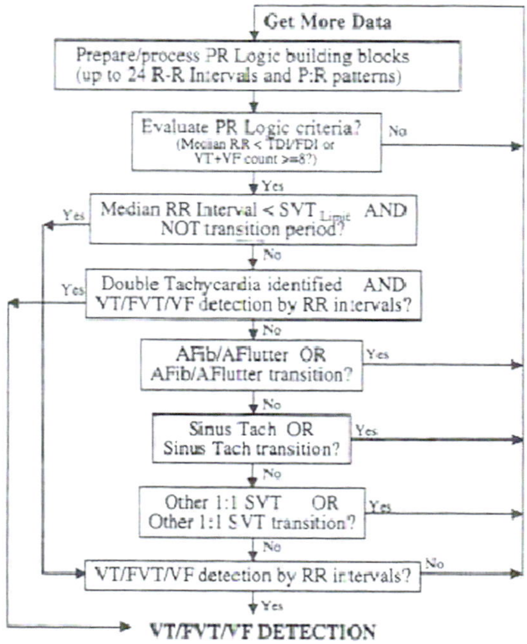

Fig 16.5 PR Logic computational flow diagram. See text for more details. (Adapted from Gillberg and Olson.[8])

4. Other 1:1 SVTs (1:1 rhythm with A:V relationship consistent with junctional tachycardia, atrial tachycardia or AVNRT)

- Median RR interval ≥ SVT limit
- Other 1:1 SVT pattern (A event recorded 80 ms before a ventricular event or l < 50 ms after a ventricular event)

5. Unknown Tachycardia (VT/FVT/VF: Therapy delivered)

If PR Logic is unable to identify a double tachycardia or an SVT, the rhythm will be classified as VT/FVT/VF and will be treated with the corresponding programmed therapy.

A new adaptive interval-based algorithm for ST detection is now available in EnTrust devices and more recent models.[10,11] This algorithm was developed in response to studies that suggested ST or atrial tachycardia (AT) with gradual onset and long PR intervals and ST or AT with intermittent atrial oversensing of far-field R waves were the most common causes of inappropriate therapy, accounting for 57% inappropriate VT/VF therapies.[1,10,12] Enhancements to the ST algorithm[12] in Gem III DR devices[8] eliminated 70% of inappropriately detected SVTs, but at the expense of a 0.8% loss in sensitivity to detect VT/VF, especially VT with 1:1 retrograde conduction.

The rationale behind this algorithm relies on the fact that a consistent pattern or slight changes in RR intervals or intrinsic PR intervals (ie, similar to sudden onset or AV dissociation, respectively) and 1:1 conduction support ST. To protect against misclassification due to intermittent ectopy, pacing interventions, and sensing errors, an expected range for RR and PR intervals is constructed based on a recent history of 1:1 AV conduction, updated on each interval which falls within twice the RR interval expected range (mean ± 2 standard deviations) (Fig 16.6). The adaptive ST algorithm operates only on P-and R-wave interval information, eliminating the need to adjust the VT/ST boundary. The algorithm uses a combination of 1:1 AV conduction pattern, gradual changes in RR intervals, and gradual changes in intrinsic PR intervals.

The **first step** is to establish whether there is *1:1 AV conduction*. Each RR interval is declared as having 1:1 AV conduction if one paced or sensed atrial event is contained in the RR interval, or if there are two paced or sensed atrial events in the RR interval with a consistent pattern of FFRWs (involving at least 4 of the last 12 RR intervals).

The **second step** is to determine whether the *current RR interval* is consistent with expectations based on the recent history of RR intervals. This step is similar to the common RR interval sudden onset criterion. The expected range is composed of a recursive estimate of the mean of RR intervals ± a recursive estimate of the variability of RR intervals, updated on each RR interval that has a recent history of 1:1 AV conduction. RR intervals that are longer than or within the range of "mean + variability" are classified as expected and increment the ST counter, whereas RR intervals shorter than this value are considered unexpected.

The **third step** is to determine whether the *current PR interval* is expected. Sudden changes in PR intervals are detected by comparing the current PR interval to an expected range. For RR intervals that contain 2 sensed atrial events, the atrial sensed event that is least likely to be oversensing of a far-field R wave is used to obtain the candidate PR interval. PR intervals that are shorter or longer than expected are evidence against ST.

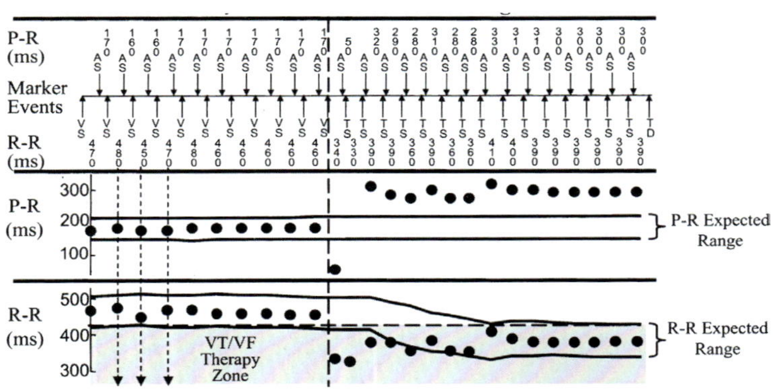

Fig 16.6 Adaptive ST algorithm behavior during spontaneous VT with 1:1 retrograde conduction arising during ST. After initiation of VT, RR and PR intervals occur outside of their expected ranges. The sudden change in RR intervals is small (460 ms to 390 ms), such that RR intervals during VT occur within the mean ± twice the variability range and adaptation of the RR interval expected range continues. Conversely, since PR intervals occur outside of twice the PR expected range, adaptation is inhibited and evidence of ST is lost by the third beat of VT. (Adapted from Stadler et al.[13])

The **fourth step** combines the determinations of *expected RR and PR intervals* into a statistic representing the accumulated evidence for ST. Strong evidence of ST exists when RR and PR intervals are classified as expected. However, evidence of ST must also be pertinent in the presence of pacing or ectopy. Therefore, the occurrence of pacing and determinations of expected RR and PR intervals are combined into 1 of 6 beat codes. Pairs of beat codes are used to build couple codes (up to 5), which are then incorporated in a pattern syntax that is continuously compared against a predefined pattern syntax for ST. Evidence for ST is maintained via an evidence counter which operates in a similar manner to the original ST algorithm.

Clinical Performance of Dual Chamber Discriminators

To assess the PR Logic detection algorithm, 933 patients with Gem DR devices were assessed, with 4867 episodes considered.[1] With ventricular cycle lengths between 305 and 400 ms, the relative sensitivity for sustained VT and/or VF was 100%, the VT/VF positive predictive value was 78.1%. The SVT positive predictive value was 100%. Enabling the algorithm reduced inappropriate therapy for SVT by 56%. Although the clinical incidence of SVT with long PR intervals is low (3%),[1,11] this may lead to inappropriately detected and treated long PR tachycardias. PR Logic was enhanced in Gem III DR and subsequent dual chamber ICDs to provide programmability in cases of "long PR SVTs."[10,12] In an analysis of 709 stored spontaneous episodes in patients with and without long PR SVT,[12] increasing the 1:1 VT:ST boundary to 66% increased the positive predictive value for VT/VF to 91%, with minimal risk of detection delay. When applied to the long PR population only, increasing the 1:1 VT:ST boundary to 66% reduced inappropriate therapies by 70%, with no loss in VT/VF sensitivity. In the overall population, the enhanced PR logic eliminated 32% of inappropriately detected SVTs, but at the cost of a 0.8% loss in sensitivity to detect VT/VF.

Relative to the original algorithm, the adaptive algorithm[13] appropriately withheld VT/VF therapy for 35% of true SVT episodes. For ST/AT with long PR intervals and ST/AT with intermittent atrial oversensing of far-field R waves, the adaptive algorithm reduced inappropriate therapy by 63.[13]

ST. JUDE MEDICAL DEVICES

Single Chamber ICDs

With ventricular-only detection, SVT/VT discriminators use (1) sudden onset, (2) interval stability, (3) morphology, and (4) bigeminal avoidance (nonprogrammable) criteria. Discriminators only affect initial detection. Importantly, a programmable parameter, "SVT upper limit," draws the highest boundary (the shortest interval) of the zone in which SVT/VT discriminators operate. It can be programmed from VT/VT1 zone + 5 ms to VF zone − 5 ms. Beyond this limit, the ventricular rate–only criterion applies, classifying and treating the arrhythmia as a VT/VF episode.

SVT/VT Discriminators

Onset
Onset is programmed as a delta in ms (fixed) or as a percent (adaptive) and measures fluctuations in interval measurements from nontachycardia interval to tachycardia interval. The onset criterion is activated when the first nonsinus interval average exceeds the cut-off value of the tachycardia zone. After each sensed event, an interval average is calculated and this value is subtracted from the average of the last 8 interval averages. If the result of *any* of the subtractions is greater than or equal to the sudden onset delta, the rhythm is determined to be sudden in onset and the qualifier posts a VT indication (Diagnosis). The sudden onset delta calculation is repeated for the interval average of all pretherapy detections of fast rhythms that are not inhibited by Bigeminal Avoidance (see later).

The window continues to shift to the right during detection until diagnosis or return to sinus. Once sudden onset is met within an episode, it remains met for the entire duration of the episode until sinus rhythm is diagnosed. It is a programmable parameter nominally set to 100 ms (or 18%), with values ranging between 30 and 500 ms (fixed) or 4% to 84% (adaptive).

Interval stability

Interval stability is programmed as a delta value. The algorithm measures the difference between the current *second* longest and the *second* shortest intervals. This feature does not use averaged intervals, but absolute values. If programmed to a nominal setting of 80 ms, a delta > 80 ms indicates that the rhythm exhibits identifiable variability among intervals, and AF is detected, whereas a delta < 80 ms indicates a regular ventricular rate (VT). The programmable values range between 30 and 500 ms. During detection, intervals within the Interval Stability Window (the nominal setting is 12) just prior to diagnosis are examined. Interval stability is re-evaluated upon each SVT diagnosis until VT diagnosis occurs.

Sinus Interval History (SIH) is a programmable parameter that provides additional evaluation of interval irregularity over time. It refines the diagnosis after the Interval Stability identifies the rhythm as VT by recognizing long intervals that have occurred during VT.

If SIH is programmed On (and Interval Stability indicates VT), then the number of sinus intervals or intervals with sinus interval averages since detection began (or since the SIH count was cleared) is counted. If this calculated SIH count is greater than or equal to the programmed value, then SIH, and therefore Interval Stability, indicates SVT; otherwise, Interval Stability indicates VT.

Morphology

Morphology is an additional parameter designed to determine whether the arrhythmia originates in atria or in ventricles. The morphology algorithm essentially operates with two indicators: the *matching score* (beat-to-beat evaluation) and the *number of matches and nonmatches* (rhythm analysis). Morphology uses a bipolar electrogram recorded from the rate sense electrodes of the ICD lead.

Matching score. The matching score requires a stored template that can be collected manually or automatically (Photon, Photon μ, Atlas [+], Epic [+], and newer devices), with auto update intervals programmable to "Off, 8 hours, 1, 3, 7, 14, or 30 days" if morphology discriminators are set to On or Passive. Automated update will not acquire a template if the ventricular interval average is faster than VT-1 cycle length or 500 ms, in Ventricular Noise Reversion, during Post Shock Detection or during pacing. If one of these conditions is present when the interval update timeout (eg, 3 d) expires, the update timer is reset with a postponement value of 8 h, after which it will try again.

Auto Update timeout verifies the current active template and keeps it active as long as more than 6/8 (80%) complexes match the template score. If not, it acquires a "Potential Template," which could become the active template if validated as representative of the baseline rhythm.

The device first tries to align the complexes by finding the dominant peak in each (largest amplitude). Complexes are considered aligned if polarities match. If the device is unable to align the complexes, the respective QRS complex is annotated as nonmatch. Once the complexes are aligned, scoring of the test beat proceeds by the summation of the surface of 4 peaks (Photon, Atlas[+], Epic[+]), or 3 peaks (Profile). To calculate the score, the areas of each of the 4 dominant peaks is calculated and the normalized differences between template and test complex are computed. A total difference is calculated, which is inversely related to the similarity percentage and reported as "% match" score (Fig 16.7). The smaller the sum of differences, the larger the % match score (ie, the more similar the complexes) and vice versa.

Number of matches and nonmatches. The number of matches and nonmatches are evaluated

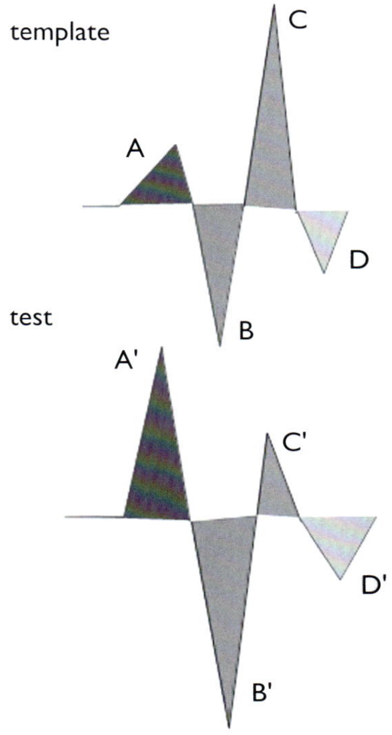

Fig 16.7 Percent match score is inversely proportional to normalized areas calculated as follow:

|area of A – area of A'| +
|area of B – area of B'| +
|area of C – area of C'| +
|area of D – area of D'|

in the Morphology Window (nominally set to 8) based on % Template Match Threshold. The number of matches is compared to the programmed threshold (nominally set to 5/8) which dictates a SVT diagnosis.

Bigeminal avoidance

Bigeminal avoidance is a nonprogrammable feature that protects against inadvertently treating ventricular bigeminy. It also prevents delivery of therapy during periods of T-wave oversensing. A particular Tach/Sinus Counter is activated, which is incremented by one for each VT/VF interval binned and decrements by one for each sinus interval and for each 2.0 s elapsed. If Tach/Sinus counter contains > 3 intervals a VT is detected and if < 3 beats are counted bigeminy is considered and therapies withheld.

Binning System

St. Jude Medical ICDs use two features for binning: the *current interval* and the *interval average*. The current interval measures the time in milliseconds between any two sensed or paced events. The interval average is the mean of the current interval and 3 prior intervals. When the current interval and average interval are the same, the interval is binned in the corresponding zone. When the current interval and interval average are classified differently, the interval is binned in the faster zone (Tables 16.2 and 16. 3).This provides a "smoothing effect" on detection. Once a sufficient number of intervals are binned according to the corresponding rate cut off, detection is satisfied. It is important to note that to satisfy tachycardia criteria, binned intervals do not need to be consecutive, so as long as sinus rhythm is not redetected, the counter will continue to increment. Because

Current Interval	Interval Average	Binned
Sinus	Sinus	Sinus
VF	Sinus	Not binned
Sinus	VF	Not binned
VF	VF	VF

Table 16.2 Binning in One-Zone Configurations with St. Jude Medical Devices

Current Interval	Interval Average	Binned
Sinus	Sinus	Sinus
Sinus	VT/VF	Not binned
VT	VT	VT
VF	VF	VF
VT	Sinus	Not binned
VF	Sinus	Not binned
VF	VT	VF
VT	VF	VF
VT-1	VT-2	VT-2
VT-2	VT-1	VT-2

Table 16.3 Binning in Two-Zone Configurations with St. Jude Medical Devices

the counters cannot decrement, the only way to reset the counter is by reestablishing sinus rhythm. Nominally, five (consecutive or non-consecutive) sinus intervals must be binned for an episode to be terminated, but this is a programmable feature that can range from three (fast termination) to seven (slow termination).

SVT Discrimination Timeout and VT Therapy Timeout

These additional counters are incorporated into detection algorithms. Exact terminology depends on the programmer version. "SVT Discrimination Timeout" (newer models) or "Maximum Time to Diagnosis (MTD)" (older terminology) is a "timer" that allows inhibition of therapy for SVTs for a programmable length of time, which starts with the first SVT diagnosis and more precisely with the first fast interval average equal to or shorter than the VT detection interval. Once this timer elapses, therapies are delivered. It has two components that can be programmed: (1) the maximum time allowed for the device to inhibit therapy due to SVT discrimination (nominally set to 30 s, range between 20 s to 60 min; it can be turned Off) and (2) the therapy that will be delivered when the timer expires, which nominally is VT Therapy. Importantly, this feature is never active in monitoring zones. SVT discrimination timeout is available only if at least one of the SVT discriminators is enabled or SVT discrimination mode is set to dual chamber. The SVT discrimination timeout timer stops and resets when it expires and therapy is initiated, when a VT diagnosis occurs or when sinus rhythm is detected.

"VT therapy timeout" (newer devices)/ "Maximum Time to Fib Therapies" (MTF) (older terminology) counter is another safety feature that pertains to VT. It is the maximum time allowed to treat VT before the device steps up to VF therapies. To trigger this counter, a diagnosis of VT must first be established. VT therapy timeout will start with first tachycardia therapy and after binning of an average interval shorter than the programmed zone, designated as the timeout zone.

If the tachycardia accelerates to fibrillation the device delivers fibrillation therapy in the normal manner, without requiring VT therapy timeout to expire. If all therapies have been delivered and the arrhythmia is not terminated, the VF therapies will only be applied after this timer expires. The VT therapy timeout timer is reset with sinus detection and it cannot be restarted during the same episode once triggered, expired, or reset. This timer is not available in two-zone configurations when VT therapies are disabled to create a monitoring zone. In three-zone configurations with VT-1 as a monitoring zone, this timer is available and starts after VT-2 therapy is delivered (Fig 16.8).

A careful appreciation of different counting principles as well as of their possible interactions is also required to avoid inappropriate ICD shocks. One common clinical scenario is binning faster intervals during ongoing SVT, during irregular rhythms such as AF or intermittent ectopy. If a pseudomonitoring zone is enabled (ie, Detection On, Therapies Off) one single

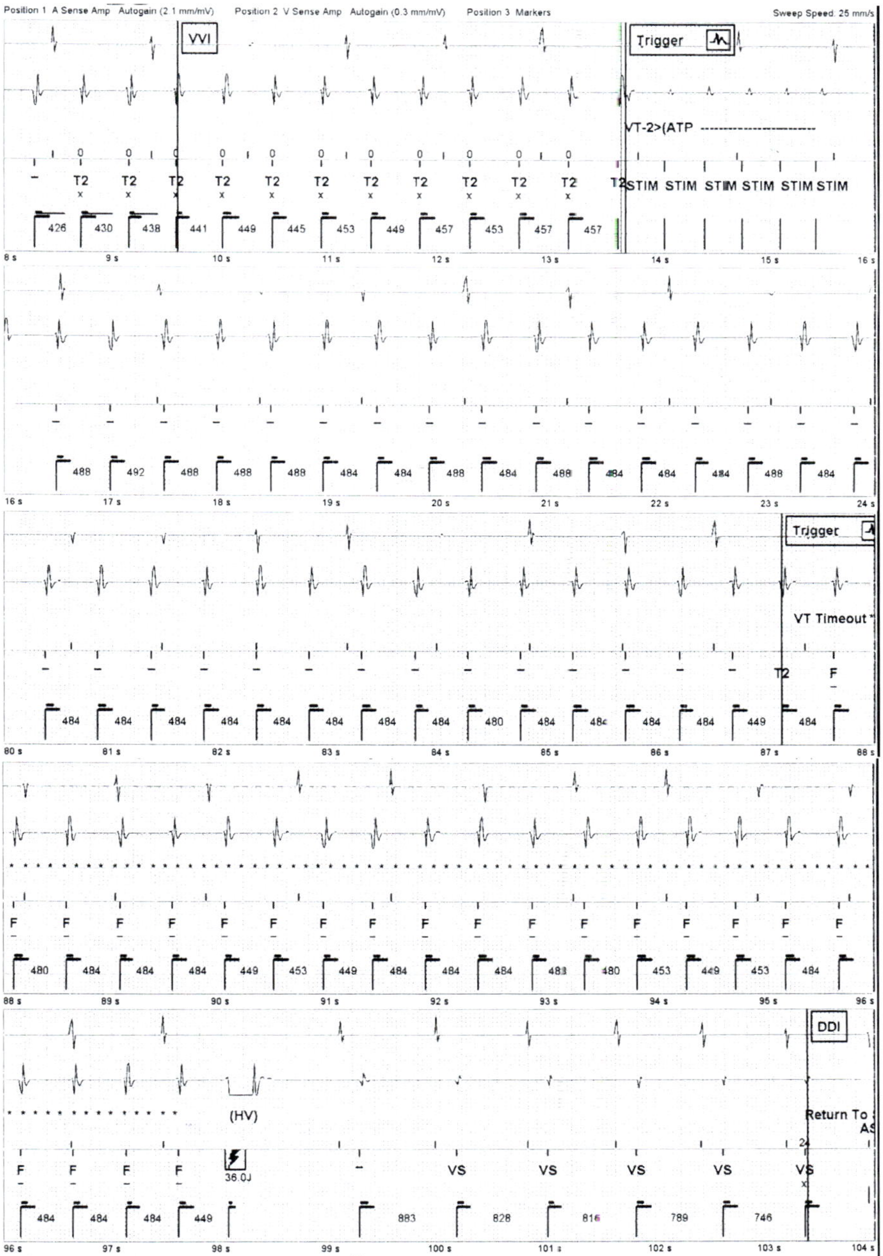

Fig 16.8 VT with AV dissociation and a mean cycle length of 455 ms. The device is programmed in a 3-zone configuration with a monitoring zone starting at 500 ms, a VT-2 limited at 460 ms, and VF for intervals < 330 ms. The ATP burst delivered to treat the detected VT-2 slows the arrhythmia into the monitoring zone, and it is therefore, nontreated. However, even if the redetection requirement to deliver therapy "Same as VT-2" was not satisfied, when the VT therapy timeout timer elapses, the device proceeds to programmed therapy for VF zone (episode annotated "F"), which restores sinus rhythm. Paper speed is 25 mm/s. The tracing is not continuous.

faster interval may trigger the MTF counter in older generations of St. Jude Medical devices resulting in an inappropriate therapy when this timer expires. For tachyarrhythmias detected in monitoring zones or for SVT following expiration of the SVT discrimination timeout, faster intervals during tachycardia (eg, intermittent ectopic beats or shorter intervals during AF) may trigger VT2 or VF counters[3] (Fig 16.9). Since these counters cannot decrement nor reset (not until five consecutive sinus interval are detected), counts continue to increment even if faster intervals are not consecutive and undesirable shocks may be delivered.

Redetection

If the arrhythmia continues after therapy was delivered, a certain number of intervals must be binned before the next therapy could be initiated (the nominal setting is 6 for VT/VF and is programmable from 6 to 20 for VT and non-programmable for VF). The post-VF/VT-2/VT-1 detection interval/rate parameter defines the new detection interval/rate required after therapy is delivered. This parameter is particularly useful in case of an ongoing arrhythmia in a higher zone that enters the monitoring zone spontaneously or following delivered therapy.

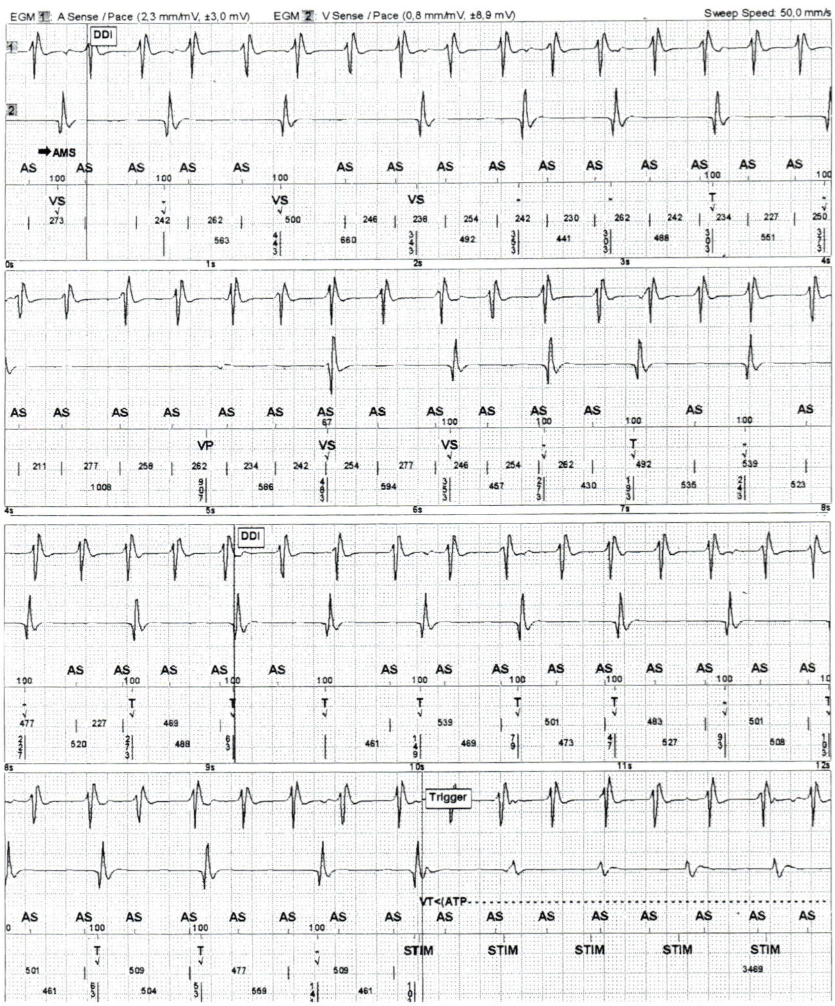

Fig 16.9 Inadvertent detection of a slow VT due to intermittent binning of faster intervals during ongoing AF. The VT timer is turned on with the first fast interval. Because the counter cannot decrement until 5 sinus beats are detected, it continues to increment. When 12 "tachy" intervals are binned, the counter is "saturated" and subsequent therapy is allowed. Paper speed is 50 mm/s.

In this case, the ICD may continue to treat the slowed arrhythmia, by delivering the next scheduled therapy in the corresponding zone if this interval has been programmed within the monitoring zone or upon expiry of VT therapy timeout (Fig 16.8). Therefore, the VF/VT-2 redetection interval/rate should be programmed "Same as VT-2" in settings with three-zone configurations and "Same as VF" in two-zone configurations.

Dual Chamber ICDs

Dual chamber ICDs operate with the following discriminators: (1) sudden onset, (2) stability, (3) morphology discrimination, (4) bigeminal avoidance, (5) sinus interval history, (6) AV association, and (7) AV interval. The principles of the first 5 parameters are similar in single chambered devices and are incorporated into a decisional algorithm along with AV interval and AV association discriminators, as depicted in Fig 16.10.

AV Association (AVA)

This function is ancillary to the stability criterion. It measures the PR interval for complexes in the "interval stability" window (default setting of 12 intervals). The calculated AVA value represents the difference between the second longest and second shortest AV interval. The algorithm compares the calculated value to the programmed AVA delta (programmable values ranging between 30 and 150 ms, in steps of 10 ms). If the calculated AVA is longer than the programmed AVA delta, the rhythm is considered dissociated (AVA "agrees" with stability), otherwise, AV association is declared.

AV Interval

This discriminator is enabled only when V = A. It operates as a "gate keeper," programmable On or Off: if set to On (nominal), fulfilling of this criterion is an absolute requirement to enter into the V = A rate branch. If the AV interval is set to On but not satisfied, or if it is set to Off, VT therapy will be delivered. This qualifier uses exactly the same algorithm as AVA but with a different programmed delta, the "AV interval delta." If this interval is longer than the programmed AV interval delta, the rhythm is dissociated and a double tachycardia VT + SVT with coincidentally similar rates is detected and treated; otherwise, ST or atrial tachycardia are considered.

Dual Chamber Algorithm Description

Dual chamber ICDs supplement the morphology discrimination (MD) criterion implemented in single chamber devices with atrial information.[14] This led to a considerable improvement in overall performance of the algorithm.[15] The AV rate branch feature was associated with significant improvements in both sensitivity (100% vs 97.9%, $p < 0.0001$) and specificity (84% vs 55.7%, $p = 0.0002$) for VT diagnosis when compared to a single chamber algorithm.[16] The system uses a hierarchical approach for tachyarrhythmia classification. After establishing the relative atrial and ventricular rate, the A/V rate branch algorithm classifies rhythms that fall within the tachycardia zone into three branches: V < A, V = A and

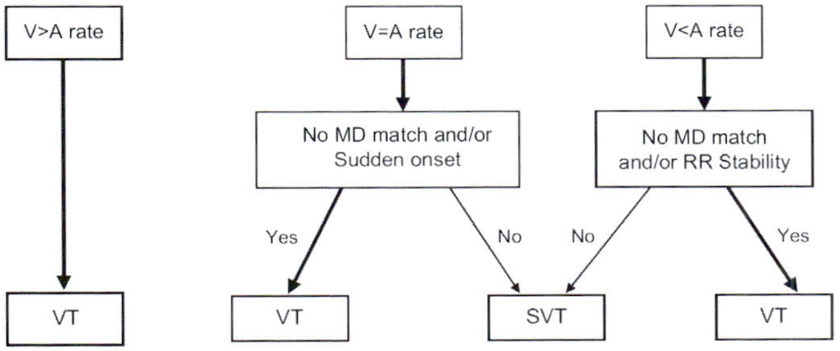

Fig 16.10 AV discrimination algorithm. Abbreviations: MD, morphology discrimination criterion; SVT, supraventricular tachycardia; VT, ventricular tachycardia.

V > A,[14,16–18] and subsequently utilize morphology analysis, onset, and stability criteria. Adequate utilization of discrimination information and overall efficacy of the algorithm is dependent on the initial sorting of the episode into one of the rate branches which, in turn, depends on accuracy of atrial sensing. Atrial sensing issues are the most common cause of failure of dual chamber discriminators,[15] occurring in up to 66%, and are predominantly due to atrial undersensing. Incorrect classification due to atrial sensing errors occur in 2%[18] to 4%[15] of episodes.

If V > A no other enhancements are applied and therapies are systematically delivered according to the corresponding zone. With V < A, the branch morphology criterion and/or RR stability will apply to distinguish between a rapidly conducted AF and a regular, morphological different VT arising during ongoing AF (double tachycardia). If V = A, morphology, sudden onset, and AV interval criteria are used to distinguish among the various diagnostic possibilities: ST, 1:1 conducted atrial tachycardia, AV nodal reentrant tachycardia, VT with 1:1 retrograde conduction, and double tachycardias (VT + SVT with nearly isorhythmic rates). If A = V or A > V, each of the two relevant discriminators may operate alone, or in combination using two types of logic:

1. ANY logic delivers VT therapy if EITHER discriminator indicates VT.
2. ALL logic delivers VT therapy only if BOTH discriminators indicate VT.

In the case of VT with 1:1 retrograde conduction, AV interval discriminators will indicate a nondissociated rhythm. Once the rhythm has been classified into the V = A branch, onset and/or morphology will determine the diagnosis. AV nodal reentrant tachycardia may be accurately diagnosed (SVT annotated) on the basis of the morphology criterion. However, the setting for this branch, including the requirement of either criterion ("ANY") for VT diagnosis, may result in misclassification as VT if sudden onset is satisfied. Therefore, careful optimization of device settings must be considered in such cases, with "ALL" criteria required for VT detection. Naturally, catheter ablation may be a reasonable alternative.

Morphology discrimination as applied in the Photon DR model has been assessed in several previous studies.[16,19] A unique feature of St. Jude Medical devices is the inclusion of the morphology criterion in the decisional tree of dual chamber algorithms. This discriminator may be fooled when used alone in single chamber devices if supraventricular arrhythmias conduct with aberrancy. The overall efficacy of the morphology discriminator to reduce inappropriate therapy without compromising device safety was assessed in both single and dual chamber devices.[19] Stored electrograms from 795 tachyarrhythmias in 106 patients (51 single chamber [Atlas VR-199 and VR-193] and 55 dual chamber [Atlas DR-241 and DR-243] ICDs) were assessed. Using the nominal template match of 60%, morphology discrimination alone provided sensitivity and specificity of 78% and 95% for single chamber ICDs and 63% and 92% for dual chamber ICDs. Combining

Parameter	VT-1 Zone	VT Zone	VF Zone
Rate (bpm)	90–200	110–220	130–250
Duration	1–60 s (nominal 2.5 s)	1–30 s (nominal 2.5 s)	1–15 s (nominal 1 s)
Redetection Duration	1–15 s	1–15 s	1 s
Post-Shock Duration	1–60 s	1–30 s	1 s

Table 16.4 Parameters for the Three Ventricular Arrhythmia Detection Zones

morphology discrimination with sudden onset and stability increased sensitivity to 98% with a specificity of 86% in single chamber devices. In dual chamber devices, the loss in sensitivity was compensated by rate branch analysis to yield an overall sensitivity of 98%.[19]

The optimal combination of discriminators to accurately distinguish between SVTs and VTs and to prevent inappropriate therapy while maintaining a high sensitivity was evaluated in a cohort study[18] that enrolled 203 patients with Photon DR ICDs. During a mean follow-up of 68 days, 596 spontaneous events were recorded and analyzed (252 SVT and 344 VT). All discriminators in the V = A and V > A branches were programmed On or Passive initially with nominal values (morphology discrimination threshold 60% [with 5 of 8 matches], interval stability 80 ms with AV association of 60, sudden onset 100 ms, and SVT upper limit same as VF). The morphology template was updated at least once every 3 days. Of 596 episodes, 11% were misclassified. The safest recommended programming to maximize specificity while maintaining a sensitivity of at least 99% was *morphology only in the V = A branch,* and stability *or* morphology *(ANY logic) in the V < A branch.*[18] This combination resulted in sensitivity, specificity, positive, and negative predictive values of 99%, 79%, 87%, and 98%, respectively.[18]

It is noteworthy that these results should not be generalized to ICD models preceding Photon DR.

BOSTON SCIENTIFIC (GUIDANT) DEVICES

With Boston Scientific single and dual chamber ICDs, algorithms proceed in the following order: Normal sinus → Detect VT/VF (8/10 beats) → Duration (6/10 beats) → Charge → Reconfirmation → Therapy delivery → Redetection

Binning System

Initial Detection and Duration

The detection window requires 8 of 10 fast intervals for zone detection to be met and 6 of 10 to remain satisfied (Table 16.4). Each interval is classified as either slow (ie, longer than the slowest VT interval) or fast (ie, shorter than the slowest VT interval) based on programmed rate thresholds. The Ventak Mini family is activated

	VT-1 Zone	VT Zone	VF Zone
Initial detection	Rate/Duration	Rate/Duration	Rate/Duration
Enhancements during initial detection	V rate > A rate AF rate threshold Stability inhibit Onset SRD RID if available	Stability accelerate	NA
Redetection	Redetection duration Stability RID if available V rate > A rate AF rate threshold	Redetection duration Stability accelerate	Redetection duration
Postshock redetection	Postshock duration Postshock V rate > A rate AF rate Postshock stability Postshock SRD	Post shock duration	Post shock duration

Table 16.5 Enhancement Criteria Applied during Initial Detection, Redetection, and Postshock Redetection. Abbreviations: RID, rhythm ID; SRD, sustained rate duration.

upon a first fast event longer than the lowest zone threshold interval. The Ventak VR/AV family, Ventak Prizm, Contak family, and Vitality initiate rhythm analysis after sensing 3 consecutive "fast" beats. Once this occurs, rhythm monitoring is in a "sliding window" of 10 ventricular intervals. Fast intervals in upper zones are also classified as being fast in lower zones and increment both counters. Every interval outside the zone threshold will decrement the counter by 1. Paced beats are considered to be slow and therefore will decrement the counter. Eight of the 10 most recent intervals must be considered fast for initial detection to be established and an episode declared. At this point, tachycardia is detected but not yet classified as sustained or nonsustained.

A second window is opened, the duration of which is programmable in seconds (see Table 16.4) and the episode timer starts. Throughout this period, if 6 of 10 intervals are considered "fast" with the last interval falling in the zone of detection, when the duration elapses, the detection is satisfied and the device proceeds to the programmed therapy. In the case of a monitoring zone, therapy is not programmed and, therefore, cannot be delivered. When the rhythm straddles two zones, for example, VT and VT-1, the highest zone where the detection window is satisfied will control therapy decisions. Whenever the sliding window no longer perceives 6 of 10 "fast" intervals, detection is no longer satisfied. At this point, another timer is enabled to confirm termination of an episode. If another 8 of 10 fast beats are not detected within this time interval (ie, 10 s if no therapy has been delivered; 10 s if ATP was delivered; 30 s after shock therapy) the episode is declared over.

Reconfirmation

Reconfirmation is the monitoring period performed during and immediately following capacitor charging. It only applies to noncommitted shocks and has two phases: during charge and after charge. During charging, the counter must maintain 6 of 10 fast intervals to deliver therapy. If 5 of 10 intervals are longer than the VT zone threshold, the shock will be diverted. Paced beats are classified as slow and therefore will decrement the counter. After charge, the 3 following intervals are analyzed. If 2 of these 3 intervals are outside the boundaries of the tachycardia zone, the shock will be diverted.[20] If there is no sensed activity within 2 s, a ventricular pacing pulse is delivered and shock is diverted (note: older models, Ventak Mini/Ventak AV, delivered the shock asynchronously in this situation).

Postshock

The programmable duration and detection enhancements available in the postshock period are listed in Tables 16.4 and 16.5. The postshock period starts 3 s after the first shock is delivered (non-programmable in newer devices; programmable from 1 to 3 s in older devices).

Redetection

The redetection period starts after the first therapy is delivered regardless of the type of therapy and is reactivated after each ventricular treatment. Similar to initial detection, 8 of 10 intervals must be detected within the VT boundaries. Once this requirement is satisfied, a second window is opened, the duration of which is programmable according to the corresponding zone (see Table 16.4). During this time interval, if at least 6 of 10 beats are classified as fast, an episode is declared sustained. Counters for fast intervals are not reset during redetection and the counting of the last 10 fast beats is made within a window that "slides" during a predefined period of time, such as 1 second for VF (see Table 16.4). Of note, if programmed in AAI mode, the atrial pacing is inhibited throughout redetection duration in order to minimize the periods of ventricular blanking which might impair VF detection; this feature might be of concern in sinus node disease patients. At the end of redetection duration therapies are delivered according to rhythm classification made during this period in a manner similar to initial duration detection. Enhancement criteria available during redetection are depicted in Table 16.5.

Overview of Rhythm ID and Detection Enhancements

Onset

This qualifier differentiates between monomorphic VT (sudden onset) and sinus activity related to exercise (gradual onset) and assesses how abruptly the cycle length changes from a "normal rhythm" to a rapid rhythm. It is available only in the lowest zone of multi-zone configurations. This feature is no longer incorporated in current Rhythm ID enhancement algorithms in newer models. It is programmable in ms or % (Table 16.6). If the clinician's intent is to deliver therapy, the programmed onset value must be set to a value lower than the measured value.

Stability

This criterion evaluates cycle length variability to differentiate stable ventricular rhythms from unstable rhythms. With the "stability-inhibit" function, if the measured value is greater than the established threshold, therapy will be withheld. The device automatically performs a stability calculation for all episodes, even if programmed Off, and reports the results in the therapy history. Programmable values are depicted in Table 16.6. Of note, stability values are fixed to 20 ms in DR Rhythm ID mode and to 30 ms in VR Rhythm ID mode. In addition, Boston Scientific devices have a specific programmable feature named "Stability-Accelerate" or "Shock if Unstable." If the measured delta value is greater than the threshold, the device will skip over remaining ATP therapies to initiate shock therapy. This is only available in the VT zone between bursts of ATP to monitor for proarrhythmia and rhythm acceleration from monomorphic (stable) VT to polymorphic (unstable) VT or VF. It cannot be programmed On

	VT-1 Zone	VT Zone#	VF Zone
3 zones configuration	RID if applicable V rate > A rate (N/A in Vitality 2) AF rate threshold (OFF/200–400 bpm)^ Stability inhibit (OFF/6–120 ms) Onset (OFF/9%–50%) SRD (OFF/10 s–60 min)	RID if applicable V rate > A rate AF rate threshold SRD	N/A
3 zones configuration (with a monitor-only zone)	N/A	RID if applicable V rate > A rate AF rate threshold Stability inhibit Onset SRD Shock if unstable*	N/A
2 zones configuration		RID if applicable V rate > A rate AF rate threshold Stability inhibit Onset SRD Shock if unstable*	N/A
1 zone configuration			N/A

Table 16.6 Detection Enhancements Available in Dual Chamber Devices. ^Exceptions: 250–400 bpm in Ventak AV models 1810/1815; 200 bpm fixed in Vitality 2; # settings are similar to VT-1 zone; * only if programmed alone (ie, it cannot be programmed On if "Stability-Inhibit" is programmed On); Abbreviations: N/A, not available; RID, Rhythm ID; SRD, sustained rate duration.

if "Stability-Inhibit" is On in the VT zone (in the case of two zone configurations) (see Table 16.6).

AF rate threshold and AF stability

The AF threshold feature is programmed in conjunction with the stability criterion (ie, Stability Inhibit) and aims to suppress inappropriate therapy for fast ventricular rates due to ventricular response to AF or Aflutter. If the ventricular rhythm is classified as unstable and the atrial rate is higher than the programmed AF threshold (200–400 bpm), therapy is withheld.

Each atrial interval is compared to the programmed AF rate threshold (Table 16.6) and classified as fast or slow. Atrial rhythm analysis begins when "Tachy Detection" is initiated (ie, after the third fast ventricular interval). In order to declare AF, 6 of the last 10 atrial intervals must be faster than the AF rate threshold at the end of "Tachy Detection" ("TRUE decision"). Atrial measurements continue throughout the duration, and as long as 4 of 10 intervals are faster than the AF limit, AF is still considered present. If therapy is not delivered, as long as 4 of 10 atrial intervals are fast throughout SRD, AF continues to be declared. If only 3 of 10 > AF Rate, AF is no longer present ("FALSE decision") and the device proceeds to programmed therapy. If the ventricular rhythm becomes stable[20] or faster than the atrial rhythm or, if SRD

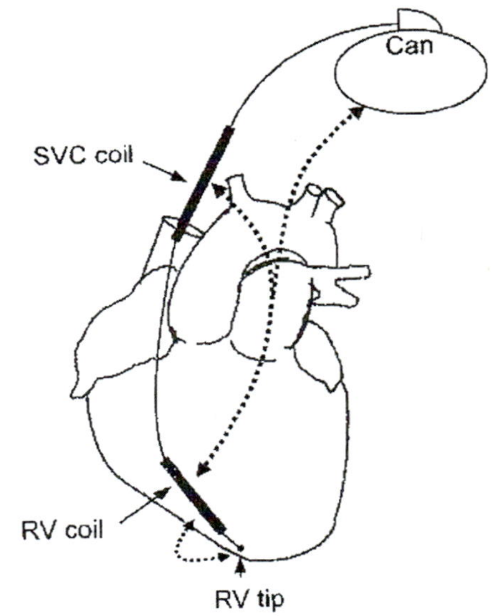

Fig 16.11 (above) Ventricular lead configuration. The rate channel signal is recorded between the right ventricular (RV) tip and the RV coil and the shock channel signal is recorded between the RV coil and the superior vena cava (SVC) coil + can. Adapted from Gold et al.[21] (Reprinted by permission of Boston Scientific Corporation.)

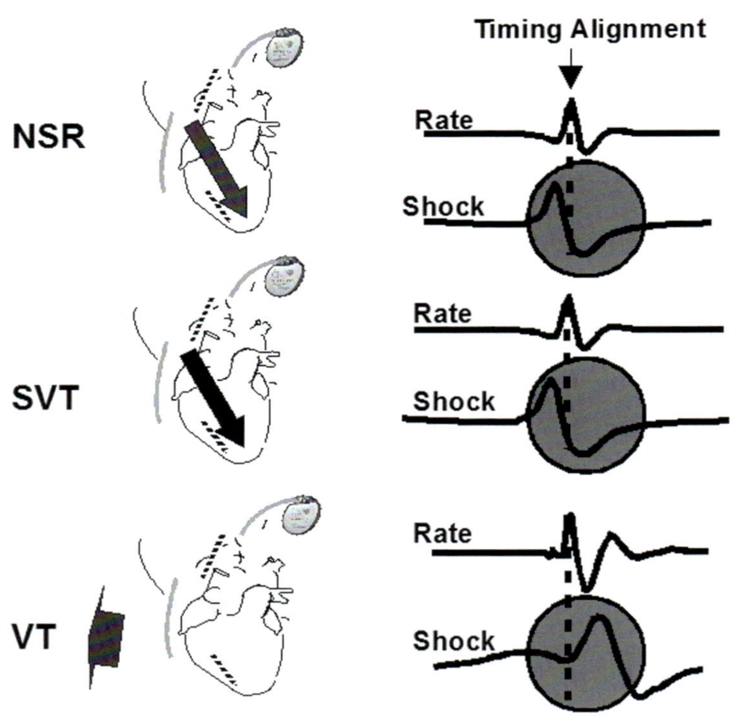

Fig 16.12 (left) Normal sinus rhythm (NSR) originates from the sinus node and has a conduction vector directed toward the apex. SVTs originate above the ventricle. The timing and shape of rate sense and shock EGMs are similar to the NSR template. For VT, the timing and shape of rate sense and shock vectors are different from the NSR template. (Reprinted by permission of Boston Scientific Corporation.)

elapses, AF is no longer confirmed and therapy is allowed.

V rate > A rate
This is a feature available only in the lowest zone configuration, when the discriminators are programmed On. Prior to the end of "duration," the device compares the average rate of the last 10 ventricular intervals to the average rate of the last 10 atrial intervals. If V Rate > A Rate by at least 10 bpm (TRUE), the other discriminators are overridden and therapy is initiated. If not (FALSE), analysis continues in a continuous running window. Therefore, therapy can be delivered any time after "duration" if the ventricular rate exceeds the atrial rate by at least 10 bpm.

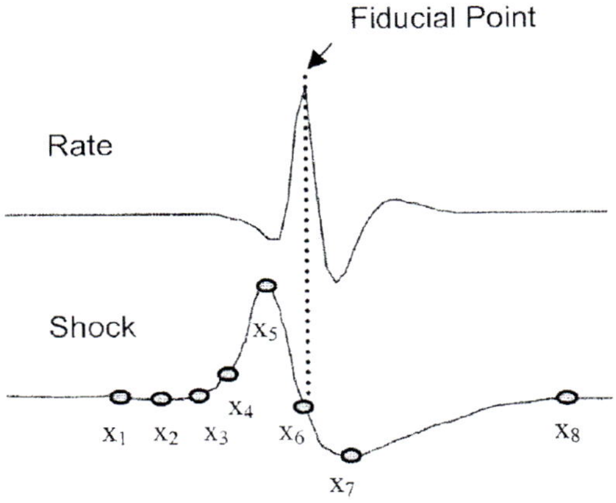

Fig 16.13 Reference vectors. (Adapted from Gold et al.[21] Reprinted by permission of Boston Scientific Corporation.)

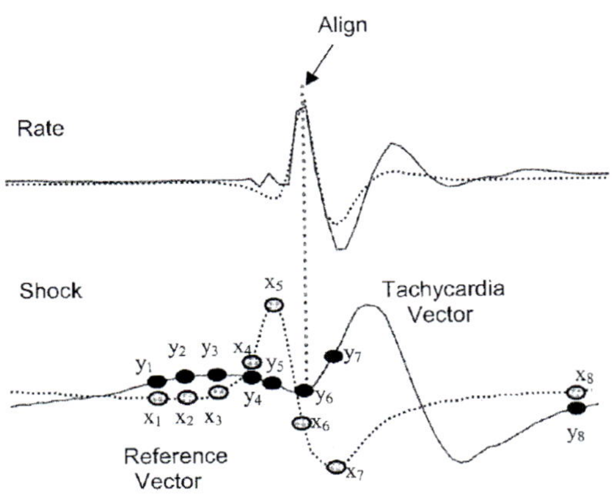

Fig 16.14 Rate sense and shock channel vectors from a template and VT complex are shown aligned by the fiducial points. Xi indicate reference vector and Yi indicate tachycardia vector. Dotted shapes indicate reference vector. Note the differences in both timing and conduction characteristics. (Adapted from Gold et al.[21] Reprinted by permission of Boston Scientific Corporation.)

Vector timing and correlation (VTC)
This is a feature designed to compare EGM signals for detected fast rhythms to stored templates collected during normal sinus rhythm. Two channels are used: local bipolar rate sense EGM (near-field) and shock EGM (far-field)[21] (Fig 16.11). The rationale behind this morphology algorithm relies on the fact that beats originating in the ventricle have different conduction vectors than sinus beats. Therefore, the timing and shape of the rate sense channel and shock channel will be different from the normal sinus template (Fig 16.12). Simultaneously collecting data from two different channels results in a more robust discrimination between normal and abnormal beats and facilitates diagnosis of ventricular arrhythmias.[21]

Three elements are incorporated in this morphology discriminator:

1. *Vector* represents the direction of the depolarization wavefront throughout the heart. The shape of the EGM on the shock lead is used as a reference.
2. *Timing* refers to the timing of the peak signal recorded on the rate sense EGM and the alignment of 8 characteristic points of the shock EGM relative to this fiducial point (including turning point, intermediate, and baseline values) (Fig 16.13).
3. *Correlation* consists in a comparison of the vector and timing of the fast rhythm to the stored template. Peaks on the rate sense EGM for each QRS of the unknown rhythm are aligned with rate sense EGM peak of the sinus template. Eight points captured on the shock EGM of the new rhythm and 8 points from the template are analyzed using a correlation equation which measures the similarity of the sinus reference conduction vectors and the suspected arrhythmia conduction vectors[21] (Fig 16.14).

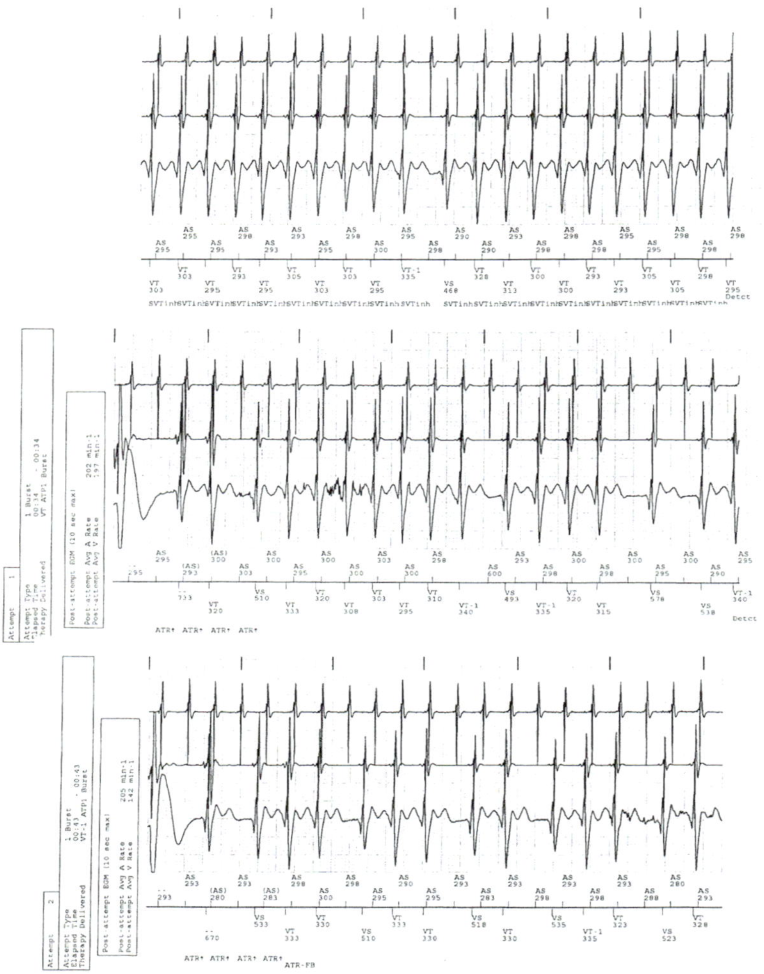

Fig 16.15 Supraventricular tachycardia with an average atrial rate of 202 bpm and average ventricular rate of 197 ms. Intermittent Wenckebach phenomenon occurs during arrhythmia. From top to bottom: atrial EGM, ventricular near-field (ventricular rate sensed), and ventricular far-field (shock channel) are shown. The device is programmed in a 3-zone configuration, with rate limits set to 140 bpm, 180 bpm, and 220 bpm, respectively. Enhancements for SVT discrimination are activated for both tachycardia zones and only during initial detection for the VT zone. The rhythm is appropriately diagnosed due to VTC correlation and annotated SVT (therapies inhibited); however, when the SRD timer elapses, the corresponding therapy is allowed. During the redetection period, which follows after the first delivered ATP burst, as SVT discrimination criteria during redetection are only applied in the lowest VT zone, as soon as 8/10 fast intervals are recorded, VT is detected and another 1-s window is opened to confirm the sustained character of the episode (6 beats within a sliding window of 10 beats). Upon delivery of the next programmed therapy (ATP burst), the rhythm slows and the rate criterion is no longer satisfied.

At the end of "duration," if at least 3 of 10 beats are correlated, the rhythm will be declared correlated and classified as SVT. If at least 8 of 10 beats are not correlated, the rhythm is annotated uncorrelated and classified as VT. VTC continues to classify rhythms on a beat-to-beat basis using a sliding window of 10 beats that begins at the end of "duration" and lasts until therapy is required.

The stored template may be updated manually or automatically. The device attempts automatic updates every 2 h 20 min. Some conditions must be met in order to successfully update the current template:

i. An intrinsic rhythm with AV conduction is required to accurately collect the new template;

ii. Ventricular-paced beats and PVCs (ie, beats with coupling intervals shorter than 85% of the average of the last four RR intervals) are excluded;

iii. Rate must be below 110 bpm and 5 bpm slower than the lowest tachycardia zone cutoff;

iv. Ventricular rate may vary within a range that extends to 150% of the RR average in order to allow updating the template during rapidly conducted AF.

If the current rhythm correlates with the template, the stored template will be retained.

If the current rhythm does not correlate with the template, a "candidate template" will be acquired using the average of the last 16 complexes. The new candidate template is then compared with the ongoing rhythm in order to verify whether it is representative of the patient's intrinsic rhythm. If a good correlation is found, the "candidate" will be stored as the new template.

Automatic update with fallback during update
This feature is initiated when automatic intrinsic rhythm update attempts have failed for 7 consecutive days. Temporary modification of pacing parameters (or Fallback) may be needed to promote the intrinsic rhythm. After verifying whether the patient is at rest, the Fallback algorithm temporarily switches off every dynamic or enhanced bradycardia parameter as well as tracking and rate response functions. It then gradually lowers the rate and makes decisions whether or not to update the template. If the Fallback attempt is unsuccessful, it will be reattempted every 27 h.

Sustained rate duration (SRD)
This feature represents the duration for which therapy is withheld by one of the described inhibition criteria (Table 16.6). The timer is initiated when a decision to inhibit therapy is made at the end of Duration. If the rhythm remains fast at the end of this programmable time period, the device will proceed to therapy (Fig 16.15). It may be reset if rate increases to a higher zone for which the detection criteria indicate VT, if any of the criteria that initially dictated therapy inhibition (ie, Stability, AF rate threshold, or V > A) is no longer satisfied or if the arrhythmia rate drops out (episode declared unsustained). It may be independently programmed during postshock period (Tables 16.5 and 16.6).

Antitachycardia pacing timeout
This function defines the maximum time permitted for antitachycardia pacing attempts prior to delivering programmed shock therapies. It is initiated once ATP is delivered and not when tachyarrhythmia is first detected. It is programmable from 10 s to 60 min or Off. ATP-timeout alone does not initiate therapies. Rate, duration, and detection enhancements must be satisfied in order to initiate shock therapy. Between each ATP burst the device analyzes the new rhythm by applying the corresponding redetection criteria while the ATP timeout counter continues to run. If the device establishes that this timer will expire before the end of the next burst, no ATP treatment will be delivered and the device will proceed directly to shock therapy.

Single Chamber Devices

In single chamber Vitality 2 VR (models T175 and T177) or dual chamber devices programmed in VR mode (eg, if atrial information is not reliable), Rhythm ID uses only two ventricular-based discriminators: (1) Vector Timing and Correlation alone for initial detection, and (2) Stability only during postshock detection (because of the concern for postshock morphology distortion) (Figs 16.16 and 16.17). In older single chamber ICDs, the available discriminators were stability and onset criteria.

Dual Chamber Devices

In the "Atrial View" algorithm implemented in Ventak AV devices (models 1821 and 1826), stability and onset discriminators were updated with atrial information ("AF rate threshold" and "ventricular to atrial rate relationship")[22] (Fig 16.18). Once a fast rhythm is detected, ventricular and atrial rates are analyzed. When "V rate > A rate," onset and stability criteria are skipped and therapy is systematically delivered. Otherwise, enhancement criteria are applied. If the ventricular rhythm is classified as unstable and the atrial rate is higher than the programmed AF threshold (200–400 bpm), therapy is withheld. If the ventricular rhythm is stable and the atrial rate is higher than the AF threshold, the device will assume that the analyzed rhythm is VT arising during ongoing AF and will deliver therapy at the end of Duration. If the atrial rate

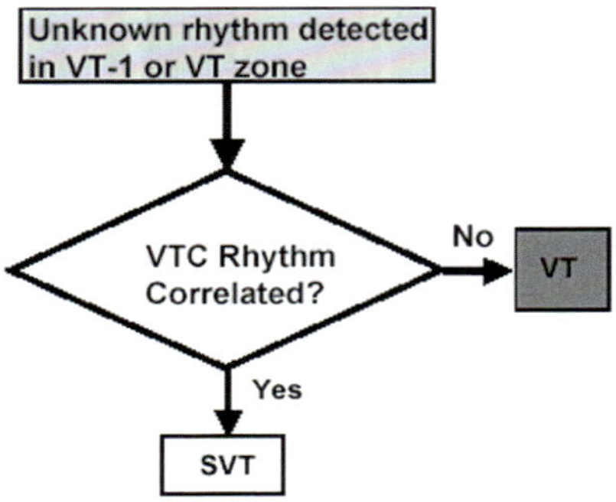

Fig 16.16 Rhythm ID VR—Initial detection. Abbreviations: SVT, supraventricular tachycardia; VT, ventricular tachycardia; VTC, vector timing and correlation. (Reprinted by permission of Boston Scientific Corporation.)

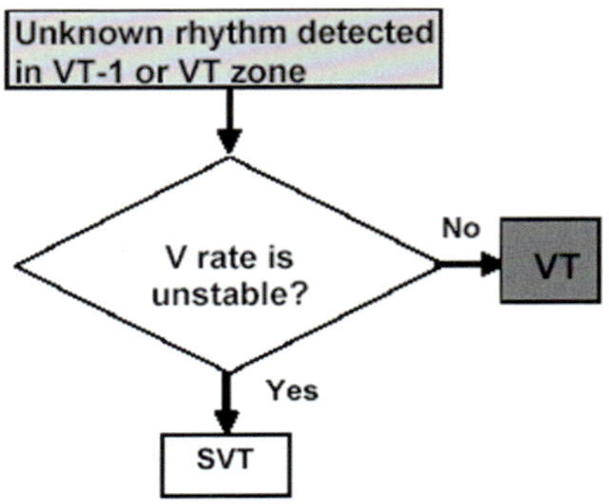

Fig 16.17 Rhythm ID VR—Postshock detection. Rhythm ID VR—Postshock uses a stability value of 30 ms alone to classify fast rhythms as SVT or VT. (Reprinted by permission of Boston Scientific Corporation.)

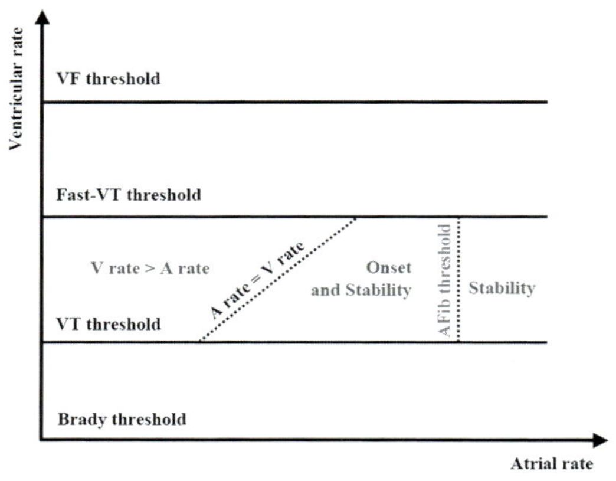

Fig 16.18 Atrial View Detection Algorithm. Note that enhancement detection criteria are available only in the VT zone. See text for more details. (Adapted from Kouakam et al.[23] Reprinted by permission of Boston Scientific Corporation.)

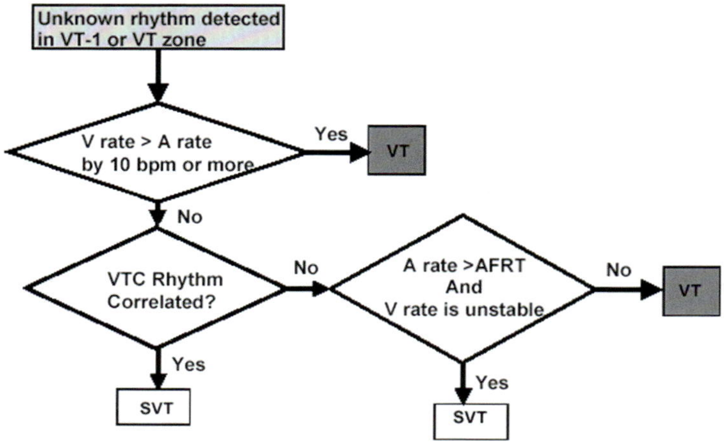

Fig 16.19 Rhythm ID DR—Initial detection Stability is fixed at 20 ms and AF rate is set to 200 bpm. Both must be met for inhibition. Abbreviations: AFRT, atrial fibrillation rate threshold; SVT, supraventricular tachycardia; VT, ventricular tachycardia; VTC, vector timing and correlation. (Reprinted by permission of Boston Scientific Corporation.)

is below the AF threshold, therapy may still be withheld if no sudden ventricular onset is detected (when onset criterion is enabled); otherwise, therapies are authorized. In a prospective study of 52 patients with Ventak AV II DR devices,[22] appropriate and successful therapies for ventricular arrhythmias were delivered in 23% during 3 months of follow-up, whereas 8% experienced inappropriate ICD therapies.

Onset and stability combinations are programmable in Ventak Mini/AV/Prizm/Prizm 2/Prizm AVT, Contak CD/CD 2/Renewal1/3/Renewal 3 RF, and Vitality AVT/DS/HE models.

Any (onset *or* stability) or both (onset *and* stability) of these criteria may be programmed. In the former case, VT will be declared if *any* of these 2 discriminators are satisfied; otherwise, therapy will be inhibited until the rhythm becomes stable, V > A, or SRD elapses. In the latter case, *both* criteria must be met to deliver therapy.

Performance of the Atrial View algorithm was further assessed in a multicenter study of 51 patients.[23] Programmed settings within the VT zone were RR stability, tachycardia onset, atrial rate, and AV relationship. Predischarge enhanced-detection algorithms were prospectively programmed as follows: stability 24 ms, onset 9%, AF threshold 200 bpm, and V > A rate. An additional sustained rate duration criterion was programmed to least at 30 s. In adjusted analyses, the algorithm had a sensitivity of 92% and specificity of 91%. However, this algorithm did not yield superior results to ventricular-only SVT discrimination.[24,25]

Boston Scientific dual chamber ICDs are now enhanced with "vector timing and correlation" (VTC), which has been implemented in the *Rhythm ID* algorithm, available in the most recent Vitality devices (Fig 16.19). Once an episode is declared and the duration has expired, Rhythm ID in DR mode uses atrial enhancements (V > A and AF rate threshold) with ventricular detection enhancement components (VTC and Stability). The algorithm first decides to treat any fast rhythm if V > A, bypassing any other enhancement criterion. If this is not the case, the morphology correlation (VTC) is assessed and a SVT is declared if the rhythm is considered correlated (at least 3 of 10 complexes correlated). If the rhythm is uncorrelated, the AF rate is analyzed. Therapy is inhibited if the atrial rate is faster than the threshold and the ventricular interval varies by more than 20 ms (AF detected). If A rate > 200 bpm, but stability dictates a ventricular rhythm, a double tachycardia is retained (AF + VT) and therapies are allowed. If the atrial rate is slower than the programmed threshold and the ventricular rhythm is unstable, therapies will be inhibited until V > A or SRD expires, or if rhythm becomes stable *and* onset was previously satisfied. This is an uncommon situation and the device assumes that the rhythm is undersensed AF and makes a decision to withhold therapies.

During Postshock Detection, Rhythm ID DR does not use VTC as a detection algorithm component because the morphology may be altered after shock delivery. V > A, AF rate threshold, and Stability are the enhancement criteria used as shown in Fig 16.20.

Performance of the VTC discriminator was previously tested in both single and dual chamber devices.[21] The VTC algorithm demonstrated accurate classification of both supraventricular and ventricular tachyarrhythmias. In a dual chamber configuration, sensitivity and specificity were 100% and 97%, respectively, with a PPV of 99% for detecting VT/ VF. All of the rhythms for which the VTC algorithm indicated that therapy should be withheld were indeed appropriately diagnosed, yielding a PPV of 100% for SVT detection. Single chamber analysis demonstrated 99% sensitivity for VT/VF detection and 97% specificity, with a PPV of 99% for VT and 97% for SVT.[21]

BIOTRONIK DEVICES

Biotronik ICD algorithms first classify RR intervals according to the programmed rate criterion. Classification is further refined using 5 adjustable functions that can be applied

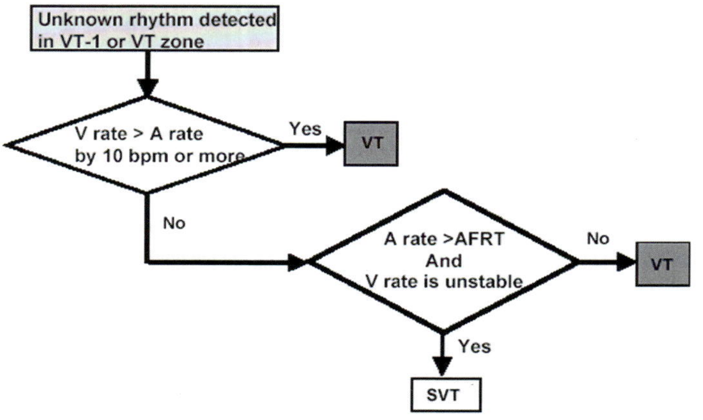

Fig 16.20 Rhythm ID DR—Postshock detection. Rhythm ID DR—Post-shock does not use Vector Timing and Correlation as a detection enhancement component. (Reprinted by permission of Boston Scientific Corporation.)

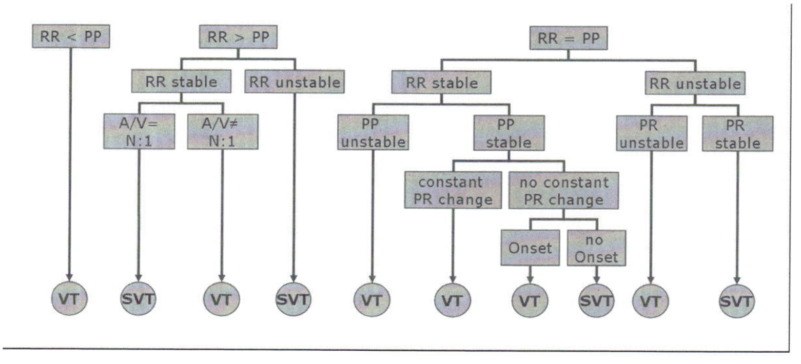

Fig 16.21 Stepwise analysis of detected tachycardia for each "branch" by the SMART detection algorithm. See text for further explanations. Abbreviations: A/V, atrial-ventricular ratio; SVT, supraventricular tachycardia; VT, ventricular tachycardia.

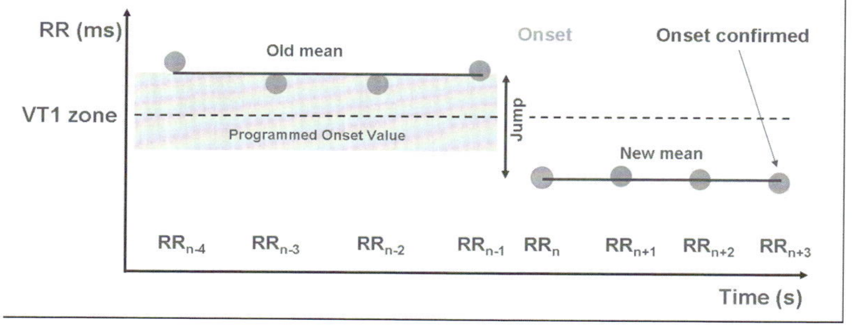

Fig 16.22 The onset criterion. Onset is considered sudden if the increase of the current average RR value (computed from the first 4 consecutive beats that fall within the VT zone) relative to previous average value (calculated from the last 4 preceding intervals) is greater than the programmed value.

depending on the type of ICD (single or dual chamber ICD): (1) detection counters; (2) onset; (3) stability; (4) sustained VT timer; and (5) SMART detection with DR and CRT devices.

Dual Chamber ICDS

Dual chamber Biotronik devices use the SMART detection algorithm to discriminate between SVT and VT. The SMART detection algorithm may be selectively applied to VT-1 and VT-2 arrhythmia classes. Any short interval for which the SMART decision is VT will increment its respective counter as well as counters set to lower levels. If SMART detection is only enabled in one zone, an interval falling in that zone for which SMART decision is VT will only increase its respective counter. The SMART detection and discrimination criteria apply only in VT zone during initial detection and redetection. This is different from single chamber devices, in which SVT discriminators (onset and stability) are only available for initial detection.

The SMART detection algorithm uses a series of six elements continuously evaluated

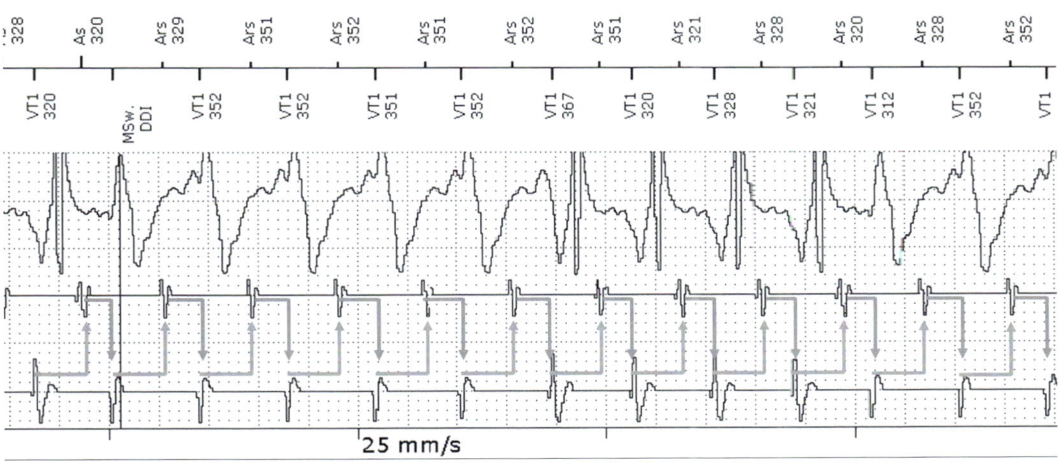

Fig 16.23 Polymorphic VT. The analyzed rhythm exhibits a 1:1 atrial to ventricular relationship and an unstable RR pattern. The stability of the PR interval is further analyzed, which in this case dictates a ventricular rhythm (unstable PR).

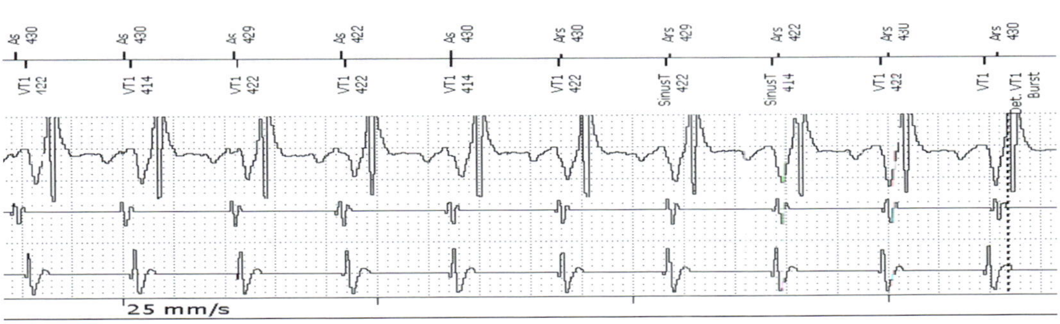

Fig 16.24 VT arising during ongoing ST. The analyzed rhythm has a 1:1 atrial to ventricular ratio with isorhythmic rates. As RR intervals and PP intervals are stable, the algorithm further applies the PR trend criterion. A monotonous decrease followed by a monotonous increase of PR intervals leads to VT diagnosis.

on a beat-to-beat basis and incorporated in a decision tree: (1) rate-interval; (2) stability; (3) onset; (4) AV regularity; (5) AV trend; and (6) multiplicity.

Rate Interval

SMART detection for VT begins when an interval falls within the VT zone as in single chamber devices. The interval average is computed as a mean of 4 most recent consecutive intervals and than updated on each interval on a beat-to-beat basis; this defines the sliding average intervals. Sliding average RR and PP intervals are continuously updated for each new event and are used to compare rates and compute adaptive parameters.

Stability

The stability applies to both the PP and RR intervals. When SMART detection is On, stability is nominally set to 12% (range: 8% to 48%). Each interval (absolute value) is compared to each of the 3 preceding intervals and the rhythm is declared stable as long as fluctuations of the last 4 fast intervals are within the predefined range of variation. The stability limit applies to both atrial PP and ventricular RR intervals. Atrial stability is only checked for 1:1 associated rhythms with stable RR (in combination with an atrial and ventricular rate comparison) (Fig 16.21). AF is essentially diagnosed using ventricular stability. Any atrial refractory-sensed event is taken into account for discrimination purposes.

Onset

Onset is considered sudden (indicating VT) if the increase of the current RR value relative to previous average value (calculated from the last 4 preceding intervals) is greater than the programmed value and is confirmed by comparing this last RR mean value with the current RR mean value (computed from the first 4 consecutive beats that fall within the VT zone) (Fig 16.22). The nominal setting is 20% (programmable between 4% and 32%). Once satisfied, it remains satisfied for the entire episode, except if there are 5 consecutive sinus/brady intervals that will reset the onset criterion.

PR Regularity

PR stability is used to check AV synchrony. A PR interval is considered regular if all 3 preceding intervals do not differ by more than a predefined limit (PR regularity limit) from the current PR interval. This feature helps differentiate the antegrade or retrograde origin of the recorded P event. This value is directly linked to the stability limit and is set by default to half the value, that is, 6%, reflecting physiological PR variations that might occur during irregular 1:1 conducted supraventricular rhythms. This feature is applied for unstable 1:1 conducted rhythms to differentiate between a SVT (relatively constant PR intervals) from a polymorphic VT arising during supraventricular arrhythmia or with 1:1 retrograde conduction (Fig 16.23).

PR Trend ("Monotonicity" of PR Intervals)

A PR trend is declared if the 4 most recently measured PR intervals are in strict increasing or decreasing order. This feature is used for 1:1 rhythms when an apparent link exists between atrial and ventricular events. If a monotonous increase or decrease of the PR interval is detected over 4 consecutive beats, the algorithm assumes that AV dissociation is present (Fig 16.24) as it is not compatible with a 1:1 conducted supraventricular arrhythmia where the PR interval is expected to be constant for a stable supraventricular rhythm. This feature may override the 20-ms tolerance of the previous rate comparison (indicating 1:1 rhythm condition). As RR and PP are both stable with 1:1 rhythms, this additional feature more precisely establishes whether the chambers are really associated or if two independent tachycardias are simultaneously running.

Multiplicity

This criterion applies for a stable tachyarrhythmia when the atrial rate is faster than the ventricular rate. Multiplicity between atrial and ventricular rates is declared when the average ventricular interval is found to be a multiple of the average atrial interval. This criterion helps differentiate a true regular VT arising during ongoing supraventricular arrhythmia from a regularly N:1 conducted Aflutter. N:1 multiplicity is met if $RR_{mean} - N \times PP_{mean} \geq$ tolerance (12 ms).

VT Sample Counter

The up-down counter is based on interval length and SMART detection decision criteria. The SMART decision is annotated for every single RR interval.

- It increments by 1 if in the VT zone and SMART detection decision criteria met
- It decrements by ¼ if ST is detected or a 1:1 interval in the VT zone
- It decrements by 4 for an AF interval in the VT zone
- It decrements by 1 if an Aflutter interval is in the VT zone
- It decrements by 1 for a sinus interval
- No change (freeze) for an interval in the VF zone

VF sample counter is independent from VT counters. An interval falling in VF zone will not increment the VT counter(s) (VT counters are frozen for 1 beat). Only when the SMART enhancement is deactivated (or with single chamber discrimination only) VF intervals will also count up the VT counter(s): if SMART is deactivated any interval falling in VT-1, VT-2, or VF zone will increment the respective counter as well as counters for zones situated at a lower level in the hierarchy.

SMART Detection Decision Tree

The SMART algorithm (see Fig 16.21) does not apply when the interval detected falls in the VF zone.[9] It can only be activated in the VT zone. The first step is the comparison of rates (or cycle lengths). The "tolerance" delta interval between the two rates (atrial and ventricular) that allows considering the two rhythms isorhythmic is 20 ms, "incorporating" physiological variations of the atrial rate and AV conduction. If the current interval is in the VT zone, the current mean of the last 4 RR intervals is computed. This value is compared with the average of the last 4 PP intervals and the rhythm is subsequently classified in 1 of 3 possible branches: (1) RR < PP; (2) RR > PP; (3) RR = PP. The 4 possible SVT SMART decisions are annotated AF, Aflut, ST, or SVT.

RR < PP (V Rate > A Rate)

Regardless of the diagnosis (ie, SR and monomorphic VT or SR and polymorphic VT) no further criteria are applied and therapy is delivered according to the corresponding zone.

RR > PP (V Rate < A Rate)

The first function analyzed is ventricular stability. If the ventricular rhythm is declared stable, diagnostic possibilities are VT and N:1 conducted Aflutter. To discriminate between these two, "multiplicity" is enabled and Aflutter with N:1 conduction is detected if this criterion is satisfied. If not, the VT counter is counted up. If the RR stability criterion is not satisfied and the V rate is slower than A rate, SVT is declared (eg, AF with irregular conduction or AT with a Wenckebach phenomenon). A higher weight of down-counting is used in this situation because of the concern for misclassifying rapidly conducted AF as a ventricular arrhythmia. Therefore, the counter decreases by 4 for 1 AF interval in VT zone.

RR = PP (V Rate = A Rate)

The first discriminator activated is ventricular RR stability. If the ventricular rhythm is stable, PP interval stability is evaluated. If RR is stable and PP is unstable, the diagnosis is not compatible with supraventricular arrhythmia (because an irregular atrial rhythm cannot drive a regular ventricular rhythm). Therefore, the device decision is VT and corresponding therapies are allowed. If the atrial and ventricular rhythms are stable and regular and there is a 1:1 relationship, the PR trend is analyzed. If a PR trend is detected (ie, an increasing or decreasing order), the device declares VT (Fig 16.24). The rationale relies on the fact that detecting a "PR trend" is not compatible with a 1:1 conducted supraventricular arrhythmia where the PR interval is expected to remain stable if the supraventricular rhythm drives tachycardia, unless a Wenckebach phenomenon occurs. With Wenckebach, a ventricular beat would be intermittently missing, leading SMART out of the 1:1 rhythm branch. In case of an atrial rate slightly slower or faster than the ventricular rate (but still within a delta tolerance zone allowing isorhythmicity), the PR interval may exhibit a consistently increasing or decreasing pattern. VT with isorhythmic AV dissociation (double tachycardia) becomes the most plausible diagnosis. Another alternative would be retrogradely conducted VT with variable Wenckebach-like VA conduction. Also in this case, an atrial beat would be intermittently missed, directing SMART out of the 1:1 rhythm branch.

With no monotonous pattern of PR changes, remaining possibilities are retrogradely conducted VT (1:1 association), or SVT with a relatively stable PR interval. Discrimination between these two entities will be made by the "onset" criterion. If sudden onset is detected, VT is diagnosed. Otherwise, an SVT is the most plausible alternative (ST or atrial tachycardia with a warm-up phenomenon and gradual onset) (Fig 16.25).

A unique feature of the SMART detection algorithm consists of delivering an active ventricular extrastimulus to determine which chamber drives the tachycardia.[14,26] ACTIVE SMART is no longer available in newer devices. If the tachycardia was atrial in origin, the PP interval will not be affected and therapy will be inhibited. If the following A event is advanced by a late PVC, VT with 1:1 retrograde conduction is the alternative. This function, however, may be fooled by a loss of ventricular capture and may theoretically be proarrhythmic.[17,26]

AV nodal reentrant tachycardia may pose difficulties. A VT diagnosis may be established, because there is a 1:1 associated stable rhythm with no AV trend and usually sudden onset. The PVC delivery may have been useful in this situation, but this feature is not available in newer devices. Catheter ablation is an option to consider.

Finally, if the ventricular rhythm is declared unstable and there is a 1:1 AV relationship, the stability of the PR interval is analyzed. A constant relationship between A and V events, reflected by a stable PR interval proves there is a linking between the two events with A triggering V, even if the resulting ventricular rhythm is irregular. SVT (ie, atrial foci with anterogradely conducted) will be declared and therapies withheld. In the opposite case, polymorphic VT (with retrograde conduction) will be diagnosed.

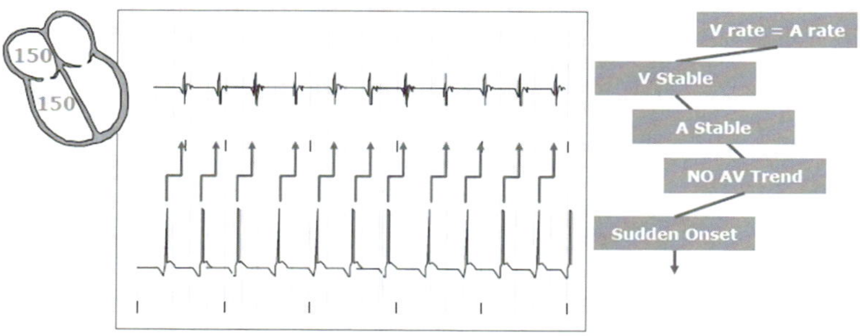

Fig 16.25 A 1:1 conducted rhythm. Both atrial and ventricular rhythms are stable. There is no monotonous increase or decrease in the AV pattern, so the onset criterion will dictate the origin of the analyzed rhythm: ventricular if sudden or sinus if gradual.

Redetection

SMART enhancements may be programmable during the redetection period. The default setting is On. This feature offers protection against additional therapies, particularly for chronic AF or for cases in which shock therapy induces AF. If SMART is deactivated during redetection, the ventricular rate–only criterion is applied with a specific redetection programmable counter. This is an up- and down-counter identical to the initial detection counter(s), with no inhibiting criteria applied, for example VT-1 and VT-2 intervals count up the corresponding redetection counters with faster zone (VT-2) intervals also incrementing the slower zone (VT-1) counter. An interval falling in the VF zone will increase VT-2 and VT-1 counters, as in single chamber discrimination, whereas sinus and brady intervals will decrement the redetection counter(s) by one.

The SMART algorithm may also be enabled during this period *after* initial VT detection if the safety timer has not expired, thus resulting in ventricular rate–only redetection. The SMART counter for redetection operates as follows:

- It increments by 1 for an interval falling in the VT zone
- It "freezes" if a given interval is in the VF zone
- It decrements by 1 if a sinus interval is detected
- It decrements by 4 for an AF interval
- It decrements by 1 for an Aflutter interval
- It decrements by ¾ for a 1:1 interval

Of note, SMART counts identically during detection and redetection, with one exception, the 1:1 branch, RR unstable, and stable PR (SVT detected). During the detection period, the counter will decrement by ¼, whereas during redetection the counter will be counted down by ¾.

The VF redetection counter is identical to the programmed "x" out of "y" VF intervals for the initial detection. VT, sinus, and brady intervals would not count up the "x," but will contribute to the "y" sliding window.

Forced Termination Timer

This additional timer applies when SMART is enabled for redetection. It is a programmable tool, by default set to 1 min and with programmable values ranging between 1 and 15 min or Off. When this timer elapses, all events are considered terminated, all therapies are reset, and the episode is annotated "Forced Termination." Forced termination is used to force termination of a ventricular episode following successful treatment of ventricular tachyarrhythmia, although termination detection (which requires 12 Sinus/Brady intervals out of a window of 16 intervals; not programmable) has not yet been fulfilled due to ongoing SVT (chronic AF) or therapy-induced SVT. This feature allows a new set of therapies to be available for the next ventricular episode. For example, if programmed Off in a chronic AF patient, after a successfully delivered therapy for a VT episode, no sinus rhythm will be redetected and the episode will not be declared over. If SMART is programmed On for redetection, the algorithm will successful discriminate and detect AF, but no termination detection would occur because the ventricular intervals (AF with irregular conduction) are not sinus intervals. If a new episode of VT occurs, it will be considered as redetection of the same episode, and the device will proceed directly to second programmed therapy. If this situation perpetuates, exhaustion of all therapies might be progressively achieved with no further therapies available for the next true ventricular episode. The most recent version of the algorithm also forces an atrial termination.

Performance of the SMART detection algorithm incorporated in the Phylax AV dual chamber ICD was assessed prospectively in 209 patients with 1245 sustained tachycardia episodes.[2] The specificity of the algorithm was 89.0%, with a sensitivity of 100%. The positive predictive value for SVT was 100% and the PPV for VF/VT was 94.5%.

Single Chamber ICDs

In single lead devices VT detection is based on rate criterion according to the programmed tachycardia zone. There are two counters acting as forward-backward counters, one for the VT1 zone and another for the VT2 zone which are enabled when the first interval enters the VT zone. The counter is reset with 5 successive slow intervals. With single chamber ICDs, Onset and Stability can be used to enhance VT discrimination. These two criteria can be used only in VT zones and only during initial detection.

When turned ON, sudden onset and stability criteria must be fulfilled for a given interval in the VT zone in order to increment the counter. If stability is programmed on, the VT-counter would be reset with every single unstable interval.

The ICD classifies intervals in the VF zone if a minimum number X of Y successive RR intervals are faster than the VF limit interval. For VF-detection, the default sliding detection window is 8 of 12 VF intervals and the respective counter cannot be decremented.

The sustained VT timer is an additional programmable safety timer available in both single and dual chamber devices that overrides the initial detection enhancements onset and stability or SMART and allows a redetection with the rate criterion only.

The timer starts with the detection of a single fast interval (VT or VF Zone) and is reset with arrhythmia termination or fulfilled initial detection. Upon expiry of the safety timer, a redetection counter is started using VT redetection counters for VT-1 and VT-2 to decide which therapy will be delivered, without inhibiting criteria (onset, stability or SMART are overridden). It applies to initial detection-only for VT zones with therapies activated and is not used during redetection.

SORIN DEVICES

The detection algorithm performs a stepwise analysis of arrhythmias. The rhythm is first classified on the basis of ventricular cycle lengths. Each tachycardia episode is then classified as supraventricular or ventricular on the basis of the stability of cycle intervals and the analysis of AV association and tachycardia onset. Therapy may be delivered if appropriate when the VT or VF persistence is reached.

Rhythm Identification

Cycle-Length Sorting

Sorin DR ICDs and CRT-D devices exclude the first 2 short ventricular cycles from analysis, in order to withdraw the unstable cycles often present at the beginning of an arrhythmia episode. Each ventricular cycle is classified according to its coupling interval into one of the following categories: SR (Slow/paced rhythm), Tachycardia, or VF. The algorithm measures the VV interval and compares it with two programmable boundaries: the VT cycle length (Tachycardia detection interval, TDI) and the VF cycle length. Each cycle is identified as follows:

1. *SR (slow rhythms) cycle* if the corresponding VV interval is longer than both the programmed VT and VF cycle lengths or ends by ventricular pacing. No therapy is available for this zone. A particular feature for Sorin devices is the possibility to program a slow VT zone in a range overlapping the upper rate limit programmed in bradycardia mode, without delaying tachycardia detection and with minimal loss in sensitivity to detect slow VTs.
2. *Tachycardia cycle* if the VV interval is longer than the programmed VF cycle length and shorter than or equal to the programmed VT cycle length; PARAD/PARAD+ discrimination only applies in this zone for dual chamber and CRT devices.

3. *VF cycle* if the intervals of the arrhythmia are shorter than or equal to the programmed VF cycle length. In the VF zone no discriminators are available, and shock therapy is the only therapy allowed.

A fast VT (FVT) zone may be defined in the VF zone, with its lower limit determined by the programmed value for the VF zone. In this zone, ventricular stability criterion allows delivering antitachycardia pacing first if the tachycardia exhibits a stable pattern (nominal setting for the stability window in this zone is 30 ms).

Majority Rhythm Identification and Persistence Counters

The "Majority Rhythm Identification" function uses two programmable parameters: (1) Y number of recent ventricular cycles taken into account and (2) X percentage of those cycles. A SR/VT/FVT/VF majority is identified if X% of the last Y cycles are within the boundaries of the respective zone. Nominal values for X and Y are 75% and 8 cycles, respectively. A majority requires at least 75% of the last 8 cycles (6) to exceed the cutoff rate zone and thus declare a tachycardia or VF rhythm. Rhythm classification is established and updated after each new cycle in a continuous running window containing the last Y cycles. Once VT majority is fulfilled, a persistence counter is turned On that requires 12 consecutive intervals. An extension was added to this counter to allow detection of AF if "search of a long ventricular interval" function is enabled (see later). The nominal setting for VF persistence is 6.

VT and VF persistence counters are independent. A VF majority increments both VF and VT persistence counters. The algorithm only resets persistence counters when it finds some other majority rhythm of a lower level (a SR or a SVT majority resets VT and VF persistence, and VT majority resets VF persistence). VT majority and persistence are required for initial detection and only a majority redetection is necessary after a first delivered therapy. The therapy for a given category (VF or VT) is only delivered when the last ventricular cycle falls within that category and if the corresponding rhythm majority is still met. This prevents delivering inappropriate therapy for a rhythm that just changed.

Sorin DR ICDs and CRT-D devices calculate the average rate over the last 4 cycles in order to apply programmed therapy for slow VTs or VTs at the end of the corresponding programmed persistence (nominal setting are 12 in both cases). If VT degenerates to VF, the device waits for VF persistence and then applies VF therapy.

Post-Therapy Detection (Redetection)

The post-therapy detection algorithm analyzes the rhythms detected after any therapy (ATP or shock). After a delivered therapy, persistence counters are not reset and the acceleration criterion is set to ventricular for the eventuality of a 1:1 VT triggered by ineffective therapy delivered on a nonaccelerated VT. Conversely, if after a therapy for dissociated VT the redetected rhythm is stable, with 1:1 association but a ventricular rate below 137 bpm, Sorin DR ICDs and CRT-D devices inhibit programmed therapies in the slow VT zone in order to prevent therapy delivery for a ST following an effective therapy. If these conditions are not satisfied and VT or VF are still confirmed post-therapy, the corresponding VT or VF therapy is triggered. An episode of tachyarrhythmia is terminated when a slow rhythm majority is detected and the corresponding episode is stored in the device's memory.

VT/SVT/ST Sorting: PARAD and PARAD+ Algorithms

Once a Tachycardia majority rhythm is identified, this diagnosis is further refined on the basis of several sequential criteria incorporated into the PARAD algorithm (P and R Arrhythmia Discrimination) (Fig 16.26). Six classification criteria are currently incorporated in the discrimination algorithm (Sorin DR ICDs and

CRT-D devices): (1) RR interval distribution; (2) PR interval distribution; (3) Long cycle occurrence; (4) AV association level; (5) Ventricular acceleration; and (6) Chamber of origin of the acceleration.

RR interval distribution and stability criterion

If a majority (X%) of the last Y cycle RR intervals is detected within the VT zone, ventricular stability is first analyzed by computing a histogram of these intervals. The RR histogram includes all RR intervals shorter than TDI contained in the last Y window (nominal 8 cycles) except for paced intervals. RR stability is present when the majority (nominal settings: 75%) of RR intervals included within the histogram do not vary by more than a programmable interval (nominal: 65 ms) and subsequent discrimination criteria are applied. Otherwise, the unstable ventricular rhythm is classified as AF, no additional discrimination criteria are required, and VT therapy is inhibited as long as AF lasts.

PR interval distribution and PR association

The algorithm uses the VV-interval histogram already constructed to assess AV association, and computes a PR-interval histogram for all cycles stored within the VV histogram. Up to 5 PR can be stored for each stored RR. Intervals < 47 ms are rejected as possible far-field R-wave oversensing. Like the VV histogram, the AV-interval histogram is scanned with a 65-ms stability window. For associated rhythms, the peak in PR histogram must contain a minimum number of intervals that must represent at least X% (75%) of the peak found in the RR interval histogram. For example, if 7 of 8 RR intervals fulfill the criteria of rate and stability, a minimum of 5 (75% × 7) PR intervals are required within the peak of PR to declare a rhythm as "associated" (Fig 16.27).

Long cycle occurrence (VT long cycle)

One of the most common clinical situations of inappropriate therapy is rapidly conducted AF, which may mimic a stable ventricular pattern

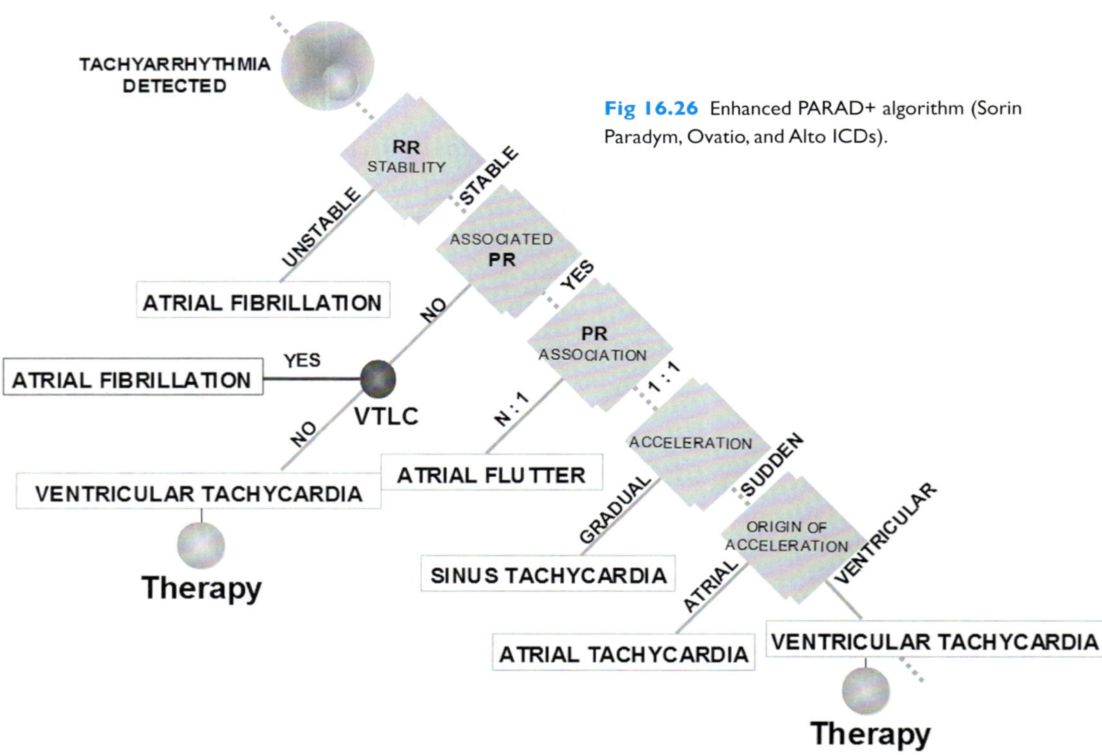

Fig 16.26 Enhanced PARAD+ algorithm (Sorin Paradym, Ovatio, and Alto ICDs).

especially at high rates. The PARAD algorithm only analyzes RR intervals exceeding the cutoff rate and thus may exclude intermittent long intervals. This feature offers protection against occasional ectopic beats with compensatory pauses, bigeminy, or intermittent under/oversensing but may prevent diagnosis of AF with fast and pseudostable ventricular rates. Careful analysis of retrieved tracings revealed a consistent finding—the occurrence of long RR cycles during AF, even in the presence of stable and relatively regular cycles lengths. This observation was exploited and added into the PARAD+ algorithm[27] available in both dual and single chamber devices (PARAD+ and Stability+/Acceleration, respectively, see Figs 16.26 and 16.28).

In dual chamber and CRT-D devices, if a stable rhythm is dissociated, VT is diagnosed unless a long cycle is detected. In the latter case, the rhythm is classified as AF with small variations in cycle length less than the programmed cutoff value and rare intermittent long RR intervals. A long VT cycle is defined as an interval longer than the average of the last 4 RR intervals within the Tachycardia or VF zone, plus a programmable interval: the Long Cycle gap (170 ms in nominal). No long cycle can be detected within the first 4 cycles of tachycardia. If the ventricular stability criterion is met and there is no AV association, the algorithm searches for a long cycle (VTLC) over the previous cycles (24 maximum, nonprogrammable). VT therapy is therefore inhibited as long as at least one VTLC is detected within the last 24 cycles.

VTLC persistence extension is a programmable number of cycles added to the VT persistence in case of VTLC search. An observation window of 24 cycles is opened, and therapy should not be delivered before the 28th tachycardia cycle, as the first 4 cycles are not analyzed. This duration is achieved with a VTLC

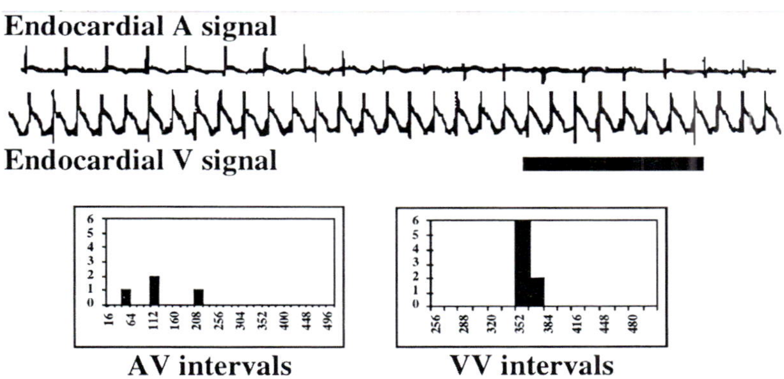

Fig 16.27 AV dissociation. The maximum number of AV intervals in any 65-ms window is three. Because the ratio of this number (3) to the number of stable VV intervals (8) is < 75%, AV dissociation is declared. (Adapted from Nair et al.[32])

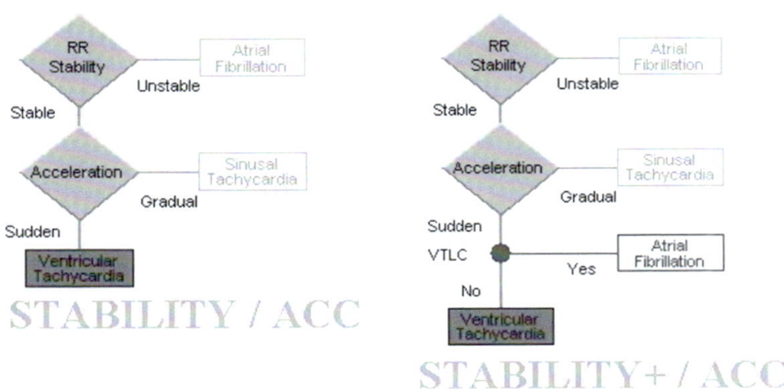

Fig 16.28 Single chamber discrimination algorithm.

persistence extension of 10 added to the nominal VT persistence of 12 and another 6 to reach a majority. The search for a long cycle is maintained until detection of SR majority, and it is also reset after therapy.

AV association level

If the rhythm is stable and associated, the level of association between atrial and ventricular events is further analyzed to differentiate between Aflutter with N:1 AV association and 1:1 associated rhythms. For example, as described previously, if 6 RR intervals are stable out of 8 stored and 5 *stable* PR intervals (< 65 ms variability between any 2 of these PR intervals) are within the peak of PR histogram, the rhythm is declared associated (5/6 > 75%). In a second step the device will look for the level of AV association. If at least X% of all PR stored intervals are included in the PR stability peak, the device concludes for a 1/1 AV association. If not, the rhythm is classified as N/1. So, in the example, if < 8 PR intervals are recorded in the PR histogram, the rhythm is classified as 1/1. If not, the rhythm is classified as 2/1 conducted Aflutter.

Ventricular acceleration

In the presence of 1:1 PR association, the algorithm examines the mode of onset in the ventricles. If the rate acceleration is gradual, ST is diagnosed. If acceleration is classified as sudden, PARAD/PARAD+ identifies the chamber of origin of onset and withholds therapy if in the atrium. A gradual acceleration is declared if RR interval prematurity is < 25% *or* if the RR interval exceeds the longest TDI, whereas a pathological acceleration is detected when RR interval prematurity is higher than 25% *and* the latest RR interval is within the tachycardia zone. In order to assess the prematurity, a given interval is compared to the acceleration reference and the difference is expressed in percentage.

In DDD mode, a ventricular beat is considered "conducted" if an atrial event is recorded in a preceding window opened between 313 ms and 31 ms (both excluded) before the recorded ventricular event. In SafeR mode, a beat is declared conducted if 1 intervening P event is recorded between 2 given R events. The acceleration reference is usually represented by the previous RR interval if it is a normal interval (conducted and nonaccelerated). When the previous RR interval is already accelerated, a ventricular pause (defined as a RR longer than 125% of previous RR) or a nonconducted beat (PVC), the acceleration reference is calculated as the average of the last 4 nonaccelerated RR intervals. A nonconducted RR interval may be included in the average if it is not accelerated (Figs 16.29 and 16.30). The algorithm requires two consecutive beats with a cycle longer than

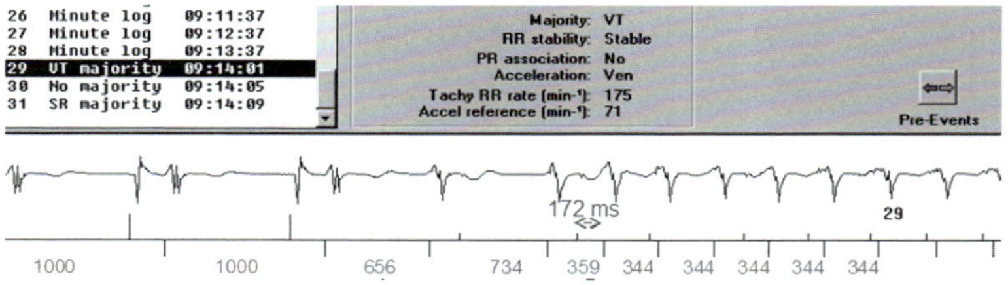

Fig 16.29 Acceleration criterion. The third (coupling interval 656 ms) and fourth beats (coupling interval 734 ms) are premature ventricular beats with no atrial event recorded within a 313 ms to 31 ms window before the ventricular event. While prematurity is more than 25% (ie, coupling intervals shorter than 750 ms), the intervals are not in the VT zone range (interval longer than TDI) and are, therefore, considered nonaccelerated. Even if these intervals are not conducted from the atrium, they may be considered when calculating the acceleration reference, because they are not accelerated. The 359-ms interval is the first accelerated beat conducted from the atrium because its coupling interval is < 75% of the average reference calculated as a mean of the last 4 previous nonaccelerating beats (ie, 734 + 656 + 2 × 1000 / 4 = 847 ms (71 bpm); 75% × 847 = 635 ms).

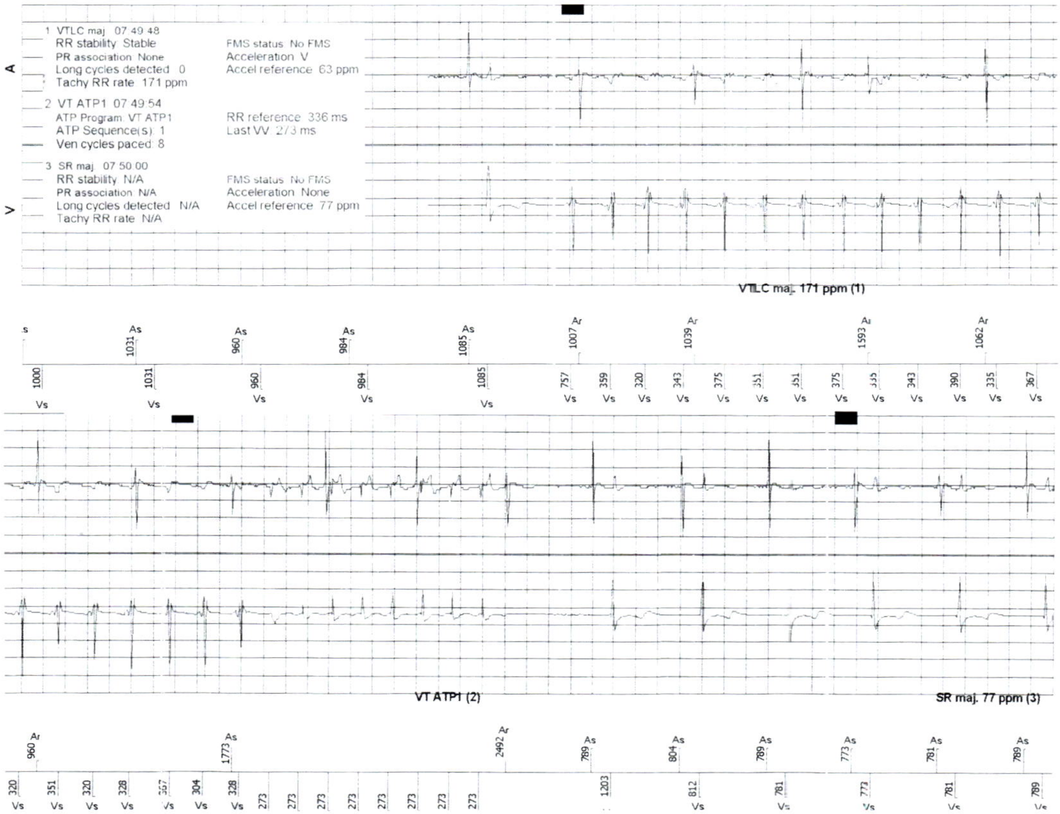

Fig 16.30 VT with AV dissociation. The rhythm is stable and dissociated so the algorithm enables VTLC search function. At the end of the persistence extension, ATP delivery establishes sinus rhythm. Of note, the acceleration reference is calculated as a mean of the last 4 nonaccelerated beats: (757 + 1085 + 984 + 960) / 4 = 946.5 ms = 63 bpm. The 757 ms interval is a nonconducted beat (PVC), thus it cannot be considered alone as a reference (it is not a normal beat), but it can be taken into account to assess the acceleration reference because it is outside the tachycardia zone.

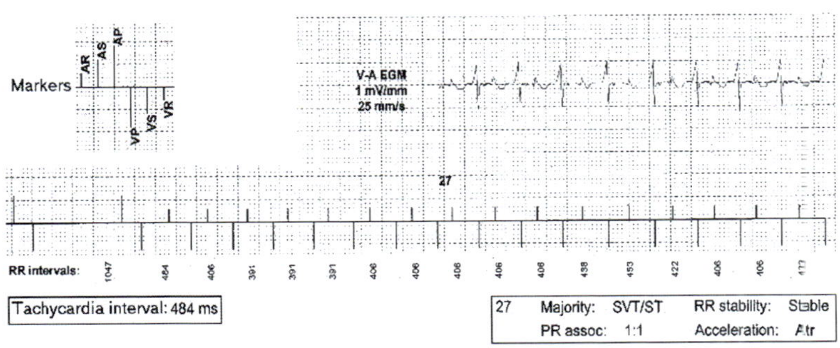

Fig 16.31 Atrial tachycardia in DDD mode. The rhythm is stable, 1 1 associated, and suddenly accelerated. The first accelerated beat (coupling interval of 484 ms) is preceded by an atrial event recorded in a predefined window opened before the ventricular event. The origin of the rhythm is declared atrial and therapies are withheld.

the longest tachycardia interval to invalidate the acceleration criterion.

Chamber of origin of the acceleration

In SafeR mode, the first accelerated cycle is classified as supraventricular if the 2 ventricular events are conducted *and* the RR interval is > 75% of the PP interval. In DDD mode, if the 2 ventricular events defining the first accelerated interval are "conducted," the origin of the acceleration will be declared at the atrial level (Fig 16.31). Conversely, if the first accelerated beat is nonconducted, this witnesses a ventricular origin for the analyzed rhythm (Fig 16.32).

In summary, a diagnosis of VT is established by PARAD/PARAD+ (Figs 16.26) if the rhythm is stable and:

- There is VA dissociation and no long ventricular cycle
  or
- 1:1 VA association and a sudden acceleration of the ventricular rhythm

AF is declared if:

- The rhythm is unstable
  or
- In the presence of stable dissociated rhythms with long ventricular cycles

Aflutter is detected if:

- The rhythm is stable
  and
- There is N:1 conduction from the atria to ventricles

Atrial tachycardia requires:

- Stable RR intervals
- 1:1 AV association
- Sudden acceleration in atria

ST will be recognized if:

- RR intervals are stable
- There is 1:1 conduction from atria to ventricles
  and
- The onset is progressive

Single Chamber Algorithms

Three classification criteria among the 6 described before are currently incorporated in the single chamber discrimination algorithm (Sorin VR ICDs): (1) RR interval distribution; (2) Long cycle occurrence; and (3) Ventricular acceleration.

In first generations of devices, the ventricular stability criterion was used to distinguish between VT and AF (Fig 16.28) with a cutoff

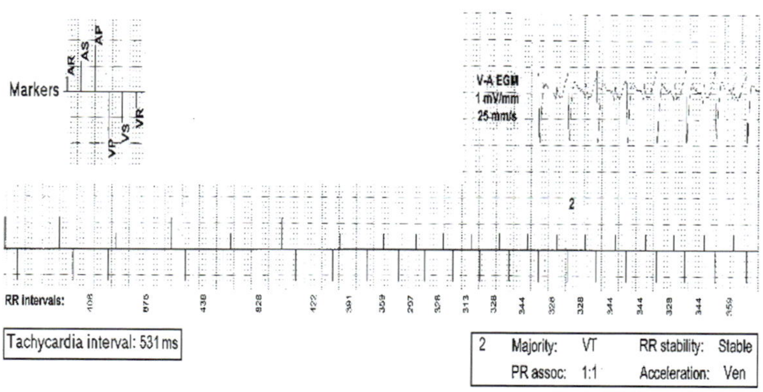

Fig 16.32 VT with 1:1 retrograde conduction. The rhythm is stable, 1:1 associated, and suddenly accelerated. The first accelerated interval (422 ms) is nonconducted because it is not preceded by an atrial event. The origin of the rhythm is, therefore, at the ventricular level.

value that could range between 16 and 125 ms (63 ms in nominal). A second level of discrimination was applied for stable rhythms by using the onset criterion (default setting for cycle length acceleration of 13%), which allowed differentiation between ST with gradual onset and VT. The enhanced Stability+/Acceleration algorithm was updated with the search of long ventricular cycles for stable, regular rhythms to discriminate between VT and AF with a fast ventricular response (Fig 16.28).

The performance of dual versus single chamber detection algorithms was assessed in a previous study,[28] which showed that programming a long TDI detection in dual chamber ICDs improved VT detection and did not increase the rate of inappropriate therapies despite a considerable increase in ST burden. The study questioned whether patients with monomorphic slow VTs benefit from a long TDI and a dual chamber detection algorithm compared with a conventionally programmed single chamber ICD. Patients with VT cycle lengths longer than 300 ms were implanted with a dual chamber ICD that was randomly programmed to a dual chamber algorithm and a TDI of 469 ms or to a single chamber algorithm with a TDI 30 to 60 ms above the slowest documented VT cycle length with enhancement criteria of cycle length variation and acceleration. A total of 1969 tachycardias were retrieved from 95 patients: 692 VTs and 1257 SVTs. Considering inappropriate therapies, number of VTs above TDI, or VTs with detection delay, a more-than-moderate superiority of the dual chamber mode was found. The sensitivity was 0.94 in the dual chamber mode and 0.82 in the single chamber mode and the specificity was 0.81 in the single chamber and 0.93 in the dual chamber mode.[28] The PARAD algorithm implemented in dual chamber ICDs was associated with a per-patient sensitivity and specificity of 99.8% and 91.6%. AF was responsible for 89% of SVT misclassified as VT. Thus, the PARAD algorithm demonstrated safety and efficacy to detect and treat life-threatening arrhythmia and maintained high specificity for SVT discrimination, particularly with respect to ST detection, while being less powerful in detecting AF.

To overcome the problem of AF underdetection, the PARAD algorithm was enhanced by adding a new discrimination criterion—long ventricular cycle search. A comparison between performance of PARAD and PARAD+ algorithms for tachycardia with ventricular rates < 150 bpm revealed a sensitivity of 96% versus 99%, specificity of 80% versus 93%, PPV of 94% versus 91%, and NPV of 86% versus 99%.[27] In the fast VT zone, the specificity and PPV of PARAD were higher than PARAD+ (95% versus 84% and 100% versus 96%). Thus, the major interest of the PARAD+ algorithm remains for the slow VT zone, where significantly increased specificity and NPV for AF were demonstrated. A frequent clinical situation remains the slow VT which may account for up to 30% of all ventricular episodes.[29,30] An accurate detection of arrhythmia in this zone requires programming a low boundary for tachycardia detection but this may lead to inappropriate detection and treatment of SVT, most commonly ST.

Specific to Sorin ICDs is the possibility offered in the detection configuration to program the lower VT detection cutoff at a value that can straddle the pacemaker upper tracking rate. Such a slow VT detection rate may be programmed even in pacemaker-dependent patients. This unique feature (BTO, Brady-Tachy Overlap) is due to the fact that paced ventricular cycles are ignored in the count of cycles necessary to fulfil the detection criteria without altering tachycardia detection.[29] Also, the maximum sensor acceleration has been limited to never be detected as pathological in case of spontaneous AV conduction.

The reported incidence of slow VT in ICD recipients varies among investigators from 8.7%[31] to 30%[30] when taking into account all episodes faster than 101 bpm and lasting more than 12 s.[30] Even if the clinical relevance and prognostic value of slow VTs does not seem alarming, they may cause symptoms such as syncope, palpitations, and congestive heart failure, leading to hospital admissions, especially in patients with a low ejection fraction.

The main concern when decreasing the detection rate is a potential loss in sensitivity causing delays in treating potentially life-threatening arrhythmias.

The safety and efficacy of the PARAD+ algorithm to detect VT with slower rates was assessed in several previous studies.[28–30] The overall specificity was 96% in a study of 374 patients, with a sensitivity that progressively increased with the tachycardia rate (93% for a cutoff rate of 101 bpm; 100% above 140 bpm).[30] Because slow VTs did not appear to be life threatening, the "low" sensitivity value was considered acceptable by the investigators. ATP efficiently terminated slow VT with a success rate of 90% and no deleterious effects. Similar data issued from a meta-analysis involving 9690 spontaneous events revealed 94% sensitivity for slow VT detection of 99.3% for VT/VF detection. The specificity for sinus rhythm/ST/SVT recognition was 94%, PPV 79.3%, and NPV 99.2%. Only 62 episodes were inappropriately treated by shocks in 40 patients, representing 5% of the overall population.

Conclusion

Over the past 20 years, ICDs have evolved into sophisticated and complex multifunctional units and are increasingly implanted for the primary and secondary prevention against sudden cardiac death. The various device companies have sought novel and creative technological solutions to appropriately detect and treat life-threatening arrhythmias, with intricate proprietary discrimination algorithms. Despite obvious and subtle differences in logic and language, the various device companies and models share a common underlying purpose: to appropriately recognize and terminate life-threatening arrhythmias while avoiding inappropriate potentially morbid therapies. Knowledge of the specific detection algorithms, their potential pitfalls, and particularities may assist caregivers in optimizing device selection, troubleshooting seemingly complex problems, and maximizing benefit while reducing associated complications.

Acknowledgments

The authors wish to thank Bernard Soucy (Medtronic), Pierre Veilleux (St. Jude Medical), Audrey Marineau (Boston Scientific), Armin Fariborz (Biotronik), Rémi Nitzsché (Sorin Group), and Marie-Claude Reid (Montreal Heart Institute) for their expert assistance.

References

1. Wilkoff BL, Kuhlkamp V, Volosin K, et al. Critical analysis of dual-chamber implantable cardioverter-defibrillator arrhythmia detection. Results and technical considerations. *Circulation.* 2001;103:381–386.
2. Sinha A-M, Stellbrink C, Schuchert A, et al, on behalf of the Phylax AV Investigator Group. Clinical experience with a new detection algorithm for differentiation of supraventricular from ventricular tachycardia in a dual-chamber defibrillator. *J Cardiovasc Electrophysiol.* 2004;15:646–652.
3. Mansour F, Khairy P. ICD monitoring zones. Intricacies, pitfalls and programming tips. *J Cardiovasc Electrophysiol.* 2008;19:568–574.
4. Wathen MS, DeGroot PJ, Sweeney MO, et al. Prospective randomized multicenter trial of empirical antitachycardia pacing versus shocks for spontaneous rapid ventricular tachycardia in patients with implantable cardioverter-defibrillators. Pacing Fast Ventricular Tachycardia Reduces Shock Therapies (PainFREE Rx II) trial results. *Circulation.* 2004;110:2591–2596.
5. Swerdlow CD, Brown ML, Lurie K, et al. Discrimination of ventricular tachycardia from supraventricular tachycardia by a downloaded wavelet-transform morphology algorithm. A paradigm for development of implantable cardioverter defibrillator detection algorithms. *J Cardiovasc Electrophysiol.* 2002;13:432–441.
6. Klein GJ, Gillberg JM, Tang A, et al, for the Worldwide Wave Investigators. Improving SVT discrimination in single-chamber ICDs. A new electrogram morphology-based algorithm. *J Cardiovasc Electrophysiol.* 2006;17:1–10.

7. Koyrakh L, Gillberg J, Wood N. Wavelet transform based algorithms for EGM morphology discrimination of implantable ICDs. *Comput Cardiol.* 2000;26:343–346.
8. Gillberg JM, Olson WH. Dual-chamber sensing and detection for implantable cardioverter defibrillators. In: Singer I, ed. *Interventional Electrophysiology,* 2nd ed. Philadelphia, PA: Lippincott Williams & Wilkins; 2001:523–569.
9. Swerdlow C, Gillberg JM, Olson WH. Sensing and detection. In: Ellenbogen KA, Kay GN, Lau C-P, Wilkoff BL, eds.. Clinical cardiac pacing, defibrillation, and resynchronization therapy. 3rd ed. Philadelphia, PA: Saunders Elsevier; 2007:75–160.
10. Wilkoff BL, Gillberg JM, DeSouza CM. The enhanced PR Logic dual chamber tachyarrhythmia detection algorithm. Retrospective analysis of supraventricular tachycardia with long PR intervals. *J Am Coll Cardiol.* 2001;37:131A. Abstract.
11. Wolpert C, Jung W, Spehl S, et al. Inappropriate therapy for sinus tachycardia with AV-block, I: incidence and implications for device programming in a new dual-chamber defibrillator. *Pacing Clin Electrophysiol.* 1999;22:A191. Abstract.
12. Gillberg JM, Wilkoff B, Cao J, et al. Enhanced PR Logic dual-chamber tachyarrhythmia detection algorithm. *Europace.* Suppl 2002;3:A253. Abstract.
13. Stadler R, Gunderson BD, Gillberg JM. An adaptive interval-based algorithm for withholding ICD therapy during sinus tachycardia. *Pacing Clin Electrophysiol.* 2003;26:1–13.
14. Aliot E, Nitzsché R, Ripart A. Arrhythmia detection by dual-chamber implantable cardioverter defibrillators. A review of current algorithms. *Europace.* 2004;6:273–286.
15. Israel CW, Gronefeld G, Iscolo N, Stoppler C, Hohnloser SH. Discrimination between ventricular and supraventricular tachycardia by dual chamber cardioverter defibrillators. Importance of the atrial sensing function. *Pacing Clin Electrophysiol.* 2001;24:183–190.
16. Bailin SJ, Niebauer M, Tomassoni G, Leman R. Clinical investigation of a new dual-chamber implantable cardioverter defibrillator with improved rhythm discrimination capabilities. *J Cardiovasc Electrophysiol.* 2003;14:144–149.
17. Swerdlow C. Supraventricular tachycardia-ventricular tachycardia discrimination algorithms in implantable cardioverter defibrillators. State-of-Art review. *J Cardiovasc Electrophysiol.* 2001;12:606–612.
18. Glikson M, Swerdlow CD, Gurevitz OT, et al. Optimal combination of discriminators for differentiating ventricular from supraventricular tachycardia by dual-chamber defibrillators. *J Cardiovasc Electrophysiol.* 2005;16:732–739.
19. Theuns DA, Rivero-Ayerza M, Goedhart DM, Van der Perk R, Jordaens LJ. Evaluation of morphology discrimination for ventricular tachycardia diagnosis in implantable cardioverter-defibrillators. *Heart Rhythm.* 2006;3:1332–1338.
20. Al-Ahmad A, Tsiperfal A, Hsia HH, Wang PJ. Inappropriate shock. A failure of SVT discriminators in a dual chamber ICD? *Pacing Clin Electrophysiol.* 2006;29:1413–1415.
21. Gold MR, Shorofsky SR, Thompson JA, et al. Advanced rhythm discrimination for implantable cardioverter defibrillators using electrogram vector timing and correlation. *J Cardiovasc Electrophysiol.* 2002;13:1092–1097.
22. Sticherling C, Schaumann A, Klingenheben T, Hohnloser SH. First worldwide clinical experience with a new dual chamber implantable cardioverter defibrillator. Advantages and complications. The Ventak AV II DR investigators. *Europace.* 1999;1:96–102.
23. Kouakam C, Kacet S, Hazard J-R, et al, on behalf of the Ventak AV Investigators. Performance of a dual-chamber implantable defibrillator algorithm for discrimination of ventricular from supraventricular tachycardia. *Europace.* 2004;6:32–42.
24. Theuns DA, Klootwijk AP, Goedhart DM, Jordaens LJ. Prevention of inappropriate therapy in implantable cardioverter-defibrillators. Results of a prospective, randomized study of tachyarrhythmia detection algorithms. *J Am Coll Cardiol.* 2004;44:2362–2367.
25. Deisenhofer I, Kolb C, Ndrepepa G, et al. Do current dual chamber cardioverter defibrillators have advantages over conventional single chamber cardioverter defibrillators in reducing inappropriate therapies? A randomized prospective

study. *J Cardiovasc Electrophysiol.* 2001;12:134–142.

26. Revishvili A. Dual-chamber implantable cardioverter-defibrillator with active discrimination of supraventricular tachycardia. *Prog Biomed Res.* 1999;2:166–171.
27. Mletzko R, Anselme F, Klug D, et al, on behalf of the "Slow VT study" investigators. Enhanced specificity of dual chamber ICD arrhythmia detection algorithm by rate stability criteria. *Pacing Clin Electrophysiol.* 2004;27:1113–1119.
28. Bänsch D, Steffgen F, Grönefeld G, et al. The 1+ 1 Trial. A prospective trial of a dual- versus a single-chamber implantable defibrillator in patients with slow ventricular tachycardias. *Circulation.* 2004;110:1022–1029.
29. Sadoul N, Mletzko R, Anselme F, et al, for the Slow VT Study Group. Incidence and clinical relevance of slow ventricular tachycardia in implantable cardioverter-defibrillator recipients. An international multicenter prospective study. *Circulation.* 2005;112:946–953.
30. Anselme F, Mletzko R, Bowes R, et al. Prevention of inappropriate shocks in ICD recipients. A review of 10,000 tachycardia episodes. *Pacing Clin Electrophysiol.* 2007;30:S128–S133.
31. Sadoul N, Jung W, Jordaens L, et al, for the Defender I and II Clinical Trials Investigators. Diagnostic performance of a dual-chamber cardioverter defibrillator programmed with nominal settings. A European prospective multicenter study. *J Cardiovasc Electrophysiol.* 2002; 13:25–32.
32. Nair M, Saoudi N, Kroiss D, Letac B, for the Participating Centers of the Automatic Recognition of Arrhythmia Study Group. Automatic arrhythmia identification using analysis of the atrioventricular association. Application to a new generation of implantable defibrillators. *Circulation.* 1997;95:967–973.

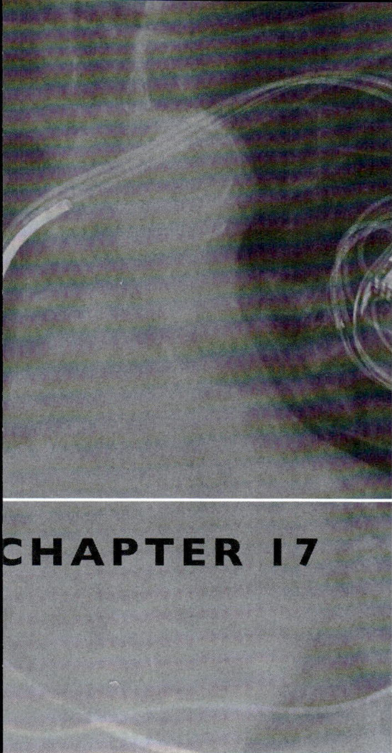

CHAPTER 17

Pacing with an ICD System

What Are the Issues?

Robert F. Rea

Introduction

Timing cycles in antibradycardia pacemakers are governed by the sometimes-competing demands of upper and lower pacing rate limits, cross-chamber sensing, pacing modes, and mode switching. In the implantable cardioverter defibrillator (ICD), complexity is added owing to the primacy of tachyarrhythmia detection and treatment in these devices. This can exert additional restraints on antibradycardia pacing algorithms. The purpose of this chapter is to review broadly pacemaker function in ICDs with a focus on timing cycle and clinical issues.

Single Chamber Pacing ICDs

ICDs in which only the right ventricle (RV) is paced and sensed account for about 25% of implants according to the National Cardiovascular Data Registry (NCDR) ICD registry. The simplest device in which the RV is paced and sensed without an activity sensor (VVI) has few limitations from a pacemaker standpoint.

Effects of Ventricular Tachycardia Detection Interval

ICDs with rate responsive right ventricular pacing (VVIR) mediated by accelerometer may have programming constraints if the upper rate limit for ventricular pacing is close to the slowest ventricular tachycardia (VT) detection zone. Such slow VTs are often seen in patients prescribed membrane-active antiarrhythmic drugs, agents that not only slow or suppress VT but also produce chronotropic insufficiency and thereby a need for rate responsive pacing.

Medtronic ICDs require that the shortest ventricular paced cycle length be at least 60 ms greater than the longest VT detection interval. Thus, VT detection set at cycle length 400 ms

Pacemakers and Implantable Cardioverter Defibrillators: An Expert's Manual. © 2010 Amin Al-Ahmad, Kenneth A. Ellenbogen, Andrea Natale, and Paul J. Wang, eds. Cardiotext Publishing, ISBN: 978-0-9790164-6-2.

would limit ventricular pacing to cycle lengths 460 ms (130 bpm) or slower.

In Boston Scientific ICDs, the fastest ventricular paced rate must be at least 5 bpm slower than the slowest VT detection rate. As in the earlier example, with VT detection set to cycle length 150 bpm (or cycle length 400 ms), the fastest ventricular paced rate would be 145 bpm (or cycle length 413 ms).

In St. Jude Medical (SJM) ICDs, the difference between the shortest pacing interval and the longest VT detection interval must be ≥ 30 ms. With a VT detection interval of 400 ms (150 bpm) the shortest paced cycle length would be 430 ms (139 bpm). A programmable discriminator designed to distinguish gradual rate increases (sinus tachycardia) from abrupt rate increases (VT) called "sudden onset" may exert an additional restraint on upper pacing rate. In SJM ICDs, if sudden onset is programmed On or Passive, the programmed value (30–500 ms [fixed] or 4%–86% [adaptive]) dictates the minimum difference between the longest VT detection interval and the shortest paced interval. Thus at the nominal sudden onset value of 100 ms (fixed) and a longest VT detection interval of 400 ms (150 bpm), the shortest paced interval would be 500 ms (120 bpm).

Sorin ICDs permit pacing at cycle lengths shorter than the ventricular tachycardia detection interval. The incidence of slow ventricular tachycardia (< 150 bpm) in ICD recipients may be as high as 30% even when there is no prior history of slow VT, (though the clinical relevance of such arrhythmias may be limited).[1] In addition, drug-induced slowing of ventricular tachycardia rates may be accompanied by sinus node suppression that can increase the need for ventricular pacing to achieve chronotropic competence. Within this algorithm (known as Brady-Tachy Overlap), slow VT is defined as rates ≥ 101 bpm but less than the programmed VT detection zone (Fig 17.1). Paced events in the slow VT zone are not counted as tachyarrhythmia intervals. If a spontaneous rhythm develops in this zone and overrides pacing, however, the device initiates rhythm analysis and therapy if indicated. A similar feature is available in Biotronik ICDs.

Effects of Ventricular Refractory Period

In addition to restraints on pacing exerted by relatively long VT detection intervals, ventricular refractory periods (VRP) initiated by pacing may limit the window for detection of VT. During such refractory periods, the device may be blind to tachyarrhythmia events.

In Medtronic ICDs, the refractory period initiated by ventricular pacing (a programmable feature) can occupy no more than 50% of the interval between paced beats. Thus at a paced cycle length of 600 ms (100 bpm) the VRP can be no more than 300 ms. Algorithms to shorten VRP at higher pacing rates circumvent some of this limitation.

In Boston Scientific ICDs, the VRP cannot be more than 50% of the programmed lower rate. In addition, the minimum sensor driven interval (or upper rate limit interval) must be at least 90 ms longer than the VRP. For example, if VRP is 300 ms (fixed) the minimum sensor driven in-

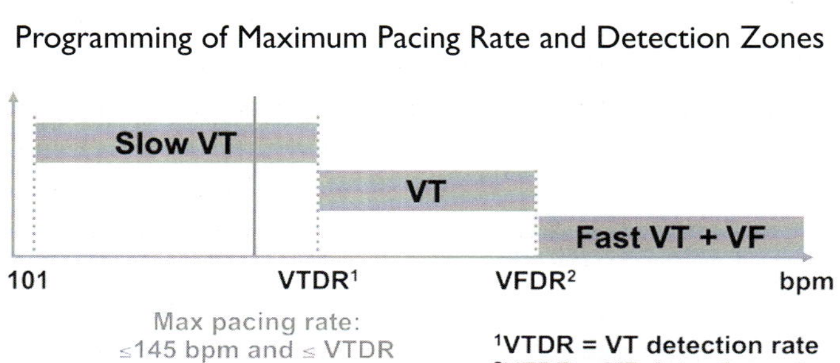

Fig 17.1 Illustration of the "Brady-Tachy Overlap" algorithm in Sorin ICDs. Ventricular-paced events in the "Slow VT" zone are sensed as slow cycles but do not initiate algorithmic analysis for discrimination of VT. When the rhythm becomes spontaneous (unpaced) in the "Slow VT" zone, the device begins algorithmic analysis to discriminate VT from SVT. (Adapted from Sorin Group with permission.)

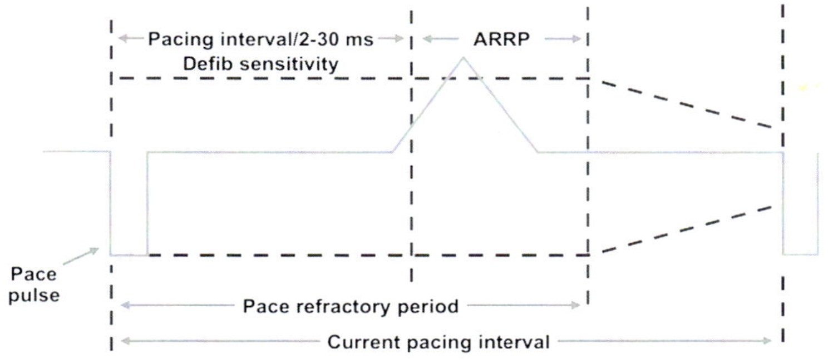

Fig 17.2 "Arrhythmia Unhiding" algorithm in St. Jude Medical ICDs. ARRP, adaptive relative refractory period. See text for discussion. (Adapted and used with permission of St. Jude Medical.)

terval is 390 ms (153 bpm). Automatic shortening of VRP as the sensor driven rate increases, however, allows higher upper rate pacing.

A feature in SJM ICDs illustrates the problem of refractory periods and tachyarrhythmia detection. The feature, called "arrhythmia unhiding" enables an adaptive relative refractory period (ARRP) to search for arrhythmias hidden by pacing (Fig 17.2). When paced ventricular rates are fast (resulting from sensor-driven ventricular pacing or tracking of atrial activity), and the paced cycle length is less than two times the longest VT detection interval, the ARRP is enabled effectively increasing the alert period for tachyarrhythmia detection. If a sensed ventricular event occurs during the ARRP, and the next event is paced, the ARRP is enabled again. If no sensed event occurs during the ARRP, or the next event is not paced, the pace refractory period returns to normal. If a specified number of intervals occur consecutively (programmable 2–13, nominal 3), the pacing cycle length is extended for six cycles in an attempt to detect or "unhide" the arrhythmia. If no arrhythmia is detected in this window of six extended pacing cycles, the ARRP is disabled for 10 cycles to prevent unnecessary truncation of upper rate pacing.

Dual Chamber Pacing ICDs

The development of dual chamber pacing ICDs obviated the need for separate ICDs and dual chamber pacemakers in the same patient. Although this eliminated unwelcome interdevice interactions, adverse intradevice interactions became manifest. This resulted, in part, from simple import of dual chamber pacemaker features into ICDs without a full appreciation for the complexities of arrhythmia surveillance.

Rate Responsiveness

With the addition of rate responsive dual chamber pacing capabilities, ICD candidates with sinus node dysfunction could be offered chronotropic support. This, however, heightened the importance of the VRP in limiting the window for arrhythmia surveillance. At high-paced rates the VRP occupies increasingly greater percentages of the cardiac cycle that might hamper VT/VF detection.

To address this issue, Ellenbogen studied 27 patients at the time of ICD implant and programmed devices to a "worst-case scenario", that is, high-rate pacing (150 bpm [DDD] or 175 bpm [DDDR]) at the time of induction of VF. With dynamic VRP set to 190 ms at the lower rate limit and 150 ms at the upper rate limit, there was no difference in VF detection time in the two groups. However, the experimental protocol had to be modified when it became clear that a programmed dynamic VRP of 250 to 240 ms would delay detection. (2) Thus long VRP setting could interfere with VF detection in these worst-case scenarios.

RR Interval Stabilization

Algorithms to stabilize oscillations in RR intervals in ICD recipients have been used in an attempt to prevent marked fluctuations in cycle length that have been associated with development of VT/VF.[3] In Guidant (now Boston Scientific) ICDs this feature, called "rate smoothing," limits the maximal increment ("rate smoothing down") and decrement ("rate smoothing up") in successive RR intervals. "Rate smoothing down" forces atrial or atrioventicular (AV) pacing as a post extrasystolic pause begins to elapse. This inserts post pace blanking intervals and VRPs into a rhythm already disturbed by premature ventricular depolarizations or the first beat(s) of VT.

Shivkumar first reported this "intradevice interaction," a term he coined to distinguish it from a device-device interaction seen in the era of separate pacemakers and ICDs in the same patient.[4] Subsequently, this phenomenon was studied systematically by Glikson[5] who noted several findings. First, detection of rapid VF or polymorphic VT (> 240 bpm) was unimpaired. Second, underdetection of VT, which could be provoked readily, depended on programming of a longer AV delay and was more common with higher pacing rates. Finally, and most importantly, impaired detection of VT/VF only occurred with programmed parameters that triggered an automatic parameter interaction warning from the programmer.

Refractory Periods and Blanking in Dual Chamber ICDs

The limitations posed by refractory and blanking in single chamber ICDs described previously are more complex in dual chamber ICDs and are exemplified next.

In current Boston Scientific ICDs, the following scenario, while admittedly contrived, illustrates the effect of blanking and refractory periods on VT detection (Fig 17.3). With a lower rate limit of 90 bpm, upper tracking or sensor driven rate at 130 bpm, a fixed AV delay of 300 ms, a postatrial ventricular blanking period of 65 ms and a VT zone at 150 bpm, VT underdetection would be predicted to occur owing to coincidence of VT events with the blanking and refractory periods.

In Medtronic dual chamber ICDs, a window for VT detection equal to the longest programmed VT detection interval plus 30 ms must be allowed after a paced or sensed ventricular event and before the next atrial-paced event. In earlier devices (prior to model D154VRC), this was achieved by disallowing certain combinations of VT detection interval, sensor rate, and paced AV delay. Attempts to program such combinations would result in an "interlock" warning (Fig 17.4). The purpose of this was to avoid inappropriate tachyarrhythmia detection if cross-chamber sensing of the atrial-pacing stimulus on the ventricular sense amplifier occurred (crosstalk).

In later devices, atrial-pacing output is moved outside the VT detection window

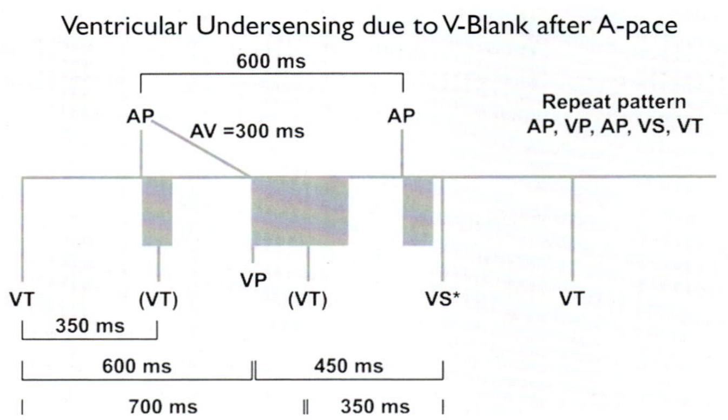

Fig 17.3 Mechanism of ventricular undersensing due to ventricular blanking after atrial pacing. The first VT event falls into the ventricular blanking period after an atrial-paced event. As this event is not sensed, the AV interval elapses and a ventricular-paced event ensues. The next VT event falls in the ventricular refractory period and is not sensed. The following two VT events are sensed but only one VT interval is logged. The pattern then repeats. (Adapted from Boston Scientific with permission.)

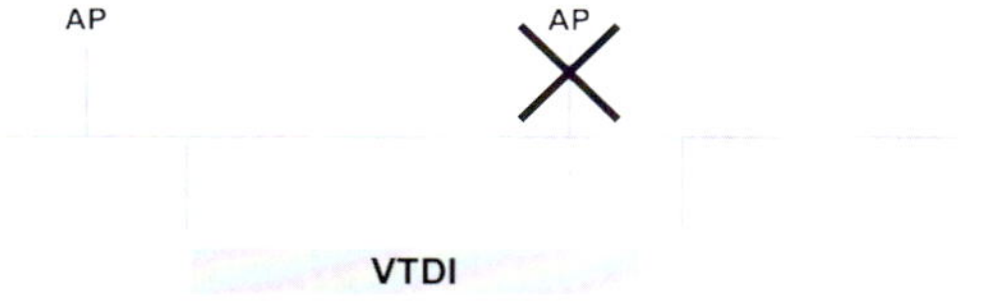

Fig 17.4 Illustration of an "interlock" in Medtronic ICDs prior to D154VRC. These devices would not permit atrial pacing in the tachyarrhythmia detection zone. For a VT detection interval of 400 ms, the maximum selectable upper rate is 100 bpm (cycle length 600 ms) with a paced AV delay of 200 ms (rate adaptive AV delay Off). (Adapted from Medtronic with permission.)

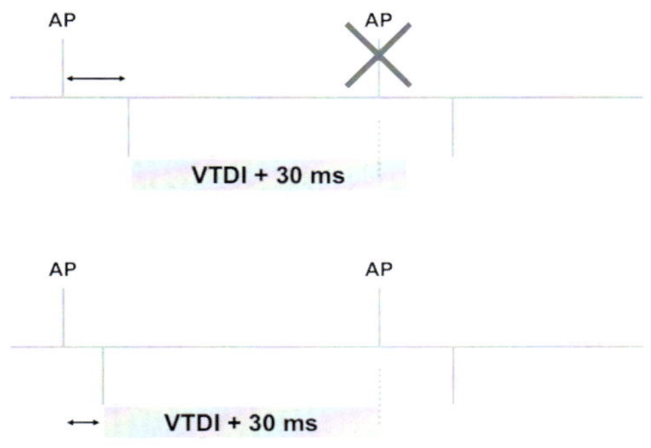

Fig 17.5 Illustration of automatic temporary paced AV delay/lower rate interval adjustment to allow detection of VT in later Medtronic ICDs. The device moves the atrial-paced event outside the VT detection interval (VTDI) if (1) the VT counter is ≥ 3 or would have been if not reset, (2) the VT + VF counter ≥ 3 or would be if not reset and there is a VF interval in the last eight beats, or (3) if a ventricular episode is in progress. (Adapted from Medtronic with permission.)

if tachyarrhythmia counters are advanced to a certain value or would be advanced if the atrial-pacing stimulus was delayed, an internal hypothesis-testing algorithm. This is achieved by automatic shortening of the paced AV delay or decreasing the pacing rate (Figs 17.5 and 17.6).

Avoiding Ventricular Pacing

Algorithms to minimize ventricular pacing are reviewed elsewhere in this book and will not be covered in this section. Two issues bear mention. First, the majority of ICD recipients have impaired ventricular function. Given this and the increasing evidence that right ventricular pacing may exacerbate left ventricular dysfunction, use of devices with these algorithms may be of greater importance in this group of patients.[6] Second, in general, avoidance of pacing (atrial and/or ventricular) limits the amount of time that blanking and refractory periods blind the device to ventricular events. An efficient algorithm to avoid ventricular pacing could enhance detection of VT.

Some algorithms to limit ventricular pacing permit one to two beats of AV block before resumption of ventricular pacing. This then sets up a short-long-short RR interval cycle length oscillation that could be proarrhythmic.[7] The concern regarding cycle length oscillations provoked by bradycardia gave rise to algorithms for RR interval stabilization as previously described. Thus the competing priorities of pacing

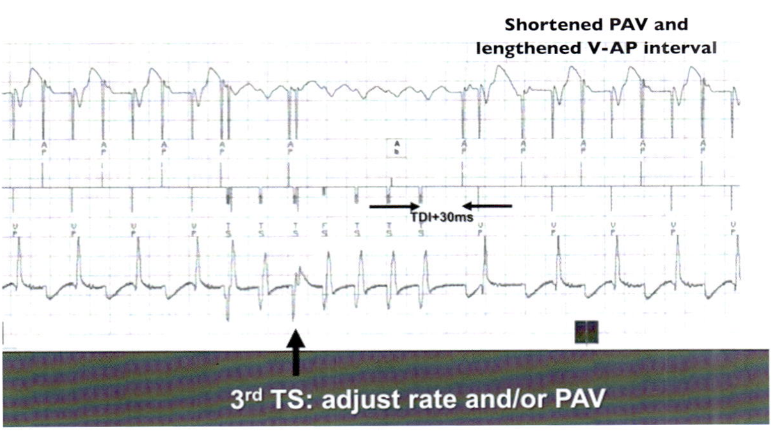

Fig 17.6 Example of automatic temporary paced AV delay/lower rate interval adjustment. The first and third VT events (TS) were potential crosstalk events but still counted as VT events. After the episode of nonsustained VT, the paced AV delay is shortened and the V to A-paced interval is lengthened for one beat as the device tries to open up a window for tachyarrhythmia sensing. (Adapted from Medtronic with permission.)

avoidance and RR interval stabilization interact at this nexus and most importantly in the ICD patient at high risk for VT/VF.

Cardiac Resynchronization Defibrillator (CRT-D)

Most of the timing cycle issues described in dual chamber ICDs are equally relevant in CRT-Ds. There, however, are some issues unique to these devices.

Unlike single and dual chamber ICDs, CRT-D pacing intervals are set to maximize ventricular pacing. Indeed, biventricular pacing < 90% of the time is a cause of inadequate improvement in heart failure symptoms. Thus, AV search hysteresis and other algorithms to maximize the chance for native AV, conduction are counterproductive.

One situation unique to CRT-D is the effect of programmed RV-LV intervals on the window for VT/VF sensing as well as the upper rate limit. This is illustrated in Fig 17.7.

In many CRT-Ds a programmable V-V interval (interventricular pace delay or IVPD) allows the provider to separate RV and LV pacing. In St. Jude Medical CRT-Ds the maximum programmable delay is 80 ms. A competing timing circuit (known as the Runaway Protection Timer), however, prevents this manufacturers' devices from delivering two ventricular pacing spikes within 400 ms of each other. In order to allow delivery of closely timed RV and LV pacing impulses, this timer is temporarily disabled during the programmed IVPD. However, the timer becomes active with the delivery of the second ventricular impulse and the 400-ms window during which V pacing cannot occur begins. If the programmed V-V interval is 80 ms, the minimum interval from the second ventricular pacing output (chamber 2) to the next ventricular pacing output (chamber 1) is 400 ms. Thus the minimum paced cycle length is 480 ms rather than 400 ms.

A similar situation is found in Medtronic CRT-Ds. When programmed LV output 80 ms before RV output, the ventricular pace blanking period must be set to 230 ms (150 ms plus the LV-RV delay). In these devices, at least one-half of the V-V interval must be available for arrhythmia surveillance. With the blanking period at 230 ms the minimum paced cycle length is then 460 ms or 130 bpm (personal communication with James Glover, Medtronic, Inc.). Some of these considerations are clearly more technical than clinically relevant because few CRT-D recipients will pace at or near the upper rate limit.

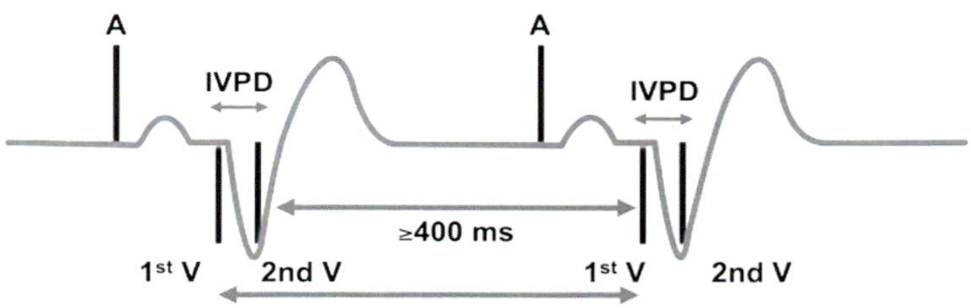

Fig 17.7 Effect of interventricular programmed delay (IVPD) on upper pacing rate in St. Jude Medical CRT-Ds. A circuit known as the Runaway Protection Timer that normally prevents delivery of two ventricular spikes within 400 ms of each other is inhibited to allow delivery of resynchronization pulses. But the timer becomes active after delivery of the second V spike and prevents delivery of the next V spike until 400 ms have elapsed. Thus the interval from the sequential first V spikes equals 400 ms plus the programmed V-V interval. (Adapted from St. Jude Medical with permission.)

References

1. Sadoul N, Mletzko R, Anselme F, et al. Incidence and clinical relevance of slow ventricular tachycardia in implantable cardioverter-defibrillator

recipients: an international multicenter prospective study. *Circulation.* 2005:112;946–953.

2. Ellenbogen KA, Edel T, Moore S, et al. A prospective randomized-controlled trial of ventricular fibrillation detection in a DDDR ventricular defibrillator. *PACE.* 2000;23:1268–1272.
3. Fromer M, Wietholt D. Algorithm for the prevention of ventricular tachycardia onset: the Prevent study. *Am J Cardiol.* 1999;83:45D–47D
4. Shivkumar K, Feliciano Z, Boyle NG, Wiener I. Intradevice interaction in dual chamber implantable cardioverter defibrillator preventing tachyarrhythmia detection. *J Cardiovasc Electrophysiol.* 2000:11;1285–1288.
5. Glikson M, Beeman AL, Luria DM, et al. Impaired detection of ventricular tachyarrhythmias by a rate-smoothing algorithm in dual-chamber implantable defibrillators: intradevice interactions. *J Cardiovasc Electrophysiol.* 2002:13;312–318.
6. The DAVID Trial Investigators. Dual-chamber pacing or ventricular backup pacing in patients with an implantable defibrillator. *JAMA.* 2002:288;3115–3123.
7. Sweeney MO, Ruetz LL, Belk P, et al. Bradycardia pacing-induced short-long-short sequences at the onset of ventricular tachyarrhythmias: a possible mechanism of proarrhythmia. *J Am Coll Cardiol.* 2007;50:614–622.

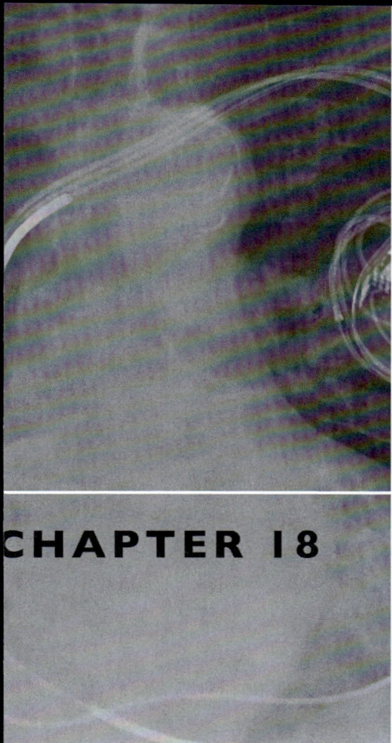

Assessing Defibrillation Efficacy at ICD Implant

CHAPTER 18

Charles D. Swerdlow and Paul J. DeGroot

Introduction

The accepted method for implantable cardioverter defibrillator (ICD) implantation includes induction of ventricular fibrillation (VF) to ensure that the ICD will sense, detect, and defibrillate VF. In an earlier era of less efficient ICDs, the value of assessing defibrillation efficacy seemed self-evident. Today, improved technology and use of ICDs for primary prevention of ventricular tachycardia (VT) or VF have led some to question the need to assess defibrillation efficacy at ICD implantation.

This chapter has four goals: (1) summarize the purpose and methods of fibrillation-defibrillation and vulnerability implant testing; (2) review the benefits, risks, and clinical utility of implant testing; (3) consider specific "how to" aspects of ICD implantation, including how to approach the patient in whom defibrillation is unreliable and how to minimize risk; and (4) provide a perspective on when implant testing is indicated and when it is not.

Pacemakers and Implantable Cardioverter Defibrillators: An Expert's Manual. © 2010 Amin Al-Ahmad, Kenneth A. Ellenbogen, Andrea Natale, and Paul J. Wang, eds. Cardiotext Publishing, ISBN: 978-0-9790164-6-2.

Background

Probabilistic Nature of Defibrillation

Clinical defibrillation is usually described by a probability-of-success curve with shock strength on the abscissa and probability of successful defibrillation on the ordinate (Fig 18.1).[1,2] The result of a series of defibrillation test shocks at the same shock strength gives an estimate of the probability of success at that shock strength. Multiple series of test shocks at different shock strengths are required to estimate the defibrillation probability-of-success curve. This curve is usually displayed as a logistic regression curve, although it may be better represented by one in which the probability of success remains at zero

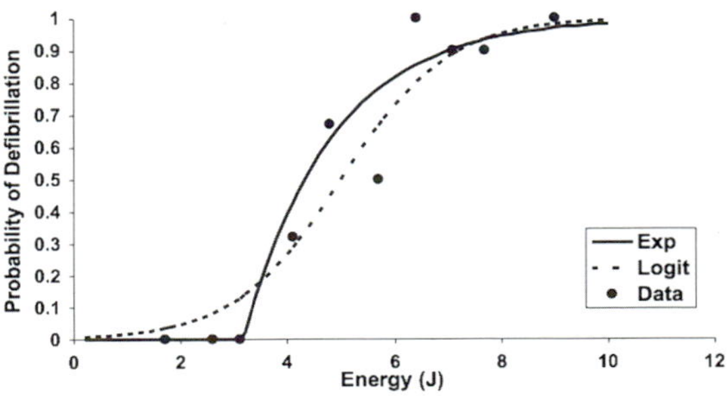

Fig 18.1 Defibrillation probability of success curve for one dog. The abscissa plots shock strength in Joules, and the ordinate plots the fraction of shocks that defibrillated at each shock strength. Each data point was computed from the results of 7 to 10 shocks. Best-fit curves are shown for exponential and logit (sigmoid-shaped) models. The exponential curve fits the data better, primarily because of the absence of successful defibrillation at shock strengths ≤ 3 J. (Adapted from Gliner et al[3].)

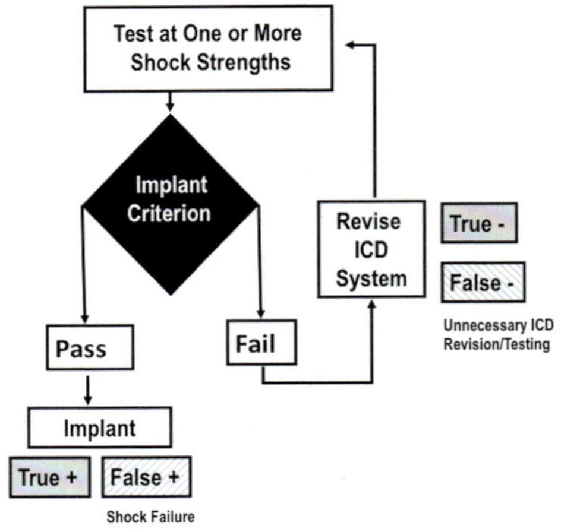

Fig 18.2 Role of the implant criterion. The implant criterion is the level of defibrillation performance predicted to result in a clinically adequate success rate for defibrillation of spontaneous VF. The implant criterion results in a true-positive result when patients who have reliable defibrillation of spontaneous VT/VF pass the test. In a false-positive result, patients who have unreliable defibrillation pass and are thereby placed at risk for unsuccessful defibrillation of spontaneous VT/VF. In a true-negative result, patients with unreliable defibrillation fail the implant criterion and may undergo indicated ICD system revision or retesting at a later date. In a false-negative test result, patients with reliable defibrillation fail the implant criterion and undergo unnecessary system revision or retesting, with their associated risks.

for very weak shocks, rises steeply from zero, and then approaches asymptotically 100%.[2–4]

The Implant Criterion

Determination of a complete defibrillation probability-of-success curve for an individual patient requires more fibrillation-defibrillation episodes than is practical or safe in humans. Thus more limited implant criteria have been developed. The fundamental principle of implant testing is illustrated in Fig 18.2. Defibrillation efficacy is assessed at one or more shock strengths. Usually, VF is induced one or more times; and each episode of VF is shocked at one or more shock strengths. The outcome of each defibrillation shock is classified as either successful or unsuccessful. Alternatively, testing based on the upper limit of vulnerability (ULV) may be used to assess defibrillation efficacy without inducing VF in most patients. In this type of testing, shocks are delivered at the most vulnerable time in the cardiac cycle. A shock strength is considered sufficient for defibrillation if VF is not induced and insufficient if VF is induced.

Whatever the method of testing, the sequence of outcomes is compared with the implant criterion, which is the level of defibrillation performance at implant predicted to result in a clinically adequate success rate for defibrillation of spontaneous VF. Performance that does not meet the implant criterion requires revising the ICD system, comprising of the leads and pulse generator.

In evaluating both the weight of the evidence supporting various implant criteria and the applicability of this evidence to present clinical practice, it is useful to consider the genesis of the most widely used criterion, reliable defibrillation at 10 J* below the ICD's maximum

*The shock waveform parameter that most directly influences defibrillation is voltage as a function of time (duration). The physics of capacitive-discharge waveforms links the energy stored in the ICD's capacitor to the shock's voltage and duration. Although shock energy is *not* a direct measure of effectiveness, it is so widely cited that we follow convention and use it unless otherwise indicated.

output. It is based on a post-hoc analysis performed in 33 patients treated with monophasic, epicardial ICDs.[5] The independent variable was the difference between ICD's maximum output and the step-down (or up) DFT. The dependent variable was defibrillation of induced VF at postoperative testing. Overall, maximum output (28 J) shocks were successful in 29 patients (88%). A maximum output shock succeeded in all 19 patients (100%) who had a safety margin of ≥ 10 J, but in only 10 of 14 patients (71%) with a safety margin < 10 J, $p < 0.04$.

The Defibrillation "Threshold" (DFT)

In physiology, a threshold stimulus is the minimum stimulus required to evoke a response. Stimuli weaker than the threshold never evoke a response, and stimuli stronger than the threshold always evoke a response. Often, the strength of the response increases as the stimulus strength increases beyond the threshold value.

The threshold concept does not apply to defibrillation. The probabilistic nature of defibrillation ensures that, over the clinically relevant range of shock strengths, the same shock strength may either succeed or fail on successive attempts. Further, with rare exceptions, the strength of the defibrillation response does not increase with increasing stimulus strength; either the stimulus defibrillates or it does not.

Nevertheless, the term *DFT* is deeply established as the minimum shock strength that defibrillates. Historically, it has been used as a patient-specific measure of defibrillation efficacy; and a DFT below a specific value has been used as a patient-specific implant criterion. Given the probabilistic nature of defibrillation, it is not surprising that clinical measurement of DFT has only fair reproducibility. In a study of 25 patients, the correlation coefficient between two successful determinations of the DFT was 0.64.[6] Two patients (8%) had differences between first and second determinations of ≥ 10 J.

Clinical Methods for Measuring the DFT

Different methods of measuring the DFT approximate different points on the probability-of-success curve. The error of estimating a point on the probability-of-success curve is a nonlinear function of the number of shocks and the specific point on the curve.[7] A multiple-reversal protocol with equal steps accurately estimates the shock energy associated with 50% defibrillation success (E_{50}), but is usually considered too rigorous for clinical testing. The Bayesian method can be used to perform an efficient estimation of an arbitrary point on the curve,[7] but it is used rarely because the nonintuitive shock sequence is generated from a computer model of an a priori estimate of the DFT probability-of-success curve. *In practice, the term DFT is used as a shorthand to mean an estimate of a point on the patient's defibrillation probability-of-success curve, usually with unknown confidence intervals.*

The most commonly used clinical DFT methods include binary search, step-down, and step-up (see Fig 18.3 on the following page). The binary search method approximates the E_{50}. The widely used, step-down DFT approximates the E_{50} to E_{70}, depending on the starting shock strength and step size; and the step-up DFT approximates the E_{30} to E_{50}, depending on the starting shock strength and step size. Step-up methods permit assessing more shock strengths with fewer episodes of VF, but they result in longer VF episodes if multiple shocks are required for defibrillation. For this reason, some investigators question their safety. In clinical practice, the binary search method gives similar results to the step-down and step-up methods. Other protocols require two or three consecutive defibrillation successes to define "enhanced" thresholds referred to as the DFT+ and DFT++, respectively.[8] They correspond to higher points on the probability-of-success curve than the DFT.

Statistical Modeling of Defibrillation Testing

Statistical modeling based on a family of estimated defibrillation probability-of-success

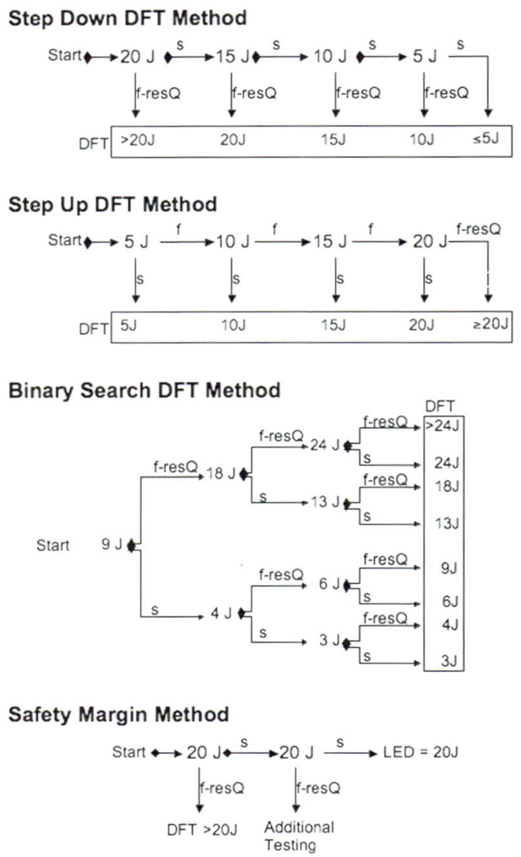

Fig 18.3 Commonly used methods for assessing defibrillation efficacy at implant of an ICD with a maximum shock strength of 30 J. The top three panels illustrate protocols to determine the patient-specific DFT. The bottom panel illustrates a method to verify a defibrillation safety margin between the maximum shock strength of the ICD and the shock strength required for consistent defibrillation. In each panel, diamonds indicate initiation of VF, "s" indicates defibrillation success, and "f-resQ" indicate defibrillation failure followed by a strong rescue shock. The rescue shock may be delivered internally from the ICD or externally from a transthoracic defibrillator. The *top panel* illustrates the step-down method in which each failed shock is followed by a rescue shock. Thus each fibrillation-defibrillation episode provides data regarding the efficacy of one shock strength. The *second panel* illustrates the step-up method. Because multiple shock strengths are tested during a single episode of VF, this method is quicker than either of the other two DFT methods. Limited available data indicate that the efficacy of a defibrillation shock is not influenced significantly by delivery of a preceding shock if the duration of VF is < 15 to 20 s. The potential for long episodes of VF is a concern regarding this method. The *third panel* illustrates the binary search method. The number of fibrillation-defibrillation episodes is fixed in the binary search method, but variable in the step-up and step-down methods. The binary search method is designed to estimate the E_{50}. Conceptually, the step-down method is more likely to result in a DFT greater than the E_{50} because it provides multiple opportunities for shocks stronger than the E_{50} to fail. In contrast, the step-up method is more likely to result in a DFT less than the E_{50} because it provides multiple opportunities for shocks weaker than the E_{50} to succeed. The magnitude by which the step-up and step-down DFTs deviate from the E_{50} depends on the starting shock strength and step size; in clinical practice, it may be small. The *bottom panel* illustrates the safety margin method. This method limits testing to the minimum necessary to determine whether there is a sufficient safety margin between the maximum shock strength of the ICD and the shock strength required for consistent defibrillation. LED indicates lowest tested energy that defibrillates. This method determines a DFT only if the DFT exceeds the tested shock strength. In all methods, the ICD system is modified if a 10-J safety margin is not achieved. The figure does not illustrate the point that success or failure of an internal rescue shock from the ICD may provide incremental information about defibrillation efficacy of the ICD system.

curves for individual patients may be used to estimate the performance of different methods for measuring the DFT. As a first step, each patient's curve is generated using logistic regression performed on a data set consisting of the few, dichotomous outcomes of the defibrillation shocks delivered at ICD implant. Often, only one shock is delivered at each shock strength, so that the calculated probability of success is either 0% or 100%. For example, if a step-down defibrillation protocol is performed with successes at 20 and 15 J and a failure at 10 J, the probability of success is calculated to be 100% at 20 J, 100% at 15 J, and 0% at 10 J. But there is a reasonable chance that the true probability of success at 15 J might be 80% and some chance that it might be 50% or lower. Similarly, there is a reasonable chance that the true probability of success at 10 J might be 20% and some chance that it might be 50% or higher.

Statistical modeling can be used to construct a probability-of-success curve that takes into account both the individual patient's defibrillation data and the pooled results from the population as a whole. The result is a family of curves representative of the population of patients.[9] See Fig 18.4.

Smits et al compared the ability of different implant criteria to identify patients with a 90% probability of a successful first shock at the maximum output of an ICD (assumed to be 35 J).[10] In a sample population in which 94% of patients had the required minimum first shock efficacy, the specificity of failing high DFT patients var-

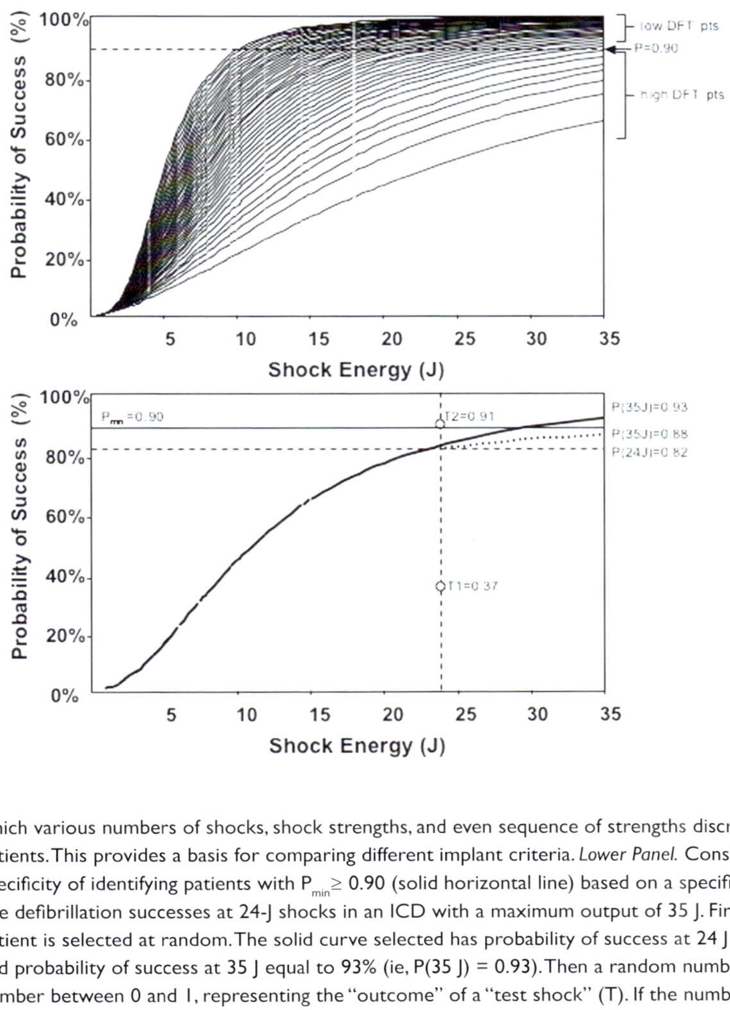

Fig 18.4 Statistical modeling of defibrillation testing. *Upper Panel.* Statistical modeling of pooled patient data is used to generate a family of probability-of-success of curves. Each curve represents an estimate of the probability-of-success curve for an individual patient. The goal of implant testing is to differentiate patients with a high probability of success ("low DFT" patients) from patients with an unacceptable probability of success ("high-DFT" patients). Thus one must first define the minimal acceptable probability (P_{min}) of success for a single, maximum output shock (eg, 35 J) at ICD implant, for example P_{min} = 0.90. Individual patient curves are divided into low-DFT groups (probability of successful defibrillation at maximum output ≥ P_{min}) and high-DFT groups (probability of successful defibrillation at maximum output < P_{min}). The model can then be used to assess the accuracy with which various numbers of shocks, shock strengths, and even sequence of strengths discriminate low-DFT from high-DFT patients. This provides a basis for comparing different implant criteria. *Lower Panel.* Consider evaluating the sensitivity and specificity of identifying patients with $P_{min} \geq 0.90$ (solid horizontal line) based on a specific implant criterion: two consecutive defibrillation successes at 24-J shocks in an ICD with a maximum output of 35 J. First, a curve representing a single patient is selected at random. The solid curve selected has probability of success at 24 J equal to 82% (ie, P(24 J) = 0.82) and probability of success at 35 J equal to 93% (ie, P(35 J) = 0.93). Then a random number generator is used to produce a number between 0 and 1, representing the "outcome" of a "test shock" (T). If the number is lower than the (P24J) on the selected curve, the outcome is classified as a success; otherwise it is classified as a failure. If the first random number (T_1) is 0.37, and the second random number (T_2) is 0.91, the first test shock is classified as a success and the second test shock is classified as a failure. Thus the patient's curve fails to meet the implant criterion. Because P(35 J) is greater than the desired P_{min} = 0.90, the result is a false-negative test. If however, the curve had P(35 J) = 0.88 (dashed upper part of curve), then the test would have produced a true-negative result. This process of selecting randomly from the family of curves and applying the chosen test shock is repeated for a large number of trials. By pooling results, the sensitivity and specificity for any proposed implant criterion combining shock strengths and shock sequence can be estimated, providing an objective measure of the criterion's performance on the test population. Generally, an implant criterion's performance depends on the family of curves used to represent the population of ICD recipients as well as the desired P_{min}, which differentiates between low- and high-DFT patients.

ied from 11% for a binary search protocol requiring DFT ≤ 24 J to 74% for a step-down protocol requiring DFT ≤ 18 J. The implant criteria had an inverse relationship between specificity of failing high DFT patients and sensitivity for passing low DFT patients. The two criteria mentioned previously had sensitivities of 100% and 91%, respectively. There was little difference in sensitivity and specificity between requiring two successes at 24 J and a single success at 15 J. Table 18.1 shows sensitivity and specificity of various implant criteria.

Fibrillation-Defibrillation Testing

In general, VF is induced one or more times by rapid pacing, direct current, or T-wave shocks; defibrillation test shocks of varying strength are delivered; and the outcome (success or failure) of the defibrillation shock or sequence of shocks is compared with the implant criterion. If the test shock is unsuccessful, a stronger rescue shock is delivered.

Test shocks. In patient-specific DFT testing, the success or failure of the first test shock usually determines the programmed strength of the next test shock: If the first test shock defibrillates, the strength of the next test shock is reduced. Alternatively, if the first test shock does not defibrillate, a stronger rescue shock is delivered, and the strength of the next test shock is increased. After a fixed or variable number of fibrillation-defibrillation episodes, a determination is made as to whether the ICD system passes or fails the implant criterion. In safety-margin testing, the outcome of the first defibrillation shock may or may not alter the strength of the second shock.

Rescue shocks. These may be delivered internally through the ICD electrodes or externally through self-adhesive patch electrodes placed prior to the procedure. Internal rescue shocks avoid skin burns associated with external shocks. Their success or failure provides incremental information about the performance of the ICD lead system. However, they may result in longer VF episodes because they are delayed by the times required for redetection of VF (unless a "commanded" shock is delivered) and charging the ICD's capacitor.

Interpreting defibrillation testing: regression to the mean

Assessment of defibrillation efficacy at ICD implantation must take the probabilistic nature of defibrillation into consideration. A defibrillation failure may be a low-probability event due to chance alone rather than evidence of substandard defibrillation performance. For example, a defibrillation system with an acceptable 95% success rate at implant testing is expected to fail to defibrillate in 5% of attempts. If a shock at the E_{95} fails to defibrillate, defibrillation of a second episode of VF at the same shock strength is likely to succeed, because it has the same 95% probability of success. To generalize, when a single measurement falls in the tails of a statis-

Protocol	Criterion	% Passing	% Sensitivity	% Specificity
2 Inductions	2/2 successes at 24 J	93	96	53
1 Induction	1/1 success at 15 J	91	94	52
1 Induction	1/1 success at 12 J	87	90	61
Step Down	DFT ≤ 24 J	96	98	32
Step Down	DFT ≤ 18 J	87	91	74
Binary Search	DFT ≤ 24 J	99	100	11
Binary Search	DFT ≤ 12 J	87	90	61

Table 18.1 Predicted Performance of Different Implant Criteria

tical distribution (ie, an unlikely defibrillation failure occurs), a repeat measurement will likely be closer to the mean. This behavior, called regression to the mean, is characteristic of parameters having a normal distribution.[11]

The clinical implication is that an ICD system should not be revised after a single defibrillation failure without other evidence that the tested shock strength is insufficient. If a system is revised after a single failure, success of a subsequent shock may merely represent regression to the mean rather than truly improved defibrillation performance: The successful shock may simply represent typical performance rather than improved performance.

Patient-specific versus safety-margin implant criteria

Both "patient-specific" and "safety-margin" implant criteria have been applied. *Patient-specific* criteria attempt to identify the minimum shock strength that defibrillates reliably so that ICD first shocks can be programmed to the lowest effective shock strength. *Safety-margin* criteria limit testing to the minimum number of induced episodes necessary to determine if there is a sufficient safety margin between the maximum shock strength of the ICD and the shock strength required for consistent defibrillation.

The objective of a patient-specific implant strategy is an accurate estimate of the minimum shock strength that achieves a specific, high probability of successful defibrillation (eg, E_{95}). Patient-specific criteria are intended to minimize the long-term potentially adverse effects of excessive programmed shock strength.

A safety-margin strategy is preferred when the principal goal is to minimize the risks of shocks and fibrillation-defibrillation testing. After safety-margin testing, the first shock usually is programmed to maximum output. Generally, safety-margin criteria are appropriate whenever a patient-specific safety margin is judged unnecessary or multiple inductions of VF are contraindicated.

Using the ULV to Assess Defibrillation Efficacy: Defibrillation Without Inducing VF

The *vulnerable period* is that portion of the cardiac cycle during which shocks induce VF. The ULV is the weakest shock strength at or above which VF is not induced when the shock is delivered at any time during the vulnerable period. There is a close correlation between the ULV and defibrillation threshold (DFT).[12] This empirical observation provided the first experimental evidence for the ULV hypothesis of defibrillation, which postulates a mechanistic relationship between the ULV—measured during sinus or paced rhythm—and the minimum shock strength that defibrillates reliably. Two related corollaries of this hypothesis have clinical relevance: (1) The ULV provides a patient-specific measure of defibrillation efficacy with a single fibrillation-defibrillation episode. (2) The safety margin for ICD shocks can be assessed without inducing VF.

The Vulnerable Zone

Definition

Shocks in the vulnerable period induce VF only if their strength is in an intermediate range, at or above the VF threshold and less than the ULV. The combination of shock coupling intervals (relative to the R wave or pacing stimulus) and shock strengths that induce VF in a regular rhythm is the *vulnerable zone*. It is displayed as a bounded, homogeneous region in a two-dimensional space defined by time (coupling interval) on the abscissa and shock strength on the ordinate (Fig 18.5).[13]

Theoretical and mechanistic considerations

Based on topological analysis, Winfree predicted that initiation of VF by shocks in the relative refractory period depends on the simultaneous occurrence in space and time of a critical degree of refractoriness and a critical shock-induced local electrical field strength (voltage gradient).[14] He predicted that the spatiotemporal coincidence of critical values of field strength

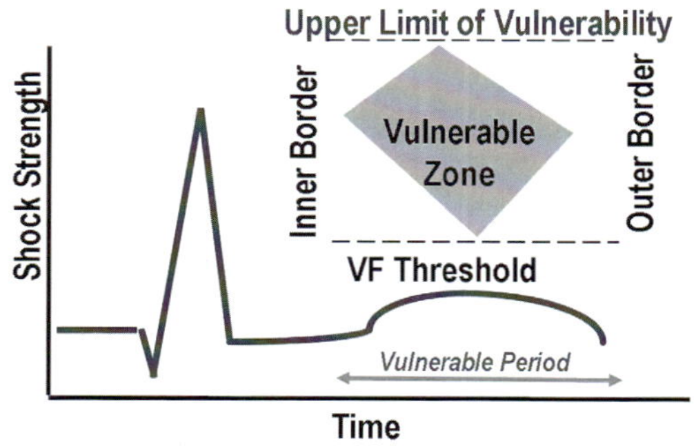

Fig 18.5 The vulnerable zone displayed as a bounded, homogeneous region in a two-dimensional space defined by time (coupling interval) on the abscissa and shock strength on the ordinate. The ULV is the weakest shock strength at or above which VF is not induced when the shock is delivered at any time during the vulnerable period. The upper border (ULV) and the lower borders (VF threshold) are defined by shock strength. The inner (left) and outer (right) borders are defined by time (coupling interval).

and refractoriness formed a "critical point" around which unidirectional block and reentry occur (field-recovery critical point). In the late 1980s and early 1990s, computer-assisted, electrode-array, activation mapping studies confirmed these critical points as the mechanism of shock-induced VF. Subsequently, a second type of critical point was predicted by bidomain theory and confirmed by optical mapping studies. This critical point occurs where the spatial derivative of the shock-induced transmembrane potential reaches a critical value (virtual-electrode critical point).[15,16]

The ULV Hypothesis of Defibrillation

This hypothesis[12] postulates a mechanistic relationship between the ULV—measured during regular rhythm—and the minimum shock strength that defibrillates reliably. It postulates both that local vulnerable periods exist during VF and that the ULV in VF is (approximately) equal to the ULV in normal rhythm. It proposes that successful defibrillation must fulfill two sequential requirements: First the shock must interrupt all VF wavefronts. Then it must not reinitiate VF. The ULV hypothesis also requires that the ULV during VF exceeds the shock strength required to stop all VF wavefronts.

According to the ULV hypothesis, a shock always defibrillates if it terminates all VF wavefronts and prevents reinitiation of VF. The latter requirement implicitly includes both spatial and temporal components: The shock must not reinitiate VF even if the spatial region of weakest field strength (lowest voltage gradient) is temporally coincident with the local vulnerable period. The minimum required shock strength is the ULV during VF. The response to a shock that stops all wavefronts but is weaker than the ULV varies depending on the unpredictable fibrillatory pattern of preshock activation and repolarization in the region of weakest field strength. If the shock times in the local vulnerable period, it reinitiates VF and is unsuccessful. Otherwise it terminates VF and is successful. Thus the ULV hypothesis predicts that defibrillation will be probabilistic on a macroscopic level.

The ULV hypothesis of defibrillation does not depend on a specific cellular or tissue mechanism for defibrillation, but rather on a class of possible mechanisms in which the failure of subthreshold defibrillation shocks is caused by shock-initiated refibrillation. Three lines of evidence support the ULV hypothesis:

1. *Empirical:* The ULV-DFT correlation has been validated in multiple animal and human studies. It remains strong and invariant, within experimental error, over almost all experimental conditions[13]: (A) changes in pacing site; (B) reversal of shock electrode polarity; (C) multiple variations in the shock waveform (monophasic vs. biphasic, time constant duration, and shape); (D) presence vs. absence of ischemia; (E) acute vs. chronic lead systems; and (F) some antiarrhythmic drugs (procainamide and amiodarone). Any successful theory of defibrillation must explain the strong ULV-DFT correlation independent of many experimental conditions.

2. *Temporal clustering of preshock intervals:* Computer-assisted activation mapping compared preshock and postshock activation patterns after unsuccessful "subthreshold" shocks, slightly weaker than the DFT.[17] Immediately

after the shock, these studies identified an isoelectric window indicating that wavefronts did not continue through the shock. In the region of earliest postshock activation, wavefronts after the shock were not a continuation of the wavefronts before the shock. Additionally, the preshock intervals at the earliest site clustered in a narrow range. These findings are best explained by the existence of a vulnerable phase during VF temporally coincident with the cluster of preshock intervals.

3. *Mapping of critical points:* Limited evidence supports postshock reinitiation of VF by critical points or virtual-electrode–induced phase singularities. Activation-mapping studies showed that—for some subthreshold shocks—critical point formation and reinitiation of VF occurs even if shocks terminate all reentrant wavefronts.[17] Optical mapping studies have documented virtual-electrode critical points as the mechanism of postshock reinitiation of VF by some, but not all, subthreshold shocks.[18] Another study found evidence supporting both voltage-gradient and virtual-electrode critical points.[19]

Developing the ULV as a Clinical Tool

For an estimate of the ULV in regular rhythm to provide a clinically useful measure of defibrillation efficacy, three conditions must be met: (1) The most vulnerable part of the human cardiac cycle corresponding to the ULV must be identified. (2) The ULV in regular rhythm must identify a specific point on the defibrillation probability of success curve. (3) The method for estimating the ULV must be efficient, accurate, and reproducible.

Timing of the peak of the human vulnerable zone. Induction of VF by a T-wave shock depends on a critical relationship between the temporal sequence of repolarization, determined by the pacing location, and the spatial region of weakest shock field, determined by the shock pathway. If the shocking configuration is kept constant, the timing of the peak of the vulnerable zone depends on the pacing vector. Accurate knowledge of this timing is required to ensure that shocks are delivered at this most vulnerable part of the cardiac cycle, which is typically measured relative to a fiducial marker of repolarization. The most common marker is the maximum absolute value of the latest peaking monophasic T wave opposite in polarity from the R wave during right ventricular apical pacing.[20,21] During endocardial pacing, the peak of the T wave represents the period of greatest transmural dispersion of repolarization[22] and can be measured with high precision.

The most vulnerable part of the human vulnerable zone is narrow, including a median of only one or two 20-ms intervals.[13,20,21,23] No single coupling interval identifies it; and a 20-ms error in coupling interval results in underestimating the ULV by up to 5 J. *Thus shocks at multiple coupling intervals are required to determine the ULV accurately.* Investigators who estimate the ULV using a single T-wave shock may underestimate the true ULV if the shock does not coincide with the most vulnerable period.

For a single-coil shock vector, a four-shock scan should be delivered at −40 ms, −20 ms, 0 ms, and +20 ms relative to the peak of the T wave.[21] For a dual-coil shock vector, a four-shock scan should be delivered at −20, 0, +20, and +40 ms relative to the peak[20] (see Figs 18.6 and 18.7[13,20,21,23]). This approach identifies the most vulnerable intervals in about 90% of patients and underestimates the ULV by ≤ 3 J in the remainder.

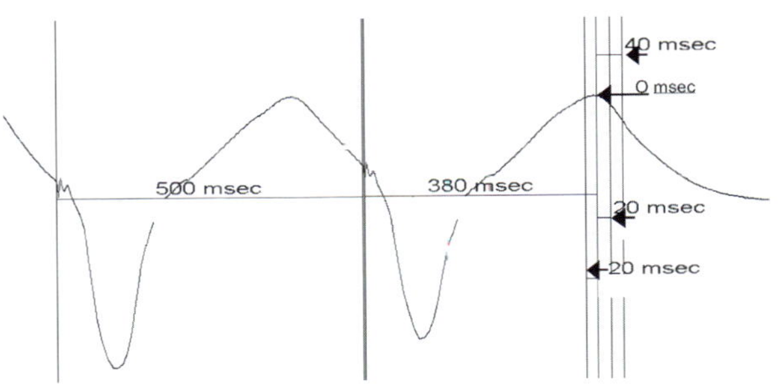

Fig 18.6 Figure shows timing of T-wave shocks for dual coil lead relative to peak of latest peaking monophasic T wave with polarity opposite to QRS during right-ventricular apical pacing at cycle length 500 ms.

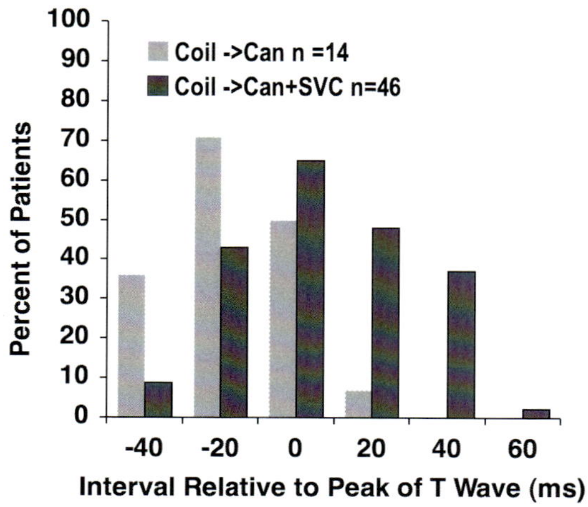

Fig 18.7 Histograms show timing of most vulnerable interval(s) (peak of vulnerable zone) relative to peak of T wave during ventricular paced rhythm at cycle length 500 ms. Separate histograms show data for 14 patients with single coil leads and 46 patients with dual coil leads. Percentages add to greater than 100% because the peak of the vulnerable zone contains a median of two coupling intervals. The distribution for single coil leads is shifted to shorter intervals relative to the distribution for dual coil leads.

Vulnerability testing would be more efficient if ICDs selected timing intervals for T-wave shocks automatically based on measurements made from intracardiac electrograms; but because these electrograms typically have biphasic T waves, their peaks are difficult to measure. An alternative to measuring the peak of the T wave is based on the recovery time, which is the maximum of the first-time derivative (dV/dt) of the T wave. For a unipolar electrogram, the recovery time is a reliable measure of local repolarization. The recovery time of the far-field (shock) electrogram has been used as a fiducial marker of global repolarization to time T-wave shocks with accuracy comparable to that provided by the peak of the T wave on the 12-lead ECG.[20] This permits an automated selection of the fiducial interval used for timing T-wave shocks.[23]

Probability of successful defibrillation at the ULV

As measured clinically, the ULV correlates closely with the shock strength that defibrillates with 90% probability (E_{90}).[24] In one study, 180 of the 200 defibrillation shocks (90%) at the ULV were successful (95% confidence interval 86%–94%). See Fig 18.8. These prospective data are consistent with retrospectively determined success rates of 89% and 92% for defibrillation shocks with strength equal to the ULV.[24,25]

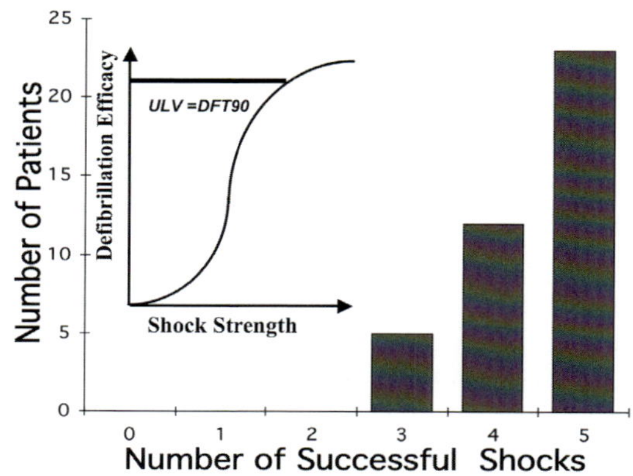

Fig 18.8 Defibrillation test shocks with strength equal to the ULV were delivered to 40 patients. The histogram shows the number of patients with successful defibrillation for 0 to 5 shocks. Overall, 90% of shocks were successful. The insert shows that the ULV thus approximates the shock strength that defibrillates with a probability of 90% (DFT90).

Acute defibrillation safety margin based on the ULV

Several single-center studies demonstrated that the acute success rate at ICD implantation for shocks with strength of 3 to 5 J above the ULV approximates 100%, providing that shocks at multiple coupling intervals are used to scan the T wave.[24,25]

Discrepancies between ULV and DFT

The ULV and DFT may be discordant for three reasons: (1) The method for estimating the ULV does not provide an accurate estimate of the true ULV, either because the method is inaccurate or because the ULV—like the DFT—is best represented as a probability-of-success curve. (2) The DFT measures an outlier point on the defibrillation probability-of-success curve. In these cases, the ULV is a more accurate estimate of the shock strength that defibrillates reliably. The ULV-DFT correlation cannot be better than the reproducibility of the clinically measured DFT.[25] (3) The ULV does not correlate with the DFT under rare conditions, such as use of lidocaine, which binds and dissociates from the sodium channel with such a short time constant that it increases the ULV relative to the DFT during rapid pacing. Gurevitz reported that major discrepancies (≥ 10 J) between ULV and DFT occurred in 8 of 167 patients (5%).[26] In all 8 patients, the ULV exceeded the DFT. However, the probabilistic nature of both ULV and DFT ensures that, in some patients, the DFT will exceed the ULV simply by chance alone.

Inductionless implantation of ICDs using only vulnerability safety margin testing

Instead of determining a patient-specific shock strength based on the ULV, a vulnerability safety margin test can be determined relative to maximum output of the ICD, analogous to a defibrillation safety margin. By definition, this shock strength equals or exceeds the ULV. *The advantage of this approach is that it does not require induction of VF to determine a safety margin for shocks that defibrillate reliably.* It has been validated prospectively in both single-center[27,28] studies and a multicenter study.[29] The multicenter study assessed acute vulnerability safety margin using a three shock T-wave scan (−20, 0, and +20 ms relative to the peak of the T wave) at 14 J in 421 patients.[29] The 77% of patients who passed vulnerability safety margin testing without induction of VF at 14 J underwent fibrillation-defibrillation testing with defibrillation shock strength of 21 J. The success rate for defibrillation of induced VF was 98.5%. Based on population estimates of the distribution of DFTs, the authors estimate that approximately 90% of ICD recipients will pass vulnerability safety margin testing at 20 J, allowing an adequate safety margin for ICDs with shock strength ≥ 30 J.[30]

How to Use Vulnerability Testing to Assess Defibrillation Safety Margin without Inducing VF.

Box 18.1 summarizes the steps of vulnerability testing for left pectoral ICDs in which the housing ("can") serves as defibrillation electrodes:

1. Record all 12-surface ECG leads at a minimum speed of 100 mm/s.

2. Deliver an R-wave synchronized 8-beat pacing train from the right ventricular apex at cycle length 500 ms. Unpublished data indicate that the method applies equally well to apical septal pacing and is insensitive to pacing cycle lengths over the range of 400 to 600 ms. In some patients with rapidly conducted atrial fibrillation, pacing must be performed at cycle length 400 ms to achieve a stable rhythm for vulnerability testing.

3. Review the pacing train to ensure capture of all 8 beats. Premature ventricular complexes or supraventricular capture beats can alter repolarization on subsequent beats. Using the last complex of the pacing train, determine the interval from the pacing stimulus to the peak of the latest peaking monophasic T wave ($S_1 - T_{peak}$) that has opposite polarity to the QRS complex. The last complex is easiest to measure because it is usually followed by a pause, which prevents superimposition of the terminal portion of a T wave with the next pacing stimulus. Measurements based on only a few leads may underestimate the $S_1 - T_{peak}$ interval. Measurements performed at slower speeds lack sufficient accuracy.

4. Select an initial test-shock strength for scanning the vulnerable zone. The optimal shock depends on the trade-off between the value of avoiding VF and that of programming the lowest effective shock strength. If maximal priority is assigned to not inducing VF, the shock strength should be 5 to 10 J below the maximum output of the ICD. If the goal is to determine the ULV—not just a safety margin, then the shock strength should be a few joules (J) higher than the population's mean DFT, usually in the 10 to 12 J range. In the authors' experience, T-wave scans at 15 J induce VF in

about 20% of patients and scans at 20 J induce VF in about 5% of patients. Because VF may be induced, vulnerability testing requires the same preparation for external, rescue defibrillation as defibrillation testing.

5. Deliver up to 4 T-wave shocks in the sequence indicated. Coupling intervals are ordered based on their probability of inducing VF.

6. Wait at least 60 s for recovery of circulation between shocks that do not induce VF. It is recommended to wait 90–120 s in the sickest patients.

7. If the 4-shock scan does not induce VF, the shock strength is greater than or equal to the ULV. *If the goal is to determine an ICD safety margin rather than the ULV, testing is complete.*

1. Ensure the R wave in native rhythm is ≥ 5 mV.
2. Record all 12-surface ECG leads at speed ≥ 100 mm/s.
3. Deliver pacing train from right ventricular apex at cycle length 500 ms.
4. Determine $S_1 - T_{peak}$ of latest peaking monophasic T wave.
5. Select the strength of the test shock.
6. Give scan of 4 T shocks:
   a. Single coil leads: 0, –20, –40, and +20 ms relative to T_{peak}
   b. Dual coil leads: 0, –20, +20, and +40 ms relative to T_{peak}
7. Wait at least 60 s between shocks.
8. If the 4-shock scan does not induce VF,
   a. If the goal is to determine a safety margin, testing is completed.
   b. If the goal is to determine the ULV, remea sure the $S_1 - T_{peak}$ interval, decrease the test shock strength, and repeat the 4-shock scan.
      i. Repeat this process until VF is induced.
      ii. If VF is induced, the previous tested shock strength is the ULV.
9. If VF is induced in step 6, the shock strength is below the ULV.
   a. Wait 4 to 5 min. Then remeasure the $S_1 - T_{peak}$ interval.
   b. Rescan the vulnerable zone using stronger shocks at the same and adjacent coupling intervals relative to the T wave.
10. Program the first ICD shock to at least 5 J ≥ the ULV or the shock strength in step 8(a).

Box 18.1 How to Perform Vulnerability Testing

Program the first ICD shock higher than the tested shock strength + 5 J. If VF is not induced in steps (6) and the goal is to determine the ULV for a patient-specific safety margin or for research, remeasure the $S_1 - T_{peak}$ interval, decrease the test-shock strength, and repeat the 4-shock scan. If VF is induced, the previous tested shock strength is the ULV. If VF is not induced, iterate the process. The lowest shock strength that ensures near 100% defibrillation success is 3 to 5 J greater than the ULV.

8. If VF is induced in step 5, the shock strength is below the ULV. Nonsustained polymorphic VT lasting longer than 3 s with cycle length < 250 ms is considered equivalent to VF for the purpose of estimating the ULV. Rarely, sustained VT is induced. Initiation of either nonsustained VF or sustained VT usually indicates that the shock strength is near a border of the vulnerable zone.

If the induced VT or VF requires defibrillation, wait 4 to 5 min. Then remeasure the $S_1 - T_{peak}$ interval and rescan the vulnerable zone using stronger shocks, starting at the same coupling interval relative to the T wave. The $S_1 - T_{peak}$ interval changes significantly in 10% to 20% of clinical ICD implants, depending on the number of shocks, number of VF episodes, and patient's autonomic tone.

Once an interval that induces VF is identified and a stronger shock at the same interval does not induce VF, the homogenous property of the vulnerable zone ensures that the scan at the higher shock strength need include only a 20-ms window on each side of the inducing interval, providing the $S_1 - T_{peak}$ interval is constant. If VF is induced at this stronger shock strength, either repeat step 8 or revise the defibrillation system.

Technical pitfalls

The observation that small errors in the coupling interval at which the ULV is determined can result in clinically significant underestimation of its value has three important corollaries: (1) *T-wave scanning.* Testing at only a single coupling interval may underestimate the ULV significantly. (2) *Selecting the coupling interval(s) for the ULV using weak shocks.* One method for clinical ULV testing scans the T wave starting with a long coupling interval using weak shocks near the VF threshold to identify a vulnerable interval. It then delivers stronger shocks at that coupling interval to determine the "ULV." This approach permits scanning with weaker shocks, rather than stronger shocks. However, because the coupling interval at the VF threshold often exceeds the coupling interval of the ULV, this method may underestimate the ULV (Box 18.2).

> Record all 12-surface ECG leads; QT dispersion may be substantial.
>
> 1. Measure at a sweep speed ≥ 100 mm/s to detect changes of ± 5 ms.
> 2. Discriminate retrograde P waves from the peaks of T waves.
> 3. Ensure that the entire pacing train of 8 stimuli capture the ventricle. Premature ventricular beats, supraventricular capture beats, or loss of capture due to failure of pacing synchronization may result in an unrepresentative value for $S_1 - T_{peak}$.
> 4. Use a validated mechanism to select coupling intervals for test shocks.

Box 18.2 Technical Pitfalls in Vulnerability Testing

Outcome of Implant Testing

Modification of the ICD System

With present active-can electrodes, efficient biphasic waveforms, and high-output (≥ ~34 J) ICDs, implant testing rarely results in modifying the ICD system. For example, in a review of 1139 consecutive patients, defibrillation testing was performed in 95%.[31] Of these, 3% had defibrillation safety margins < 10 J despite use of high-output pulse generators. The incidence of system modification based on implant testing varies from 0% to 5% in studies. No study has tested the hypothesis that system modification improves clinical outcomes, although all recognize the potentially fatal consequences of failed defibrillation of spontaneous VT/VF.

Advantages of a Low DFT

A large defibrillation safety margin (eg, DFT ≤ 15 J) can be achieved in ~ 90% of ICD recipients with present technology, although system revision may be required in ~ 10% of patients.[32] Presently, excluding patients considered too sick to test, mean DFTs for fixed-tilt waveforms are in the range of 8 to 10 J for dual-coil leads and 10 to 12 J for single-coil leads, with standard deviations of about 4 J.[32]

Time-dependent increases in DFT

Studies of patients with active-can biphasic waveform ICDs report time-dependent increases in DFT that compromise defibrillation in up to 15% of patients who are programmed to a 10-J safety margin.[8] However, the standard deviation of DFTs also increases with time so that the increase is often greater for patients with higher initial DFTs.

Drug-dependent increases in DFT

Postimplant addition of new drugs that may increase the DFT, chiefly amiodarone, is an important consideration. ICD patients are often treated with noncardiac drugs. These drugs usually are withheld at the time of ICD implantation, and little is known about their effects on defibrillation efficacy postimplant.

Advantages of a Lower Programmed First-Shock Strength

Programming a low first-shock strength on the basis of a low patient-specific implant criterion minimizes the potential, long-term adverse effects of excessive programmed shock strength. It reduces battery depletion if the ICD charges frequently for delivered or aborted shocks in the setting of "VT storm," repetitive nonsustained VT, lead failure, or repetitive inappropriate detection of SVT. Postshock depression of myocardial contractility depends on shock strength,[33] and avoiding unnecessarily strong shocks may reduce this phenomenon. But most ICD shocks are programmed to maximum output, and it is not known if patient-specific programming reduces the incidence of fatal postshock electromechanical dissociation.[34] Because the time required to charge an ICD capacitor is longer for stronger shocks and increases as most ICDs age, the risk of syncope with resultant trauma may be lower when the first shock is programmed to a low patient-specific value rather than to maximum output. Although this consideration is less important for some modern ICDs, programming a long duration to detect VF and a low patient-specific shock strength may be preferable in some patients with rapid, self-terminating VT/VF (eg, long QT syndrome) to permit prompt therapy without aborted charges. Finally, postimplant shocks may increase mortality in ICD patients [Daubert 2008, Poole 2008, Sweeney 2008]; lower shock strengths may attenuate any adverse effect of shocks on mortality.[35–37]

ICD-system factors

- Defibrillation electrode size, shape, and surface area
  Active can
  Subcutaneous electrode or array
- Defibrillation electrode location (including right- or left-sided pectoral implant)
- Single versus dual coil leads
- Shock waveform and polarity

Testing methods

- Duration of VF
- Defibrillation protocol (eg, step-down, step-up, binary search)
- Number of VF inductions
- Type of anesthesia
- Circadian variations

Patient-specific factors

- Left-ventricular ejection fraction, size, and mass
- Congestive heart failure class
- Gender
- Body surface area
- Ischemia
- Type of underlying heart disease (eg, hypertrophic cardiomyopathy)
- Drugs (eg, amiodarone)

Box 18.3 Factors That Influence the DFT

Factors That Influence Shock Strength Required for Defibrillation

Four types of factors influence the shock strength required for defibrillation: patient-specific factors, factors related to the ICD system (leads, shock waveform, defibrillation pathway), drug effects, and implant-related factors and complications (see Box 18.3).

Patient-specific Factors

If DFT could be predicted by clinical variables, testing could be restricted to a subset of patients. Common correlates of higher DFTs have been identified in multiple studies[31,38]: (1) lower left-ventricular ejection fraction, greater left-ventricular size or mass, and worse clinical heart failure; (2) male gender; (3) greater body surface area; and (4) specific cardiac diseases such as hypertrophic cardiomyopathy or Brugada Syndrome. However, the strength of these correlations has varied.

Further, most patients with risk factors for high DFTs have adequate safety margins. To date, no variable is a strong predictor of high DFT; there is no consensus on the relative influence of different variables on DFT; and no study has reported an accurate discriminator to identify either high-DFT or low-DFT patients. Thus no specific guidelines exist on how to use the correlates of high DFTs to plan defibrillation testing. Nevertheless, most experts consider testing of greater importance in patients with multiple risk factors for high DFTs.

Data regarding DFTs in cardiac resynchronization patients are limited. One study reported DFTs generally comparable to those reported for other ICD patients, but 11% of patients were either not stable enough to undergo testing or had unacceptable DFTs.[39] In another study, 9% of patients could not undergo defibrillation testing, and 12% of the remainder had high DFTs.[40] QRS duration was the only predictor of a high defibrillation threshold.

ICD System Factors

Factors related to the shock waveform, shock vector, and high voltage leads can be altered directly or indirectly at implant. Thus familiarity with their effects is important in the management of high-DFT patients.

Shock waveform

The key characteristics of ICD biphasic defibrillation waveforms include time constant (the product of capacitance and pathway resistance) and the duration of each phase.[41] Shock efficacy can be altered by changing waveform truncation based either on tilt or duration. For commercial ICDs with fixed duration waveforms, initial recommended programming is based on an estimated cardiac membrane time constant of 3.5 ms. High DFTs may be reduced by reprogramming waveform duration, but the relative contributions of improved defibrillation efficacy and regression to the mean have not been determined.

Shock polarity

Basic science studies support programming the right ventricular electrode as the anode in the first phase of biphasic waveforms.[41] This is associated with a moderately lower DFT for an inefficient biphasic waveform, but little or no benefit for efficient biphasic waveforms.[41] Within statistical uncertainty,[6] reversing polarity does not improve defibrillation efficacy[42,43] and should be abandoned as a troubleshooting step in high DFT patients.[41]

Shock vector and leads

Ideally, the three-dimensional orientation of the shock vector should provide a uniform field throughout the left ventricle. This vector depends on the position of the high-voltage coils and the active can in relation the heart. Low DFTs have been reported with leads placed near the apex, outflow tract, or septum. Alternatively, a rate-sensing lead may be placed in a different right ventricular location.

For fixed tilt waveforms, dual-coil leads reduce left pectoral DFTs by 10% to 20% compared with single-coil leads, provided the proximal coil is positioned high enough to prevent shunting of current through the right atrial blood pool.[32] The reduction in DFT provided by superior vena cava or subcutaneous electrodes may be caused by creation of a more uniform field in the left ventricle and/or shortening of fixed-tilt waveforms secondary to reduced pathway resistance. Conversely, the advantage of dual-coil leads is less when waveform duration is optimized for pathway resistance of a single-coil lead. If the proximal coil must be positioned low in the atrium, it should be excluded from the circuit or a single-coil lead should be used. An alternative to a dual-coil lead is a proximal coil on a second lead that can be positioned independently of the first lead, usually in the superior vena cava, innominate vein, or left subclavian vein. Less commonly, proximal coils are positioned in the coronary sinus, brachiocephalic vein, azygous vein, or inferior vena cava.

Right-sided pectoral implants require stronger defibrillation shocks than left-sided implants. The average increase in DFT is ~50%. Removing the pulse generator can from the pathway may reduce DFT in some right-sided implants. This may be accomplished either by using a pulse generator with an inactive can or by electronic programming (some manufacturers). A coil electrode in the innominate vein may be especially useful in right-sided implants to provide a leftward shock vector.

A subcutaneous electrode or electrode array is the most effective of commonly used methods for reducing DFTs. Limitations include potential long-term risks of infection, erosion, and chronic pain.

Drug Effects

Drug-ICD interactions have been reviewed extensively.[44]

Antiarrhythmic drugs

Antiarrhythmic drugs are prescribed to 22% to 67% of patients with ICDs.[38] Of these, the most widely studied is oral amiodarone, which increases DFTs by 15% to 48% in unselected patients. A meta-analysis reported that amiodarone increased DFT by a mean of 35%, but it increased variance of DFT by 52%, thus having a disproportionate effect on patients with high DFTs. If the DFT is known to be low (≤ 15 J), the risk of an increase sufficient to prevent defibrillation with maximum output is adequately low that repeat defibrillation testing is not required.[47] However, if the defibrillation safety margin at implant is small or unknown, follow-up defibrillation testing is usually recommended after the loading phase of amiodarone therapy. Patients taking amiodarone are three times more likely to have high DFTs than patients not taking amiodarone.[31]

In general, sodium channel blocking drugs increase DFTs.[44] Lidocaine has a profound effect. Conversely, potassium channel blocking drugs (sotalol, dofetilide, and azimilide) reduce DFTs and have been prescribed to reduce high DFTs.[45,46]

Anesthetics

Several studies address the effect of modern anesthetics. A randomized, prospective study reported no difference in DFTs among patients treated with either isoflurane or propofol.[48] Another study reported that DFT was lower when implants were performed using local anesthesia with lidocaine followed by propofol for defibrillation testing than when they were performed using general anesthesia with halothane, isoflurane, or fentanyl plus nitrous oxide.[49] However, systemic concentrations of lidocaine and marked elevation of DFTs have been reported after use of lidocaine during ICD implantation. Lidocaine may be administered intravenously to reduce local pain at the propofol infusion site. It should not be infused with propofol immediately prior to defibrillation testing. Some implanters prefer bupivicaine to lidocaine for local anesthetic during ICD implantation. It provides longer analgesia and may have less of an effect on DFT. Additionally, anesthetics may have secondary effects on DFT related to myocardial depression, hypoxia or hypercapnea.

Cardiac drugs

Most beta blockers have no significant effect on DFT, but limited data indicate that carvedilol can increase DFT. Angiotensin-converting enzyme inhibitors and angiotensin receptor blockers have no effects. Verapamil increases DFTs. It is prescribed to improve diastolic function in patients with hypertrophic cardiomyopathy and severe hypertrophy, who may independently be at risk for high DFTs.

Implant-related Factors and Complications

If defibrillation is unsuccessful, high-voltage connections to the pulse generator should be checked. Inspection of routine tip-to-ring and high-voltage electrograms does not identify switched high-voltage connections. Comparison of the electrogram between the can and right ventricular coil with the electrogram between the can and proximal coil will detect a reversed connection if lead markings are hard to identify at generator replacement. Retained guide wires or fragments of old electrodes may shunt current through parallel intrathoracic current paths and away from the heart. Pleural or pericardial effusions also create parallel current paths. Pneumothorax increases pathway resistance and DFT by placing insulating air in the current path. It may cause a marked increase in resistance between right ventricular coil and pectoral can.

DFTs may be elevated by prolonged procedures or many VF episodes with insufficient intervening time for recovery.[40] One clue that prolonged testing may be the problem is failure of a shock strength that defibrillated reliably earlier in the case.

Management of High DFT Patients

Our stepwise approach is summarized in Box 18.4. Attention to preventing high DFTs (Step 0) probably reduces the need to troubleshoot high DFTs. These include positioning the distal defibrillation coil accurately in the right ventricular apex (possibly against the septum) and use of a high-output ICD generator (≥ ~ 34 J). Confirm that high-voltage connections are correct and have nominal impedances measured by low-voltage pulses.

Before beginning to troubleshoot a high DFT, the diagnosis should be confirmed. Failure of a test shock at ≥ 20 J and a maximum output rescue shock is sufficient, if detection of VF is rapid and the charge time to maximum output is ≤ 10 s. But a single failed defibrillation can occur by chance alone. Thus, if a test shock fails but a maximum output shock succeeds, the test shock should be repeated, preferably with a measure related to ULV. Unreliable defibrillation at the minimum desirable safety margin should prompt an effort to improve defibrillation efficacy.

Once a high DFT is established, the first step is to identify and correct acutely reversible causes according to the check list in Step 1: Exclude ischemia, metabolic causes (including hypercapnea and acidemia which may occur after deep sedation in the absence of intubation), alternate current paths, and sources of increased resistance such as pneumothorax.

If the defibrillation system does not pass the implant criterion but the DFT is below maximum output, consider reprogramming the shock waveform if this is an option (Step 2). If this is unsuccessful or not an option, alter the transvenous shock vector if practical (Step 3). If this is impractical or unsuccessful, insert a subcutaneous electrode or array (Step 4). Inserting a subcutaneous array should be the first step if the DFT exceeds the maximum output of the ICD, because programming or alterations of a well-placed transvenous lead system are unlikely to produce a sufficient reduction in DFT.[40]

At intervals, consider whether a reversible factor cannot be corrected acutely, such as myocardial depression, pharmacological effect, or left pleural effusion. If so, testing may be better performed on another day after the problem has been resolved. If no potentially reversible factors are present, consider an epicardial lead system (Step 5).

STEP 0: Prevent High DFTs

Before implant
- Consider risk/benefit of continuing or withdrawing drugs that may increase DFT
- Optimize medical therapy of heart failure
- Drain left pleural effusion

At implant
- Position RV electrode tip at apex (before testing)
- Ensure appropriate position of proximal coil in high SVC or innominate vein; exclude proximal coil if low in atrium
- Set right-ventricular polarity to anode for phase 1 if not nominal
- Optimize waveform duration for shock pathway impedance if programmable
- Use a high-output generator (≥ ~ 34 J)
- Confirm high-voltage connections
- Correct connections of RV and SVC electrodes
- Integrity of current paths (nominal impedance assessed by low-voltage pulses)

STEP 1: Identify and Correct Acutely Reversible Causes

Correctable at implant
- Metabolic: hyperkalemia, hypoxemia
- Ischemia
- Alternate current paths
- Retained guide wire
- Fragments of old intracardiac or intravascular electrodes
- Pneumothorax

Not correctable at implant
- Myocardial depression
- Pharmacological (eg, amiodarone, verapamil, lidocaine)
- Prolonged procedure with multiple fibrillation-defibrillation episodes
- Left, pleural effusion or hemothorax; pericardial effusion or hemopericardium

STEP 2: [Optional] Change Shock Waveform if Programmable

Reprogram pulse durations for a different time constant

Chronic amiodarone: program shorter phase 2

STEP 3: [if Defibrillation Succeeds at Maximum Output] Alter Transvenous Shock Vector

Proximal coil in SVC, innominate vein, or high right atrium (exclude proximal coil if low)

Right-sided implant: exclude can or use cold can

Add separate coil (eg innominate vein or left subclavian vein)

STEP 4: Implant Subcutaneous Electrode or Electrode Array

STEP 5: Consider Epicardial System

Box 18.4 Stepwise Approach to the Patient with High DFTs

Predictive Value of Implant Testing

Assessing the value of implant testing requires considering four questions: (1) Does it predict shock success for induced VF? (2) Does it predict shock success for spontaneous VT/VF? (3) Does it predict conversion of spontaneous ventricular tachyarrhythmias? (4) Does it predict total mortality or sudden death? The value may differ in various patient populations.

Bayes' theorem and the implanter's dilemma

Bayes' theorem of conditional probability theory combines the a priori estimate of the probability that a condition is present with measures of test performance to derive an a posteriori estimate. The test in question is the implant criterion. The condition being estimated is the probability of successful defibrillation at a given shock strength for either induced or spontaneous VF.

Bayes' Theorem shows that testing provides limited incremental information if the a priori probability is very high or very low. For modern left pectoral ICDs and high-output pulse generators, the probability of passing a 10-J safety margin is sufficiently high (95%) that testing provides little incremental information. Most patients who fail the implant criteria do so because of false-negative tests.[9] Although rigorous testing recommends unnecessary system revision in a significant minority of patients, occasionally implant testing results in a system revision that saves a patient's life. This is the implanter's dilemma.

Prediction of shock success for induced VF

Passing implant criteria results in an extremely high success rate for defibrillation of induced VF. The LESS trial, performed in patients who had DFTs ≤ 15 J, applied a strict, patient-specific implant measure referred to as the DFT++ (the weakest shock strength that defibrillated on three consecutive trials).[8] At implant, the defibrillation success rate was 91% for shocks at the DFT++ and > 99% for shocks 4 to 6 J above the DFT++. Similarly, shocks programmed to the patient-specific ULV+5 J defibrillate acutely with near 100% success. In defibrillation safety margin testing, a single defibrillation success at 10 to 15 J predicts success for maximum output shocks with an accuracy of ~ 99%. However, modern defibrillation waveforms are sufficiently effective that maximum output shocks defibrillate all patients in some populations. In primary prevention patients with single-chamber ICDs, maximum output shocks successfully defibrillated all 717 patients who underwent testing in the SCD-HeFT trial.[50]

Prediction of shock success for spontaneous arrhythmias in the programmed VF zone of ICDs

The VF zone of ICDs is a rate- or cycle length-based zone that includes all arrhythmias with cycle lengths shorter than a boundary value between about 320 ms and 240 ms. Most arrhythmias in this zone are monomorphic VT. First shock success rates for spontaneous rapid VT or VF range from 83% to 93%,[38] lower than rates for induced VF.

This consistent observation suggests that shocks for spontaneous VT/VF fail for reasons that are not evaluated at implant. This is not surprising: Defibrillation testing is performed on sedated patients after clinical variables have been optimized. In contrast, spontaneous VT/VF occur in a less "controlled" environment that may include variations in multiple variables known to reduce defibrillation efficacy: autonomic tone, hyperkalemia, exacerbation of heart failure, drugs prescribed in follow-up, or progression of cardiac disease. DFTs are also higher in the upright than supine position. Durations of VT/VF > 15 seconds may increase DFT.[51] This is relevant either when undersensing occurs or when prolonged charge times occur due to aging effects on ICD batteries or failure to reform capacitors at adequate intervals. Circadian variation may be another factor: A morning peak in DFT corresponds to a morning peak in failed first shocks for spontaneous VT/VF.

Prediction of overall conversion of spontaneous VT/VF

Presently, the first-shock success rate for spontaneous VT/VF has at best a weak relationship with the overall conversion rate for VT/VF. Two factors account for this disparity. First antitachycardia pacing terminates 60% to 70% of fast VT in the traditional VF zone of ICDs and all episodes of VT in about 60% of ICD recipients (see Chapter 14). Second, ICDs deliver multiple shocks for VT/VF; subsequent shocks may succeed if the first fails.

Prediction of sudden death and total mortality

The central question is whether better implant testing can reduce sudden cardiac death and total mortality in ICD patients. Meta-analyses of randomized clinical trials indicate that ICD therapy reduces the risk of sudden cardiac death by about 60%.[52] VT/VF is the most common initial rhythm when ICD patients die suddenly.[34] The two largest studies of postmortem interrogation of ICDs indicate that 25% of sudden deaths in ICD patients are caused by failure to defibrillate VF.[34] Postdefibrillation electromechanical dissociation accounts for 29% of these deaths,[34,52] and multiple shocks were required to defibrillate VF in many of these episodes. Thus failure to defibrillate spontaneous VF remains a major cause of sudden death in ICD patients and failure to defibrillate promptly may be equally or more important.

Older data regarding the relationship between implant criteria and either total mortality or arrhythmic death are both limited and difficult to interpret. Blatt[50] reported no correlation between defibrillation safety margin and mortality in the SCD-HeFT study, but only 2% of patients had defibrillation safety margins ≤ 10 J.

Gula et al[53] used a decision-analysis model to estimate the benefit of assessing defibrillation efficacy at ICD implant. They found that the benefit of testing was highest in patients who had high risk of both VT/VF and a high DFT. Although almost no patients who meet present indications for ICDs had lower risk without testing, there was no meaningful predicted survival benefit in the vast majority of primary prevention patients.

This analysis combined with post-hoc analysis of the SCD-HeFT study[50] suggests that most primary prevention patients with cardiomyopathy and left-pectoral, single chamber ICDs do not benefit from implant testing. However, this conclusion does not necessarily apply to secondary prevention patients or primary prevention patients at high risk for unsuccessful defibrillation.

Only prospective, randomized trials on implant testing versus no implant testing will once and for all address the implanter's dilemma and are currently underway. The SAFE-ICD trial is a prospective observational study of the SAFEty of Two Strategies of ICD Management at Implantation. The investigators estimate enrollment of 1568 patients randomized to ICD implantation with and without VF induction with the primary outcome measure being a composite of (1) severe intraoperative complications at ICD implant, (2) events during a 2-year follow-up and secondary outcome being severe intraoperative complications occurring as a consequence of DFT testing (www.clinicaltrials.gov, Trial Identifier: NCT00661047). A similar ongoing study is Shockless Implant Evaluation (SIMPLE) planning on enrollment of 2500 patients and with a primary outcome of failed first appropriate clinical shock from the ICD or arrhythmic death with 2-year follow-up, with a secondary outcome being the 30-day complication rate (www.clinicaltrials.gov, Trial Identifier: NCT00800384).

Implant Testing at Pulse Generator Replacement

The principal considerations at generator change are integrity of the lead system and possible changes in ICD safety margin since implant caused by progression of heart disease, changes in drug therapy, and possibly lead maturation. In one study, generator replacement or "upgrade" (to dual chamber or cardiac resynchronization ICDs) was an independent risk factor for needing to modify the defibrillation electrodes to achieve reliable defibrillation.[31] The authors suggest that defibrillation efficacy be assessed (by either defibrillation or vulnerability testing) if structural heart disease has progressed significantly or if the safety margin was low or not tested at implant, especially if drugs known to affect the DFT (eg, amiodarone) have been added.

In some coaxial defibrillation leads, most notably the Medtronic Model 6936, inner insulation failure may be undetected by standard noninvasive diagnostics and present as postshock oversensing.[54] Some leads with insulation abrasion in the pocket may provide sufficient dielectric to measure nominal lead impedance when assessed by a low-voltage pulse but fail catastrophically when a high-voltage shock is delivered. Both phenomena can be identified by a maximum output shock in normal rhythm without inducing VF.

Risks of Assessing Defibrillation Efficacy at Implant

The risks of DFT testing are related to VF, shocks alone, and anesthesia required for shocks. Birnie et al reported on 19,067 patients who underwent ICD implant, of whom about 80% had limited fibrillation-defibrillation testing.[55] Death or life-altering complications from defibrillation testing occurred in 5 patients (0.026%). These risks must be weighed against the likelihood that postimplant sudden death (caused by failure to defibrillate or postdefibrillation electromechanical dissociation)[34,52,56] can be prevented by implant testing. Box 18.5 summarizes contraindications to implant testing.

Absolute

- Risk of thromboembolism
  - —Left-atrial thrombus
  - —Left-ventricular thrombus without systemic anticoagulation
  - —Atrial fibrillation without systemic anticoagulation*
- Inadequate anesthesia or anesthesia support
- Known inadequate external defibrillation
- Severe aortic stenosis
- Unstable angina
- Severe, unrevascularized coronary artery disease with jeopardized myocardium
- Hemodynamic instability requiring inotropic support

Relative

- Left-ventricular mural thrombus with adequate systemic anticoagulation
- Questionable external defibrillation (eg, massive obesity)
- Severe unrevascularized coronary artery disease
- Recent coronary stent
- Hemodynamic instability
- Recent stroke or transient ischemic attack
- Questionable stability of coronary venous lead

*Unless transesophageal echocardiography demonstrates no thrombus and anticoagulation initiated postoperatively.

Box 18.5 Contraindications to ICD Implant Testing

Risks of VF

Central nervous system hypoperfusion

Intraoperative electroencephalographic (EEG) monitoring during DFT testing frequently shows EEG "slowing" consistent with cerebral ischemia, and cerebral blood flow may be depressed for several minutes after normalization of mean arterial pressure and EEG.[57] Thus these changes may have a cumulative depressant effect on the EEG if repeated VF inductions are performed without sufficient recovery time.

Myocardial ischemia

In patients with coronary artery disease, hypotension due to prolonged VF may result in myocardial ischemia. Perioperative myocardial infarction is difficult to diagnose because shocks delivered for routine defibrillation testing may cause both elevation of troponin and nonspecific ECG changes. In patients with recent coronary stents, acute stent thrombosis is a potential consequence of VF-induced hypotension.

Electromechanical dissociation

Pulseless electrical activity caused by true electromechanical dissociation is the most common fatal or life-altering complication of fibrillation-defibrillation testing. In the largest reported series of complications associated with defibrillation testing, postdefibrillation electromechanical dissociation caused 2 of 3 deaths and both life-altering complications (hemodynamic collapse requiring urgent cardiac transplantation and anoxic encephalopathy in 1 patient each).[55]

Shocks alone may depress myocardial contractility, and the magnitude of shock-induced myocardial depression correlates with shock strength.[33] However, myocardial depression is greater after the fibrillation and defibrillation than after shocks alone, and significant hypotension is more common after a single fibrillation-defibrillation episode than after three T-wave shocks that do not induce VF (8% vs. 2%, $p = 0.006$).[58]

Fatal electromechanical dissociation has been reported only after defibrillation from VF,[31,39,55,59] but not after shocks alone. It should be noted that this distinction applies both during implant testing and follow-up. Although postshock electromechanical dissociation is a leading cause of sudden death in patients treated with ICDs,[34] it has not been reported after inappropriate shocks. Some patients who had fatal electromechanical dissociation during defibrillation testing had severe left ventricular dysfunction[59] or underwent many fibrillation-defibrillation episodes, but it has also been reported in stable patients during the first or second fibrillation-defibrillation episode.[55]

Prolonged resuscitation and refractory VF

One study reported that all tested ICD shocks failed and ≥ 3 external rescue shocks were required in 0.5% of patients.[60] Birnie et al[55] reported an incidence of prolonged resuscitation from pulseless electrical activity or refractory VF of 0.14%. No patient died from refractory VF.

Risks of Shocks Alone

Thromboembolic complications

Shocks may cause arterial thromboembolism if intracardiac thrombus is present. In patients with atrial fibrillation and left atrial appendage thrombus, either T-wave shocks or defibrillation shocks may cause thromboembolism. This risk is analogous to the well-studied risk of thromboembolism associated with atrial cardioversion. Anticoagulation is typically discontinued before and after ICD implantation, potentially increasing the risk of left atrial appendage thrombus formation in patients with atrial fibrillation. Birnie et al reported that stroke or transient ischemic attack occurred with an overall incidence of 0.026%.[55] All 5 patients had atrial fibrillation; all received warfarin and/or heparin, but the duration of warfarin therapy was not reported. In 4 of these 5 patients, defibrillation shocks cardioverted AF. Left ventricular thrombus may also be a source of thromboembolism in patients undergoing defibrillation implant testing, but the magnitude of this risk is less established.

Risks at Implantation of Cardiac Resynchronization ICDs

Patients undergoing implants of cardiac resynchronization ICDs are some of the sickest patients in whom defibrillation testing is considered, and they undergo some of the longest implant procedures. Shocks may dislodge passive coronary venous electrodes. Further, improvement in left ventricular function by cardiac resynchronization pacing may reduce the DFT over time. Some experts have suggested deferring testing for 1 to 3 months because of procedure duration, left ventricular lead stability, or the likelihood of future reverse remodeling. Others argue that a lead dislodged by a shock will probably dislodge during follow-up and that, for efficiency testing should be done at implant.

Anesthesia-related Complications

A common technique is local anesthesia for insertion of leads and pulse generator combined with short-acting, deep intravenous sedation for defibrillation testing. This method reduces implant time and may reduce anesthesia-related complications in comparison with endotracheal intubation, but it requires careful monitoring of airway and ventilatory status. The most commonly used drugs are midazolam, fentanyl, and propofol. Etomidate has also been recommended because it has minimal or no effect on cardiac or vascular function. General anesthesia may be preferred in patients with Brugada syndrome in whom local anesthetics may be proarrhythmic. Anesthetics with direct depressant effect on myocardial contractility typically are avoided, peripheral vascular effects often cause hypotension; and all anesthetics may have secondary effects if respiratory depression leads to hypoxia or hypercapnea, especially in patients with lung disease or sleep apnea.

Risks of Vulnerability Testing versus Safety of Defibrillation Testing

Vulnerability safety margin testing avoids the risks associated with VF or circulatory arrest in up to 90% of patients, including the most common fatal problem of postshock electromechanical dissociation. Vulnerability testing does not reduce risks caused by shock-induced thromboembolism or anesthesia. Although defibrillation testing has a good safety record, vulnerability testing probably is safer. See Table 18.2.

Sensing and Detection of VF

In addition to testing the adequacy of the programmed shock strength, VF is induced at ICD implantation to assess electrical integrity of the connections between leads and pulse generator and reliable sensing, detection, and redetection in VF. Low voltage pulses or shocks in normal rhythm can achieve the first goal.

Undersensing during VF was an important clinical problem for early ICD leads and sensing amplifiers. To ensure adequate sensing during VF, maximum sensitivity has traditionally been programmed to an insensitive setting (~ 1 mV) during fibrillation-defibrillation testing. Conceptually, reliable sensing of VF at this setting ensures an adequate safety margin either for sensing of "fine" VF with nominal sensitivity (~ 0.3 mV) or for programming a less-sensitive setting to avoid T-wave oversensing.

Vulnerability safety margin testing does not verify sensing of VF. Because of the correlation between R-wave amplitude in native rhythm and VF,[61] the first studies using this method required patients to have an adequate R wave (≥ 5–7 mV) in native rhythm.[27] Using this approach, VF was not undersensed at implant[23,27,29,62] or follow-up.[27]

Even if R waves are small, modern ICDs rarely undersense VF.[63] When it occurs, undersensing usually is caused by either transient

	Defibrillation Testing	Vulnerability Testing
Risks of VF		
Prolonged resuscitation	+	±
Postshock EMD	+	0
Risks of Shocks Alone		
Thromboembolism if intracardiac thrombus	+	+
Anesthesia required	+	+

Table 18.2 Risks of Vulnerability Testing (Shocks Alone) versus Defibrillation Testing (Shocks + VF) at ICD Implant Testing

effects that reduce the slew rate of local electrograms (eg, ischemia, drug, or hyperkalemia) or electrogram amplitudes that vary faster than automatically adjusting sensitivity can react. Unfortunately, neither is reproducible in the electrophysiology lab,[38,64] and both can occur with adequate baseline R waves. Ruetz et al reported no correlation between baseline R-wave amplitude and sensing of induced VF in modern true-bipolar sensing leads with sensitivity programmed to 1.2 mV.[65] Undersensing in VF was caused by variations in signal amplitude or low-frequency electrograms in 36 of 1177 patients (3%). Detection delay occurred in only 1 episode (0.08%) with a sinus R wave of 13.7 mV. Thus, while there are valid reasons to ensure an adequate R wave in baseline rhythm (eg, prevention of T-wave oversensing and excluding lead perforation), VF undersensing at implant cannot be predicted by R-wave amplitude for presently used true-bipolar sensing leads.

Sensing and redetection of VF after unsuccessful defibrillation is the most difficult case for detection of VF. Early-model, integrated bipolar leads with short tip-coil spacing (eg, 6 mm) were prone to postshock undersensing. Postshock redetection of VF may be tested if a chronically implanted system uses such an electrode. Testing of sensing during VF is also indicated if patients have separate electrical devices that may interfere with ICD sensing, such as neurostimulators or cardiac-contractility modulation devices. The most important of these is failure to sense VF due to resetting of auto-adjusting sensitivity or automatic gain control by the electrical stimuli from the other device. In dual chamber ICDs, detection of VF may be delayed or prevented by "intra-device" interactions, such as one caused by ventricular blanking periods related to rate-smoothing pacing.[66]

Minimizing Risks of Implant Testing

Most disasters are avoided before the first shock is delivered by following safety guidelines:

Preoperatively:

1. Assess oxygenation, the airway (including ease of endotracheal intubation). Review drugs that might alter the DFT; review laboratory data with attention to hyperkalemia. Ensure heart failure is compensated. Assess the native rhythm to determine the need for postshock pacing. Exclude active ischemia and aortic stenosis. Review the chest X-ray for left pleural effusion that may elevate DFTs.
2. Patients with morbid obesity or diabetic neuropathy may need to fast more than 6 hours to ensure gastric emptying and minimize the risk of aspiration.
3. In patients with atrial fibrillation, perform a transesophageal echo if adequate duration or level of anticoagulation cannot be confirmed for at least 3 weeks.
4. Test the external defibrillator and its connections to self-adhesive defibrillation electrode pads; confirm proper location of defibrillation pads. Have a back-up external defibrillator. Unreliable transvenous defibrillation will occur eventually. Unreliable external defibrillation is a complication that has not yet happened.

In the electrophysiology lab before testing:

5. Exclude mechanical complications such as hemopericardium and pneumothorax.
6. Confirm sensing and pacing functions in baseline rhythm.
7. Confirm integrity of the high-voltage leads by measuring lead impedance using low-voltage pulses. Proceed only if the impedance is in a range that excludes both a short circuit and an open circuit or inadequate lead connection (desired range: 20–80 Ω).
8. Recheck the airway and level of sedation during testing.
9. Wait between VF inductions: at least 1 min between shocks that do not induce VF and 4 to 5 min between shocks that induce VF. Recovery of cardiac output and cerebral perfusion lags recovery of arterial pressure by several minutes.

10. Monitor respiratory status, including respiratory rate, tidal volume, oxygen saturation, and expired pCO_2. If acidosis is a concern, draw an arterial blood gas.
11. If atrial fibrillation is cardioverted inadvertently, consider refibrillating the atrium using the ICD's atrial lead or a separate catheter.
12. If acute hypotension occurs, assess for acute reversible surgical complications (tension pneumothorax, hemothorax, pericardial tamponade); assess the ECG for ST segment changes or other signs of ischemia; and assess for anesthetic or metabolic complications.
13. After each shock, reassess the patient for hemodynamic effects and respiratory status. Determine whether it is safe to proceed.

Noninvasive Postoperative Testing of ICDs

Noninvasive postoperative testing, either predischarge or a few months after implant, is an alternative to testing at implantation. Postoperative testing is not influenced by some factors that affect defibrillation efficacy at implant, it may be performed after contraindications to vulnerability or fibrillation-defibrillation testing have resolved, and it may identify problems that occur between implant and testing. However, it is less convenient than intraoperative testing and it adds cost to ICD therapy. Further, if the need for system revision is identified at noninvasive testing, a separate reoperation is required. With a few exceptions, most data regarding postoperative testing relates to its role as a supplement to intraoperative testing, rather than a substitute for it.

Perspective and Recommendations

Implant testing is evolving, but its goal is unchanged—to find the optimal balance between implant safety and long-term benefits of ICD therapy. Experts consider testing less critical now than they did 10 years ago. Clinically, true DFT testing is performed rarely. Most testing is limited, defibrillation safety-margin testing. A minor trend is toward substitution of vulnerability testing for defibrillation testing. As discussed, limited modeling[53] and retrospective[50] data indicate no benefit of testing in primary prevention patients without risk factors for high DFTs. Although no prospective data support the value of testing, most implanters, patients, and families have near-zero tolerance for sudden cardiac death caused by preventable, failed defibrillation. In this context, we offer the following considerations:

Sensing and detection of VF should be tested if required to evaluate device-device interactions. Conventional wisdom recommends testing if the baseline R wave is $\leq$ 5 mV, but this may not be necessary in new implants with true-bipolar leads. Overall, sensing and detection issues require induction of VF in < 5% of ICD recipients.

Defibrillation or vulnerability should be used to assess a defibrillation safety margin if the a priori estimate of the shock strength required for reliable defibrillation is high. See Box 18.3. The fraction of patients varies, but may range from 20% to 40%.

A patient-specific implant criterion should be used if long detection times are advisable in patients with frequent, long episodes of nonsustained VT/VF to prevent unnecessary aborted or delivered shocks while preventing syncope with short charge times. This includes about 5% of ICD recipients.

Contraindications to implant testing are critical for patient safety. Absolute contraindications occur in about 5% of ICD recipients; and a relative contraindication occurs in 10% to 30%.

Legal and regulatory considerations. Presently, assessing defibrillation efficacy at implantation of ICDs is the legal standard of practice. The labeling on all U.S.-manufactured ICDs recommends assessment of defibrillation efficacy at implant and programming the first VF shock with a 10-J safety margin. The Heart Rhythm Society also recommends implant defibrillation testing.[67] If testing is not performed, it is recommended to document both the specific contraindication and whether postimplant testing is planned.

In summary, VF should be induced to assess sensing in < 5% of ICD recipients. Defibrillation or vulnerability testing is indicated in 20% to 40% of recipients who can be identified as having a higher-than-usual probability of an inadequate defibrillation safety margin based on patient-specific factors. At least one maximum output shock usually should be delivered at the time of generator replacement to assure lead integrity. Implant testing is too risky in ~ 5% of ICD recipients and may not be worth the risks in 10% to 30% more. In 25% to 50% of ICD recipients, implant testing cannot be identified as either critical or contraindicated.

References

1. McDaniel WC, Schuder JC. The cardiac ventricular defibrillation threshold: inherent limitations in its application and interpretation. *Med Instrum.* 1987;21(3):170–176.
2. Davy JM, Fain ES, Dorian P, et al. The relationship between successful defibrillation and delivered energy in open-chest dogs: reappraisal of the "defibrillation threshold" concept. *Am Heart J.* 1987;113:77–84.
3. Gliner BE, Murakawa Y, Thakor NV. The defibrillation success rate versus energy relationship: Part I—Curve fitting and the most efficient defibrillation energy. *Pacing Clin Electrophysiol.* 1990;13(3):326–338.
4. Malkin RA, Souza JJ, Ideker RE. The ventricular defibrillation and upper limit of vulnerability dose-response curves. *J Cardiovasc Electrophysiol.* 1997;8(8):895–903.
5. Marchlinski FE, Flores B, Miller JM, et al. Relation of the intraoperative defibrillation threshold to successful postoperative defibrillation with an automatic implantable cardioverter defibrillator. *Am J Cardiol.* 1988;62(7):393–398.
6. Swerdlow CD, Davie S, Ahern T, et al. Comparative reproducibility of defibrillation threshold and upper limit of vulnerability. *Pacing Clin Electrophysiol.* 1996;19(12 Pt 1):2103–2111.
7. Li H, Malkin RA. An approximate bayesian up-down method for estimating a percentage point on a dose-response curve. *J Appl Stat.* 2000;27(5):579–587.
8. Gold MR, Higgins S, Klein R, et al. Efficacy and temporal stability of reduced safety margins for ventricular defibrillation: primary results from the Low Energy Safety Study (LESS). *Circulation.* 2002;105(17):2043–2048.
9. DeGroot PJ, Church TR, Mehra R, et al. Derivation of a defibrillator implant criterion based on probability of successful defibrillation. *Pacing Clin Electrophysiol.* 1997;20(8 Pt 1):1924–1935.
10. Smits K, DeGroot P. A Bayesian approach to reduced implant testing of a ventricular defibrillator: a computer simulation. *Europace.* 2004;6(s1):S97 Abstract.
11. Barnett AG, van der Pols JC, Dobson AJ. Regression to the mean: what it is and how to deal with it. *Int J Epidemiol.* 2005;34(1):215–220.
12. Chen P-S, Shibata N, Dixon E, et al. Comparison of the defibrillation threshold and the upper limit of ventricular vulnerability. *Circulation.* 1986;73:1022–1028.
13. Swerdlow CD, Shehata M, Chen PS. Using the upper limit of vulnerability to assess defibrillation efficacy at implantation of ICDs. *Pacing Clin Electrophysiol.* 2007;30(2):258–270.
14. Winfree AT. Sudden cardiac death: A problem in topology. *Sci Am.* 1983;248:144–149.
15. Yamanouchi Y, Cheng Y, Tchou PJ, et al. The mechanisms of the vulnerable window: the role of virtual electrodes and shock polarity. *Can J Physiol Pharmacol.* 2001;79(1):25–33.
16. Efimov IR, Gray RA, Roth BJ. Virtual electrodes and deexcitation: new insights into fibrillation induction and defibrillation. *J Cardiovasc Electrophysiol.* 2000;11(3):339–353.
17. Chen P-S, Wolf PD, Ideker RE. The mechanism of cardiac defibrillation: a different point of view. *Circulation.* 1991;84:913–919.
18. Efimov IR, Cheng Y, Yamanouchi Y, et al. Direct evidence of the role of virtual electrode-induced phase singularity in success and failure of defibrillation. *J Cardiovasc Electrophysiol.* 2000;11(8):861–868.

19. Evans FG, Ideker RE, Gray RA. Effect of shock-induced changes in transmembrane potential on reentrant waves and outcome during cardioversion of isolated rabbit hearts. *J Cardiovasc Electrophysiol.* 2002;13(11):1118–1127.
20. Swerdlow C, Shivkumar K, Zhang J. Determination of the upper limit of vulnerability using implantable cardioverter-defibrillator electrograms. *Circulation.* 2003;107(24):3028–3033.
21. Swerdlow CD, Martin DJ, Kass RM, et al. The zone of vulnerability to T wave shocks in humans. *J Cardiovasc Electrophysiol.* 1997;8(2):145–154.
22. Yan GX, Antzelevitch C. Cellular basis for the normal T wave and the electrocardiographic manifestations of the long-QT syndrome. *Circulation.* 1998;98(18):1928–1936.
23. Shehata M, Belk P, Kremers M, et al. Automatic determination of timing intervals for upper limit of vulnerability using ICD electrograms. *Pacing Clin Electrophysiol.* 2008;31(6):691–700.
24. Swerdlow CD, Ahern T, Kass RM, et al. Upper limit of vulnerability is a good estimator of shock strength associated with 90% probability of successful defibrillation in humans with transvenous implantable cardioverter-defibrillators. *J Am Coll Cardiol.* 1996;27(5):1112–1118.
25. Swerdlow C, Ahern T, Chen P-S. Comparative reproducibility of defibrillation threshold and upper limit of vulnerability. *Pacing Clin Electrophysiol.* 1996;19:2103–2111.
26. Gurevitz OT, Friedman PA, Glikson M, et al. Discrepancies between the upper limit of vulnerability and defibrillation threshold: prevalence and clinical predictors. *J Cardiovasc Electrophysiol.* 2003;14(7):728–732.
27. Swerdlow CD. Implantation of cardioverter defibrillators without induction of ventricular fibrillation. *Circulation.* 2001;103(17):2159–2164.
28. Green UB, Garg A, Al-Kandari F, et al. Successful implantation of cardiac defibrillators without induction of ventricular fibrillation using upper limit of vulnerability testing. *J Interv Card Electrophysiol.* 2003;8(1):71–75.
29. Day JD, Doshi RN, Belott P, et al. Inductionless or limited shock testing is possible in most patients with implantable cardioverter-defibrillators/cardiac resynchronization therapy defibrillators: results of the multicenter ASSURE Study (Arrhythmia Single Shock Defibrillation Threshold Testing Versus Upper Limit of Vulnerability: Risk Reduction Evaluation With Implantable Cardioverter-Defibrillator Implantations). *Circulation.* 2007;115(18):2382–2389.
30. Ruetz L, Belk B, Stromberg K. A model of defibrillation efficacy for comparing upper limit of vulnerability testing to conventional implant testing. *Heart Rhythm.* 2008;5(5):S240.
31. Russo AM, Sauer W, Gerstenfeld EP, et al. Defibrillation threshold testing: is it really necessary at the time of implantable cardioverter-defibrillator insertion? *Heart Rhythm.* 2005;2(5):456–461.
32. Gold MR, Olsovsky MR, DeGroot PJ, et al. Optimization of transvenous coil position for active can defibrillation thresholds. *J Cardiovasc Electrophysiol.* 2000;11(1):25–29.
33. Tokano T, Bach D, Chang J, et al. Effect of ventricular shock strength on cardiac hemodynamics. *J Cardiovasc Electrophysiol.* 1998;9(8):791–797.
34. Mitchell LB, Pineda EA, Titus JL, et al. Sudden death in patients with implantable cardioverter defibrillators: the importance of post-shock electromechanical dissociation. *J Am Coll Cardiol.* 2002;39(8):1323–1328.
35. Daubert JP, Zareba W, Cannom DS, et al. Inappropriate implantable cardioverter-defibrillator shocks in MADIT II: frequency, mechanisms, predictors, and survival impact. *J Am Coll Cardiol.* 2008;51(14):1357–1365.
36. Poole JE, Johnson GW, Hellkamp AS, et al. Prognostic importance of defibrillator shocks in patients with heart failure. *N Engl J Med.* 2008;359(10):1009–1017.
37. Sweeney MO, Sherfesee L, DeGroot PJ, et al. Differences in effects of electrical therapy type for ventricular arrhythmias on mortality in implantable cardioverter-defibrillator patients. *Heart Rhythm.* 2010;7(3):353–60.
38. Swerdlow CD, Russo AM, DeGroot PJ. The dilemma of ICD implant testing. *Pacing Clin Electrophysiol.* 2007;30(5):675–700.
39. Schuger C, Ellenbogen KA, Faddis M, et al. Defibrillation energy requirements in an ICD population receiving cardiac resynchronization

therapy. *J Cardiovasc Electrophysiol.* 2006;17(3): 247–250.

40. Mainigi SK, Callans DJ. How to manage the patient with a high defibrillation threshold. *Heart Rhythm.* 2006;3(4):492–495.
41. Kroll M, Swerdlow C. Optimizing defibrillation waveforms for ICDs. *J Interv Card Electrophysiol.* 2007;18(3):247–263.
42. Narasimhan C, Panotopoulos PT, Deshpande S, et al. Reversing the initial phase polarity in biphasic shocks: is the polarity benefit reproducible? *Pacing Clin Electrophysiol.* 1999;22(1 Pt 1):60–64.
43. Kroll MW, Efimov IR, Tchou PJ. Present understanding of shock polarity for internal defibrillation: the obvious and non-obvious clinical implications. *Pacing Clin Electrophysiol.* 2006;29(8):885–891.
44. Goldschlager N, Epstein A, Friedman P, et al. Environmental and drug effects on patients with pacemakers and implantable cardioverter/defibrillators: a practical guide to patient treatment. *Arch Intern Med.* 2001;161(5):649–655.
45. Dorian P, Newman D, Sheahan R, et al. d-Sotalol decreases defibrillation energy requirements in humans: A novel indication for drug therapy. *J Cardiovasc Electrophysiol.* 1996;7:952–961.
46. Qi XQ, Newman D, Dorian P. Azimilide decreases defibrillation voltage requirements and increases spatial organization during ventricular fibrillation. *J Interv Card Electrophysiol.* 1999;3:61–67.
47. Hohnloser SH, Dorian P, Roberts R, et al. Effect of amiodarone and sotalol on ventricular defibrillation threshold: the optimal pharmacological therapy in cardioverter defibrillator patients (OPTIC) trial. *Circulation.* 2006;114(2):104–109.
48. Moerman A, Herregods L, Tavernier R, et al. Influence of anaesthesia on defibrillation threshold. *Anaesthesia.* 1998;53(12):1156–1159.
49. Weinbroum AA, Glick A, Copperman Y, et al. Halothane, isoflurane, and fentanyl increase the minimally effective defibrillation threshold of an implantable cardioverter defibrillator: first report in humans. *Anesth Analg.* 2002;95(5):1147–1153, table of contents.
50. Blatt JA, Poole JE, Johnson GW, et al. No benefit from defibrillation threshold testing in the SCD-HeFT (Sudden Cardiac Death in Heart Failure Trial). *J Am Coll Cardiol.* 2008;52(7):551–556.
51. Gradaus R, Bode-Schnurbus L, Weber M, et al. Effect of ventricular fibrillation duration on the defibrillation threshold in humans. *Pacing Clin Electrophysiol.* 2002;25(1):14–19.
52. Anderson KP. Sudden cardiac death unresponsive to implantable defibrillator therapy: an urgent target for clinicians, industry and government. *J Interv Cardiol Electrophysiol.* 2005;14(2):71–78.
53. Gula LJ, Massel D, Krahn AD, et al. Is defibrillation testing still necessary? A decision analysis and Markov model. *J Cardiovasc Electrophysiol.* 2008;19(4):400–405.
54. Ellenbogen KA, Wood MA, Shepard RK, et al. Detection and management of an implantable cardioverter defibrillator lead failure: incidence and clinical implications. *J Am Coll Cardiol.* 2003;41(1):73–80.
55. Birnie D, Tung S, Simpson C, et al. Complications associated with defibrillation threshold testing: the Canadian experience. *Heart Rhythm.* 2008;5(3):387–390.
56. Pires LA, Hull ML, Nino CL, et al. Sudden death in recipients of transvenous implantable cardioverter defibrillator systems: terminal events, predictors, and potential mechanisms. *J Cardiovasc Electrophysiol.* 1999;10(8):1049–1056.
57. de Vries JW, Bakker PF, Visser GH, et al. Changes in cerebral oxygen uptake and cerebral electrical activity during defibrillation threshold testing. *Anesth Analg.* 1998;87(1):16–20.
58. Day J, Freedman R, Zubair I, et al. Most patients may safely undergo inductionless ICD implants *Circulation.* 2003;108:IV–324 abstract.
59. Frame R, Brodman R, Furman S, et al. Clinical evaluation of the safety of repetitive intraoperative defibrillation threshold testing. *Pacing Clin Electrophysiol.* 1992;15(6):870–877.
60. Alter P, Waldhans S, Plachta E, et al. Complications of implantable cardioverter defibrillator therapy in 440 consecutive patients. *Pacing Clin Electrophysiol.* 2005;28(9):926–932.
61. Ellenbogen KA, Wood MA, Stambler BS, et al. Measurement of ventricular electrogram amplitude during intraoperative induction of

ventricular tachyarrhythmias. *Am J Cardiol.* 1992;70(11):1017–1022.

62. Birgersdotter-Green U, Garg A, Al-Kandari F, et al. Successful implantation of cardiac defibrillators without induction of ventricular fibrillation using upper limit of vulnerability testing. *J Interv Cardiol Electrophysiol.* 2003;8(1):71–75.
63. Kenigsberg DN, Mirchandani S, Dover AN, et al. Sensing failure associated with the Medtronic Sprint Fidelis defibrillator lead. *J Cardiovasc Electrophysiol.* 2008;19(3):270–274.
64. Dekker LR, Schrama TA, Steinmetz FH, et al. Undersensing of VF in a patient with optimal R wave sensing during sinus rhythm. *Pacing Clin Electrophysiol.* 2004;27(6 Pt 1):833–834.
65. Ruetz L, Koehler J, Jackson T, et al. Sinus-rhythm R-wave amplitude does not predict undersensing of ventricular fibrillation by implantable cardioverter-defibrillators. *Circulation.* 2009; 120(18 Supp2):S650.
66. Glikson M, Beeman AL, Luria DM, et al. Impaired detection of ventricular tachyarrhythmias by a rate-smoothing algorithm in dual-chamber implantable defibrillators: intradevice interactions. *J Cardiovasc Electrophysiol.* 2002; 13(4):312–318.
67. Curtis AB, Ellenbogen KA, Hammill SC, et al. Clinical competency statement: Training pathways for implantation of cardioverter defibrillators and cardiac resynchronization devices. *Heart Rhythm.* 2004;1(3):371–375.

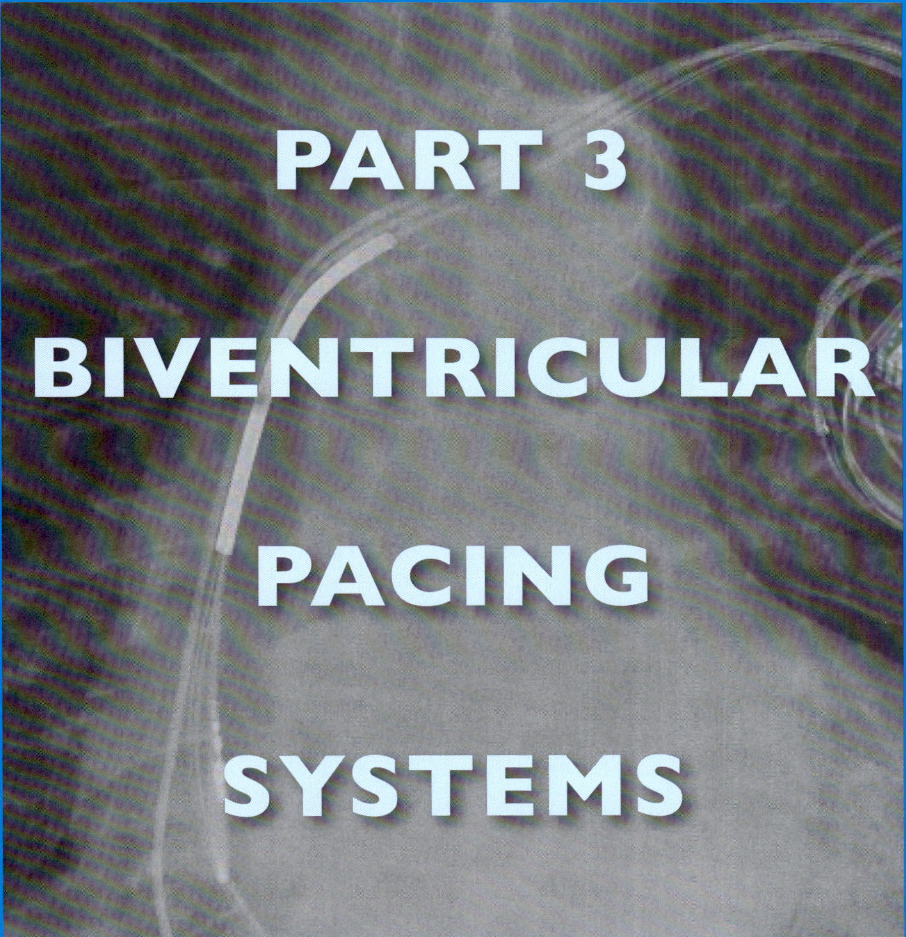

PART 3

BIVENTRICULAR PACING SYSTEMS

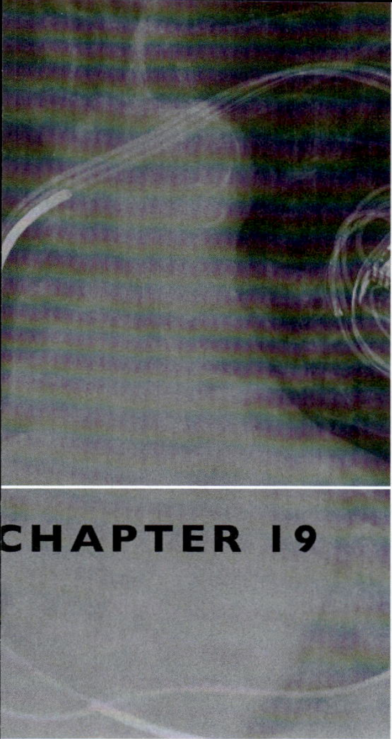

CHAPTER 19

Basics of Biventricular Pacing Systems

Principles and Timing Cycles

Ravi Ranjan and Joseph E. Marine

Overview

Over the past decade, biventricular pacing (also called cardiac resynchronization therapy) has become an important treatment for selected patients with congestive heart failure (CHF). The main indication for biventricular pacing is the presence of chronic CHF refractory to medical therapy and left ventricular dyssynchrony. Left ventricular dyssynchrony has been shown to exacerbate CHF through inefficient ventricular contraction, ventricular dilatation, increased wall stress, and increased mitral regurgitation.[1,2] Despite advances in echocardiography-based criteria, a prolonged QRS duration (> 120–130 ms) is still the most widely used measure for dyssynchrony.[3]

The primary goal of biventricular pacing is to achieve synchronized left ventricular contraction. This is usually achieved by placement of a lead in the right ventricle against the interventricular septum and another lead in the coronary sinus by the lateral wall of the left ventricle. By pacing these two sites, left ventricular dyssynchrony is reduced leading to a more efficient ventricular contraction, reduced left ventricular dilatation, and decreased mitral regurgitation.[4,5] Studies have shown that appropriately selected patients treated with biventricular pacing have improved exercise tolerance, reduced heart failure class, fewer hospitalizations, and better quality of life.[6,7]

The value of biventricular pacing has been established in a number of randomized clinical trials, two of the most important being COMPANION and CARE-HF.[8,9] COMPANION enrolled 1520 patients with NYHA Class III to IV heart failure, QRS duration > 120 ms, and left ventricular ejection fraction < 35%. The patients were randomized to optimal medical therapy, biventricular pacemaker, or biventricular pacemaker with ICD. The risk of combined end point of death or hospitalization for heart failure was significantly reduced in both

Pacemakers and Implantable Cardioverter Defibrillators: An Expert's Manual. © 2010 Amin Al-Ahmad, Kenneth A. Ellenbogen, Andrea Natale, and Paul J. Wang, eds. Cardiotext Publishing, ISBN: 978-0-9790164-6-2.

the biventricular pacemaker and biventricular pacemaker with ICD group.[8] In CARE-HF, 813 patients in NYHA class III or IV heart failure with evidence of left ventricular dyssynchrony on standard medical therapy were randomized to medical therapy or biventricular pacing. In this study, the primary end point was death or hospitalization for a major cardiovascular event and again the group with a biventricular pacemaker had a significantly better outcome.[9]

Physical Components of a Biventricular Pacing System

The primary goal of a biventricular pacing system is to have synchronized left ventricular contraction. Theoretically, this could be best achieved by pacing the left ventricle simultaneously at multiple sites.[10] Practically, this is achieved by pacing the interventricular septum (via a lead in the right ventricle) and the lateral wall of the left ventricle (usually with a lead in the coronary sinus). The practical difficulty of pacing the lateral wall of the left ventricle is circumvented by using the branches of the coronary sinus (Fig 19.1). The branch locations are highly variable but there is a lateral branch suitable for LV pacing in almost all patients. Patients who have had prior cardiac surgical procedures, especially mitral valve repair or replacement, are more likely to have alteration of coronary sinus anatomy that may render left ventricular lead placement very difficult.

The steps for implantation of a biventricular pacing or ICD system are similar to that used for standard dual chamber systems, with the additional steps required to place the left ventricular lead. After an infraclavicular incision is made, a prepectoral pocket is created and cephalic and/or axillary vein access is obtained. The right ventricular lead is usually placed first, as patients getting biventricular devices often have complete left bundle branch block, and coronary sinus cannulation may lead to transient block in the right bundle and asystole. Once the right ventricular lead has been placed, backup VVI pacing is established.

Successful placement of left ventricular pacing leads through the coronary sinus is a substantially more complicated procedure, and a full discussion is beyond the scope of this chapter.[11] The first step is gaining access to the coronary sinus with a guiding sheath. Next, a balloon-tipped catheter is passed through the sheath into the mid-coronary sinus and contrast venography is performed in multiple views (Fig 19.1). Adequate venography is important to establish all potential targets for left ventricular lead placement. In general, a lateral coronary sinus tributary is most optimal, followed by posterolateral, then anterolateral locations. LV pacing in the anterior interventricular vein may produce limited cardiac resynchronization and should generally be avoided.[12] Once a tributary has been chosen, an 0.014 soft-tipped wire is guided into the vein and then the lead is passed over the wire and passively fixed in place. A large variety of leads, most with bipolar pacing capability, are now available (Fig

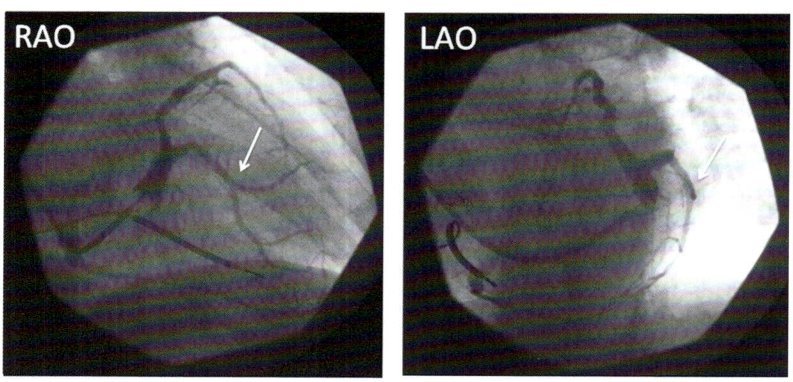

Fig 19.1 RAO and LAO views of coronary sinus venography. The right ventricular ICD lead is already in place. A large branching lateral coronary sinus tributary is visible (arrow).

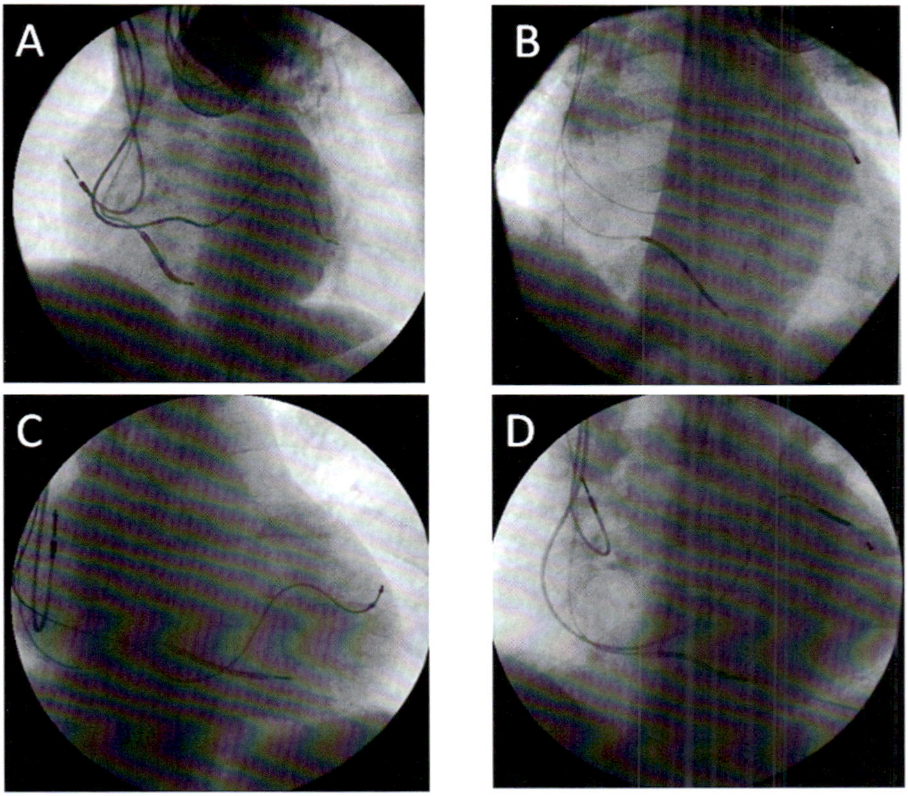

Fig 19.2 Fluoroscopic views of four different biventricular pacing systems each using a different type of left ventricular lead placed in the coronary sinus.

19.2). Their diameter generally ranges from 4 to 6 Fr. Some have a natural curve or coil formed into the tip of the lead to improve stability in larger veins.

Once the lead has been placed, sensing and capture threshold testing are performed. For sensing, the local electrogram amplitude is less important than ensuring that local activation is late in the intrinsic QRS. (Fig 19.3). Pacing threshold should be established in each lead configuration (tip and ring electrodes, when present, in both unipolar and bipolar configuration), and maximum-output pacing performed to exclude phrenic nerve or chest wall capture. Pacing from the left ventricular lead should result in a QRS complex with RBBB morphology. If LBBB morphology is seen, then the lead is likely placed too anteriorly and is capturing the interventricular septum rather than the left ventricular free wall, and poor resynchronization is likely to result. Pacing right ventricular and left ventricular leads will likely show a narrower QRS complex, although this is not an absolute prerequisite for successful cardiac resynchronization (Fig 19.4).[13]

Once adequate sensing and pacing parameters are established, the coronary sinus sheath is removed and the lead is anchored to the prepectoral fascia. The right atrial lead is then implanted with standard approach, except in cases of permanent atrial fibrillation where it is unnecessary. The leads are then connected to the biventricular pacemaker or ICD generator, which is placed in the pocket, and the incision is closed (Fig 19.5). Testing of ICD function is then generally performed with standard single or dual chamber ICD implantations.

With currently available equipment, long-term successful left ventricular lead placement can be accomplished from an endocardial approach in > 90% of cases, with some centers reporting > 95% success.[6,11] In those cases where

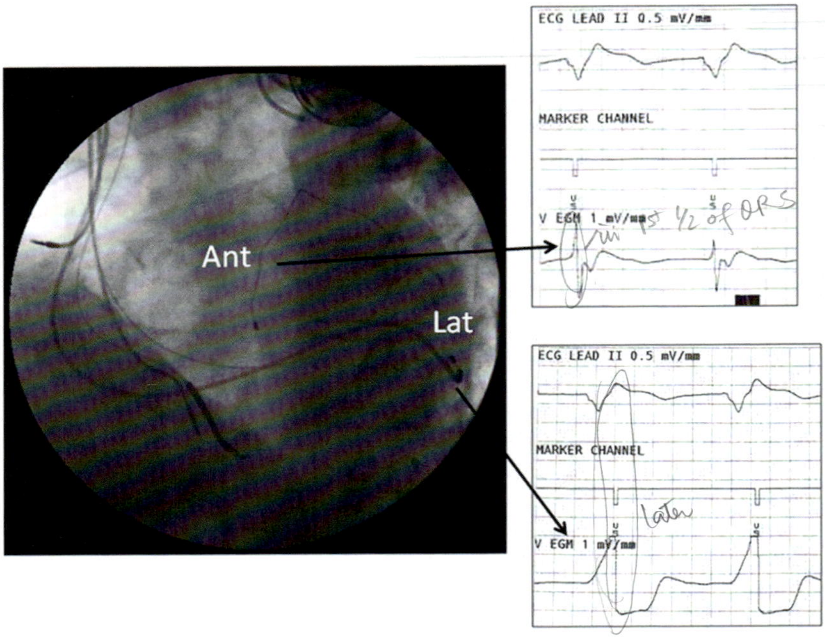

Fig 19.3 LAO fluoroscopic view of a biventricular pacing system after revision to an ICD model. The original left ventricular lead was placed in the anterior interventricular vein (Ant), where local activation is seen to occur in the first half of the QRS complex. During revision to biventricular ICD, in addition to adding an ICD lead in the right ventricle, a new pacing lead was placed in a lateral tributary of the coronary sinus (Lat), where much later local activation was observed. Pacing at this location is more likely to lead to reduced dyssynchrony and better hemodynamics.

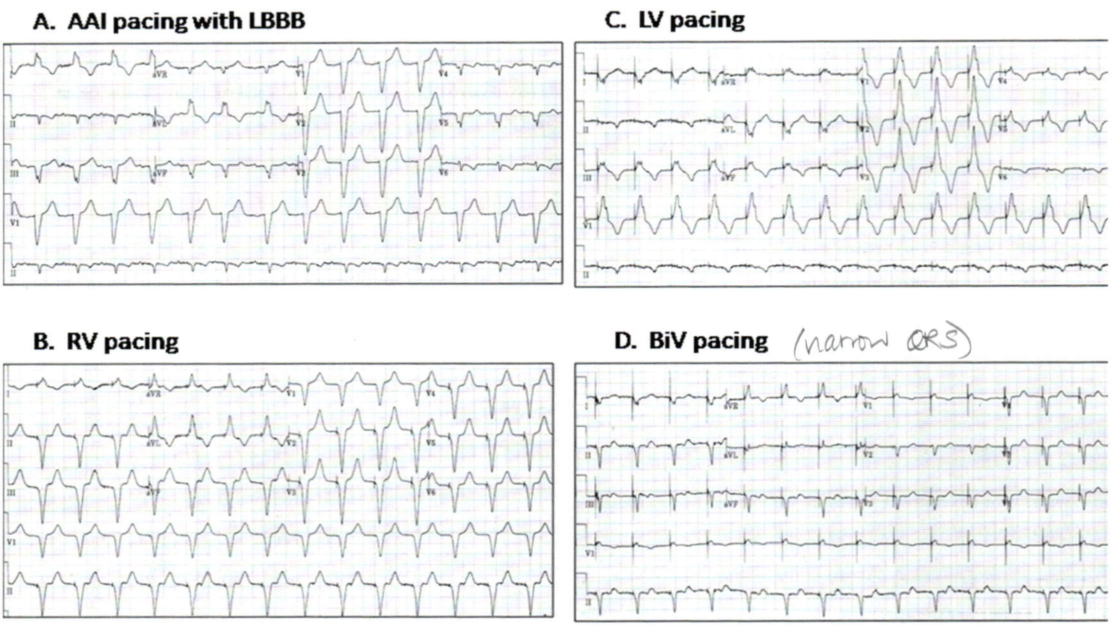

Fig 19.4 Four 12-lead ECGs from the same patient pacing different components of a biventricular pacing system with resultant changes in the QRS complex. **A**: AAI pacing showed intrinsic QRS with LBBB morphology. **B**: VVI pacing from the right ventricular (RV) lead only. **C**: VVI pacing from left ventricular (LV) lead only, demonstrating a RBBB QRS morphology. **D**: VVI pacing from RV and LV leads simultaneously. Note the relatively narrow QRS complex.

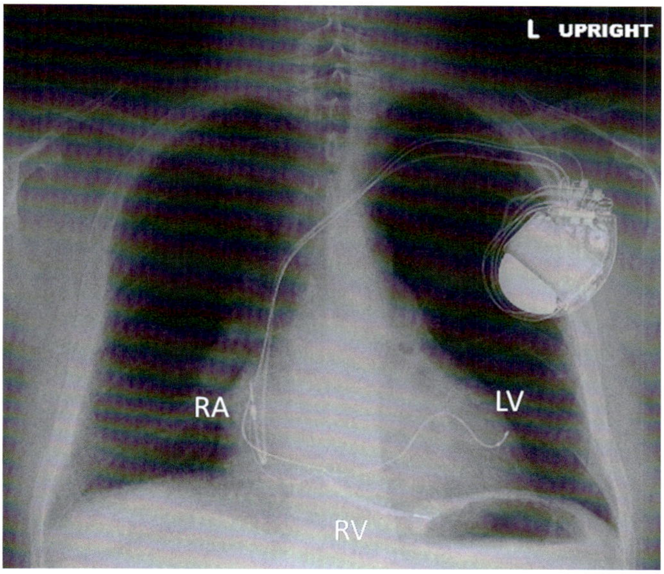

Fig 19.5 Posteroanterior chest X-ray after implantation of a new biventricular ICD system. Right atrial (RA), right ventricular (RV), and left ventricular (LV) leads are in standard locations.

anatomy is unsuitable for endocardial left ventricular lead placement, epicardial leads can be implanted with surgical techniques, often with a minimally invasive thoracoscopic approach. The surgical epicardial approach has the advantage of allowing placement of the lead to the desired left ventricular site unrestricted by the vagaries of coronary sinus anatomy.[14] Direct visualization of the left phrenic nerve allows avoidance of diaphragmatic stimulation. Disadvantages of the surgical approach include longer recovery time and greater potential for increase in chronic pacing thresholds. Some potential complications of biventricular device implantation are listed in Box 19.1.

- Subclavian vein thrombosis
- Pneumothorax
- Pocket hematoma
- Hemothorax
- Cardiac perforation and tamponade
- Coronary sinus dissection or perforation
- Contrast nephropathy
- Asystole from transient injury to right bundle branch
- Lead dislodgement

Box 19.1 Complications of Biventricular Pacemaker or ICD Implantation

Principles of Biventricular Pacing and Sensing

The basic principles of biventricular pacing and sensing are similar to those for standard single and dual chamber pacing systems, with several important modifications. The first leads designed for coronary sinus pacing were all unipolar. Before dedicated biventricular generators were commercially available to accommodate the third lead, implanters would yoke the coronary sinus lead to the right ventricular lead with a Y-adaptor, and then connect the single pin of the Y-adaptor into the single ventricular port of the generator. In this situation, stimulation could occur either through a wide bipole configuration, in which the RV tip serves as the cathode and the LV tip as the anode, or, more commonly, a split cathode in which both RV and LV tips split the cathodal output and either the RV ring/RV coil or the pulse generator serves as the anode. The first generation of dedicated biventricular pacemaker and ICD generators effectively Y-adapted the RV and LV leads together in the header, producing similar electrical configuration, albeit with simpler hardware.

There are several problems with the Y-adapted RV-LV lead configuration. For sensing, the Y-adapted configuration will produce a composite electrogram with two components (RV and LV) originating from opposite sides of the heart. If timing of the second component of the composite electrogram exceeds the ventricular blanking period, then the single ventricular event could be counted twice.[15] Unfortunately, this would be most likely to occur in patients with a very wide left bundle branch block and with a well-positioned coronary sinus lead (ie, the most suitable candidates for the therapy), in which the RV-LV interval would be expected to exceed 120 ms. The most common scenarios in which double sensing could occur are during slow ventricular tachycardias (Fig 19.6) and during sinus or atrial tachycardias during which the atrial rate exceeds the programmed upper tracking rate. In biventricular ICDs, such events frequently resulted in inappropriate ICD therapies, as ventricular blanking periods are generally fixed at 120 ms and not programmable, and were a major limitation of the technology. In both biventricular pacemakers and ICDs programmed in DDD mode, the second ventricular sensed event will reset the postventricular atrial refractory period (PVARP), potentially resulting in the next P wave falling into the PVARP, thus perpetuating loss of biventricular pacing with resultant deleterious hemodynamic effects and continuation of ventricular double counting.

Biventricular pacing through a Y-adapted configuration has several additional pitfalls. First, pacing impedance through this configuration is generally lower, resulting in greater current drain and shorter battery longevity. Second, the ventricular output must be programmed above the higher of the two ventricular lead thresholds (generally the LV). Because separate testing of the leads through the pulse generator cannot be performed, assessment of individual pacing capture thresholds is more difficult, and assessment of separate pacing impedances is not possible. Detection of occult fracture is therefore more challenging, as impedance changes may be masked and "noise" cannot be clearly attributed to one lead or the other.

Because of these numerous limitations to Y-adapted lead configuration, manufacturers moved quickly to introduce biventricular pacemaker and ICD generators with separate, dedicated pacing and sensing circuits for the LV lead, and all currently marketed systems are so configured. Separate, dedicated LV sensing channels have virtually eliminated double counting as a clinical problem. Follow-up assessment and troubleshooting of the ventricular leads is greatly simplified. In addition, numerous models of dedicated bipolar coronary sinus (CS) pacing leads have been introduced, allowing true bipolar LV pacing and sensing. Coupled with changes in pulse generator programmability, bipolar LV leads allow up to six different pacing configurations, utilizing LV tip or LV ring as the cathode and the alternate LV pole, the RV

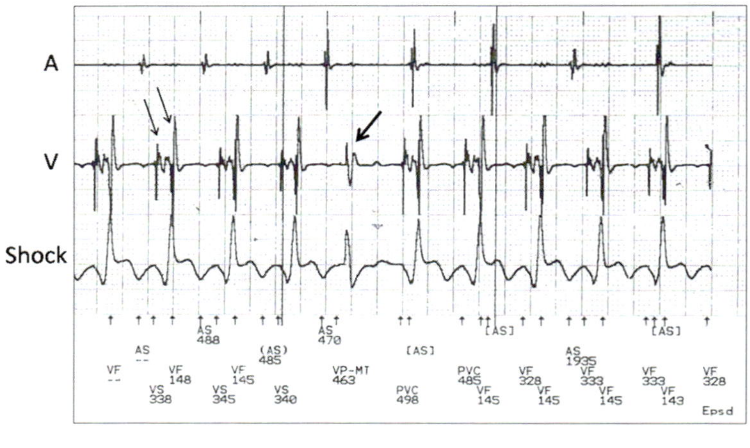

Fig 19.6 Stored electrogram from a first-generation biventricular ICD showing a slow ventricular tachycardia (CL 480–490 ms) with double sensing by the ICD (thin double arrows). After the first three beats of VT, the next QRS is not double counted, and the retrograde P wave is tracked with a resulting ventricular-paced event (VP-MT). The ventricular tachycardia then accelerates slightly so that each ventricular-sensed event falls into the programmed VF zone (180 bpm), resulting in a detected episode (Epsd). A, atrial channel; V, dual RV-LV channel; Shock, shock electrogram channel showing far-field electrogram.

ring/coil, or pulse generator as the anode, in various combinations. The ability to alter the LV pacing configuration noninvasively can be helpful in follow-up, when increase in LV capture threshold and/or development of diaphragmatic stimulation may occur with the originally programmed LV pacing configuration.

Biventricular Timing Cycles

The general principles of biventricular timing cycles are similar to those of standard single and dual chamber pacemakers described in previous chapters. However, given the additional lead in the coronary sinus and the need to have synchronized left ventricular contraction and maximal percentage of biventricular pacing, the biventricular pacing system has its own timing cycle requirements as well as some unique timing cycle issues.[16]

Pacing Modes

For patients in sinus rhythm, biventricular devices are usually programmed to pace in the DDD mode with or without rate responsiveness. DDDR mode is an atrial tracking mode where after an atrial event is sensed, a ventricular event is scheduled based on the programmed sensed AV delay. If there is no atrial sensed event after the VA interval times out, then the atrium is paced, initiating the AV delay. If no ventricular sensed event occurs before the AV delay times out, then ventricular pacing occurs. The DDDR mode is used to preserve the beneficial effect of atrial contraction on ventricular filling.

It should be noted that original trials of biventricular pacing generally utilized the VDD mode, in which there is no atrial pacing and no paced AV delay, and a lower rate limit of 30 to 40 bpm. Because DDDR mode has not been formally tested in the biventricular pacing trials, the most appropriate lower rate limit in this mode is not known. Most cardiologists program biventricular pacing systems in DDDR mode with a lower rate of 50 to 60 bpm, due to frequent coexistence of sinus node dysfunction and/or need for beta blockers and/or antiarrhythmic drugs in the heart failure population. However, the hemodynamics of A-V sequential pacing may differ from those of VDD pacing, and the optimal paced AV delay may be much longer than the optimal sensed AV delay. This complex subject will be covered in more detail in Chapter 21.

If a patient is in permanent atrial fibrillation there is no benefit in tracking the atrial activity, in which case the device is usually programmed in the VVIR mode. For VVIR mode to be effective in atrial fibrillation, there should be enough nodal block so that electrical activity is not proceeding down the normal conduction system (AV node and His-Purkinje system), and the pacing rate exceeds the intrinsic ventricular rate. If there is conduction down the AV node, then there is no pre-excitation of the left ventricle and the potential benefit of biventricular pacing may be lost. In some cases, adequate nodal blockade cannot be achieved by pharmacotherapy, as patients with heart failure may not be able to tolerate these medications at the required doses. In such cases, the AV node may be ablated, resulting in complete AV block and pacemaker dependence.[17] For patients with AF and preserved AV conduction, biventricular pacemaker and ICD models also increasingly possess features designed to maximize percentage of LV pacing during AF. Two of these features, LV triggering after RV sensing, and ventricular rate smoothing algorithms, are discussed in later sections.

AV Delay

With the goal to have synchronized ventricular contraction, it is important to pre-excite the left ventricle. This pre-excitation is accomplished by ensuring that the programmed AV delay is substantially shorter than the intrinsic AV interval. In contrast, most standard dual chamber pacemakers with leads in the right atrium and right ventricle implanted for sinus node dysfunction are programmed in a fashion that will minimize ventricular pacing (DDI, AAI with mode switch to DDD, or DDD with a long programmed AV delay). These programming modes are generally inappropriate for biventricular pacing systems, where the goal is to maximize ventricular pacing to resynchronize left ventricular contraction.

An important difference also exists in programmed AV interval for sensed and paced atrial events. The AV interval for paced atrial events (often referred to as the AV delay) should be programmed longer than the AV interval for sensed atrial events (referred to as the PV delay), similar to the situation for standard dual chamber pacemakers. The AV delay should be longer than the PV delay because with an atrial-sensed event, the atrial activity has already begun before it is sensed by the atrial lead. In contrast, with an atrial-paced event the atrial activity begins when the atrium is paced by the pacemaker. Hence, to have similar atrial to ventricular mechanical delay the AV delay is made longer than the PV delay, usually by 30 to 70 ms.

Another important feature of the programmed AV delay, similar to standard dual chamber pacemakers, is rate-responsive AV delay. AV conduction is sensitive to autonomic tone and so the AV delay (or the PV delay) may be decreased as the sinus rate increases to mimic normal physiology and in the case of biventricular pacemaker to preserve LV pre-excitation. In biventricular pacemakers, if the AV delay is set for a lower heart rate and is not rate-responsive then at higher heart rates the AV conduction might improve to the point that LV pre-excitation from the pacemaker is diminished. On the other hand, if one programs the AV delay (or PV delay) to be too short to preempt this problem, then the AV delay might be too short to maximize the benefit of atrial contraction.

The complexity of programming of the AV and PV delays in biventricular pacemakers is rendered more complex by the additional problem of interatrial conduction delay, which is often present in patients with cardiomyopathy. The most important mechanical AV relationship is that between left atrial and left ventricular contraction. In general, however, atrial sensing and pacing is usually accomplished in the right atrium, typically in the right atrial appendage region or lateral wall. However, the conduction time from the right atrial lead to the lateral wall of the left atrium may vary substantially among patients. A variety of techniques have been proposed to optimize the AV delay and RV-LV timing using echocardiographic and electrophysiologic criteria.[18]

Upper Rate Behavior and PVARP

In the DDD mode, atrial events are tracked. This is the best mode to achieve AV coordination, but during atrial tachy-arrhythmias this becomes a problem. Tracking such high atrial rates could lead to hemodynamic impairment and ventricular arrhythmias. Therefore, for the biventricular pacemakers just as in other dual chamber pacemakers, there is a maximum tracking rate. In a typical dual chamber pacemaker this determines the maximum rate at which the ventricle is paced in response to an atrial-sensed event. Typical upper rate behavior is to increase the AV delay for consecutive atrial events until there is pseudo-Wenckebach and an atrial event is dropped (or not followed by a ventricular event as it falls in the PVARP) and the cycle resets (Fig 19.7A).

In biventricular pacing, because native AV conduction is often intact, an important potential complication of upper rate behavior is persistent loss of biventricular pacing. In biventricular devices, as the AV delay is prolonged there is progressive fusion between the paced and intrinsically conducted beat and ultimately the AV delay is so long that all atrial beats are conducted intrinsically. Because of the intact AV conduction with each beat the cycle is reset and there is no further prolongation of the AV delay (Fig 19.7B). Once this occurs there may be complete loss of biventricular pacing (and hence resynchronization).

At high atrial rates, depending on the programmed PVARP, it is possible that the atrial events might continuously fall in the PVARP (Fig 19.8A). This will occur when the atrial cycle length is shorter than the total atrial refractory period (TARP = PVARP + sensed AV

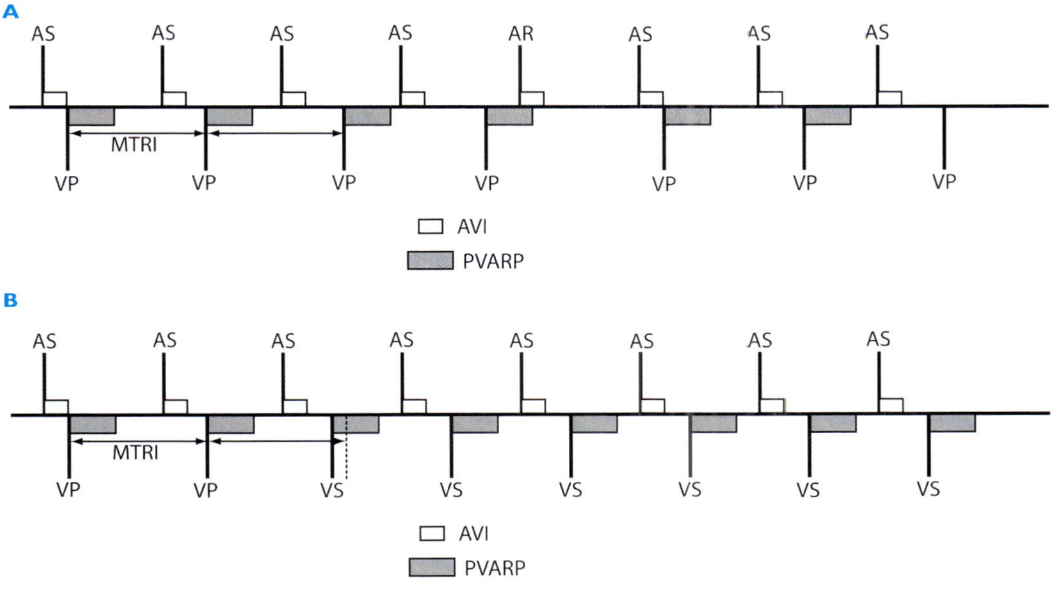

Fig 19.7A-B Upper rate behavior in (**A**) a standard dual chamber pacemaker in a patient with AV block and (**B**) a biventricular pacemaker with intact AV conduction. In a dual chamber pacemaker (**A**) when the atrial rate is above the maximum tracking rate the PV delay is prolonged to maximum track rate interval. With the prolongation of the PV delay, one of the atrial events falls in the PVARP and is not tracked. With the next atrial event the cycle repeats itself. In (**B**) a biventricular pacemaker again the PV delay is prolonged to reach the maximum track rate interval (MTRI) but due to intact AV conduction the ventricular event is sensed before the MTRI is timed out in the second beat. This happens with each subsequent beat and there is complete loss of biventricular pacing. AS, atrial-sensed event; AR, atrial event in the refractory period; VP, ventricular-paced event; AVI, AV interval; PVARP, postventricular atrial refractory period; MTRI, maximum track rate interval.

delay). In this case the atrial events will not be tracked and if native conduction is intact there will be complete loss of biventricular pacing.[19] In addition, once the atrial events fall in the PVARP, loss of biventricular pacing is likely to continue until the atrial cycle length increases to less than the intrinsic TARP (PVARP + intrinsic PR interval). If the intrinsic PR interval is much longer than the programmed sensed AV delay, then the patient could be "locked in" to ventricular sensing for long periods of time, with resultant hemodynamic deterioration and/or loss of exercise tolerance.

An analogous situation may occur after a PVC, if PVARP-extension is programmed On. In conventional dual chamber pacing systems, this feature extends PVARP after a PVC, because this is the usual situation in which pacemaker-mediated tachycardia (PMT) is initiated. If the next sinus P wave falls into the extended PVARP, and the atrial cycle length is shorter than the intrinsic TARP, biventricular pacing may be lost until the atrial rate slows. A similar problem may occur with PMT-termination algorithms, which transiently extend PVARP or interrupt atrial tracking when atrial-tracked ventricular pacing is occurring at or near the upper tracking rate.

These problems can be overcome several ways. First, it is important to program the highest upper tracking rate that the patient is likely to tolerate. If in follow-up numerous episodes of PMT are detected by the device, it is likely that the patient's intrinsic sinus rate frequently exceeds the upper tracking rate, and increasing the upper tracking rate further and/or increasing beta blockade should be considered. Next, it is important to program the shortest possible PVARP compatible with the patient's VA conduction. Many devices allow programming of an automatically adjusted PVARP, during which PVARP will shorten at higher atrial rates. In addition, some devices in the setting of atrial events in PVARP followed by ventricular-sensed events below the maximum tracking rate briefly shorten the PVARP. This allows the atrial event to fall outside the PVARP leading to an atrial-sensed event that is then tracked (Fig 19.8B). Finally, for reasons noted previously, PVARP-extension and PMT-termination algorithms should generally be programmed Off unless clearly required by individual patient circumstances.

V-V Timing Issues

With two ventricular leads (RV and LV) one can imagine potentially complex timing cycles depending on the chambers sensed, chambers paced, and then potentially also changing the delay between the pacing in the two chambers. But most current devices use only RV sensing to determine the timing cycle, which simplifies the algorithm. In most devices there is an option to add a delay in the LV-RV pacing (or pre-excite the LV) as it can potentially improve hemodynamics. Figure 19.9 shows the three possible pacing outcomes when adjusting the LV-RV delay. Here the timing is based on RV sensing only so the AV interval between the atrial-paced event (AP) and the RV-paced event (RVP) remains the same. For the first cycle the LV-paced event (LVP) comes before the RV-paced event. For the second cycle there is no delay and both the LV- and RV-paced events happen at the same time. In the third cycle the delay is pro-

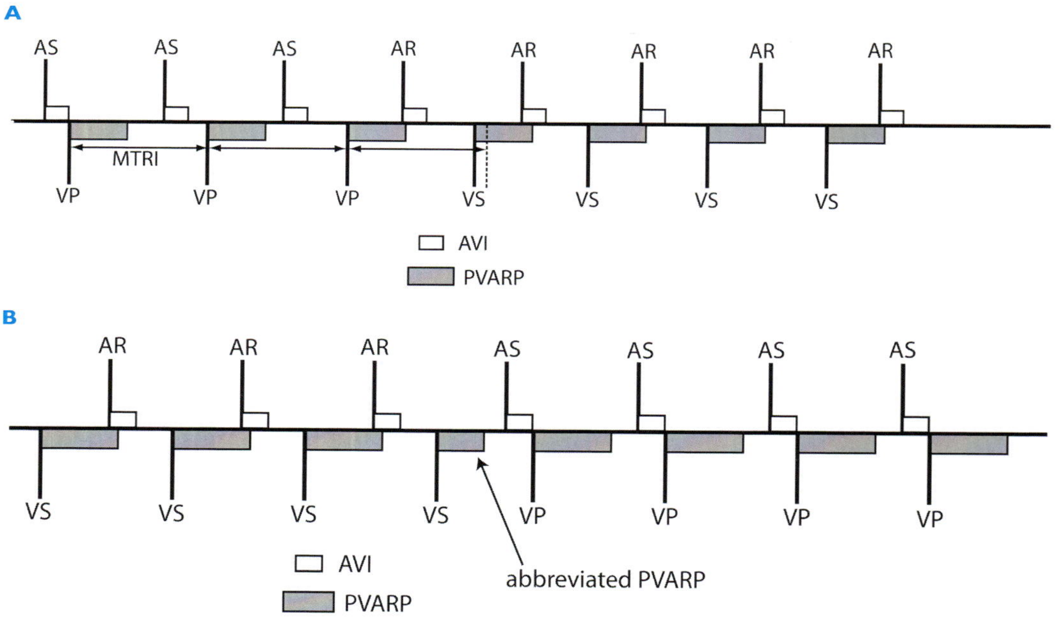

Fig 19.8A-B Upper rate behavior in a biventricular pacemaker resulting in (A) "locked-in" ventricular sense mode and (B) abbreviation of PVARP to interrupt the locked-in phenomenon. In (A) the PV delay is prolonged to reach the maximum track rate interval (MTRI) but due to intact AV conduction the ventricular event is sensed before the MTRI is timed out in the fourth beat. This happens with each subsequent beat and there is complete loss of biventricular pacing. Moreover, the atrial event occurs during PVARP. Depending on PVARP it is possible that even with atrial rate falling below the maximum track rate the atrial event continues to fall in PVARP and not to be tracked with complete loss of biventricular pacing. (B) To interrupt this locked-in phenomenon, the PVARP is abbreviated for a beat. The next atrial event is a sensed event and is tracked because it is below the maximum track rate. This results in restoration of biventricular pacing. AS, atrial-sensed event; AR, atrial event that falls during PVARP; VP, ventricular-paced event; VS, ventricular-sensed event; AVI, AV interval; PVARP, postventricular atrial refractory period; MTRI, maximum track rate interval.

grammed such that the RV-paced event comes before the LV-paced event. In clinical practice, the most common scenario is intrinsic left bundle branch block and in those cases programming the delay to pre-excite the LV ventricle generally is most appropriate.

If the AV delay is set too long then due to native AV conduction there will be an RV-sensed event during the atrioventricular interval (AVI) requiring that the AV delay be reduced as shown in Fig 19.10. Here the first atrial-paced event is followed by an LV-paced and RV-sensed event. The LV is paced after the preprogrammed AV delay minus the LV-RV delay. Here the AV delay was too long which leads to an RV-sensed event before the end of AVI when the RV would have been paced. For the next atrial-paced event the AV delay is reduced. As a result the LV is paced sooner and this time the AV delay is short enough that the RV is also paced resulting in biventricular pacing. The third atrial event is a sensed event but the AV delay is short enough that both ventricles are paced.

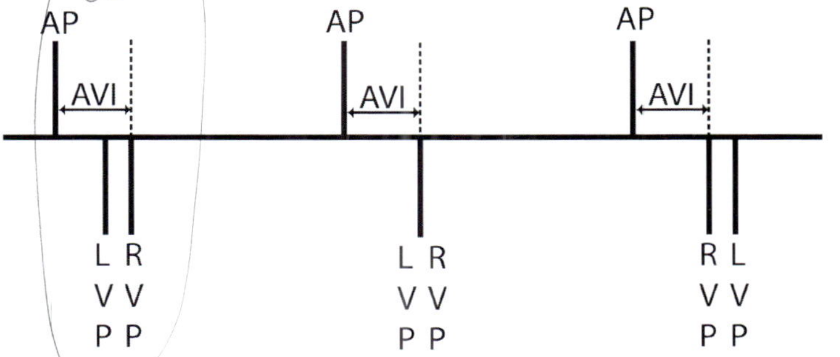

Fig 19.9 (right) Effect of LV-RV pacing delay on biventricular timing cycle based on RV sensing only. Because the timing cycle is based on RV sense only the RV pacing comes at the end of the AVI. Here the first beat is programmed to pace with a positive LV to RV delay (LVP precedes RVP) and hence the LVP occurs within the AVI. For the second beat the LV to RV delay is set to zero so both LVP and RVP occur at the same time, that is, at the end of the AVI. For the third beat the LV to RV delay is negative hence the LVP occurs after the AVI. AP, atrial-paced event; LVP, left ventricular-paced event; RVP, right ventricular-paced event; AVI, AV interval.

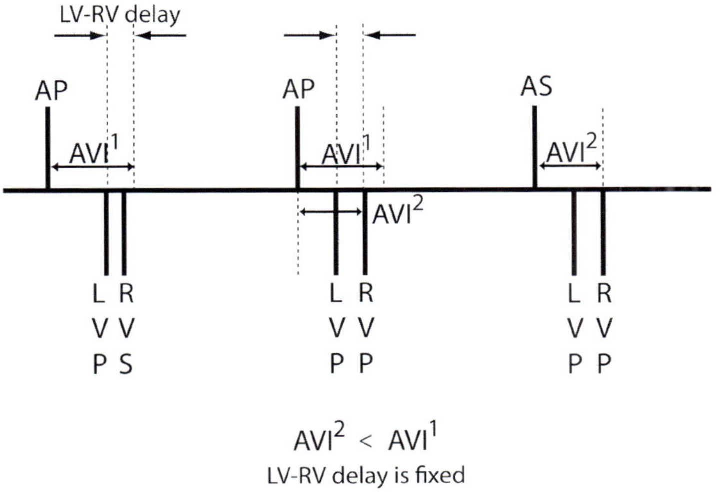

Fig 19.10 (left) AV delay in biventricular timing cycle. For this figure the LV to RV delay was positive and AVI timing is based on RV sense only. After the first atrial event there is a LVP event and a RVS event. The RV pacing is inhibited as the RVS happened before the AVI (labeled AVI[1]) was timed out. For the next beat the AVI is reduced (labeled AVI[2]) and now the LVP event occurs earlier within the AVI. The AVI times out before a RVS event leading to RVP event and hence biventricular pacing. The third beat is an atrial-sensed event but the shortened AV delay (AVI[2]) delay is still short enough such that both ventricles are paced. AP, atrial-paced event; AS, atrial-sensed event; LVP, left ventricular-paced event; RVS, right ventricular-sensed event; RVP, right ventricular-paced event; AVI, AV interval.

Sensing in RV versus Both RV and LV

With leads in the two ventricles each chamber can be sensed and paced. With sensing in both chambers a sensed event may inhibit pacing in that chamber. Theoretically, this avoids pacing during a vulnerable period in that chamber and reduces the risk of initiating a tachycardia. On a more practical note even if dual RV-LV sensing is not present, as long as the LV-RV delay is not too long, any pacing event even if it happens asynchronously in one of the chambers is likely to be in the refractory period and hence poses little increased risk of initiating a tachycardia. Fig 19.11 shows several possible combinations of paced and sensed events in the two chambers when sensing and pacing in the two ventricles. Here the first atrial-paced event is followed by pacing in both the right and left ventricles after the termination of the paced AV interval. No delay occurs in the LV and RV pacing events. After the second atrial-paced event an LV event is sensed which leads to inhibition in that chamber and the RV is paced at the end of the programmed AV interval. For the third atrial-paced event an RV event is sensed before the termination of the AV interval and hence leads to inhibition of RV pacing. The LV is paced at the termination of the programmed AV interval. After the fourth atrial-paced beat events are sensed in both the ventricles before the termination of the programmed AV interval and leads to inhibition of pacing in both chambers. Today very few devices use the sensed events in both the RV and the LV for timing cycle purposes and is restricted mostly to certain biventricular pacemakers.

In the Frontier II biventricular pacemaker manufactured by St. Jude Medical, there is sensing in both the ventricles and a sensed event in either of the ventricles is used to reset the V-V timing interval. A sensed event in the RV does not lead to inhibition in RV only but resets the timing for both the chambers. This device also may be programmed in the triggered mode when any sensed ventricular activity during the alert period leads to pacing in both the ventricles.

In the InSync III device manufactured by Medtronic, sensing may be programmed from RV tip to LV tip. Depending on the interventricular conduction delay this sensing configuration can lead to a separate ventricular-sensed event in the left ventricle for each paced beat in

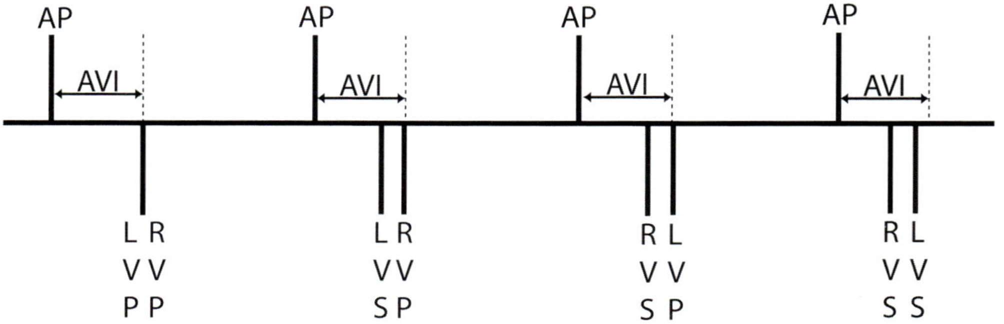

Fig 19.11 Sensing in RV versus both RV and LV. Biventricular timing cycle with sensing in each ventricle. For this figure the LV to RV delay is set to zero. After the first atrial-paced beat there is biventricular pacing at the end of the AVI. After the second atrial-paced beat a LVS event occurs during the AVI which inhibits LV pacing. The RV is paced at the end of the AVI. After the third atrial-paced beat a RVS event occurs during the AVI and inhibits RV pacing. The LV is paced at the end of the AVI. After the fourth atrial-paced event both LVS and RVS event occurs during the AVI inhibiting pacing in both the chambers. AP, atrial-paced event; LVP, left ventricular-paced event; RVP, right ventricular-paced event; LVS, left ventricular-sensed event; RVS, right ventricular-sensed event; AVI, AV interval.

the right ventricle. A separate sensed event in the left ventricle leads to resetting of the ventriculoatrial interval and all the other refractory periods such as PVARP. To prevent this from happening the device allows for programming of a separate interventricular refractory period. As long as the interventricular refractory period is set longer than the depolarization interval between the two ventricles for a RV-paced event there is no double counting of ventricular events and the timing cycle is not affected.

With sensing in both ventricles there are additional possibilities of resetting the VA interval. The most straightforward scenario is when there is no AV conduction then a pacing event in the RV resets the VA interval. The reset could be timed with an LV-paced event. The possibilities increase with AV conduction. The VA interval can be reset with a sensed event in either ventricle or the VA interval can still be timed to the expiration of the AV interval from the atrial-sensed event irrespective of the sensed event in the ventricles. For current biventricular ICD devices, this is not as relevant because most of the devices use a timing cycle based on RV sensing only.

Ventricular-Sensed Response and Rate-Smoothing Algorithms

Given the importance of maintaining maximal biventricular pacing in achieving cardiac resynchronization and amelioration of heart failure symptoms, manufacturers have increasingly incorporated complex timing cycle algorithms to maximize biventricular pacing during episodes of atrial fibrillation, periods of accelerated AV conduction, and in patients with frequent premature ventricular depolarizations. In one such algorithm, an LV or biventricular pacing stimulus is triggered by a right ventricular sensed event. The stimulus is triggered within 1 to 10 ms of the sensed event. The sensed ventricular event could be a premature ventricular depolarization, a conducted complex during atrial fibrillation or flutter, or a conducted beat in sinus rhythm where native AV conduction unexpectedly improves and precedes the programmed AV delay. Proprietary names for this feature include Biventricular Trigger (Boston Scientific) and Ventricular Sense Response (Medtronic). In most devices the sensing is only in the right ventricle and hence the response is essentially an immediate triggered pacing of the left ventricle, as long as the timing does not violate the upper tracking rate or another programmable upper rate tied to this feature. The clinical benefit to this form of triggered pacing has not been established, but nonetheless has been increasingly utilized due to theoretical benefit and reports demonstrating worse outcomes in patients with lower percentage of biventricular pacing.

Another programmable feature present in most current biventricular devices is designed to smooth out variability in RR intervals and increase percentage biventricular pacing in patients when mode switched to VVIR, DDIR, or VDIR during atrial fibrillation or flutter. These proprietary features, for which detailed algorithms are not published, are designed to produce 40% to 80% biventricular pacing during atrial fibrillation or flutter with normal AV conduction, depending on the settings programmed. The basic principle is that intrinsic RR intervals/ventricular rates are continuously measured and the programmed lower rate limit for ventricular pacing is continuously adjusted based on a weighted average of intrinsic RR intervals in an attempt to maintain the pacing rate just above the intrinsic rate. These features have a programmable upper rate limit to prevent excessively short RR intervals. As with triggered biventricular pacing, there is as yet little published evidence for clinical benefit of these algorithms, and the basis for their use is largely theoretical and should be individualized to each patient's clinical situation.

Programmable LV Refractory Period

In devices that sense only in the right ventricle it is possible to imagine a scenario in which a late-coupled premature ventricular depolarization originating in the left ventricle conducts with enough delay toward the right ventricle such that it is not sensed and hence does not inhibit a timed ventricular paced event. In this scenario, LV pacing (which is often programmed to high output to overcome higher thresholds on the LV epicardium) could potentially occur during local phase 3 of the action potential, with induction of ventricular arrhythmia. Such an event would require critical timing, such that the LV paced event occurs after the absolute refractory period but before full repolarization, and the preceding premature ventricular depolarization conducts with enough delay that it is not detected in the RV and hence does not inhibit ventricular pacing.

To prevent this scenario, one device manufacturer (Boston Scientific) has incorporated a feature that utilizes sensing in the left ventricle solely to inhibit LV pacing during this vulnerable period, creating an LV refractory period. The duration of this LV refractory period is programmable, but nominally set to 400 ms after a sensed LV event. For obvious reasons, the LV refractory period cannot be programmed in a way that would prevent biventricular pacing at the programmed upper tracking rate or upper sensing rate of the device. The LV refractory period is reset after every paced or sensed event in the LV. The timing cycle is shown in Fig 19.12.

Physicians using this feature should be aware of its potential to inhibit biventricular pacing in patients with frequent premature ventricular depolarizations, especially when they are late coupled and the sinus rate is relatively rapid. In such cases, the feature may have to be programmed Off, or ventricular premature depolarizations suppressed with antiarrhythmic drugs or catheter ablation. Another troublesome interaction may occur during LV threshold testing, whereby inhibition of LV pacing output may occur in the absence of loss of capture. This may happen if the LV refractory period is programmed relatively long in the setting of rapid intrinsic rate or frequent ventricu-

DDDR or VDDR mode if in sinus rhythm

- Lowest tolerable lower rate limit
- Highest tolerable upper track rate
- Shortest acceptable PVARP/auto-PVARP
- Program PVARP-extension and PMT-termination algorithms Off

VVIR mode if in permanent atrial fibrillation

- Use higher lower rate limit to increase pacing frequency
- Activate features that trigger pacing upon ventricular-sensed event
- Consider ventricular rate smoothing algorithms

Box 19.2 Programming Considerations to Optimize Biventricular Pacing

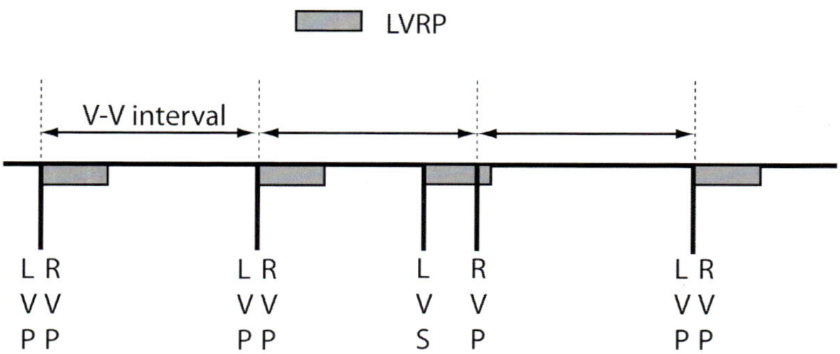

Fig 19.12 Left ventricular refractory period. After any LV-paced or LV-sensed event there is a left ventricular refractory period (LVRP). There is no pacing in the LV during this LVRP. Here the first two are biventricular-paced events. The third event is an LV-sensed event likely from a PVC. The next V-V interval times out during the LVRP from this PVC and as a result there is no LVP but only a RVP event. The next cycle is again normal with biventricular pacing as when the V-V interval times outside the LVRP. LVP, left ventricular-paced event; RVP, right ventricular-paced event; LVS, left ventricular-sensed event.

lar premature depolarizations. In such cases, the LV refractory period may need to be shortened or turned Off in order to properly test the LV threshold.

Summary

Biventricular pacing is an important advance in the treatment of CHF. Successful application of biventricular pacing requires appropriate patient selection, choice of hardware, implantation technique, selection of LV lead pacing site, and programming of the pulse generator. Knowledge of the patient's medical history, rhythm status, and indication for pacing is important for properly tailored programming (Box 19.2). The implanting and following physicians should be aware of the increasing number of special features of biventricular devices and how they vary among manufacturers and models. Although the basic features of timing cycles apply across the spectrum of cardiac pacemakers and defibrillators, knowledge of specific features of the device being used in the individual patient is very important to achieving the best possible outcome.

References

1. Hunt SA, Abraham WT, Chin MH, et al. 2009 Focused update incorporated into the ACC/AHA 2005 Guidelines for the Diagnosis and Management of Heart Failure in Adults: A Report of the American College of Cardiology Foundation/American Heart Association Task Force on Practice Guidelines Developed in Collaboration With the International Society for Heart and Lung Transplantation. *J Am Coll Cardiol.* 2009;53:e1–e90.
2. Kass DA. Cardiac resynchronization therapy. *J Cardiovasc Electrophysiol.* 2005; 16 Suppl1:S35–S41.
3. Chung ES, Leon AR, Tavazzi L, et al. Results of the Predictors of Response to CRT (PROSPECT) trial. *Circulation.* 2008;117:2608–2616.
4. St John Sutton MG, Plappert T, Abraham WT, et al. Effect of cardiac resynchronization therapy on left ventricular size and function in chronic heart failure. *Circulation.* 2003;107:1985–1990.
5. Yu CM, Chau E, Sanderson JE, et al. Tissue Doppler echocardiographic evidence of reverse remodeling and improved synchronicity by simultaneously delaying regional contraction after biventricular pacing therapy in heart failure. *Circulation.* 2002;105:438–445.
6. Burkhardt JD, Wilkoff BL. Interventional electrophysiology and cardiac resynchronization therapy: delivering electrical therapies for heart failure. *Circulation.* 2007;115:2208–2220.
7. McAlister FA, Ezekowitz J, Hooton N, et al. Cardiac resynchronization therapy for patients with left ventricular systolic dysfunction: a systematic review. *JAMA.* 2007;297:2502–2514.
8. Bristow MR, Saxon LA, Boehmer J, et al. Cardiac-resynchronization therapy with or without an implantable defibrillator in advanced chronic heart failure. *N Engl J Med.* 2004;350:2140–2150.
9. Cleland JG, Daubert JC, Erdmann E, et al. The effect of cardiac resynchronization on morbidity and mortality in heart failure. *N Engl J Med.* 2005;352:1539–1549.
10. Leclerq C, Gadler F, Kranig W, et al. A randomized comparison of triple-site versus dual-site ventricular stimulation in patients with congestive heart failure. *J Am Coll Cardiol.* 2008;51:1455–1462.
11. Worley S. Left ventricular lead implantation. In: Ellenbogen KA, Kay GN, Lau CP, et al., eds. *Clinical Cardiac Pacing, Defibrillation, and Resynchronization Therapy.* Philadelphia, PA: Saunders Elsevier; 2007:653–826.
12. Butter C, Auricchio A, Stellbrink C, et al. Effect of resynchronization therapy stimulation site on the systolic function of heart failure patients. *Circulation.* 2001;104:3026–3029.
13. Barold SS, Giudici MC, Herweg B, et al. Diagnostic value of the 12-lead electrocardiogram during conventional and biventricular pacing for cardiac resynchronization. *Cardiol Clin.* Aug 2006;24:471–490.
14. DeRose JJ, Ashton RC, Belsley S, et al. Robotically assisted left ventricular epicardial lead

implantation for biventricular pacing. *J Am Coll Cardiol.* 2003;41:1414–1419.

15. Barold SS, Herweg B, Gallardo I. Double counting of the ventricular electrogram in biventricular pacemakers and ICDs. *Pacing Clin Electrophysiol.* 2003;26:1645–1648.
16. Wang P, Kramer A, Estes NAM, Hayes DL. Timing cycles for biventricular pacing. *Pacing Clin Electrophysiol.* 2002;25:62–75.
17. Ferreira AM, Adragao P, Cavaco DM, et al. Benefit of cardiac resynchronization therapy in atrial fibrillation patients vs. patients in sinus rhythm: the role of atrioventricular junction ablation. *Europace.* 2008;10:809–815.
18. Gorcsan J, Abraham T, Agler DA, et al. Echocardiography for cardiac resynchronization therapy: Recommendations for performance and reporting—A report from the American Society of Echocardiography Dyssynchrony Writing Group. *J Am Soc Echocardio.* 2008;21:191–213.
19. Barold SS, Herweg B. Upper rate response of biventricular pacing devices. *J Intervent Cardiovasc Electrophysiol.* 2005;12:129–136.

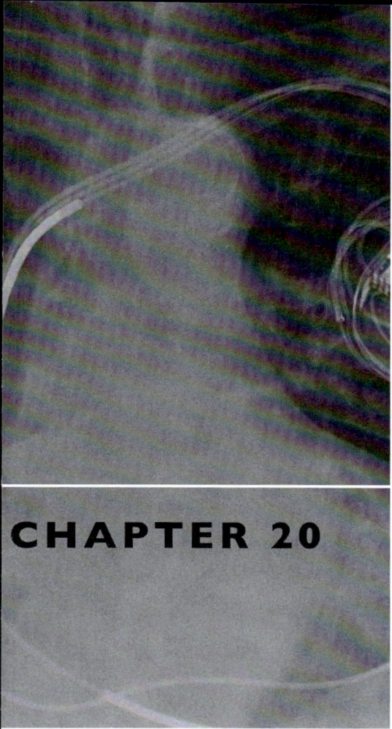

Programming to Avoid Phrenic Nerve Stimulation during Left Ventricular Pacing

CHAPTER 20

Paul J. Wang, Amin Al-Ahmad, Henry H. Hsia, Paul C. Zei, and Mintu P. Turakhia

Introduction

Biventricular pacing, utilizing a left ventricular pacing lead in a branch in the cardiac venous system, has been an important therapy in patients with left ventricular dysfunction, heart failure, and ventricular conduction abnormalities. Because the lateral aspect of the left ventricle is commonly targeted in biventricular pacing, stimulation of the left phrenic nerve, which lies in this region, is common. Because phrenic nerve stimulation is particularly uncomfortable due to vigorous left diaphragmatic contraction, every attempt should be made to avoid this phenomenon. Testing is performed at maximal output during implant to detect any evidence of phrenic nerve stimulation. In general, if phrenic nerve stimulation occurs while the patient is supine, phrenic nerve stimulation will occur when the patient sits up. During lead implantation, the presence of phrenic nerve stimulation necessitates an attempt to reposition the lead.

Programming Electrode Configurations

Several programming strategies are employed to avoid phrenic nerve stimulation. The most common strategy is the use of programming differing electrode pairs for left ventricular pacing. Gurevitz et al demonstrated that using programmable left ventricular pacing configurations could resolve phrenic nerve stimulation. The left ventricular electrode used for stimulation may be the distal or proximal electrode in a bipolar electrode left ventricular lead or the distal electrode in a unipolar left ventricular lead. The other electrode may be the other left ventricular electrode (true bipolar configuration) or a nonleft ventricular electrode such as the

Pacemakers and Implantable Cardioverter Defibrillators: An Expert's Manual. © 2010 Amin Al-Ahmad, Kenneth A. Ellenbogen, Andrea Natale, and Paul J. Wang, eds. Cardiotext Publishing, ISBN: 978-0-9790164-6-2.

distal shock coil, the right ventricular tip electrode, the right ventricular ring electrode (in so-called true bipolar ICD leads), and the can. Selection of these electrode pairs will alter the capture threshold current vector, and the ability to avoid phrenic nerve stimulation. The basic principle in avoiding phrenic nerve stimulation is to direct the stimulation field away from the phrenic nerve. In some cases bipolar pacing between the distal and proximal left ventricular electrodes may prevent phrenic nerve stimulation that was present with distal electrode stimulation and a more remote anode.

The distal left ventricular electrode frequently serves as the cathode and the distal shock coil or can serves as the anode.

Programming Left Ventricular Outputs

In addition to selecting the optimal pacing pairs, managing the left ventricular output is a method of avoiding phrenic nerve stimulation. If phrenic nerve stimulation is present despite using multiple lead configurations, it still may be possible to avoid phrenic nerve stimulation when there is an adequate separation between the left ventricular capture threshold and the phrenic threshold. In practice, the left ventricular output is programmed just above the threshold value, a practice that also optimizes battery longevity. The extension of the pacing pulse width also may be used to avoid phrenic stimulation. If a left ventricular automatic capture algorithm is available, this feature can also be used to adjust the left ventricular output above the threshold. However, if the left ventricular threshold increases, but the output threshold for phrenic nerve does not increase similarly, the patient may suddenly develop diaphragmatic stimulation.

Device- and System-specific Left Ventricular Pacing Electrode Configurations

Medtronic

The Consulta CRT-D device has the following programmable left ventricular pacing configurations: LV tip to RV coil, LV ring to RV coil, and LV tip to LV ring. The nominal configuration is LV tip to RV coil. See Table 20.1.

Using the Attain 4194 bipolar ventricular lead and a CRT-D device, the following configurations are possible: LV tip to RV coil, LV ring to RV coil, and LV tip to LV ring. The Attain Ability 4196 bipolar left ventricular lead and a Consulta CRT-D are used with the following configurations: LV tip to RV coil, LV ring to RV coil. Using this lead, the LV tip to LV ring configuration is generally avoided because it may result in elevated thresholds and produce anodal stimulation. Using the Attain 4193 unipolar left ventricular lead and a CRT-D device, the LV tip to RV coil configuration is possible.

Using the InSync III 8042 CRT-P device and the Attain 4194 bipolar ventricular lead, the

DEVICE	Bipolar Lead Attain 4194, Attain Ability 4196*	Unipolar Lead Attain 4193, Attain StarFix 4195
Consulta CRT-D	LV tip to RV coil, LV ring to RV coil, and LV tip to LV ring*	LV tip to RV coil
InSync III 8042 CRT-P	LV tip to RV ring, LV tip to LV ring,* and LV tip to can	LV tip to RV ring and LV tip to can

Table 20.1 Medtronic Left Ventricular Pacing Configurations.
*LV tip to LV ring generally should be avoided for Attain Ability 4196, which may have elevated thresholds and produce anodal stimulation.

following configurations are possible: LV tip to RV ring, LV tip to LV ring, and LV tip to can. Using Attain Ability 4196 bipolar and a CRT-P device, the LV tip to RV ring and LV tip to can configurations are used and the LV ring to LV ring is generally avoided because of high thresholds. Using the Attain 4193 unipolar left ventricular lead and a CRT-P device, the LV tip to RV ring and LV tip to can configurations are possible.

Boston Scientific

The COGNIS CRT-D device has the ability to achieve six pacing configurations with a bipolar left ventricular lead and two pacing configurations with a unipolar left ventricular lead. See Table 20.2. The six bipolar configurations for CRT-D include LV tip to LV ring, LV tip to RV coil, LV ring to RV coil, LV tip to can, LV ring to can, and LV ring to LV tip. If the device is attached to an integrated bipolar ICD lead, bipolar pacing is to RV coil. If the device is attached to a dedicated bipolar ICD lead, bipolar pacing is to RV ring. The two unipolar configurations are LV tip to RV ring and LV tip to can. The six bipolar configurations for Contak Renewal TR CRT-P include LV tip to LV ring, LV tip to RV ring, LV tip to can, LV ring to RV ring, LV ring to can, and LV ring to LV tip. The two unipolar configurations are LV tip to RV ring and LV tip to can.

St. Jude Medical

Promote™ RF CRT-D has three left ventricular pacing configurations for bipolar leads that may help avoid phrenic nerve stimulation and diaphragmatic stimulation. See Table 20.3 These

DEVICE	Bipolar Lead Easytrak 2, Easytrak 3, Acuity Steerable	Unipolar Lead Easytrak, Acuity Spiral
COGNIS CRT-D	LV tip to LV ring, LV tip to RV coil,* LV ring to RV coil,* LV tip to can, LV ring to can, and LV ring to LV tip	LV tip to RV coil, LV tip to can
Contak Renewal TR CRT-P	LV tip to LV ring, LV tip to RV ring, LV tip to can, LV ring to RV ring, LV ring to can, and LV ring to LV tip	LV tip to RV ring and LV tip to can

Table 20.2 Boston Scientific Left Ventricular Pacing Configurations.
*If the device is attached to an integrated bipolar ICD lead, pacing is to RV coil. If the device is attached to a dedicated bipolar ICD lead, pacing is to RV ring.

DEVICE	Bipolar Lead QuickFlex; QuickSite Bipolar	Unipolar Lead QuickSite Unipolar
Promote RF CRT-D	LV tip to LV ring, LV tip to RV coil, and LV ring to RV coil	LV tip to RV coil
Epic II HF	LV tip to LV ring and LV tip to RV coil	LV tip to RV coil
Anthem CRT-P	LV tip to LV ring, LV tip to RV ring, LV tip to can, and LV ring to RV ring	LV tip to RV ring and LV tip to can

Table 20.3 St. Jude Medical Left Ventricular Pacing Configurations.

configurations are LV tip to LV ring, LV tip to RV coil, and LV ring to RV coil. Epic™ II HF has two pacing configurations: LV tip to LV ring and LV tip to RV coil. For unipolar leads and the CRT-D devices, the configuration LV tip to RV coil is available. The Anthem™ CRT pacemakers can pace LV tip to LV ring, LV tip to can, LV tip to RV ring, and LV ring to RV ring. Using unipolar leads and CRT-P devices the configurations LV tip to RV ring and LV tip to can are available.

Biotronik

The Lumax 540 HF-T CRT-D has the following left ventricular pacing configurations: LV tip to LV ring, LV tip to RV ring, LV ring to LV tip, and LV ring to RV ring. See Table 20.4.

The Stratos™ 338 200 LV-T CRT-P uses the LV tip to LV ring left ventricular pacing configuration for a bipolar lead. Stratos 338 200 CRT-P has the following left ventricular pacing configuration for a unipolar lead: LV tip to can.

Reference

1. Gurevitz O, Nof E, Carasso S, et al. Programmable multiple pacing configurations help to overcome high left ventricular pacing thresholds and avoid phrenic nerve stimulation. *PACE* 2005;28:1255–1259.

DEVICE	Bipolar Lead Corox Bipolar	Unipolar Lead Corox
Lumax 540 HF-T CRT-D	LV tip to LV ring, LV tip to RV ring,* LV ring to LV tip, and LV ring to RV ring*	LV tip to RV ring*
Stratos 338 200 LV-T CRT-P	LV tip to LV ring	LV tip to can

Table 20.4 Biotronik Left Ventricular Pacing Configurations.
*If the device is attached to an integrated bipolar ICD lead, pacing is to RV coil. If the device is attached to a dedicated bipolar ICD lead, pacing is to RV ring.

AV and VV Optimization

CHAPTER 21

Jeffrey H. Chung, Robert J. Kim, and Kenneth M. Stein

Introduction

Since their introduction in 1972, programmable permanent pacemakers have undergone countless improvements, and remain a proven life-saving therapy for patients with bradyarrhythmias. More recently, cardiac resynchronization therapy (CRT) has emerged as a beneficial treatment for patients with intraventricular dyssynchrony and moderate-to-severe medically refractory heart failure.[1,2] Proper programming of pacemakers and CRT devices may be critical in maximizing their therapeutic benefit. This chapter focuses on methodologies for the optimization of the atrioventricular ("AV") interval and left ventricular-right ventricular offset ("VV interval") for the initial and ongoing stages of therapy with pacemakers and CRT, including techniques based on echocardiography, manufacturer-specific algorithms, and other novel modalities (Box 21.1).

At the outset, several points regarding AV and VV optimization bear consideration. First,

Echocardiographic Techniques

- Ritter's Method (AV)
- Iterative Method (AV)
- Transmitral, LVOT, or transaortic VTI (AV, VV)
- Doppler-derived left ventricular dP/dt (AV, VV)

Electrogram-based Techniques

- Boston Scientific SmartDelay (AV)
- St. Jude Medical QuickOpt (AV/VV)

Other Techniques

- Continuous finger photoplethysmography (AV)
- Acoustic cardiography (AV/VV)

Box 21.1 AV/VV Optimization Techniques.
AV: Suitable for AV optimization
VV: Suitable for VV optimization

Pacemakers and Implantable Cardioverter Defibrillators: An Expert's Manual. Cardiotext Publishing, ISBN: 978-0-9790164-6-2.

the existence of a fixed "optimum" AV or VV interval is questionable. The ideal AV interval may vary with changes in posture, activity, volume status, and even autonomic tone.[3,4] Therefore, the best values derived at rest in a supine position may not correspond to the settings that would yield the most relief of symptoms during activity.[5,6] It is also certainly the case that the optimum AV interval during atrial pacing may differ substantially from that during an atrial-sensed rhythm, necessitating separate optimizations for these two different situations.[3,7] Moreover, based on the Frank-Starling relationship, the AV and VV intervals that best reduce left atrial filling pressures are likely to differ from the intervals that best increase cardiac output. The selection of an optimum AV or VV delay may depend on whether any given patient's symptoms predominantly reflect poor forward flow (eg, fatigue) versus elevated pulmonary pressures (eg, dyspnea). Finally, with LV remodeling, optimal AV and VV intervals may change with time and periodic reprogramming may be indicated.[8–10] It should also be recognized that although a number of small-scale studies indicated benefit, as of yet, no large-scale randomized clinical trials have established a significant advantage to routine AV or VV optimization.[11–13] One of these positive studies was a randomized, prospective trial of 40 patients with severe heart failure referred for CRT. The study revealed that immediately following CRT, there was a difference in the improvement of LVEF [7.8 ± 6.2% vs. 3.4 ± 4.4% ($p < 0.02$)], and at 3 months, in the improvements in New York Heart Association (NYHA) Classification [1.0 ± 0.5 vs. 0.4 ± 0.6 class points ($p < 0.01$)] and Quality of Life (QOL) score [23 ± 13 vs. 13 ± 11 points ($p < 0.03$)], between the respective groups of AV delay optimized by Doppler echocardiography versus AV delay empirically set to 120 ms.[14] Similar promising results from AV optimization (albeit using a different echocardiographic technique) were observed at 6-month follow-up by other investigators.[13]

The question of whether there is a benefit to systematic AV optimization is currently being addressed on a larger scale in the SMART-AV [www.clinicaltrials.gov/ct2/show/NCT00677014] and FREEDOM [www.clinicaltrials.gov/ct2/show/NCT00418314] clinical trials. However, all of the major randomized clinical trials demonstrating a benefit to CRT used some form of AV optimization: echocardiographic assessment of mitral inflow ("iterative technique") in the MIRACLE trials[15,16] and CARE-HF[17]; electrocardiogram/electrogram-based techniques in CONTAK-CD[18] and COMPANION.[19] Therefore, physicians who do not routinely optimize patients postimplant should strongly consider optimization for patients who are under-responders or nonresponders to CRT. Even patients who have already been optimized may gain from reoptimization if they experience a subsequent heart failure decompensation.

AV Optimization

Although optimization of the AV delay is applicable to both dual chamber pacemakers and CRT, particular focus has been put on biventricular pacing, as the effects are more readily apparent. There are also different considerations when programming a dual chamber pacemaker versus a CRT device, which will be reviewed. In terms of hemodynamics, the AV interval determines the degree of preload at the time of ventricular systole. The optimal AV delay will best augment the filling of the left ventricle from the left atrium, resulting in increased diastolic filling time, increased stroke volume, and shortened isovolemic contraction time. However, the AV delay should *not* be prolonged to the point it causes diastolic mitral regurgitation, as this would compromise stroke volume. In both dual chamber pacemakers and CRT devices, suboptimal programming of the AV delay can result in as much as a 10% to 15% decline in cardiac output.[20,21]

In CRT patients, particular care should be made to allow biventricular pacing and maintain LV pre-excitation. These two goals of maximizing diastolic filling and providing biventricular pacing may be incompatible in patients with an intrinsically short PR interval (especially those < 150 ms) or those with a long intra-atrial conduction delay and intact AV conduction. Hence, in rare cases, AV node ablation may be required to fully realize the benefits of resynchronization therapy.

Rate adaptation programming of AV delay may also need to be different between a dual chamber pacemaker and a CRT device. Numerous studies and physiologic correlates have proven the benefits of a shortened AV delay with increased heart rates and exercise for patients with traditional dual chamber pacemakers (DDDR). In these patients, rate adaptive AV shortening mirrors the normal physiologic shortening of the PR interval from increased sympathetic tone. In CRT patients, however, there have been conflicting data suggesting that the relationship may not be so direct.[4,6] Although one investigation of 15 patients with CRT suggests improvement of echocardiographic hemodynamics during exercise with rate adaptive shortening of the AV delay,[6] other studies have not borne this out. In fact, a larger study suggests that increased heart rates from both programmed pacing and physical exercise required a longer AV delay from baseline to maximize cardiac output as measured by left ventricular outflow tract velocity time integral (LVOT VTI) on echocardiography.[4] The difference may be attributed to the CRT patient demographics, which primarily include patients with severe cardiomyopathy, often with associated diastolic dysfunction and ventricular dilatation. The response to increased stress may in fact, necessitate an increased filling time to increase stroke volume in these cardiac patients with severely depressed LV function and abnormal LV relaxation. Therefore, CRT patients may actually benefit from an "inverse" rate adaptive programming protocol that gradually increases AV delay based on heart rate,[22] and predetermined parameters set by the protocol used in the aforementioned study.[4,5] Of note, if the AV delay becomes sufficiently prolonged based on this programming, intrinsic conduction may become the predominant rhythm, and obviate the advantage of CRT at higher heart rates. More research will be required before definitive guidelines can be formulated, but the conflicting preliminary data on rate adaptive AV interval programming in CRT, signifies that for the time being, this issues bears thoughtful consideration on a case-by-case basis.

VV Optimization

VV optimization still occupies an unclear role in improving outcomes with CRT. Modern CRT devices allow VV interval programming, with up to 80 ms of offset between left and right ventricular pacing. By convention based on the benefits of LV-RV sequential pacing, a VV interval of "+80 ms" corresponds to an LV pre-excitation of 80 ms, and "–80 ms" corresponds to an RV pre-excitation of 80 ms prior to LV pacing. The most common programming is simultaneous LV-RV timing (VV interval = 0) or a 20-ms LV pre-excitation, given that most patients who undergo CRT have a baseline left bundle branch block. RV pre-excitation is generally avoided, due to its association with decreased LV function.[23]

Thus far, two randomized trials have both demonstrated no long-term benefit from routine VV interval optimization in patients who underwent routine AV optimization.[11,12] Although most CRT patients seem to experience little benefit with VV interval optimization, there may be a small group of patients who respond with significant improvements in their LV dyssynchrony, resulting in increased diastolic filling, LV function, and decrease in functional mitral regurgitation and heart failure symptoms.[24] The adjustment in the VV interval may be counteracting suboptimal LV lead placement, and substantial areas of scar with slow conduction properties. As with the optimal AV delay, the optimal VV interval is highly patient specific and variable, and without reliable clinical predictors.[23,25] In addition, the optimal VV interval is also a dynamic factor that changes based on the patient's level of activity,[24] and frequently over time on follow-up.[10,26] The InSync III study of 433 patients who underwent CRT demonstrated a median increase in stroke volume of approximately 7%, among the 77% of patients who were CRT responders.[27] Although at 6 months, greater exercise capacity was noted in the sequential paced group versus the simultaneous paced group, there were no differences in quality of life or NYHA heart failure class symptoms.[27]

Echocardiographic Techniques

The most commonly utilized modality for AV/VV delay programming in dual chamber pacemakers and CRT remains Doppler echocardiography. Different techniques use different measures within Doppler echocardiography as a surrogate for optimized AV hemodynamics. These include aortic Doppler velocity-time integral (VTI), LVOT VTI, mitral inflow profiles, and changes in LV systolic pressures.

The Ritter technique, which was originally developed for AV optimization in dual chamber pacemakers over a decade ago, has also been used in CRT with success.[28,29] The underlying postulate is that coordinating the end of the mitral A wave to the closure of the mitral valve from LV systole maximizes LV diastolic filling. The first step is to program a nonphysiologically short AV interval (AV_{short}) and measure the interval between the ventricular contraction spike from pacing and the end of the mitral A wave (QA_{short}). The second step is to program a long AV interval (AV_{long}), and once again measure the same interval from ventricular contraction to the end of the mitral A wave (QA_{long}). The difference between (AV_{long}) and (QA_{long}) represents the maximal diastolic left ventricular filling time. Ultimately, the optimal AV delay is equal to the set long AV interval reduced by the difference between QA_{short} and QA_{long} or as follows:

$AV(optimal) = AV_{short} + [(AV_{long} + QA_{long}) - (AV_{short} + QA_{short})]$, which is then reduced to: $AV(optimal) = (AV_{long}) - [(QA_{short}) - (QA_{long})]$

The Ritter method works well in patients with dual chamber pacemakers, but cannot always be applied to patients with CRT devices, and tends to produce shorter AV delay settings.[7,30] In CRT device patients with a normal or short PR interval, obtaining the AV_{long} parameter may be technically impossible, because intrinsic conduction would take place prior to the interval measurement. Furthermore, patients with elevated LVEDP who exhibit distorted mitral A waves on Doppler echocardiography are not ideal candidates, due to technical limitations. The Ritter technique can be used for AV optimization, but not for VV optimization.

The Iterative technique (Fig 21.1) also uses the mitral inflow profile and the A wave to extend the diastolic filling time and is the technique currently endorsed by the American Society of Echocardiography for AV optimization in CRT devices.[31] First a "long" AV delay slightly shorter than the intrinsic AV interval is set. The AV delay is then subsequently shortened in 20-ms increments, until the mitral valve A wave becomes truncated by premature mitral valve closure. Finally, the AV delay is increased in 10-ms increments until the mitral valve A wave truncation disappears.[32] As with the Ritter method, the Iterative technique only applies to AV optimization.

In addition to using the mitral inflow profiles to maximize diastolic filling time, one can calculate the Doppler-derived VTI of the diastolic transmitral flow, LV outflow, or transaortic flow as surrogates for cardiac output. The longest AV delay that still results in biventricular excitation is programmed. The AV delay is then decreased in 20-ms increments after at least 20 cardiac cycles, to a minimum AV delay of 60 ms. Aortic VTI is measured after 10 cardiac cycles at each programmed AV delay and the optimized AV delay is defined as the AV delay that resulted in the greatest increase in aortic VTI from baseline. The CRT-AVO trial found that the optimal AV delay obtained by maximizing the VTI of diastolic transmitral flow was superior to the Ritter method in optimizing acute hemodynamics (as measured by peak LV dP/dt determined invasively).[33] However, consistent and accurate VTI measurements are time-consuming and technically demanding, limiting their widespread application. The VTI technique can be used for both AV and VV optimization. In general, VV optimization is performed once the optimum AV delay has been programmed.

When significant mitral regurgitation is

Fig 21.1 (A–D) AV optimization using the iterative technique. **A**: First, a "long" AV delay (AVD) slightly shorter than the intrinsic AV interval is set (160 ms). **B–D**: AV delay is subsequently shortened in 20-ms increments, until the mitral valve A wave becomes truncated by premature mitral valve closure. In this example, an AV delay of 140 ms appears to lack truncation of the mitral valve A wave, and maximizes the separation of the E and A waves.

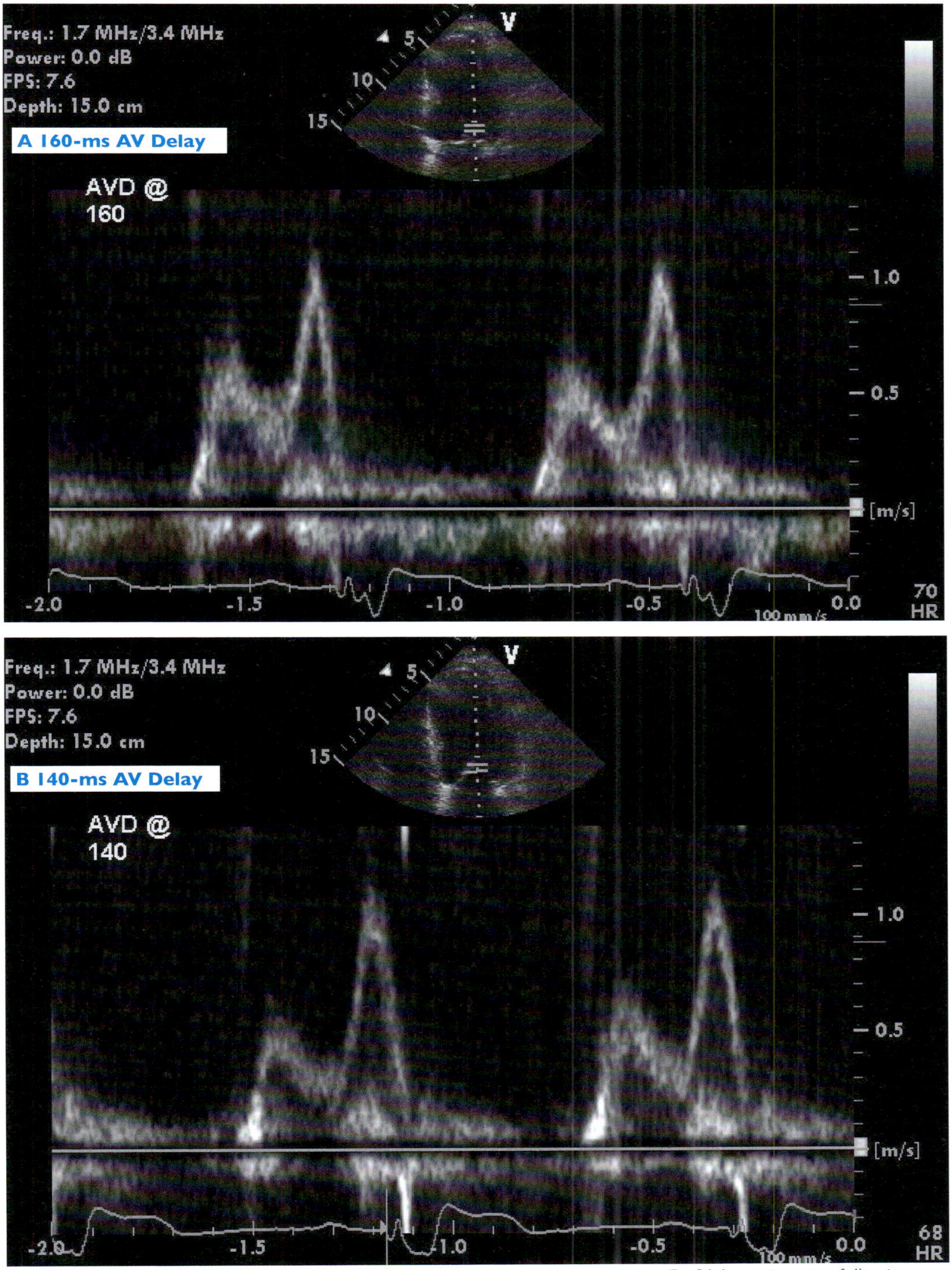

Fig 21.1 continues on following page

Fig 21.1 (*continued*)

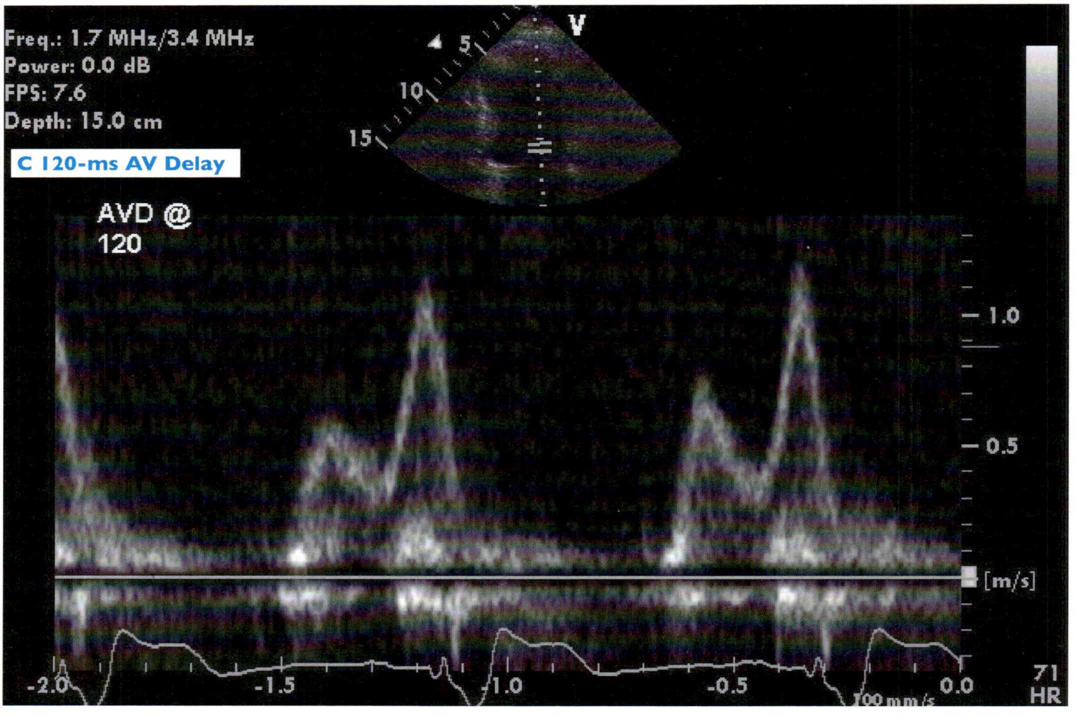

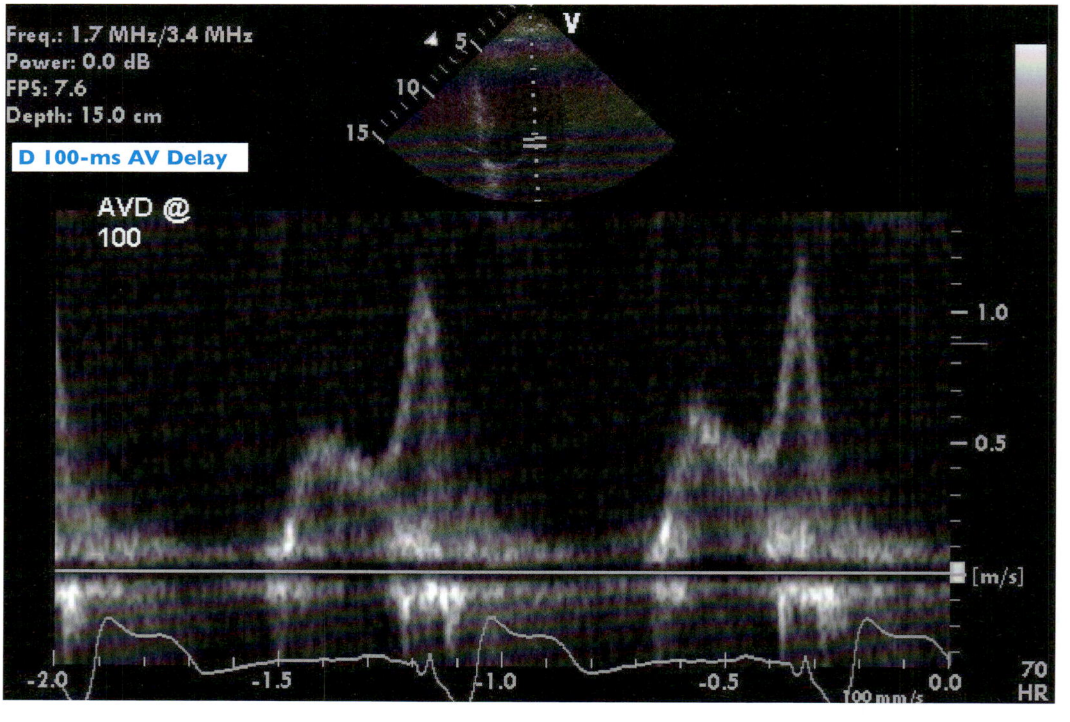

present, continuous spectral Doppler measurements of mitral velocity can be used to calculate LV dP/dt max, and the programmed AV delay that maximizes dP/dt max can be chosen. For example, the time difference between two points on the continuous wave Doppler measurement from 2 m/s to 3 m/s would represent the time difference corresponding to an LV-LA pressure gradient change from 16 mm Hg to 36 mm Hg, based on the modified Bernoulli equation. Assuming a constant LA pressure, this pressure difference of 20 mm Hg over the measured time difference represents LV dP/dt. A confounding factor in this technique is that the improvement of CRT programming may lead to decreased functional mitral regurgitation. Even so, this physiologic improvement is usually attributed more to VV optimization than AV optimization. The Doppler-derived LV dP/dt technique can be used for both AV and VV optimization in a manner analogous to the VTI technique.

Electrogram-based Techniques

Although Doppler echocardiography serves as a popular modality to optimize AV programming, other techniques exist. Boston Scientific and St. Jude Medical have both developed proprietary algorithms that use intracardiac electrogram timing (IEGM) to predict which programmed delays result in the greatest hemodynamic improvement.

The Boston Scientific programmer-based SmartDelay algorithm (Fig 21.2) monitors

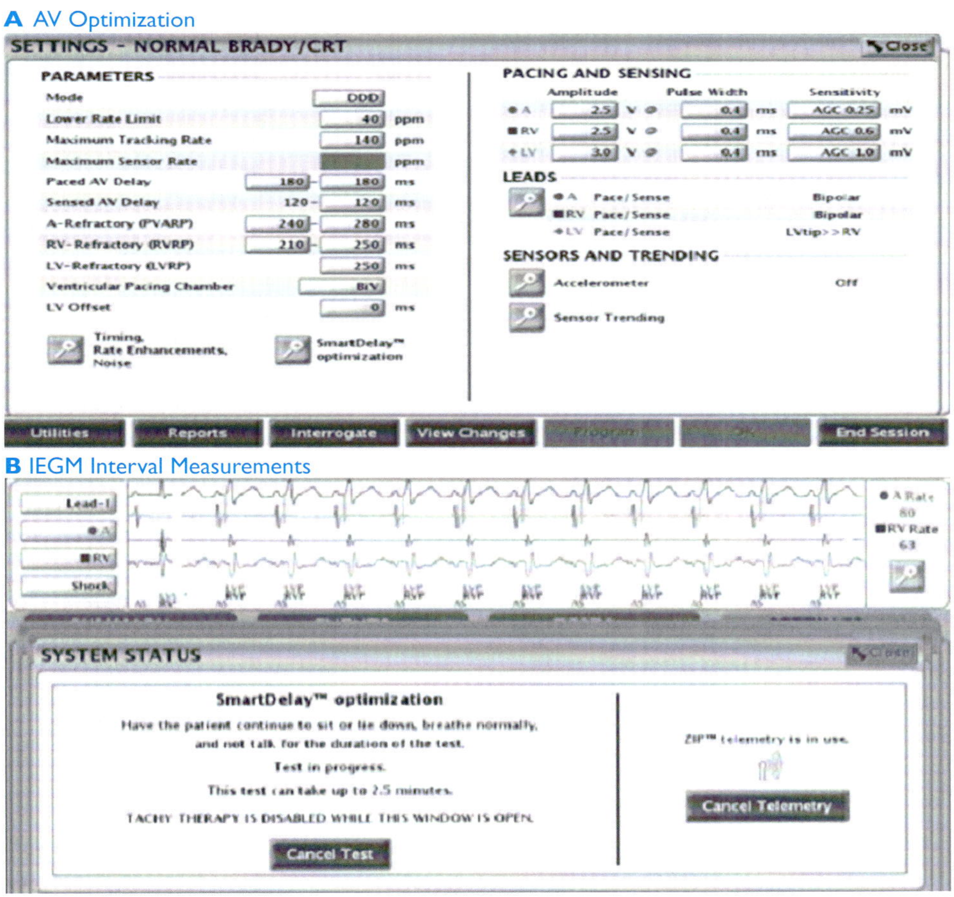

Fig 21.2 (A–B) SmartDelay optimization. The algorithm attempts to improve the fusion of intrinsic activation of RV septum with LV-paced complex. Optimal sensed and paced AV delays are calculated separately. **A**: Programming screen showing SmartDelay option. **B**: Programming screen during optimization. (Courtesy of Boston Scientific)

the conduction delays, and adjusts the timing of ventricular activation to attempt to best improve fusion of the LV-paced complex with intrinsic activation of the RV septum, based on the AVsensed-RVsensed, AVsensed-LVsensed, AVpaced-RVsensed, and AVpaced-LVsensed intervals, as well as lead position. Optimal sensed and paced AV delays are calculated separately. This technique generates a suggested AV delay, but does not provide VV optimization. In fact, if VV optimization is to be performed, the manufacturer recommends determining the VV offset and programming it independently prior to employing SmartDelay. In the CRT-AVO trial, SmartDelay was at least as good as the echocardiographic VTI technique for acute optimization of hemodynamics. This algorithm is only appropriate for CRT patients in sinus rhythm with intact AV nodal conduction.[7]

QuickOpt is the proprietary programmer-

Fig 21.3 (A–D) QuickOpt AV and VV optimization algorithm. If LV is more delayed and needs to be paced first, Δ is a positive value, but if the RV is to be paced first, Δ is a negative value. The optimal VV interval equals the average of Δ and ε or $VV_{optimal} = (\Delta + \varepsilon)/2$. (Courtesy of St. Jude Medical.)

A

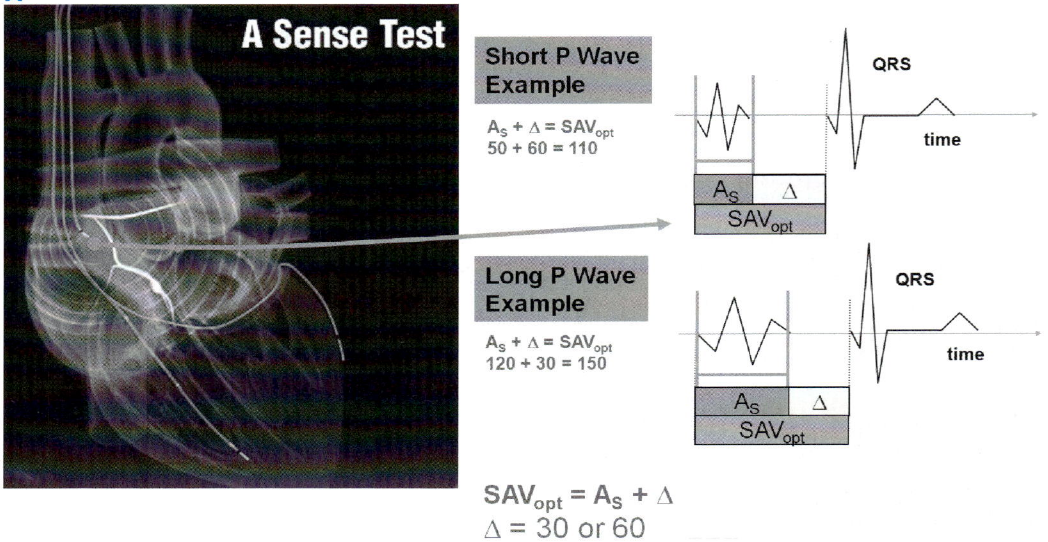

B

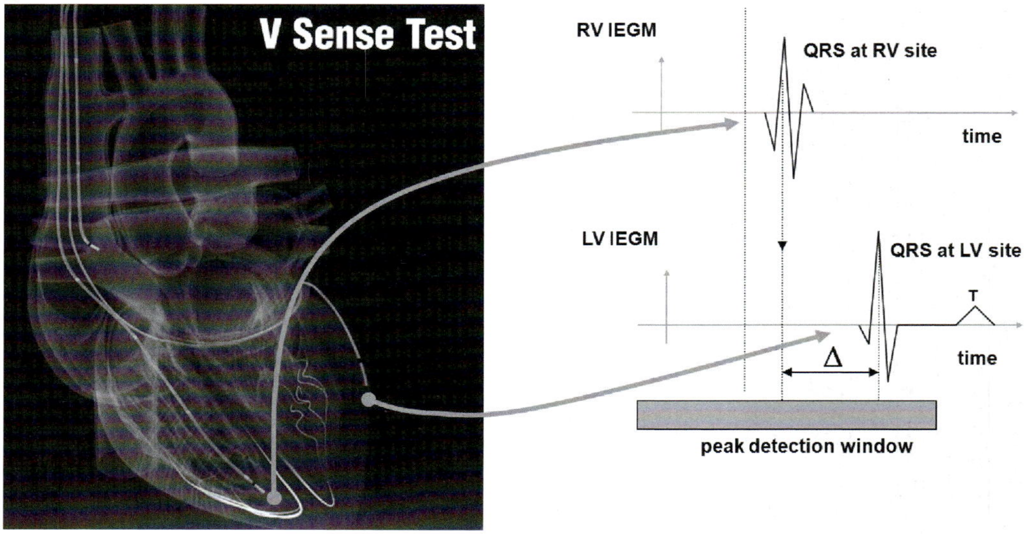

based system from St. Jude Medical for AV and VV optimization (Fig 21.3). The device first goes through a sensing test between the atrium and ventricle (AVsensed-RVsensed, AVsensed-LVsensed, AVpaced-RVsensed, and AVpaced-LVsensed intervals), and identifies the precise delay prior to intrinsic ventricular activation for AV optimization, as well as the ventricle with the more delayed depolarization. This first step sets the AV delay, measures the intrinsic depolarization delay (Δ), and establishes which ventricle will be paced first. If the LV is more delayed, and is to be paced first, an arbitrary sign of "positive" is assigned by the programmer to the intrinsic depolarization delay (Δ). If the RV is to be paced first, then the sign is "negative." The automatic sequence then obtains a comparison of the IEGM of the left and right ventricles with an analysis of the intraventricular conduction delays for VV optimization. The LV paced–RV sensed and RV paced–LV sensed intervals are measured, and their difference generates a value epsilon (ε), which is the interventricular conduction delay. If the LV paced–RV sensed interval is greater than the RV paced–LV sensed interval, the epsilon (ε) value is positive. The

C

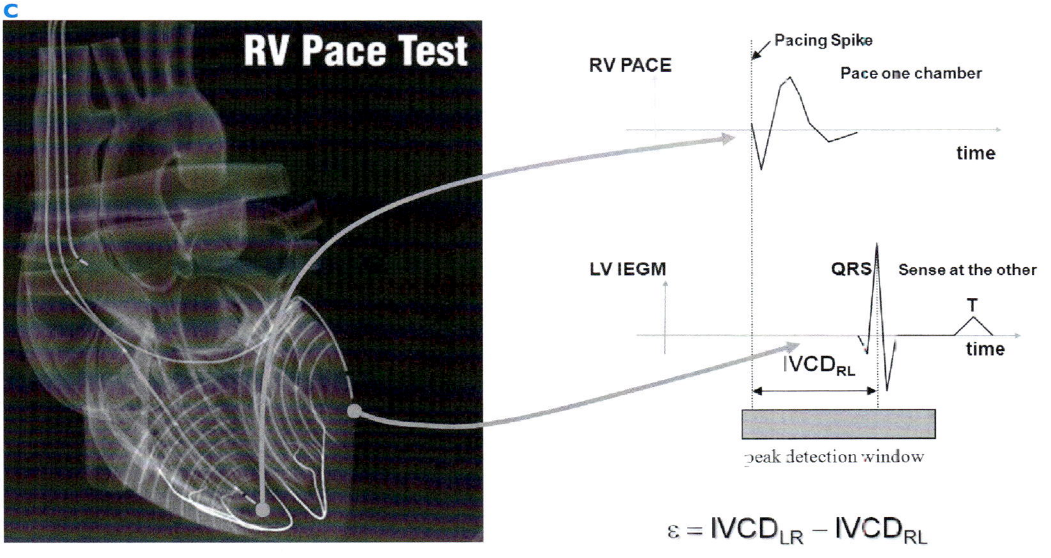

D

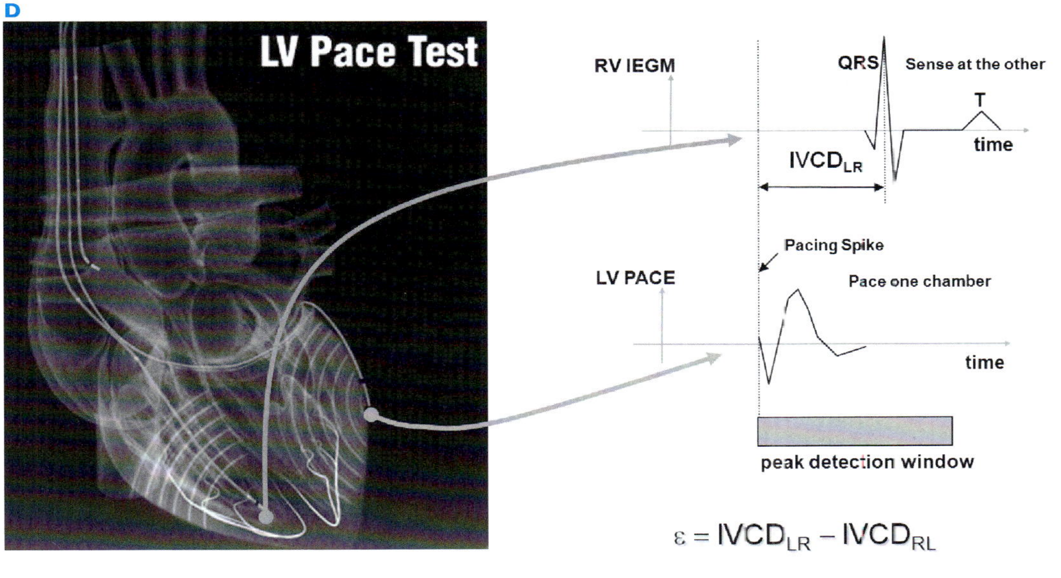

algorithm uses an optimal VV offset that equals the average of the intrinsic depolarization delay and interventricular conduction delay or $(\Delta + \varepsilon)/2$.[34] A small study of 32 heart failure patients who underwent CRT followed by invasive monitoring of their LV dP/dt with QuickOpt programming, and with simultaneous biventricular pacing failed to establish an immediate difference in hemodynamic results.[35] However, a larger clinical trial (FREEDOM) is currently investigating the long-term clinical response to using frequent QuickOpt CRT optimization compared to empiric programming or a one-time optimization using a non–IEGM-based technique.

Photoplethysmography-based Technique

Sophisticated noninvasive blood pressure monitoring has also been developed for optimization of CRT, although its use has largely been limited to Europe. The Finapres system produced by the Finapres Medical Systems (Arnhem, Netherlands) incorporates continuous finger photoplethysmography (FPPG) to measure hemodynamic responses to subtle changes in the AV delay. Consequently, AV programming resulting in the maximal distal pulse pressure would also logically correlate with the maximal aortic pressure, and represent the optimal setting. A comparison of invasive aortic pressure data and FPPG obtained simultaneously in 57 heart failure patients during both intrinsic and paced rhythm revealed that this technique correctly identified 78% of patients with increased aortic pulse pressure following CRT optimization, as well as determined the associated AV delay responsible for maximal aortic pulse pressure change.[36] The sensitivity of this technique was 71% (95% CI: 60%–80%) for a positive change in the aortic pulse pressure, and just 57% (95% CI: 44%–69%) for a negative change. However, the specificity was 90% (95% CI: 84%–94%) for a positive pulse pressure change, and 96% for a negative change (95% CI: 91%–98%).[36] Based on these limited findings, FPPG still remains an emerging technology that may in the future provide a simple, noninvasive method for AV optimization. Its limited sensitivity for pulse pressure changes makes its systematic application problematic. Many patients with CRT may not have any hemodynamic change measureable by FPPG with changes in AV programming. However, if hemodynamic changes are detected by this system, they are highly reproducible, and more pronounced at higher heart rates.[37] Although this technique could in principle, be applied to both AV and VV optimization, thus far, only AV programming has been validated.

Acoustic Cardiographic Technique

On the other end of the spectrum, acoustic cardiography relies on changes in the acoustic properties of heart sounds to monitor and trend hemodynamic alterations, and even progression of heart failure. This technology has been primarily promoted by Inovise Medical, Inc. through its proprietary Audicor system, first introduced in 2003. The optimal AV delay is determined using simultaneous acquisition of ECG and acoustic cardiographic parameters via special sensors, most commonly placed in the V3 and V4 positions. The period from the beginning of the Q wave on the ECG to the mitral component of the S1 heart sound represents the electromechanical activation time (EMAT). The Audicor system possesses enough sensitivity to distinguish the prominent higher frequency of the mitral valve closure secondary to the elevated pressure and flow velocities, compared to the tricuspid component of S1.[38] The EMAT interval, calculated in this manner, reflects the amount of time necessary for the left ventricle to generate enough pressure to close the mitral valve. EMAT correlates with peak LV dP/dt and therefore acts as a load-independent measure of effective contractility (Fig 21.4A). Therefore, AV and VV settings that produce the shortest EMAT time are considered optimal for maximizing contractility and heart function. The system can also measure the intensity of the S3 heart sound, a correlate of left atrial end-diastolic pressure as well

A

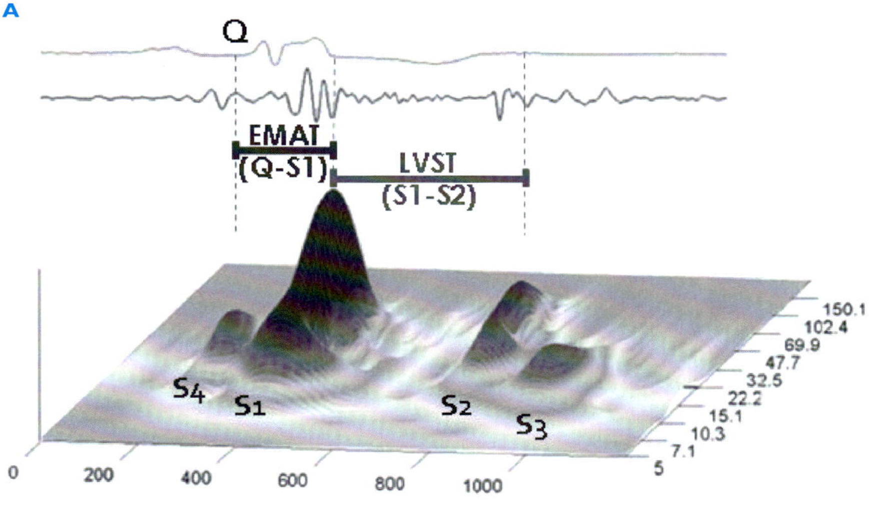

B AV Optimization

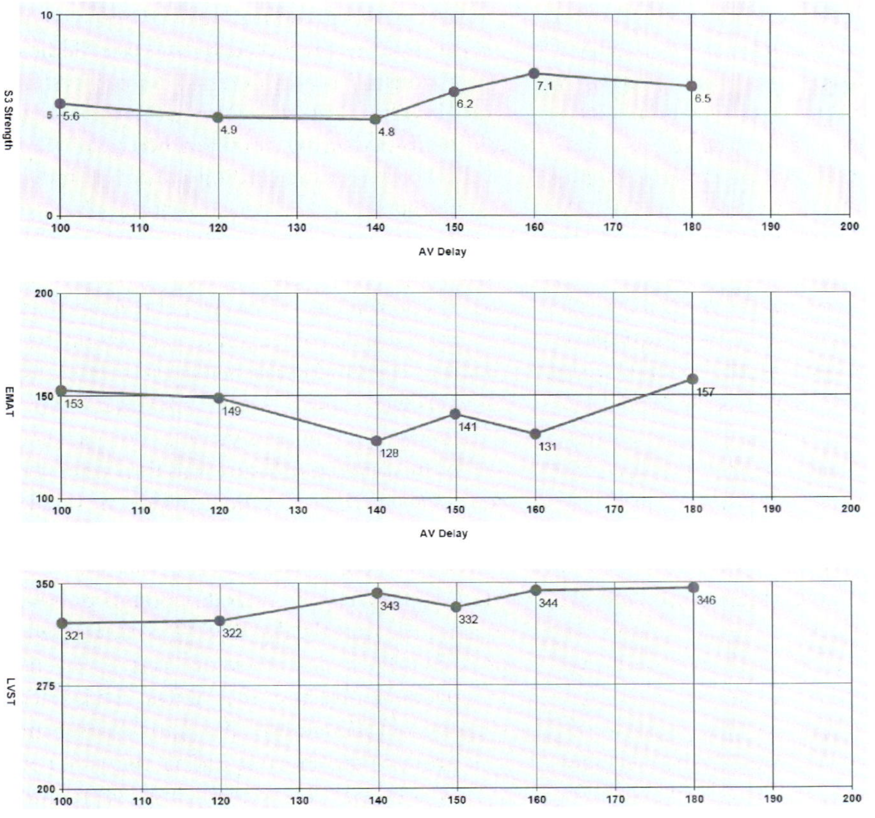

Fig 21.4 (A–B) AV optimization via acoustic cardiography using the Audicor system. **A**: Measurement of EMAT, S3, and LVST using the surface electrocardiogram and spectral analysis of heart sounds. The interval from the Q wave on the ECG to the mitral component of S1 (Q-S1) represents the electromechanical activation time (EMAT), a correlate of peak LV dP/dt. S3 amplitude reflects left atrial end-diastolic pressure. The time period from mitral valve closure to aortic valve closure (S1-S2) represents the left ventricular systolic time (LVST). **B**: Example of AV optimization using acoustic cardiography. In this example, a programmed AV delay of 140 s minimizes EMAT while resulting in an S3 signal strength below 5.0 units. (Courtesy of Inovise Medical, Inc.)

as LVST (left ventricular systolic time). CRT optimization using the Audicor system aims to first minimize the intensity of S3 (to below 5 arbitrary units) and then to minimize EMAT (Fig 21.4B).

In a study of 14 patients at a single center in Lucerne, Switzerland, AV and VV optimization using the EMAT calculated by the Audicor system demonstrated significant improvements in objective clinical and hemodynamic parameters in comparison to typical settings of a fixed AV delay of 120 ms and VV offset of 0 ms.[38] At 6 weeks follow-up from initial CRT optimization, echocardiographic parameters of LV ejection fraction, LV end-systolic volume, and left ventricular outflow tract VTI, as well as clinical cardiac performance measures of work capacity, and maximum oxygen uptake were found to be improved on the Audicor arm versus the group on the baseline "out-of-the-box" settings. Furthermore, small studies comparing Audicor to echocardiographic methods of CRT optimization suggest similar intraobserver variability, but superior reproducibility of optimal programming by acoustic cardiography.[39]

The advantage of acoustic cardiography over other modalities may be its ease of use, given the main barriers to routine or systematic AV or VV optimization remain the extensive time and resources required for the procedure.[40] Echocardiographic-based CRT optimization may take anywhere from 30 min to 2 h, but the Audicor system only requires 10-s intervals of data acquisition in between analyses, and the entire process can usually be completed in < 15 min.[41] However, further studies with larger patient populations will be necessary to determine the efficacy of acoustic cardiography compared to the current standard of echocardiography.

Conclusion

For patients with dual chamber pacemakers and CRT devices, optimal pacing programming provides an avenue for improved clinical outcomes. In particular, for CRT patients with suboptimal response to therapy, AV and VV programming may be the key to unlocking the benefits of their devices. Thus far, although the indications for CRT are becoming more defined, and its use has experienced explosive growth, there are still no evidence-based uniform guidelines for the use of AV and VV optimization. Ongoing clinical trials hope to better elucidate the proper role of AV and VV optimization, as well as to establish a hierarchy of technologies based on their efficacy and accuracy. Until then, one must navigate through the various available techniques to determine the most appropriate modality for AV and VV optimization for both the physician and each individual patient.

References

1. Epstein AE, DiMarco JP, Ellenbogen KA, et al. (2008). ACC/AHA/HRS 2008 Guidelines for Device-Based Therapy of Cardiac Rhythm Abnormalities: a report of the American College of Cardiology/American Heart Association Task Force on Practice Guidelines (Writing Committee to Revise the ACC/AHA/NASPE 2002 Guideline Update for Implantation of Cardiac Pacemakers and Antiarrhythmia Devices) developed in collaboration with the American Association for Thoracic Surgery and Society of Thoracic Surgeons. *J Am Coll Cardiol.* 51(21):e1–62.
2. Vardas PE, Auricchio A, Blanc J-J, et al. (2007). Guidelines for cardiac pacing and cardiac resynchronization therapy: The Task Force for Cardiac Pacing and Cardiac Resynchronization Therapy of the European Society of Cardiology. Developed in collaboration with the European Heart Rhythm Association. *Eur Heart J.* 28(18):2256–2295.
3. Bax JJ, Abraham T, Barold SS, et al. (2005). Cardiac resynchronization therapy: Part 2—issues during and after device implantation and unresolved questions. *J Am Coll Cardiol.* 46(12):2168–2182.
4. Scharf C, Li P, Muntwyler J, et al. (2005). Rate-dependent AV delay optimization in cardiac resynchronization therapy. *Pacing Clin Electrophysiol.* 28(4):279–284.

5. Whinnett ZI, Briscoe C, Davies J, et al. (2008). The atrioventricular delay of cardiac resynchronization can be optimized hemodynamically during exercise and predicted from resting measurements. *Heart Rhythm.* 5(3):378–386.
6. Grimm RA, Sun JP, Agler D, et al. (2009). Shorter AV delays provide improved echocardiographic hemodynamics during exercise in patients receiving cardiac resynchronization therapy. *Pacing Clin Electrophysiol.* 32(4):457–465.
7. Gold MR, Niazi I, Giudici M, et al. (2007). A prospective comparison of AV delay programming methods for hemodynamic optimization during cardiac resynchronization therapy. *J Cardiovasc Electrophysiol.* 18(5):490–496.
8. Boriani G, Biffi M, Müller CP, et al. (2009). A prospective randomized evaluation of VV delay optimization in CRT-D recipients: echocardiographic observations from the RHYTHM II ICD study. *Pacing Clin Electrophysiol.* 32 Suppl 1:S120–S25.
9. Zhang Q, Fung JW-H, Chan, Y-S, et al. (2008). The role of repeating optimization of atrioventricular interval during interim and long-term follow-up after cardiac resynchronization therapy. *Int J Cardiol.* 124(2):211–217.
10. Porciani MC, Dondina C, Macioce G, et al. (2006). Temporal variation in optimal atrioventricular and interventricular delay during cardiac resynchronization therapy. *J Card Fail.* 12(9):715–719.
11. Boriani G, Muller CP, Seidi KH, et al. (2006). Randomized comparison of simultaneous biventricular stimulation versus optimized interventricular delay in cardiac resynchronization therapy. The Resynchronization for the HemodYnamic Treatment for Heart Failure Management II implantable cardioverter defibrillator (RHYTHM II ICD) study. *Am Heart J.* 151(5):1050–1058.
12. Rao RK, Kumar UN, Schafer J, et al. (2007). Reduced ventricular volumes and improved systolic function with cardiac resynchronization therapy: a randomized trial comparing simultaneous biventricular pacing, sequential biventricular pacing, and left ventricular pacing. *Circulation* 115(16):2136–2144.
13. Morales MA, Startari U, Panchetti L, et al. (2006). Atrioventricular delay optimization by Doppler-derived left ventricular dP/dt improves 6-month outcome of resynchronized patients. *Pacing Clin Electrophysiol.* 29(6):564–568.
14. Sawhney NS, Waggoner AD, Garhwal S, et al. (2004). Randomized prospective trial of atrioventricular delay programming for cardiac resynchronization therapy. *Heart Rhythm.* 1(5):562–567.
15. Abraham WT, Fisher WG, Smith AL, et al. (2002). Cardiac resynchronization in chronic heart failure. *N Engl J Med.* 346(24):1845–1853.
16. Young JB, Abraham WT, Smith AL, et al. (2003). Combined cardiac resynchronization and implantable cardioversion defibrillation in advanced chronic heart failure: the MIRACLE ICD Trial. *JAMA.* 289(20):2685–2694.
17. Cleland JG, Daubert JC, Erdmann N, et al. (2005). The effect of cardiac resynchronization on morbidity and mortality in heart failure. *N Engl J Med.* 352(15):1539–1549.
18. Higgins SL, Hummel JD, Niazi IK, et al. (2003). Cardiac resynchronization therapy for the treatment of heart failure in patients with intraventricular conduction delay and malignant ventricular tachyarrhythmias. *J Am Coll Cardiol.* 42 (8):1454–1459.
19. Bristow MR, Saxon LA, Boehmer J, et al. (2004). Cardiac-resynchronization therapy with or without an implantable defibrillator in advanced chronic heart failure. *N Engl J Med.* 350 (21):2140–2150.
20. Inoue N, Ishikawa T, Sumita S, et al. (2005). Long-term follow-up of atrioventricular delay optimization in patients with biventricular pacing. *Circ J.* 69(2):201–204.
21. Meisner JS, McQueen DM, Ishida Y, et al. (1985). Effects of timing of atrial systole on LV filling and mitral valve closure: computer and dog studies. *Am J Physiol.* 249(3 Pt 2):H604–H619.
22. Tse HF, Siu CW, Lee KLF, et al. (2005). The incremental benefit of rate-adaptive pacing on exercise performance during cardiac resynchronization therapy. *J Am Coll Cardiol.* 46(12):2292–2297.
23. Sogaard P, Egeblad H, Pedersen AK, et al. (2002). Sequential versus simultaneous biventricular resynchronization for severe heart

failure: evaluation by tissue Doppler imaging. *Circulation.* 106(16):2078–2084.

24. Bordachar P, Lafitte S, Reuter S, et al. (2006). Echocardiographic assessment during exercise of heart failure patients with cardiac resynchronization therapy. *Am J Cardiol.* 97(11):1622–1625.
25. Burri H, Sunthorn H, Dipen S, et al. (2006). Optimization of device programming for cardiac resynchronization therapy. *Pacing Clin Electrophysiol.* 29(12):141–1425.
26. O'Donnell D, Nadurata V, Hamer A, et al. (2005). Long-term variations in optimal programming of cardiac resynchronization therapy devices. *Pacing Clin Electrophysiol.* 28 Suppl 1:S24–S26.
27. Leon AR, Abraham WT, Brozena S, et al. (2005). Cardiac resynchronization with sequential biventricular pacing for the treatment of moderate-to-severe heart failure. *J Am Coll Cardiol.* 46(12):2298–2304.
28. Ritter P, Daubert C, Mabo P, et al. (1989). Haemodynamic benefit of a rate-adapted A-V delay in dual chamber pacing. *Eur Heart J.* 10(7):637–646.
29. Kindermann M, Fröhlig G, Doerr T, et al. (1997). Optimizing the AV delay in DDD pacemaker patients with high degree AV block: mitral valve Doppler versus impedance cardiography. *Pacing Clin Electrophysiol.* 20(10 Pt 1):2453–2462.
30. Kerlan JE, Sawhney NS, Waggoner AD, et al. (2006). Prospective comparison of echocardiographic atrioventricular delay optimization methods for cardiac resynchronization therapy. *Heart Rhythm.* 3(2):148–154.
31. Gorcsan J, 3rd, Abraham T, Agler DA, et al. (2008). Echocardiography for cardiac resynchronization therapy: recommendations for performance and reporting—a report from the American Society of Echocardiography Dyssynchrony Writing Group endorsed by the Heart Rhythm Society. *J Am Soc Echocardiogr.* 21(3):191–213.
32. Lane RE, Chow AWC, Chin D, et al. (2004). Selection and optimisation of biventricular pacing: the role of echocardiography. *Heart.* 90 Suppl 6:vi10–vi16.
33. Jansen AH, Bracke FA, Van Dantzig JM, et al. (2006). Correlation of echo-Doppler optimization of atrioventricular delay in cardiac resynchronization therapy with invasive hemodynamics in patients with heart failure secondary to ischemic or idiopathic dilated cardiomyopathy. *Am J Cardiol.* 97(4):552–557.
34. Baker JH, 2nd, McKenzie J 3rd, Beau S, et al. (2007). Acute evaluation of programmer-guided AV/PV and VV delay optimization comparing an IEGM method and echocardiogram for cardiac resynchronization therapy in heart failure patients and dual-chamber ICD implants. *J Cardiovasc Electrophysiol.* 18(2):185–191.
35. van Gelder BM, Meijer A, Bracke FA. (2008). The optimized V-V interval determined by interventricular conduction times versus invasive measurement by LVdP/dtMAX. *J Cardiovasc Electrophysiol.* 19(9):939–944.
36. Butter C, Stellbrink C, Belalcazar, A, et al. (2004). Cardiac resynchronization therapy optimization by finger plethysmography. *Heart Rhythm.* 1(5):568–575.
37. Whinnett ZI, Davies JER, Willson K, et al. (2006). Determination of optimal atrioventricular delay for cardiac resynchronization therapy using acute non-invasive blood pressure. *Europace.* 8(5):358–366.
38. Toggweiler S, Zuber M, Kobza R, et al. (2007). Improved response to cardiac resynchronization therapy through optimization of atrioventricular and interventricular delays using acoustic cardiography: a pilot study. *J Card Fail.* 13(8):637–642.
39. Zuber M, Toggweiler S, Quinn-Tate L, et al. (2008). A comparison of acoustic cardiography and echocardiography for optimizing pacemaker settings in cardiac resynchronization therapy. *Pacing Clin Electrophysiol.* 31(7):802–811.
40. Gras D, Gupta MS, Boulogne E, et al. (2009). Optimization of AV and VV delays in the real-world CRT patient population: an international survey on current clinical practice. *Pacing Clin Electrophysiol.* 32 Suppl 1:S236–S239.
41. Hasan A, Abraham WT, Quinn-Tate L, et al. (2006). Optimization of cardiac resynchronization devices using acoustic cardiography: a comparison to echocardiography. *Congest Heart Fail.* 12 Suppl 1:25–31.

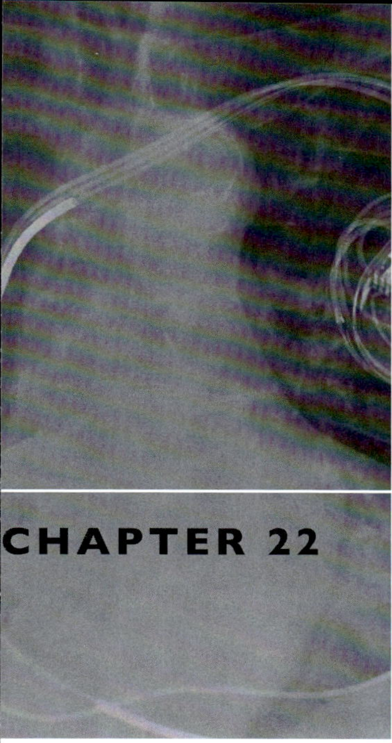

Electromagnetic Interactions from Magnetic Resonance Imaging in Patients with Implantable Arrhythmia Devices

CHAPTER 22

Saman Nazarian and Henry R. Halperin

Introduction

Compared to other diagnostic modalities, magnetic resonance imaging (MRI) provides superior soft tissue resolution and multi-planar imaging capabilities. The unique capability of cardiac MRI for identification of scar fibrosis and fat deposition makes it an ideal imaging modality for the evaluation of patients presenting with arrhythmia. In addition, the absence of X-ray radiation makes MRI suitable for follow-up of chronic disease and imaging in young patients and women of childbearing age. Due to the ever-expanding indications for implantation of permanent pacemakers and implantable cardioverter defibrillators (ICDs), advancing severity of disease and age of the population, and advances in device technology, the number of patients with implantable cardiac devices will continue to increase. It has been estimated that patients with a pacemaker or ICD have a 50% to 75% likelihood of developing a clinical indication for MRI over the lifetime of their device.

Catastrophic complications have been reported when MRI is performed on patients with older implantable devices. However, many studies over the past 10 years have reported the safety of MRI with selected pacemaker and ICD systems when imaging is performed with appropriate supervision and following a protocol for safety. Familiarity with potential MRI and implanted device electromagnetic interactions is essential for arrhythmia professionals who wish to safely provide pacemaker or ICD recipients with MRI when it is medically necessary.

Potential Electromagnetic Interactions

The static and gradient magnetic fields and radiofrequency energy of MRI may result in

Pacemakers and Implantable Cardioverter Defibrillators: An Expert's Manual. © 2010 Amin Al-Ahmad, Kenneth A. Ellenbogen, Andrea Natale, and Paul J. Wang, eds. Cardiotext Publishing, ISBN: 978-0-9790164-6-2.

several potential interactions with implanted pacemakers and ICDs.

Force and Torque

Ferromagnetic implants are subject to static and gradient magnetic field induced force and torque in the MRI environment. The potential for movement of an implanted device due to these forces depends upon the magnetic field strength, ferromagnetic properties and size of the device, the implant distance from the magnet bore, and the stability of the implant. In an in vitro analysis of modern permanent pacemakers (manufactured after 1996) and ICDs (manufactured after 2000), we found that the maximal force acting upon devices was < 100 g in a 1.5 Tesla MRI scanner.[1] This amount of force is unlikely to dislodge a chronic device which is adherent to the surrounding tissue. However, this observation led to the adaptation of a 6-wk waiting period prior to MRI after device implantation.

Current induction

The radiofrequency and pulsed gradient magnetic fields in the MRI environment may induce electrical currents in leads within the field. The lead length in relation to the radiofrequency wavelength, and conformations such as loops favor improved transition of energy to the implanted device. A study from the laboratory assessed the magnitude of MRI-induced current using a current recorder connected in series to single chamber permanent pacemakers programmed to subthreshold asynchronous output during unipolar and bipolar pacing. Under conventional implant conditions, without additional lead loops, the magnitude of induced current was < 0.5 mA and no myocardial capture was observed. With the addition of 5 lead loops current induction at > 30 mA was possible and resulted in myocardial capture. Importantly, breaking the return pathway by electrically isolating the pulse generator case from the circuit abolished low frequency–induced current.[2]

Heating

The extent of radiofrequency energy deposition in tissues is described by the specific absorption rate (SAR, units of Watts per kg). Metallic devices and leads can act as an antenna thus amplifying local radiofrequency energy deposition, which may lead to heating and tissue damage at the device–tissue interface. Fractured leads or lead loop configurations may increase the potential for heating. Epicardial leads, which are not cooled by blood flow, may also be prone to increased heating. In the in vivo analysis of modern permanent pacemakers and ICDs, when performing clinical MRI protocols (SAR < 2.0 W/kg), temperature changes were limited to 0.5°C.[1] It is important to note, however, that due to poor correlation of heating at different SAR of sequences across different scanners even within the same manufacturer, the SAR limits from each study should not be directly applied to other MRI systems.

Inappropriate Pacing and Shocks or Inhibition of Therapies

Pacemakers and ICDs have the potential for receiving electromagnetic interference in the MRI environment, resulting in radiofrequency noise tracking, asynchronous pacing, inhibition of demand pacing, delivery of ICD therapies, programming changes, or loss of function. The static magnetic field of the MRI scanner can also alter device function by inducing unexpected reed switch opening or closure.

Such potential risks have led to concerns from device manufacturers and MRI authorities regarding the performance of MRI procedures in cardiac implantable device recipients. However, several studies have assessed techniques to safely perform MRI in recipients of implanted cardiac devices.

Implantable Monitors

Patients with an implantable loop recorder (Reveal, Medtronic Inc.) can be safely scanned.[3]

However, the device may record MRI electromagnetic interference artifacts as arrhythmia. Care should be taken to clear episodes recorded during MRI to prevent future misinterpretation of artifact as clinically significant arrhythmia.

Temporary Pacemakers

The majority of temporary pacemakers (implanted outside of the electrophysiology laboratory) have no fixation leads that are prone to movement. Furthermore, the leads are longer, and potentially more susceptible to induction of lead currents and heating. An in vitro study of temporary transvenous pacing leads showed that lead heating exceeding 15°C is common, and temperature rises up to 63.1°C are possible.[4] Such a temperature rise would be capable of producing an ablation lesion at the lead tip resulting in failure to capture and local myocardial damage. Additionally, the electronic platform of external temporary pacemakers is less sophisticated and has less filtering compared to modern permanent pacemakers. Therefore such devices are likely more susceptible to electromagnetic interference in the MRI environment, and imaging of patients with temporary pacemakers cannot be recommended.

Permanent Pacemakers

Previous studies of clinical MRI in the setting of implanted devices have been reviewed in Table 22.1 (see following page). At our institution we began the process of imaging patients with permanent pacemakers by extensive in vitro testing. Roguin et al tested in vitro and in vivo lead heating, device function, torque, and image distortion at 1.5 Tesla.[1] Based upon our in vitro and in vivo analyses, we then developed a protocol including (a) device selection based on previous testing, (b) device programming to minimize inappropriate activation or inhibition of brady/tachyarrhythmia therapies, and (c) limitation of the specific absorption rate of MRI sequences (< 2.0 W/Kg).[5] The protocol is discussed in detail later. Using this protocol MRI has been successfully performed on more than 200 patients with implantable devices. The initial report of safety included 31 patients with permanent pacemakers, 22% of whom were pacemaker dependent. Pacing mode was changed to an asynchronous mode for pacemaker-dependent patients, and to demand mode for others. Blood pressure, ECG, oximetry, and symptoms were monitored. In this initial study the system-estimated whole-body average SAR was successfully limited to 2.0 W/kg in more than 99% of sequences, while maintaining the diagnostic capability of MRI. No episodes of inappropriate inhibition or activation of pacing were observed, and there were no significant differences between baseline and immediate or long-term (median 99 days after MRI) sensing amplitudes, lead impedances, or pacing thresholds.[5]

Implantable Cardioverter Defibrillators

During in vitro testing of ICDs several generators (manufactured before 2000) were found to be damaged by MRI. Therefore we focused our in vivo testing to ICDs manufactured after 2000. Such systems from the three major manufacturers were implanted in 18 dogs, and after 4 wk, 3- to 4-h MRI scans were performed under worst-case-scenario conditions (imaging over the region containing the generator, and SAR up to 3.5 W/kg). No device dysfunction occurred. After 8 wk of follow-up, pacing threshold and intracardiac electrogram amplitude were unchanged, with exception of 1 animal with transient (< 12 h) capture failure. Due to this observation, we currently do not perform MRI on pacemaker-dependent ICD patients. ICD leads are generally longer than pacemaker leads and may therefore be at higher risk for heating at the lead tip. Pathological data of the scanned animals revealed very limited necrosis or fibrosis at the tip of the lead area, which was not different from controls not subjected to MRI.[1]

Based upon our prior in vitro and in vivo testing, the safety protocol has now been used to safely scan more than 75 patients with ICDs. Our initial report of safety included 24 patients

Source	Number of Patients	Device Type	Finding
Gimbel et al[7]	5 (1 pacemaker dependent)	Permanent pacemaker	No device abnormalities were noted after MRI (0.5 Tesla). A 2-s pause was noted on pulse oximetry in the pacemaker-dependent patient whose device (with unipolar leads) was programmed to dual chamber asynchronous pacing. Patients were otherwise asymptomatic and did not report any feeling of torque or heat.
Sommer et al[8]	44	Permanent pacemaker	MRI at 0.5 Tesla did not inhibit pacing output or cause pacemaker malfunction.
Vahlhaus et al[9]	32	Permanent pacemaker	Lead impedance and sensing and stimulation thresholds did not change immediately or 3 mon after MRI at 0.5 Tesla. However, diminished battery voltage was noted immediately after MRI with recovery 3 months later. Reed switch temporary deactivation was seen in 12 of 32 patients when positioned in the center of the magnetic field.
Martin et al[10]	54	Permanent pacemaker	Cardiac, vascular, and general 1.5 Tesla MRI studies were performed. Significant changes were reported in 9.4% of leads, however only 1.9% required a change in programmed output.
Del Ojo et al[11]	13	Permanent pacemaker	MRI at 2.0 Tesla was unassociated with pacemaker inhibition, inappropriate rapid pacing, or significant changes in device parameters.
Gimbel et al[12]	7	ICD	No changes in pacing, sensing, impedances, charge times, or battery status were observed with MRI at 1.5 Tesla. However, one implantable cardioverter defibrillator (Medtronic 7227Cx, lumbar spine MRI) experienced a "power-on-reset."
Sommer et al[13]	82	Permanent pacemaker	MRI at 1.5 Tesla was unassociated with inhibition of pacemaker output or induction of arrhythmias. However, increased capture threshold was noted post-MRI. In 4 of 114 examinations, troponin increased from a normal baseline value to above normal after MRI (one was associated with a significant increase in capture threshold).
Nazarian et al[5]	55	31 Permanent pacemaker/24 ICD	MRI at 1.5 Tesla was not associated with any inappropriate inhibition or activation of pacing. There were no significant differences between baseline and immediate or long-term (median 99 days after MRI) sensing amplitudes, lead impedances, or pacing thresholds.
Naehle et al[14]	44	Permanent pacemaker	MRI at 3 Tesla using a transmit-receive head coil was performed safely in all patients without changes in lead parameters or serum troponin I level.

Table 22.1 Previous Studies of Clinical MRI in the Setting of Permanent Pacemakers and ICDs.

with ICDs. No episodes of inappropriate inhibition or activation of pacing were observed, and there were no significant differences between baseline and immediate or long-term sensing amplitudes, lead impedances, or pacing thresholds.[5]

Retained Leads

There have been no systematic studies to assess the potential risks associated with retained permanent pacemaker and ICD leads. Retained leads are prone to previously described risks of movement, heating, and current induction. Depending upon the lead length and configuration, retained segments may be prone to significantly higher temperature rises than those attached to pulse generators. It has been our practice to exclude from MRI those patients with retained lead fragments and unused capped leads. More studies to delineate risks in this patient group are warranted.

Safety Protocol for MRI of Patients with Implanted Devices

The safety protocol followed at our institution (Fig 22.1) is based upon selection of device generators previously tested under worst-case-scenario (prolonged imaging over the region containing the generator and SAR up to 3.5 W/kg) MRI conditions.[1] To perform MRI on patients with implanted devices, it is recommended that device generators prone to electromagnetic interference (generally older devices not on the tested devices list in the protocol, Fig 22.1) be excluded. Despite the low risk for lead and generator movement, conservative measures to exclude patients with leads that are more prone to movement are recommended. Therefore, we recommend avoiding MRI in patients with < 6 weeks' time since device implant or patients with no fixation (superior vena cava coils) leads. However, in our experience, patients with mature active and passive fixation endocardial (and coronary sinus) leads of any diameter can safely undergo MRI. We do recommend avoidance of MRI when device leads that are prone to heating such as nontransvenous epicardial and abandoned (capped) leads are present. To reduce the risk of inappropriate inhibition of pacing due to detection of radiofrequency pulses, we prefer device programming to an asynchronous, dedicated pacing mode in pacemaker-dependent patients. Also, given the lack of asynchronous pacing programming capability and transient loss of pacing capture after worst-case-scenario (SAR 3.5 W/kg for 3 h) in vivo testing of 1 of 15 animals implanted with an ICD,[1] we recommend excluding pacemaker-dependent patients with ICDs. To avoid inappropriate activation of pacing due to tracking of radiofrequency pulses, device programming to a nontracking ventricular or dual chamber inhibited pacing mode in patients without pacemaker dependence is suggested. We also recommend deactivation of rate response, premature ventricular contraction response, ventricular sense response, and conducted atrial fibrillation response to ensure that sensing of vibrations or radiofrequency pulses does not lead to unwarranted pacing. Although asynchronous pacing for short time periods is typically well-tolerated, it is preferable to reduce the already-minimal chance of inducing arrhythmia or causing AV dyssynchrony by minimizing asynchronous pacing in patients without pacemaker dependence through deactivation of the magnet mode when possible. Tachyarrhythmia monitoring is typically deactivated to avoid battery drainage that results from recording of multiple radiofrequency pulse sequences as arrhythmic episodes. Reed switch activation in ICD systems disables tachyarrhythmia therapies. However, reed switch function in the periphery versus the bore of the magnet is unpredictable; therefore therapies should be disabled to avoid unwarranted antitachycardia pacing or shocks. Finally, to reduce the risk of thermal injury and changes in lead threshold and impedance, limit the estimated whole body averaged SAR of MRI sequences (< 2.0 W/kg when possible). Blood pressure, ECG, pulse oximetry, and symptoms should be monitored for

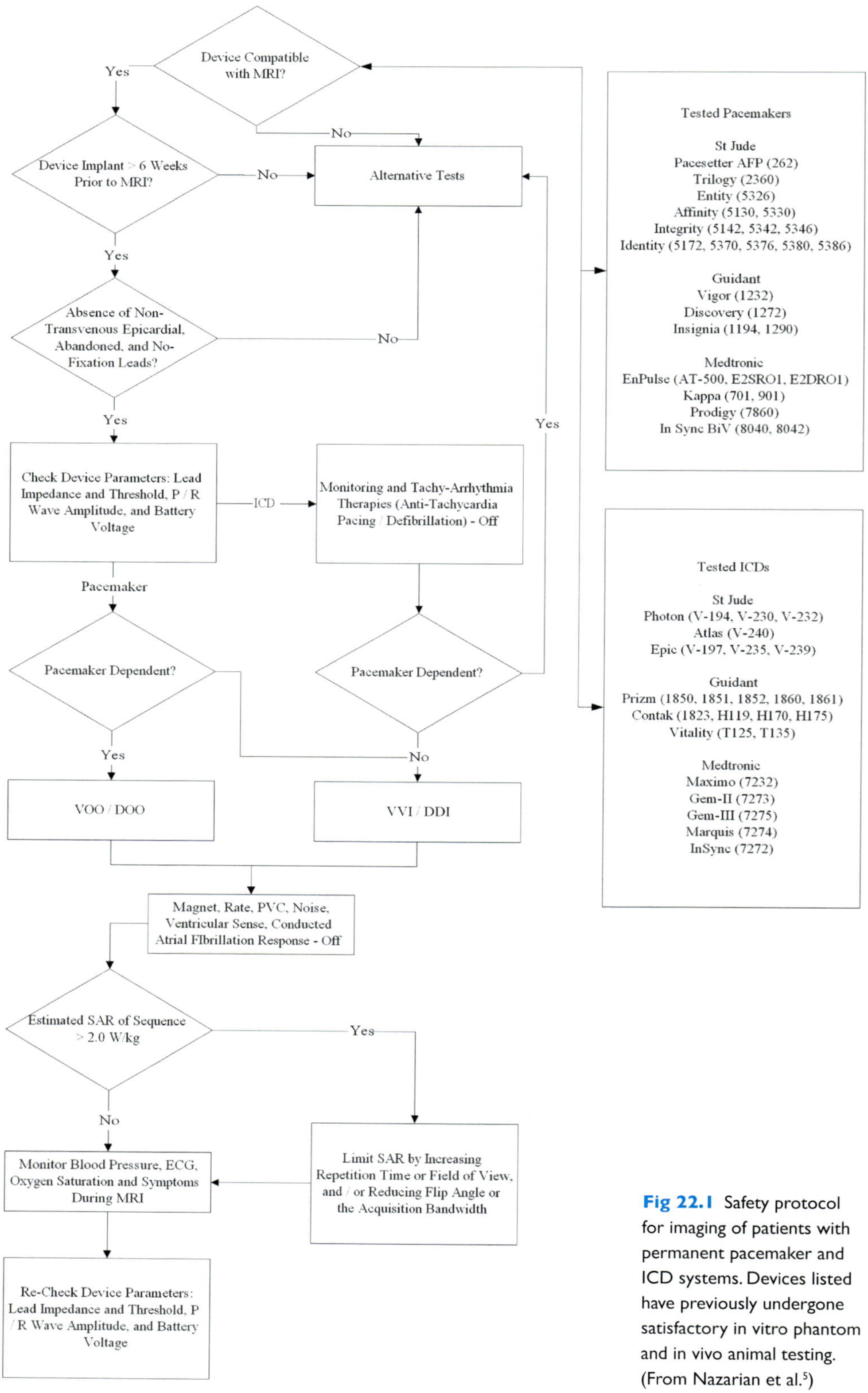

Fig 22.1 Safety protocol for imaging of patients with permanent pacemaker and ICD systems. Devices listed have previously undergone satisfactory in vitro phantom and in vivo animal testing. (From Nazarian et al.[5])

the duration of the examination. It is favorable to have a radiologist and cardiac electrophysiologist, or advanced cardiac life support trained individual familiar with device programming and trouble shooting present during all scans.[5] At the end of the examination all device parameters should be checked and programming should be restored to pre-MRI settings.

Image Artifacts

The presence of ferromagnetic materials can cause variations in the surrounding magnetic field resulting in image distortion, signal voids or bright areas, and poor fat suppression. Susceptibility artifacts appear to be most pronounced on inversion recovery and steady-state free precession sequences (Fig 22.2). In our experience, artifacts on inversion recovery prepared delayed cardiac MRI show high signal intensity and can mimic areas of delayed enhancement, which would otherwise indicate myocardial scar. Correlation of suspect areas on different pulse sequences can help avoid misidentification of artifact as scar. Using imaging planes perpendicular to the plane of the device generator, shortening of the echo time, and using spin echo and fast spin echo sequences appears to reduce the qualitative extent of artifact. Figure 22.3 is a short axis inversion recovery gradient echo image showing midwall septal scarring in a patient with a biventricular pacemaker and defibrillator system, and demonstrates the feasibility of diagnostic quality cardiac imaging in device recipients. In an initial report of imaging patients with permanent pacemakers and implantable cardioverter defibrillators, diagnostic questions were answered in 100% of nonthoracic and 93% of thoracic studies. Clinical findings included diagnosis of vascular abnormalities (9 patients), diagnosis or staging of malignancy (9 patients), and assessment of cardiac viability prior to surgical ventricular reconstruction (13 patients).[5]

Summary

Due to its superior spatial resolution, multiplanar capabilities, and lack of ionizing radiation, MRI is the preferred imaging technique in many clinical scenarios. The decision to perform MRI in patients with potential contraindi-

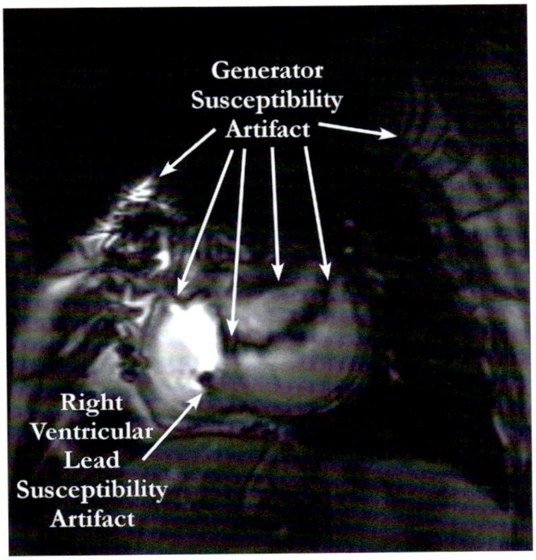

Fig 22.2 Extensive susceptibility artifact on a short axis steady-state free precession image in a patient with an implantable cardioverter defibrillator.

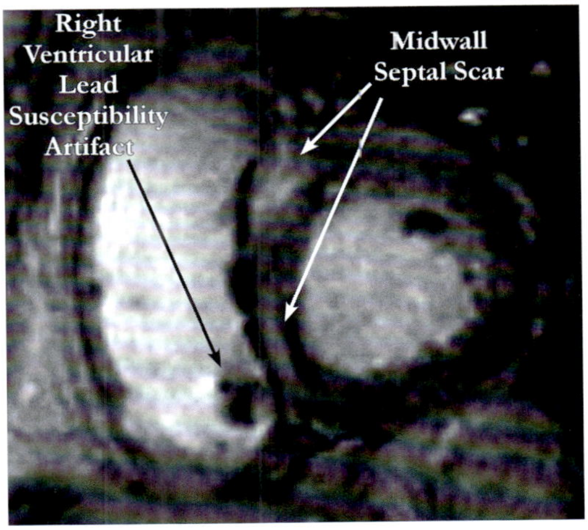

Fig 22.3 Minimal susceptibility artifact on a short axis inversion prepared gradient echo image. Areas of late gadolinium enhancement consistent with scar are visible in the midwall region of the left ventricular septum. A small susceptibility artifact associated with the distal right ventricular coil is visible in the lower right ventricle.

cations is frequently made by considering possible benefits of MRI relative to the attendant risks. Given the potential risks, it is important to conduct a systematic review of the patient's condition and implanted devices prior to proceeding with MRI. In addition to usual MRI facility protocols and questionnaires for patient safety, safety protocols designed for implantable cardiac device recipients, such as that in Fig 22.1, are likely to reduce complications. The reader is encouraged to consult other resources such as the American Heart Association Scientific Statement,[6] and web sites that provide more specific information regarding individual devices (eg, www.mrisafety.com) for specific device testing details.

Disclosure

Dr. Halperin is a scientific advisor for Boston Scientific, Inc. The Johns Hopkins University Advisory Committee on Conflict of Interest manages all commercial arrangements.

References

1. Roguin A, Zviman MM, Meininger GR, et al. Modern pacemaker and implantable cardioverter/defibrillator systems can be magnetic resonance imaging safe: in vitro and in vivo assessment of safety and function at 1.5 T. *Circulation.* 2004;110:475–482.
2. Tandri H, Zviman MM, Wedan SR, et al. Determinants of gradient field-induced current in a pacemaker lead system in a magnetic resonance imaging environment. *Heart Rhythm.* 2008;5: 462–468.
3. Gimbel JR, Zarghami J, Machado C, Wilkoff BL. Safe scanning, but frequent artifacts mimicking bradycardia and tachycardia during magnetic resonance imaging (MRI) in patients with an implantable loop recorder (ILR). *Ann Noninvasive Electrocardiol.* 2005;10:404–408.
4. Achenbach S, Moshage W, Diem B, et al. Effects of magnetic resonance imaging on cardiac pacemakers and electrodes. *Am Heart J.* 1997; 134:467–473.
5. Nazarian S, Roguin A, Zviman MM, et al. Clinical utility and safety of a protocol for noncardiac and cardiac magnetic resonance imaging of patients with permanent pacemakers and implantable-cardioverter defibrillators at 1.5 Tesla. *Circulation.* 2006;114:1277–1284.
6. Levine GN, Gomes AS, Arai AE, et al. Safety of magnetic resonance imaging in patients with cardiovascular devices: an American Heart Association scientific statement from the Committee on Diagnostic and Interventional Cardiac Catheterization, Council on Clinical Cardiology, and the Council on Cardiovascular Radiology and Intervention: endorsed by the American College of Cardiology Foundation, the North American Society for Cardiac Imaging, and the Society for Cardiovascular Magnetic Resonance. *Circulation.* 2007;116:2878–2891.
7. Gimbel JR, Johnson D, Levine PA, Wilkoff BL. Safe performance of magnetic resonance imaging on five patients with permanent cardiac pacemakers. *Pacing Clin Electrophysiol.* 1996;19:913–919.
8. Sommer T, Vahlhaus C, Lauck G, et al. MR imaging and cardiac pacemakers: in-vitro evaluation and in-vivo studies in 51 patients at 0.5 T. *Radiology.* 2000;215:869–879.
9. Vahlhaus C, Sommer T, Lewalter T, et al. Interference with cardiac pacemakers by magnetic resonance imaging: are there irreversible changes at 0.5 Tesla? *Pacing Clin Electrophysiol.* 2001;24:489–495.
10. Martin ET, Coman JA, Shellock FG, Pulling CC, Fair R, Jenkins K. Magnetic resonance imaging and cardiac pacemaker safety at 1.5-Tesla. *J Am Coll Cardiol.* 2004;43:1315–1324.
11. Del Ojo JL, Moya F, Villalba J, et al. Is magnetic resonance imaging safe in cardiac pacemaker recipients? *Pacing Clin Electrophysiol.* 2005;28:274–278.
12. Gimbel JR, Kanal E, Schwartz KM, Wilkoff BL. Outcome of magnetic resonance imaging (MRI) in selected patients with implantable cardioverter defibrillators (ICDs). *Pacing Clin Electrophysiol.* 2005;28:270–273.
13. Sommer T, Naehle CP, Yang A, et al. Strategy for safe performance of extrathoracic magnetic

resonance imaging at 1.5 tesla in the presence of cardiac pacemakers in non-pacemaker-dependent patients: a prospective study with 115 examinations. *Circulation.* 2006;114:1285–1292.

14. Naehle CP, Meyer C, Thomas D, et al. Safety of brain 3-T MR imaging with transmit-receive head coil in patients with cardiac pacemakers: pilot prospective study with 51 examinations. *Radiology.* 2008;249:991–1001.

INDEX

Boxes are indicated by b, *figures by* f, *and tables by* t *following the page number.*

316LMV (Fort Wayne Metals), 245

AAIsafeR (ELA Medical), 95t
ACap Confirm (St. Jude Medical), 172
Accufix leads (Telectronics), 26–27
ACE inhibitors, 384
acoustic cardiography, 428, 429f, 430
Activitrax (Medtronic), 184
ADIR pacing mode, 95t, 100–101, 101f–102f
Advanced Hysteresis (St. Jude Medical), 159–60
AF. *See* atrial fibrillation (AF)
AF Suppression (St. Jude Medical), 151
Affinity device (St. Jude Medical), 185–86
algorithms. *See also under* specific manufacturers' names
  arrhythmia detection, dual chamber ICDs
    Biotronik SMART detection algorithm, 344f, 345–50, 345f
    Boston Scientific/Guidant devices, 341, 342f, 343
    Medtronic devices, 321–27
    Sorin devices, 350–56
    St. Jude Medical devices, 333–35, 333f, 334t
  arrhythmia detection, single chamber ICDs
    Biotronik SMART detection algorithm, 350
    Boston Scientific/Guidant devices, 341, 342f
    Medtronic devices, 317–21
    Sorin devices, 356–58
    St. Jude Medical devices, 327–33
  atrial overdrive, battery drain and, 9
  automatic amplitude, pacing pulses, 11
  automatic sensing, 138–44
  binning systems
    Boston Scientific/Guidant devices, 335–43, 335t
    St. Jude Medical devices, 329–30, 329t, 330t
  dual chamber minimal ventricular pacing, 102, 103f, 104
  intracardiac electrogram timing, 425–28, 425f–427f
  minimizing right ventricular pacing (*See* right ventricular pacing)
  rate drop pacing, 159–60, 160f
  rate-smoothing, in biventricular pacing, 411
  threshold measuring (*See* automatic threshold measuring algorithms)

algorithms (*continued*)
  timing cycle, abnormalities vs. pacemaker malfunction, 65
amiodarone, 165, 383–84
amplifier saturation, 137, 137f
amplitude of pacing pulses, 10–12, 11f
anesthetics, 384, 389–90
angiotensin-converting enzyme (ACE) inhibitors, 384
anode, 20, 20f
Anthem CRT-P (St. Jude Medical), 417t, 418
antiarrhythmic drugs
  cardiac signal amplitudes and, 124
  defibrillation threshold and, 383–84
  myocardial thresholds and, 165
antitachycardia pacing (ATP), 295–306
  atrial, 152–53
  burst, 296f
  clinical trials, 298–99, 298f, 299f
  efficacy of, 297–99, 297f
  programming options, 301–6
    autoswitch schemes, 304, 304t
    differences in ICD models, 302t
    variables, 303–4
  safety of, 296–97
  as shock reduction strategy, 295
  success factors in, 299–306
    burst vs. ramp pacing, 301, 301f, 304f
    fast VT therapy, 304–6, 305f
    increased detection intervals, 300–301
    progression of therapies, 306
AorTech Biomaterials, 246–47
AP-VS interval, 87–88, 88f
ARP (atrial refractory period), 66
arrhythmias, endless loop, 90–92, 91f
asystole, 285
AT (atrial tachycardia), 147, 152–53
AT/AF burden
  atrial antitachycardia pacing and, 151
  definition, 148, 148f
  pacing and reduction of, 151–52
Atlas ICDs (St. Jude Medical), 205f, 275f, 334
ATP. *See* antitachycardia pacing (ATP)
ATP During Charging (Medtronic), 306
ATP One Shot (Biotronik), 306
atrial arrhythmias
  AT/AF burden, 148, 148f
  pacemaker management of, 147–56
    antitachycardia pacing, 152–53
    arrhythmia counting features, 148–49
    automatic mode switching, 149–50, 149f
    initial interrogation, 148–49, 148f
    programmable parameters, 149
    rate drop response, 153, 159
    rate smoothing therapy, 153
    single chamber device limitations, 148
  pacing and prevention of, 151–52
  tachyarrhythmia types, 150–51, 150f
  types of, 147
Atrial Capture Management (Medtronic), 169t, 174–75, 174f
atrial escape interval, 69–70, 69f
atrial fibrillation (AF), 147. *See also* implantable cardioverter defibrillators (ICD)
  atrial rate histogram, 148, 148f
  battery drain and, 10
  defibrillation therapies, 153
  other atrial tachyarrhythmia types vs., 150–51, 150f
  pacing and prevention of, 151
  paroxysmal, atrial rate histogram, 148, 148f
  permanent, emergence of, 111
atrial flutter, 147
  atrial rate histogram, 148, 148f
  other atrial tachyarrhythmia types vs., 150–51, 150f
atrial overdrive pacing
  atrial fibrillation prevention, 151
  automatic mode switching, 150
  battery drain and, 9
atrial pacing, single chamber, 80
atrial refractory period (ARP), 66
atrial tachycardia (AT), 147, 152–53. *See also* antitachycardia pacing (ATP)
atrioventricular association, 333, 333f, 354
atrioventricular block, 79, 110–11
atrioventricular conduction disturbances, 109–11
atrioventricular coupling
  AV interval as surrogate for, 104
  in minimal ventricular pacing
    decoupling as clinical concern, 111
    timing disruptions and, 104–7, 105f–106f
atrioventricular delay
  battery current drain and, 9
  in biventricular pacing, 405–6, 420–21
  dual chamber pacemaker vs. CRT rate adaptation programming, 421

optimization of
clinical trials, 420
introduction to, 419–21
techniques, 419b, 422–30
atrioventricular desynchronization arrhythmia, 90, 91f, 92
atrioventricular interval (AV interval). *See also* atrioventricular delay; paced atrioventricular interval (PAVI)
in atrial pacing, 87, 88f
as AV coupling surrogate, 104
baseline, in atrial sensing, 87
in dual chamber pacing, 67–68
continuously operational, 80–85
intermittently operational, 94–102
histograms, 217–18
none in single-chamber atrial pacing, 80
optimization in biventricular pacing, 419–30
St. Jude Medical algorithm for, 333, 333f
timing disruptions, 104–7, 105f–106f
atrioventricular nodal reentrant tachycardia (AVNRT), 147, 150f, 151
atrioventricular reciprocating tachycardia (AVRT), 147, 150–51
atrioventricular synchrony, 179–80
Attain Ability (Medtronic), 416–17, 416t
Attain StarFix (Medtronic), 44f, 45
Audicor system (Inovise Medical), 428, 429f, 430
Auto Sense (Boston Scientific), 139, 141, 141f
AutoCapture (St. Jude Medical), 11, 166, 170–72, 171f, 176
AutoIntrinsic Conduction Search (AICS), PAVI extensions (St. Jude Medical), 84, 85t, 86f
Automatic Capture Control (Biotronik), 169t, 175–76
Automatic Capture Verification (Boston Scientific), 169t, 173–74
Automatic Mode Conversion (DDD/AMC) (ELA Medical), 85
automatic mode switching, 149–50, 149f
automatic threshold measuring algorithms
introduction, 165–66
ACap Confirm (St. Jude Medical), 172
Atrial Capture Management (Medtronic), 169t, 174–75, 174f
AutoCapture (St. Jude Medical), 11, 166, 170–72, 171f, 176
Automatic Capture Control (Biotronik), 175–76
Automatic Capture Verification (Boston Scientific), 173–74
automatic verification of capture (AVC), 165, 166–68
characteristics, 158, 169t, 170
clinical outcomes, 176
device longevity, 176, 176f
Left Ventricular Capture Management (Medtronic), 175
limitations of, 176–77, 176f
programmability of devices, 169t, 170
Right Ventricular Capture Management (Medtronic), 173–74
Ventricular Autothreshold (ELA Medical), 169, 176
automatic verification of capture
clinical goals, 165
clinical outcomes, 176
in dual chamber devices, 168
evoked response measurement, 166, 167f, 168
independent pace/sense configuration, 166
limitations of, 176–77
method in threshold testing algorithms, 168, 169t
physiologic response, 168
autonomic tone, 217
AV delay. *See* atrioventricular delay
AV Hysteresis, PAVI extensions (Biotronik), 84
AV Search Hysteresis (Boston Scientific), 83, 83t, 86
AVNRT (atrioventricular nodal reentrant tachycardia), 147, 150f, 151
AVRT (atrioventricular reciprocating tachycardia), 147, 150–51
azimilide, 384

backup safety pulse, 170, 170f
batteries. *See also* elective replacement indicator (ERI)
amplitude of pacing pulses, 10–12
chemistry, 6–7, 204
components, 230, 230f
current drain, 8–10, 207
diagnostic information, 204–9
electrolyte, 230
ICD, 207–9, 230–33
ideal design, 6, 230
lithium-based, 6–8, 230–33
longevity, 7–8, 12f

batteries (*continued*)
estimated, 207, 209
ICD, service life, 233
internal resistance, 206, 207f
lead impedance and, 12–13
voltage curve, 204, 206, 206t
nickel cadmium, 6–7
nuclear powered, 7
pacemakers, 6–8, 204–7
pulse width of pacing pulses, 12
QMR technology, 7
safety of, 233
zinc mercuric oxide, 6
Bayes' theorem, 386
beat-to-beat capture assessment, 168, 169t, 170
BEST sensor rate adaptive pacemakers (Sorin), 191, 192, 192f
binning systems
Boston Scientific/Guidant, 335–43, 335t
St. Jude Medical, 329–30, 329t, 330t
Biotronik devices
algorithms
arrhythmia detection, single chamber ICDs, 350
ATP One Shot, 306
Automatic Capture Control, 169t, 175–76
automatic sensitivity adjustment, 139, 140f
AV Hysteresis, PAVI extensions, 84
Burst + PES, 301
forced termination timer, 349
redirection, 349
SMART arrhythmia detection, 344f, 345–50, 345f, 348f
AT/AF histograms, 218
atrial-based timing cycles, 71
biventricular pacing
Corox lead, 44f
Lumax 540 HF-T CRT-D, 267t, 418, 418t
LV pacing leads, specifications, 64t
stored events, 224
Stratos 338 200 LV-T CRT-P, 418, 418t
ventricular sensitivity after pacing, 267t, 418t
blanking periods, 75
closed loop stimulation sensors, 190–91
crosstalk inhibition, 285
electrode pullback specifications, 61t
ICDs
batteries, 233
dual chamber, SMART arrhythmia detection, 344f, 345–50, 348f
Phylax dual chamber ICD, 349
stored events, 224
magnet response, 76–77, 207, 208t
mean heart rate reporting, 219
pacemaker event storage, 222
sensor rate reporting, 219
bipolar pacing systems, 20–21, 20f
integrated vs. dedicated lead design, 266, 269, 269f
lead conductors, 23
oversensing and, 129
Bisping leads (Medtronic), 26, 26f
bit flips (RAM failure), 5
biventricular pacing. *See also* cardiac resynchronization therapy (CRT)
atrioventricular delay, 405–6
AV / VV delay optimization, 419–30, 419b
introduction, 419–20
acoustic cardiographic techniques, 428, 429f, 430
AV delay optimization, 420–21
echocardiography for, 422, 423–24f, 425
intracardiac electrogram timing algorithms for, 425–28, 425f–427f
photoplethysmography techniques, 428
VV delay optimization, 421–22
avoiding phrenic nerve stimulation, 415–16
basics of, 399–413
for congestive heart failure, 399
coronary sinus branches for, 400, 400f
goals of, 399, 400
indications for, 43, 419
leads for, 43–46, 44f, 403–5
left ventricular refractory period, programmable, 411–13, 412f
LV-RV timing issues, 408–9, 409f
pacing modes, 405
pacing sites, 43
principles of, 403–5
programming
Biotronik devices, 418, 418t
Boston Scientific devices, 417, 417t
electrode configurations, 415–16
left ventricular outputs, 416
Medtronic devices, 416–17, 416t
optimal, 412b

St. Jude Medical devices, 417–18, 417t
rate-smoothing algorithms, 411
sensing
double sensing, 404, 404f
right ventricle vs. both chambers, 410–11, 410f
ventricular-sensed response, 411
system components, 400–403
system implantation
complications, 403b
procedures, 400–403, 401f–403f
risks in, 389
timing cycles, 405–13
upper rate behavior and PVARP, 406–8, 407f, 408f
value of, 399–400
Biventricular Trigger (Boston Scientific), 411
blanking periods. *See also* postventricular atrial blanking period (PVAB)
cross-chamber, and VT detection delays, 89–90, 89f, 90f
dual chamber pacing, 73–76, 364–65, 365f
ICD sensing, 269–70, 270t
long PAVI programming conflicts, 89–90, 89f, 90f
pacemaker sensing, 123–24, 123f
programmable ranges by manufacturer, 74t
programming strategies by manufacturer, 75f
Boston Scientific devices
activity sensing and accelerometer-based devices, 186
algorithms
Auto Sense, 139, 141, 141f
Automatic Capture Verification, 169t, 173–74
AV Search Hysteresis (AVSH), 83, 83t, 86
Biventricular Trigger, 411
Capture pulse amplitude, 11
Dynamic Noise, 283
mediated pacemaker tachycardia management, 158
Quick Convert ATP, 305–6
SmartDelay, 425–26, 425f
Sudden Brady Response, 159
atrial-based timing cycles, 71
biventricular pacing
batteries, 208
COGNIS CRT-D, 267t, 281f, 417, 417t
Contak Renewal TR CRT-P, 417, 417t
left ventricular refractory period programming, 412, 412f
LV pacing leads, specifications, 62t
Teligen CRT-D, 267t
ventricular sensitivity after sensing, 267t
blanking periods, 74
diaphragmatic potentials oversensing, 283–84, 284f
ICDs
batteries, 208, 233
paced T-wave oversensing adjustments, 276
smart blanking function, 285
stored events, 224–25
ventricular refractory period, 362–63
VT detection interval, 362
noise response, 162
pacemakers
dual sensor, 194–95, 194t
event storage, 222
magnet response, 76, 162, 207
minute ventilation sensor, 188
Wenckebach counter, 216
patient-activated memory storage, 223
subcutaneous array, 37, 253f
Boston Scientific/Guidant devices
algorithms
arrhythmia detection, ICD, 334t, 335–43, 335t; dual chamber device, 341, 342f, 343; enhancements, 337–41, 337t, 338–40f; initial and duration, 334t, 335–36, 335t; single chamber device, 341, 342f
binning system, 335–43, 335t
paced T-wave oversensing, 278
CPIs
defibrillation leads, specifications, 52t–53t
electrode pullback specifications, 61t
ENDOTAK leads, 37, 42, 257
ICD leads, 33
ICDs
Insignia, 186, 188, 194t
Pulsar Max, 186, 188, 194t
Ventak devices, 337f, 343, 2335–336
loss of hermetic seal, 16
LV pacing leads, specifications, 62t
pacemakers
generator recalls, 15t
Meridian, 16
Pulsar AFR system, 154–55

Boston Scientific/Guidant pacemakers (*continued*)
recalls, 16
Reliance leads, 30f, 242t, 245, 251, 256f, 288
Brady-Tachy Overlap (Sorin), 362, 362f
Brugada syndrome, 271, 390
Burst + PES (Biotronik), 301
burst pacing, 301, 301f

capacitance, 234
capacitors, ICD, 233–35, 234f
CapSure SP (Medtronic), 13, 26, 26f
Capture Management pulse amplitude (Medtronic), 11
Capture pulse amplitude (Boston Scientific), 11
carbon monofluoride (CFx) lithium batteries, 7
cardiac activity, intrinsic. *See also* sensing, pacemaker
exercise and signal amplitudes, 124, 125f
lead performance and sensing of, 36–37
pulse generators and sensing of, 4
size vs. sensing threshold, 122
Cardiac Compass reports (Medtronic), 220, 220f
cardiac drugs, defibrillation threshold and, 384
cardiac events, low rate timer response, 65, 66
cardiac implantable electronic devices (CIED), 19
cardiac output, 179–80
cardiac resynchronization therapy (CRT). *See also* biventricular pacing
bipolar LV lead and pacing options, 45, 45f
chronotropic incompetence, 180
defibrillation threshold in, 382
defibrillator implantation risk, 389
defibrillator pacing, 366, 366f
diaphragmatic pacing complications, 45
heart failure monitoring, 220–21, 220f
indications for, 43, 419
lead dislodgment rates, 45
leads for, 43–46, 44f
LV pacing sites, 43
steroid elution, 45–46
stored events, evaluation, 225
true bipolar leads and clinical response to, 252
ventricular pacing, 9
ventricular sensing, 212–13, 225
cardiac sarcoidosis, 271
cardiography, acoustic, 428, 429f, 430
cardiomyopathy, diffuse, 165
cathode, 20, 20f
central nervous system hypoperfusion, 388
charge time, 234
ChargeSaver (Medtronic), 306
charging circuit, high-output, 235, 235f, 236f
Chorus (Sorin), 188, 195
chronotropic incompetence
CLS pacing for, 191
definition, 196–97
exercise response in heart failure, 179
prevalence, 179, 196, 196f
cladding, 247
closed-loop stimulation (CLS) sensors, 182
advantages and limitations, 191
sensor and algorithm, 189–90, 190f
COGNIS CRT-D (Boston Scientific), 267t, 281f, 417, 417t
cold flow, 246
communication, wireless, 5
Concerto ICD (Medtronic), 267t, 268f
conductors
drawn filled tube, 31, 31f, 245, 245f
fractures and lead failure, 41
ICD leads, materials for, 241, 245, 245f
pacemaker leads, 23–27, 23f
congestive heart failure, 399
connectors
ICD leads, 34–35, 35f, 247
pacemaker leads, 26
Consulta CRT-D (Medtronic), 267t, 416, 416t
Contak Renewal TR CRT-P (Boston Scientific), 417, 417t
coronary sinus branches, in biventricular pacing, 400, 400f
Corox lead (Biotronik), 44f
coupling, atrioventricular (AV-C)
AV interval as surrogate for, 104
minimal ventricular pacing and timing disruptions, 104–7, 105f–106f
CPI devices
BT-10 failures, 42
defibrillation leads, specifications, 52t–53t
electrode pullback specifications, 61t
ENDOTAK-C failures, 42, 257
critical mass, in shock therapy, 310
crosstalk
in atrial antitachycardia pacing, 152
definition, 160

in dual chamber pacing, 67–68, 73–74
inhibition in ICDs, 284–85
noise control mechanisms, 161–62
prevention of, 160–62
ventricular oversensing as, 136f, 137
ventricular safety pacing algorithms, 160–61
CRT. *See* cardiac resynchronization therapy (CRT)
current drain, battery, 8–10
current consumption vs. pacing rate, 9f
device diagnostics and, 207
current induction, 433–34

DDDR pacing mode, 405
DDIR pacing mode, 92, 92t, 93f
defibrillation. *See also* implantable cardioverter defibrillators (ICD)
adverse effects of shocks, 295
atrial, 153
efficiency and lead design, 254
probability of success curve, 369–70, 370f
upper limit of vulnerability hypothesis, 376–77
defibrillation coils
design and construction, 248–49
materials, 247
single vs. dual coil ICD leads, 29–30, 248–49, 252–53
defibrillation implant testing, 369–93
Bayes' theorem, 386
defibrillation threshold
definition and measurement of, 371
discrepancies with upper limit of vulnerability, 378–79
factors influencing, 382–85, 382b
high DFT patient management, 384–85, 385b
low, advantages of, 381
fibrillation-defibrillation testing, 374–75
first-shock strength; advantages of lowering, 381–82
implant criteria, 370–71, 370f, 375
interpretation and regression to the mean, 374–75
minimizing risks of, 391–92
noninvasive postoperative, 392
outcomes of, 381–82
predictive value of, 386–87
at pulse generator replacement, 387–88
recommendations for, 392–93
risks and contraindications, 388b
anesthesia-related, 389–90
implantation of CRT-Ds, 389
thromboembolism, 389
ventricular fibrillation, 388–89
sensing and ventricular fibrillation detection, 390–91
statistical modeling in, 371–74, 373f, 374t
sudden cardiac and, 386
upper limit of vulnerability
as clinical tool, 377–81, 377f, 378f
in defibrillation efficacy assessment, 375–77
discrepancies with defibrillation threshold, 378–79
implant criterion and, 370
ventricular fibrillation induction, 369
vulnerability safety margin testing
how to perform, 379–80, 380b
safety of defibrillation testing vs., 390, 390t
technical pitfalls, 380–81, 381b
defibrillation threshold (DFT)
biphasic shock waveforms and, 311–12, 312f
in cardiac resynchronization therapy, 382
clinical methods for measuring, 371, 372f
current delivery location and, 38, 39f
electrode efficiency and, 39
electrode pullback, 38, 38f, 61t
energy loss in lead and, 38
factors influencing, 382b
drug effects, 383–84
ICD system factors, 383
implant-related factors, 384
patient-specific, 382–83
high DFT patient management, 384–85, 385b
in implant efficacy testing, 371
IS-4 connector and, 35
lead design determinants of, 37–39
low, advantages of, 381
multiple defibrillator electrodes and, 37
subcutaneous electrodes and, 37
upper limit of vulnerability discrepancies from, 378–79
depolarization
progressive, 311, 311f
retrograde atrial, 90
virtual electrode, 311–12, 312f
device diagnostics. *See also* elective replacement indicator (ERI)

device diagnostics (*continued*)
clinical status vs. pacemaker dysfunction, 216
ICD batteries
charge times, 207f, 209
chemistry and life cycle, 207–8, 207f
longevity estimation, 209
lead measurements
in CRT devices, 209, 210–11t
high-voltage impedance, 213–14
lead impedance, 213–14
marker channels, 209, 210t–211t
performance trends, 214, 215f
sensing, 209, 212–13, 212f
threshold, 213
magnet rate, pacemakers, 207, 208t
pacemaker batteries, 205f
current drain and longevity, 207
internal resistance, 206, 207f
voltage, 204, 206, 206t
patient diagnostics
atrial and ventricular paced and sensed events, 214–15
atrial arrhythmia trends and AT/AF histograms, 218–19
atrial refractory events as sensed, 215–16
availability of information, 203
heart failure monitoring, ICD and CRT, 220–21, 220f
heart rate at rest, 219
heart rate histograms, 216–18, 217f
pacemaker counts vs. ECG analysis, 216
patient activity monitoring, ICD, 219
percent pacing counters, 214–16
premature ventricular contraction counters, 215
sensor rate reporting, 219
underlying rhythm and pacemaker dependency, 214
ventricular rate counters during AT/AF events, 219
power supply, 204
programmed parameters, 203–4, 205f
stored event evaluation
electrograms, 221–22
ICDs and CRTs, 224–25
marker channels display, 222
mode switch vs. high rate episodes, 222, 223f
pacemaker events, 222–24
pacemaker memory, 224, 224t
patient-activated memory storage, 223–24
device failure
CPI devices, 42
ICD leads, 40–43, 259–60
pacemakers
FDA reporting requirements, 13–14
insulation failure and atrial oversensing, 131, 133f, 134t
return of devices to manufacturer, 13
sensing failures and electromagnetic interference, 134t, 137–38, 137f
Pellethane 80A insulation, 24, 30, 246
dexamethasone sodium phosphate, 26
DFT. *See* defibrillation threshold (DFT)
diagnostic information. *See* device diagnostics
diaphragmatic myopotentials and oversensing, 282–84, 282f
diaphragmatic pacing, 45
dielectrics, 234
Discovery pacemaker (Guidant), 16
dofetilide, 384
double sensing
in biventricular pacing, 404, 404f
P-wave, in atrial oversensing, 131, 132f
drawn brazed strand wire, 31, 31f, 245, 245f
drawn filled tube conductors, 31, 31f, 245, 245f
drug effects, on defibrillation threshold, 383–84
dual chamber pacing
automatic verification of capture, 168
AV decoupling, clinical concerns, 111
AV interval
continuously operational, 80–85
intermittently operational, 94–102; ELA Medical AAIsafeR (versions 1 and 2), 95t, 100–101, 101f–102f; Medtronic MVP devices, 95–96, 95t, 96f–100f
in timing cycles, 67–68
blanking periods, 67f, 73–76, 364–65, 365f
crosstalk management, 67–68, 73–74
with ICDs, 363–66
low rate timer, 68–72
managed ventricular pacing algorithms, 102, 103f, 104
programmable values by manufacturer, 68t
rate responsiveness, ICD, 363
refractory periods, 67f, 72–73, 73f, 364–65, 365f
RR interval stabilization, 364

safety-pacing period, 68
timing cycles, 66–76
upper rate limit, 72
Durata leads (St. Jude Medical), 241, 247, 248, 250
Dynamic Noise Algorithm (DNA) (Boston Scientific), 283
dyssynchrony, left ventricular, 421

ECG. *See* electrocardiogram (ECG)
echocardiography
for AV / VV delay optimization, 422–25
Iterative technique, 422, 423–24f, 425
Ritter technique, 422
ELA Medical devices. *See also* Sorin devices
AAIsafeR (versions 1 and 2), 95t, 100–101, 101f–102f, 222
Automatic Mode Conversion (DDD/AMC), 85
ICDs
power supply, 208
stored events, 224
mode switching storage, 222
pacemaker generator recalls, 15t
Ventricular Autothreshold, 169, 176
Elast-Eon (AorTech Biomaterials), 246–47
elective replacement indicator (ERI)
as battery voltage indicator, 8
ICD batteries, 208t, 209
pacemaker batteries
diagnostics, 204, 206, 206t
function and, 162
electrocardiogram (ECG)
impedance pulse sensing, 189
intracardiac electrogram vs., 117
pacing event counters and, 216
refractory period vs. atrial undersensing, 124
unipolar vs. bipolar pacing spikes, 21
ventricular safety pacing, 137
electrodes
efficiency and defibrillation threshold, 39
ICD leads, 31–32, 31f, 247
materials for, 23
pullback and defibrillation threshold, 38, 38f, 61t
size and impedance, 21
subcutaneous, 37
electrograms, intracardiac
definition, 117
evaluation of stored events, 221–22
far-field, 118
filtering of, 118–20, 118f, 120f
printout after electrode implantation, 120f, 121
retention when storage memory is full, 222
shape of, 117–18, 118f
timing algorithms for AV / VV optimization, 425–28, 425f–427f
ventricular, in sensor-driven pacing, 182–83
electrolyte, battery, 230
electromagnetic interference (EMI)
atrial oversensing and, 131, 133f, 134t
feed-through filters preventing, 137, 138f
ICD sensing and, 288–89, 288f
MRI and implantable cardiac devices, 433–40
pacemaker sensing failure and, 134t, 137–38, 137f
potential interactions with implanted devices, 433–34
risks of, 138
electromechanical activation time (EMAT), 428, 429f, 430
electromechanical dissociation, 388–89
Encor leads (Telectronics), 26, 27, 236f
end of life (EOL), battery. *See also* batteries, longevity
battery service life, 233
internal resistance and, 206
pacemaker charges by manufacturer, 206t
voltage indicators, 8
endless loop tachycardia, 85, 90, 91f, 93f
endocardial acceleration, peak, 183, 191–93, 192f
endocardial ICD lead systems, 29–43
advantages, 29
coaxial vs. multilumen construction, 32–34, 33f
complications, 40–41
conductors and electrodes, 31–32, 31f, 32f
connectors, 34–35, 35f
implantation mortality and morbidity, 239–40, 255
implantation sites, 34, 34f
insulation, 30–31f
lead failure, 40–43
leads
adapters and extenders, 35
coating, 39–40
defibrillation threshold determinants, 37–39
design, 32–34, 33f
extraction, 40
fixation, 35, 36f

endocardial ICD lead systems (*continued*)
integrated vs. dedicated bipolar, 29, 29f
performance and sensing function, 36–37
single vs. dual coil defibrillation, 29–30
size and surface area, 34, 34f
steroid elution, 35–36
subcutaneous electrodes, 37
ENDOTAK leads (Boston Scientific/Guidant), 37, 42, 257
EnPulse (Medtronic), 184
EnRhythm (Medtronic), 142, 142f, 143t, 184
EnTrust devices (Medtronic), 326
Epic II HF (St. Jude Medical), 417t, 418
epicardial ICD lead systems, 27–29, 28f
lead malfunctions, 28
morbidity and mortality, 28, 239
patch systems, 27–28, 240–41, 241f, 253–54
ERI. *See* elective replacement indicator (ERI)
ethylene tetrafluoroethylene (ETFE), 23
etomidate, 390
evoked potentials, 122, 122f
evoked response, 166, 167f, 168
exercise
battery drain and, 9–10
cardiac signal amplitudes and, 124, 125f
heart failure and, 180

failure of devices. *See* device failure
fentanyl, 390
fibrillation-defibrillation testing, 374–75
Finapres Medical Systems, 428
firmware, pulse generators, 4–5
fixation mechanisms
active fixation, 25, 25f
ICD leads, 35, 36f
pacemaker leads, 25–26
passive fixation, 25–26
fluoropolymers, 30, 246
force, as MRI effect, 433–34
Fort Wayne Metals
316LMV, 245
MP35N, 31, 31f, 241, 245
Frontier II (St. Jude Medical), 410
functional undersensing, 128–29, 128f, 129f

gain control, 252
Gem DR devices (Medtronic), 323, 324, 327
Gem III AT (Medtronic), 153
Gore-Tex, 247
Guidant devices. *See* Boston Scientific/Guidant devices

heart disease, shock therapy for, 313–14
heart failure
exercise response in, 180
ICD and CRT monitoring of, 220–21, 220f
heart rate
histograms, 216–18, 217f
resting, 219
variation in, 180, 220, 221f
heating, as MRI effect, 433–34
hermetic seal, loss of, 16
histograms, heart rate, 216–18, 217f
home monitoring of pacemakers, 5–6
housekeeping current, 8
hyperkalemia, 272
hysteresis algorithms, battery drain and, 10

ICD. *See* implantable cardioverter defibrillators (ICD)
Identity device (St. Jude Medical), 185
impedance. *See under* leads
implant testing. *See* defibrillation implant testing
implantable cardioverter defibrillators (ICD)
adverse effects of shocks, 295
antitachycardia pacing, 295–306
for atrial defibrillation, 153
basic system components, 229–36
batteries, 207–9, 230–33, 230f
capacitors, 233–35, 234f
charging circuit, high-output, 235, 235f, 236f
pulse generator, 230
device sensitivity programming, 122
endocardial systems (*See* endocardial ICD lead systems)
epicardial systems (*See* epicardial ICD lead systems)
heart failure monitoring, 220–21, 221f
history of, 229–30
implant testing (*See* defibrillation implant testing)
leads (*See* leads, ICD)
MRI interactions with, 435, 436f, 437

- pacing with
  - complexities of, 361
  - dual chamber, 363–66
  - single chamber, 361–63
  - ventricular, avoidance of, 365–66
- patient activity monitoring, 219
- PAVI programming conflicts in, 89–90, 89f, 90f
- potential MRI interactions with, 433–34
- programmed parameters, 203–4, 205f
- sensing (*See* sensing, ICD)
- shock therapy, 309–14
- stored events, evaluation, 224–25
- sudden cardiac death prevention, 309, 309f

inappropriate shocks
- conductor fractures and, 42
- CRT-ICDs and, 45
- electromechanical dissociation not reported with, 389
- lead failure and, 256, 257, 258, 259, 287f
- mortality risk and, 295, 314
- oversensing and, 36, 41, 42, 265, 281
- as potential MRI interaction with implanted device, 314
- rapid ventricular rate and, 219
- significance of, 314

independent pace/sensing, 166

inductive telemetry, 5

injury current, 121, 121f

Inos CLS sensor (Biotronik), 190–91

Inovise Medical devices, Audiocor system, 428, 429f, 430

Insignia device (Boston Scientific/Guidant), 186, 188, 194t

insulation
- failure of
  - atrial oversensing and, 131, 133f, 134t
  - lead failure and, 41
  - Pellethane 55D vs. Pellethane 80A, 24–25, 30, 246
- ICD capacitors, 234
- ICD leads, 30–31f, 246–47, 246f
- pacemaker leads, 23, 24–25

InSync III 8042 CRT-P (Medtronic), 410–11, 416–17, 416t

integrated bipolar sensing, 118

integrated circuits, in pulse generators, 4

interrogation report
- AT/AF burden, 148–49, 148f
- initial, and atrial arrhythmias, 148–49, 148f

iridium oxide, 39

IS-4 connectors, 35

Jewel AF (Medtronic), 153

Kappa devices (Medtronic)
- Blanked Flutter Search, 155
- Kappa 400, 187–88, 193–94, 194t
- recalls, 16

leads
- biventricular pacing, 403–5
- conductors, 23–27, 23f
- design, introduction, 19
- device diagnostics, 209–14
- extraction of, 40, 254–55, 254f, 255f
- impedance
  - battery longevity and, 12–13, 13f
  - definition, 213
  - electrode size and, 21
  - high-voltage, 214
  - measurement, 213–14
- performance trends, 214, 215f
- retained, MRI interactions with, 437
- sensing
  - in CRT devices, 209, 210t–211t
  - function of, 36–37
  - marker channels, 209, 210t–211t
  - performance measurements, 209, 212–13, 213f
- threshold testing, 168, 169t, 213

leads, ICD, 27–43. *See also* endocardial ICD lead systems; epicardial ICD lead systems
- for cardiac resynchronization therapy, 43–46
- conductors
  - design and construction, 248, 248f
  - materials, 241, 245, 245f
- connectors, 247, 249, 249f
- defibrillation coils
  - design and construction, 248–49
  - materials, 247
  - single vs. dual designs, 29–30, 252–53
- defibrillation threshold and, 383
- design principles

leads, ICD (*continued*)
basic concepts, 240–41, 240f
engineering design and construction, 247–52
functional concepts, 252–55
materials, 241–47
design specifications
Boston Scientific (Guidant), 52t–53t, 242t
electrode pullback, 61t
LV pacing leads, 62t–64t
Medtronic, 54t–60t, 243t
St. Jude Medical, 244t
displacement and T-wave oversensing, 272
electrodes, 247
evolution of, 239, 240b
fixation mechanisms, 35, 36f
functional issues, 27
bipolar leads, integrated vs. dedicated, 252, 266, 269, 269f
defibrillation efficiency, 254
lead extraction, 254–55, 254f, 255f
oversensing and design of, 252
pullback distance, 252
single vs. dual coil, 252–53
future outlook for, 46
history of, 27
hybrid systems, 253–54
implantation
mortality and morbidity, 239–40, 255
sites for, 34, 34f
technique, 255–56, 255f, 256f
insulation, 246–47, 246f
lead design and construction
cable distribution, symmetric vs. asymmetric, 249–50
coaxial, 249, 249f
compression lumens, 250f, 251
connection methods, 250–51, 251f
integrated bipolar vs. true bipolar leads, 250, 250f
lead diameter and, 251–52, 251f
multilumen, 249–50, 250f
lead failure mechanisms and recalls, 256–59, 256b
ENDOTAK DSP (model 0125) (Guidant/CPI), 257
following pulse generator replacement, 256
manifestations of, 256
Medtronic Sprint Fidelis, 42–43, 212f, 251, 258–59, 258f, 269, 286f
Medtronic Transvene (model 6936), 257–58
metallurgical incompatibility, 251
monitoring and reporting, 259–60
subcutaneous systems and arrays, 253–54, 253f
leads, pacemaker, 20–27
advisories and recalls, 26–27
components, 20, 20f
conductors, 23–27, 23f
connectors, 26
design and engineering, 20–22
electrodes
design, 22
materials, 23
porous, 22, 22f
size and impedance, 21
fixation mechanisms, 25–26, 25f
influences on performance, 20
insulation, 23, 24–25
polarity, 20–21
polarization, 21–22
steroid-eluting, 26
unipolar vs. bipolar, 20–21, 20f
lead-tissue interference, 213
Left Ventricular Capture Management (Medtronic), 175
left ventricular contraction, synchronized, 399, 400
left ventricular dyssynchrony, 421
left ventricular ejection fraction (LVEF), 299
left ventricular–right ventricular offset. *See* VV interval
lidocaine, 384
lithium batteries
lithium carbon monofluoride (Li/CF_x), 7, 233, 233f
lithium iodine, 6–8, 230–31
lithium manganese dioxide (LI/MnO_2), 232–33
lithium silver vanadium oxide (Li/SVO), 7, 231–32, 231f
voltage decay curve, 7–8, 7f, 231, 231f
long QT syndrome, 271, 272, 273
low rate timer
in dual chamber pacing
atrial-based timing, 69f, 70–72
nomenclature and methods by manufacturer, 69t
timing strategies by manufacturer, 71–72
ventricular-based timing, 69–70, 69f
in single chamber pacing, 65, 66

- Lumax 540 HF-T CRT-D (Biotronik), 267t, 418, 418t
- LVEF (left ventricular ejection fraction), 299

- magnet response
  - Biotronik devices, 76–77, 207
  - Boston Scientific devices, 76, 162, 207
  - Medtronic devices, 76, 162
  - pacemaker, 77t, 207, 208t
  - pacemakers vs. ICDs, 162
  - Sorin devices, 77–78
  - St. Jude Medical devices, 76, 162, 207
  - timing cycles and, 76–78
- magnetic resonance imaging (MRI)
  - electromagnetic interactions with implanted devices, 433–40
    - ICDs, 435, 437
    - implantable monitors, 434–35
    - permanent pacemakers, 435–37, 436t
    - potential types of, 433–34
    - retained leads, 437
    - temporary pacemakers, 433–34
  - image artifacts, 439
  - safety protocols for implanted devices, 437, 438f, 439
- managed ventricular pacing (MVP)
  - atrial-based timing, 71
  - Medtronic devices, 71, 95–96, 95t, 96f–100f
  - performance, clinical trials, 102, 103f, 104
- Manufacturer and User Device Experience (MAUDE) database, 259
- marker channels, 209, 210t–211t, 222
- Marquis DR ICD (Medtronic), 323
- matching score, 328
- Medtronic devices
  - activity sensing and accelerometer-based devices, 184–85, 185f
  - algorithms
    - arrhythmia detection: dual chamber ICDs, 321–27; single chamber ICD, 317–21
    - ATP During Charging, 306
    - Atrial Capture Management, 169t, 174–75, 174f
    - Capture Management pulse amplitude, 11
    - EnRhythm pacemaker sensing, 142, 142f, 143t
    - Kappa Blanked Flutter Search, 155
    - Left Ventricular Capture Management, 175
    - pacemaker mediated tachycardia management, 157–58
    - PR Logic, 321–27, 322f, 325f, 326f
    - Ramp+, 303, 304f
    - Rate Drop Response, 153, 159
    - Right Ventricular Capture Management, 173–74
    - Search AV / Search AV+ , PAVI extensions, 81–83, 82f, 82t, 86–87, 86f, 87f
    - Sensing Assurance, 141–42, 141f
    - Ventricular Sense Response, 411
  - atrial-based timing cycles, 71
  - AV interval histograms, 217–18
  - Bisping leads, 26, 26f
  - biventricular devices
    - Consulta CRT-D, 267t, 416, 416t
    - defibrillator pacing, 366
    - InSync III 8042 CRT-P, 410–11, 416–17, 416t
    - stored events, 225
    - ventricular sensitivity after pacing, 267t
  - CapSure SP, 13, 26, 26f
  - electrode pullback specifications, 61t
  - fast VT therapy, 305
  - heart failure monitoring, 220, 220f
  - ICD leads
    - Sprint Fidelis, failure of, 42–43, 212f, 251, 258–59, 258f, 269, 286f
    - Sprint Quattro Secure, 30f, 240f, 243t
    - Sprint Quattro Secure Model 6947, 34f
    - Tensi-Lock technology, 255
  - ICDs
    - batteries, 233
    - charge time-optimized battery, 208
    - Concerto, 257t, 268f
    - Gem DR devices, 323, 324, 327
    - Gem III AT, 153
    - Jewel AF, 153
    - lead design specifications, 54t–60t, 243t
    - lead failures, 41–42
    - Marquis DR, 323
    - refractory and blanking periods, 364–65, 365f
    - sensing vectors, 269, 269f
    - single chamber, arrhythmia detection algorithms, 317–21
    - stored events, 225
    - ventricular refractory period, 362
    - VT detection interval, 361–62
  - interconnect wire problems, 16

Medtronic devices (*continued*)
left ventricular pacing electrode configurations, 416–17, 416t
left ventricular pacing leads, specifications, 63t
magnet response, 76, 162
managed ventricular pacing (MVP), 71, 95–96, 95t, 96f–100f
Model 4012 lead insulation failure, 24
night heart rate reporting, 219
noise reversion, 161–62
paced T-wave oversensing prevention, 277, 277f, 278–79
pacemakers
EnPulse, 184
EnRhythm, 142f, 143t, 184
EnTrust devices, 326
generator recalls, 15t
Kappa 400 dual sensor, 193–94, 194t
Kappa 400 minute ventilation sensor, 187–88
recalls, 16
sensor-driven, 184–85
patient-activated memory storage, 223–24
patient-device interaction problems, 16
sensor rate reporting, 219
subcutaneous array electrodes, 37
Transvene leads, 33, 41, 249f, 257–58
ventricular rate counters during AT/AF events, 219
ventricular safety pacing, 161
ventricular sensitivity settings, 273
MedWatch (FDA), 259
Meridian pacemaker (Boston Scientific/Guidant), 16
metal-induced oxidation, 24
midazolam, 390
MiniLiving devices (Sorin), 186, 192
modesum, 323
monitors, implantable, 434–35
mortality and morbidity
defibrillation implant testing predicting, 386
epicardial ICD lead systems, 28, 239
ICD leads implantation and, 239–40, 255
inappropriate shocks and, 295, 314
sudden cardiac death, 229
MP35N (Fort Wayne Metals), 241, 245
MVP mode. *See* managed ventricular pacing (MVP)
myocardial fibrosis, 25
myocardial infarction, 165
myocardial ischemia, 313, 388
myocardial thresholds, 165–66
myopotential oversensing
diaphragmatic, 282–84, 282f
unipolar atrial leads, 131, 132f
ventricular, 134, 135f

neurocardiogenic syncope, 158–60, 190
nickel cadmium batteries, 6–7
noise response algorithms, 161–62
noise reversion, 137, 138f, 161–62
nuclear powered pacemakers, 7

Ohm's law, 21
Omnisense accelerometer (St. Jude Medical), 185
Optim Insulation (St. Jude Medical), 247
OptiVol fluid index (Medtronic), 220
Opus devices (Sorin), 186, 188
oversensing
atrial
causes of, 129–30, 130t, 131f, 280–81, 281f
electromagnetic interference and, 131, 133f, 134t
inappropriate pacing inhibition in, 131
insulation failure and, 131, 133f, 134t
unipolar lead myopotentials and, 131, 132f
ventricular far-field oversensing, testing and reprogramming, 133–34, 133f, 135t
causes of, 129, 130t
diaphragmatic myopotentials, 282–84, 282f
ICD (*See under* sensing, ICD)
integrated bipolar. vs. dedicated bipolar leads, 252
in pacemakers, 129–37
T waves
after paced beats, 273, 274f–275f, 276–79
after sensed beats, 271–73, 271f, 272f
operative intervention, 279
pacemakers vs. ICDs, 270–71
site specificity of, 279, 279f
ventricular
causes of, 134, 134t, 136f
crosstalk, 136f, 137
myopotential oversensing, 134, 135f
oxidation, metal-induced, 24

P waves
double sensing in atrial oversensing, 131, 132f
oversensing, ICD, 279–81, 280f
paced atrioventricular interval (PAVI)
algorithm performance, 85–87
automatic extensions, operational characteristics, 81–85
Biotronik AV Hysteresis, 84
Boston Scientific AV Search Hysteresis (AVSH), 83, 83t, 86
ELA Automatic Mode Conversion (DDD/AMC), 85
long fixed and dynamic
DDIR mode reducing timing cycle conflicts, 92, 92t, 93f
delayed VT detection and, 89–90, 89f. 90f
dynamic, performance characteristics, 81
endless loop arrhythmias and, 90–92, 91f
limitations for minimizing ventricular pacing, 87–89, 88f, 89f
programming conflicts in ICD platforms, 89–90, 89f
risks of, 89–101
static, effectiveness of, 81
timing cycle conflicts, 89t
ventricular pararrhythmia from, 92, 94, 94f
manipulation in ventricular pacing, 80–85
Medtronic Search AV and Search AV+, 81–83, 82f, 82t, 86–87, 86f, 87f
St. Jude Medical devices
AutoIntrinsic Conduction Search (AICS), 84, 85t, 86d
Ventricular Intrinsic Preference (VIP), 84, 85t
Vitatron Refined Ventricular Pacing (RVP), 84–85
pacemaker alternans, 285
pacemaker mediated tachycardia, 157–58
pacemaker syndrome, 90
pacemakers
components, 3
dependency on, 214
device recalls
hierarchies for, 14
loss of hermetic seal, 15t
pacemaker generators, 15t
pacemaker leads, 26–27
failure of, 13–16
hardware, 4–6
MRI interactions with
permanent pacemakers, 435, 436f
temporary pacemakers, 435
types of, 433–34
nuclear powered, 7
potential advances in, 6
programmed parameters, 203–4, 205f
sensing (*See* sensing, pacemaker)
pacing capture thresholds, 285
pacing modes
ADIR, 95t, 100–101, 101f–102f
automatic mode switching, 149–50, 149f
biventricular pacing, 405
DDDR, 405
DDIR, 92, 92t, 93f
rate adaptive, 198–99, 198f
single chamber pacing, 65–66
pacing pulses
amplitude of, 10–12
automatic amplitude algorithms, 11
current drain and, 8–9
current drain vs. pulse width, 12f
energy vs. lead impedance, 12–13, 13f
pulse width, 12
pacing site, and ATP success, 299–300
pacing thresholds. *See also* automatic threshold measuring algorithms
changes in, 165–66
device diagnostics, 213
testing triggers in algorithms, 169t, 170
PARAD and PARAD+ (Sorin), 277, 350, 351–56, 352f, 353f, 357, 358
passive fixation leads
ICDs, 35, 36f
myocardial fibrosis and, 25
pacemakers, 25–26
patch systems, ICD leads, 27–28, 240–41, 241f, 253–54
patient diagnostics. *See under* device diagnostics
PAVI. *See* paced atrioventricular interval (PAVI)
peak endocardial acceleration, 183, 191–93, 192f
Pellethane 55D insulation , 24–25, 30, 246
Pellethane 80A insulation, 24, 30, 246
Photon DR ICD (St. Jude Medical), 334–35
photoplethysmography, 428
phrenic nerve stimulation, 415–16
Phylax dual chamber ICD (Biotronik), 349
plutonium-238 (isotope), 7

polarization
  artifacts, in pacemaker sensing, 122, 122f
  myocardial, vs. evoked response, 166, 167f
  pacemaker leads and, 21–22
polytetrafluoroethylene polymers, 40, 247
polyurethanes, for lead insulation, 24–25, 30, 246
Post-Paced Delay Decay (St. Jude Medical), 277
posture, detection by CLS sensors, 191
postventricular atrial blanking period (PVAB)
  in atrial arrhythmia management, 154, 154f
  atrial tachycardia sensing and, 74, 75f
  function, 73, 154
postventricular atrial refractory period (PVARP)
  in atrial arrhythmia management, 154, 154f
  function, 72–73, 73f
  minimal ventricular pacing strategies and, 90–92, 91f
  mode switching algorithm and, 154–55
  upper rate behavior and, in biventricular pacing, 406–8, 407f, 408f
potassium channel blockers, 384
power supply, pacemaker vs. ICD, 204
PR interval
  AV association and, 333
  AV interval mimicking, 67
  in AV optimization, 420, 421, 422
  baseline, 111
  minimal ventricular pacing strategies and, 104, 105, 105f
  oversensing and, 280
  in PARAD algorithms, 352
  in PR Logic algorithms, 322, 323, 327
  regularity of, 346
  in SMART algorithm, 348
  in supraventricular tachycardia detection algorithms, 326–27, 326f
  trends in, 346
PR Logic (Medtronic), 321–27, 322f, 325f, 326f
premature ventricular contraction (PVC)
  AV interval and, 68
  counters for, 215
  pacemaker response to, 70–71, 70f
probability of success curve, defibrillation, 369–70, 370f
Promote RF CRT-D (St. Jude Medical), 267t, 417–18, 417t
propofol, 390
Protos CLS sensor (Biotronik), 190–91
pullback, electrode, 38, 38f, 61t
pullback distance, 252
Pulsar devices (Boston Scientific/Guidant)
  AFR system, 155
  Pulsar Max, 186, 188, 194t
pulse generators, 3–16
  battery, 6–8
  cardiac sensing of, 4
  firmware, 4–5
  functions, 3
  hardware, 4–6
  hybrid circuit, 3, 4
  for ICDs, 230
  implant testing at replacement, 387–88
  inductive telemetry, 5
  integrated circuits, 4
  lead impedance and longevity, 12–13, 13f
  structure, 3f
  telemetry control, 5
  transtelephonic monitoring, 5–6
  wireless communication, 5
PVAB. *See* postventricular atrial blanking period (PVAB)
PVARP. *See* postventricular atrial refractory period (PVARP)
PVC. *See* premature ventricular contraction (PVC)

QMR battery, 7
Quick Convert ATP (Boston Scientific), 305–6
QuickOpt (St. Jude Medical), 426–27f, 426–28
quiescent current, 8

R waves, double-counting of, 281–82
radiofrequency (RF) telemetry, 5
RAM (random access memory), 4–5
Ramp+ algorithm (Medtronic), 303, 304f
ramp pacing, 301, 301f
rate adaptive pacing modes, 198–99, 198f
rate drop pacing
  algorithms, 159–60, 160f
  in atrial arrhythmia management, 153
  clinical trials, 158–59
  for neurocardiogenic syncope, 158–60
Rate Drop Response (Medtronic), 153, 159
rate responsiveness, 363–64
rate smoothing therapy, 153

reduced coupling capacitor (RCC), 166
Refined Ventricular Pacing (RVP), PAVI extensions (Vitatron), 84–85
refractory periods
  in dual chamber pacing, 67f, 72–73, 73f, 364–65, 365f
  extension theory for ICD shock therapy, 311, 311f
  ICD sensing and, 269–70, 270t
  left ventricular, 411–13, 412f
  pacemaker sensing and, 123f, 124, 124f
  postventricular atrial, 72–73, 73f, 90–92, 91f
  programmable ranges by manufacturer, 74t
  programming strategies by manufacturer, 75f
  in single chamber pacing, 66, 362–63
  total atrial, 72–73, 73f
regression to mean, 374–75
Reliance leads (Boston Scientific/Guidant), 30f, 242t, 245, 251, 256f, 288
rescue shocks, 374
rest rate, pacemaker, 10
resting heart rate, 219
resuscitation, prolonged, 388–89
retrograde atrial depolarization, 90
returned product analysis, 43
RF telemetry, 5
Rhapsody devices (Sorin), 188, 195
Riata leads (St. Jude Medical), 33f, 34f, 36f, 241, 250f
Right Ventricular Capture Management (Medtronic), 173–74
right ventricular pacing, 79–111
  adverse effects, chronic, 79–80
  avoidance in ICD recipients, 365–66
  with ICDs, 361–63
  minimal pacing strategies
    algorithm performance, 85–87
    AV interval continuously operational, 80–85
    AV interval intermittently operational, 94–102
    constraints on long-term use, 109
    dual chamber algorithms, performance of, 102, 103f, 104
    limitations and risks: AV timing disruptions, 104–5, 105f–106f, 107; long PAVIs, 87–89; ventricular proarrhythmia, 107–9, 107f, 108f
    no AV interval, 80
    PAVI manipulation, 80–85
    single-chamber atrial pacing, 80
    survivability of, 111
  permanent atrial fibrillation, emergence of, 111
  sinus node dysfunction, AV conduction stability in, 109–11
Ritter technique (echocardiography), 422
ROM (read-only memory), 4–5
RR intervals
  analysis in dual chamber ICDs, 321
  analysis in single chamber ICDs, 317–19, 318f
  stabilization of, 318, 364
Runaway Protection Timer (St. Jude Medical), 366
R-wave voltage, in T-wave oversensing, 271–72

safety pacing, ventricular, 68, 129, 129f, 137
Search AV / Search AV+ (Medtronic), 81–83, 82f, 82t, 86–87, 86f, 87f
SenseAbility (St. Jude Medical), 142–43, 144f
sensing, biventricular pacing
  double sensing, 404, 404f
  rate-smoothing algorithms, 411
  right ventricle vs. both chambers, 410–11, 410f
  ventricular-sensed response, 411
sensing, ICD, 265–89
  introduction to, 265–70
  bipolar lead design, integrated vs. dedicated, 266, 269, 269f
  blanking periods, 269–70, 270t
  crosstalk inhibition, 284–85
  defined, 265
  diaphragmatic myopotentials, oversensing of, 282–84, 282f
  electromagnetic interference, 288–89, 288f
  hardware problems
    contact between leads, 288
    defective connections, 285–86, 287f
    lead conductor fracture, 285, 286f
    seal plug damage, 286–88, 287f
  oversensing
    autoadjusting algorithms, 265, 266f
    inappropriate shock episodes, incidence, 265
    P-wave, 279–81, 280f
  R waves, double-counting of, 281–82
  refractory periods in, 269–70, 270t
  T-wave oversensing, 270–81
    after paced beats, 273, 274f, 275f, 276–79
    after sensed beats, 271–73, 271f

sensing, ICD/T-wave oversensing (*continued*)
causes of, 271–72
operative intervention for, 279
programmable paced blanking and, 277–78
R-wave voltage and, 271–72
sensitivity settings programming to avoid, 272–73, 272f
site specificity of, 279, 279f
ventricular channel sensitivity, 266, 267t, 268f
ventricular fibrillation detection, 265–66, 266f
sensing, pacemaker, 117–44
antiarrhythmic drugs and cardiac signal amplitude, 124
automatic sensing algorithms, 138–44
Biotronik devices, 139, 140f
Boston Scientific devices, 139, 141, 141f
Medtronic devices, 141–42, 141f, 142f, 143t
St. Jude Medical SenseAbility algorithm, 142–43, 144f
blanking periods, 123–24, 123f
device sensitivity programming, 122–23
electromagnetic interference and, 134t, 137–38, 137f
exercise and, 124, 125f
feed-through EMI filters, 137, 138f
at implantation, 120–21, 121f
injury current, 121, 121f
lead performance in, 36–37
lead polarity and bipolar spacing, 118–24, 119f
noise reversion, 137, 138f
normal sensing, 117–18
oversensing, 129–37
polarization artifacts and evoked potentials, 122, 122f
pulse generators and, 4
refractory periods, 123f, 124, 124f
sensing circuit, 118, 118f, 120, 120f
sensing over time, 124
sensing threshold vs. cardiac signal size, 122
undersensing, 124–27
Sensing Assurance (Medtronic), 141–42, 141f
sensor-driven pacing
activity sensing and accelerometer-based pacemakers, 181, 182t, 184–87, 184f
Boston Scientific devices, 186
clinical results, 186–87
limitations of, 187
Medtronic devices, 184–85, 185f
Sorin devices, 186
St. Jude Medical devices, 185–86
classification of sensors, 180–83, 182t
clinical benefits, 196–99
patient factors affecting, 196–98, 196b, 197f
rate adaptive pacing modes and, 198–99, 198f
ventricular pacing site and, 199, 199f
dual sensor devices, 193–96, 194t
Boston Scientific devices, 194–95, 194t
indications for, 195, 196b
Medtronic Kappa 400 device, 193–94
sensor blending vs. sensor cross-checking, 193
Sorin devices, 194t, 195, 195f
impedance in, 181–82
peak endocardial acceleration sensing, 191–93, 192f
physiological basis of, 179–80
sensor characteristics, ideal, 180
sensor performance, relative, 183, 183t
ventricular impedance sensing devices, unipolar, 182t
advantages and limitations of, 191
Biotronik CLS devices, 190–91
closed-loop stimulation (CLS) sensors, 189–91
minute ventilation sensor devices, 187–88
shock polarity, 383
shock therapy, ICD. *See also* inappropriate shocks
biphasic shock waveforms and defibrillation threshold, 311–12, 312f
critical mass in, 310
heart disease prognosis and use of, 313–14
progressive depolarization in, 311, 311f
upper limits of vulnerability, 310–11, 310f, 311f
virtual electrode depolarization, 311–12, 312f
shock vector, 383
shock waveform, 383
short QT syndrome, 272
Sigma devices (Medtronic), recalls, 16
silicone insulation, 24, 246, 246f
silver vanadium oxide (SVO) batteries, 7
single chamber pacing
atrial, for minimizing ventricular pacing, 80
cardiac event response, 65
with ICDs, 361–63
pacing mode, 65–66
programmable values by manufacturer, 67t

timing cycles, 65–66, 66f
ventricular refractory period, 66, 362–63
ventricular tachycardia detection interval, 361–62
sinus node dysfunction (SND)
adverse effects of right ventricular pacing, 79
AV conduction stability with minimal pacing algorithms, 109–11
chronotropic incompetence, prevalence, 179
pacemaker optimization goals, 80
pacing and prevention of, 151
permanent atrial fibrillation in, 111
single chamber atrial pacing, 80
SMART arrhythmia detection (Biotronik), 344f, 345–50, 345f, 348f
SmartDelay (Boston Scientific), 425–26, 425f
sodium channel blockers, 384
sonR sensor (Sorin), 192
Sorin devices. *See also* ELA Medical devices
activity sensing and accelerometer-based devices, 186
arrhythmia detection algorithms, dual chamber ICDs, 350–58
AV association, 354
cycle-length sorting, 350–51
long cycle occurrence, 352–54
majority rhythm identification and persistence counters, 351
PARAD and PARAD+ algorithms, 277, 350, 351–56, 352f, 353f, 357, 358
PR interval distribution, 352, 353f
RR interval distribution, 352
ventricular acceleration, 354, 354f–355f, 356
arrhythmia detection algorithms, single chamber ICDs, 353f, 356–58
atrial-based timing cycles, 71–72
BEST sensor rate adaptive pacemakers, 191, 192, 192f
blanking periods, 76
Brady-Tachy Overlap, 362, 362f
Chorus, 188, 195
dual sensor pacemakers, 194t, 195, 195f
fast VT therapy, 305
magnet response, 77–78
MiniLiving, 186, 192
minute ventilation sensor pacemakers, 188
Opus devices, 186, 188
Rhapsody, 188, 195
sensor-driven pacing, 188–89, 195
sonR sensor, 192
Swing sensor, 186
Symphony, 188, 195
Talent, 188, 195
VT detection interval, ICD, 362
sotalol, 384
Sprint Fidelis ICD lead (Medtronic), 42–43, 251, 258–59, 258f, 269, 286f
Sprint Quattro Secure ICD lead (Medtronic), 30f, 212f, 240f, 243t
Sprint Secure ICD lead, Model 6947 (Medtronic), 34f
St. Jude Medical devices. *See also* Telectronics devices
activity sensing and accelerometer-based devices, 185–86
algorithms
ACap Confirm, 172
Advanced Hysteresis, 159–60
AF Suppression, 151
arrhythmia detection, dual chamber ICDs, 333–35, 333f, 334t
arrhythmia detection, single chamber ICDs, 327–33
AutoCapture 11, 166, 170–72, 171f, 176
AutoIntrinsic Conduction Search (AICS), PAVI extensions, 84, 85t, 86f
AV association, 333, 333f
AV interval histograms, 217, 218f
binning system, 329–30, 329t, 330t
pacemaker mediated tachycardia management, 158
Post-Paced Delay Decay, 277
QuickOpt, 426–27f, 426–28
redetection, 332–33
Runaway Protection Timer, 366
SenseAbility, 142–43, 144f
SVT and VT therapy discrimination timeout, 330–32, 331f
SVT/VT discriminators, 327–29
Ventricular Intrinsic Preference (VIP), PAVI extensions, 84, 85t
Ventricular Post-Paced Start, 277
VT Therapy Timeout, 304, 330–33, 331f, 332f
arrhythmia "unhiding" function, 278, 278f
atrial arrhythmia histograms, 218–19

St. Jude Medical devices (*continued*)
biventricular pacing
Anthem CRT-P, 417t, 418
defibrillator pacing, 366, 366f
Epic II HF, 417t, 418
Frontier II device, 410
LV pacing leads, specifications, 64t
Promote RF CRT-D, 267t, 417–18, 417t
ventricular sensitivity after pacing, 267t, 366f
blanking periods, 74–75
crosstalk detection window, 160–61
electrode pullback specifications, 61t
ICD leads
design specifications, 244t
Durata, 241, 247, 248, 250
Optim Insulation, 247
Riata, 33f, 34f, 36f, 241, 250f
Ventritex, 33, 61t, 249
ICDs
Atlas devices, 205f, 275f, 334
batteries, 233
Photon DR, 334–35
stored events, 225
ventricular refractory period, 363, 363f
Vitality devices, 185–86, 341, 343
VT detection interval, 362
magnet response, 76, 162, 207
noise response, 161
paced T-wave oversensing, troubleshooting, 276f
pacemakers
event storage, 222
generator recalls, 15t
patient-activated memory storage, 223
sensor rate reporting, 219
Tendril lead, 25f
ventricular rate counters during AT/AF events, 219
Zephyr XL, pacing energy vs. longevity, 12
statistical modeling in defibrillation testing, 371–74, 373f, 374t
steroid elution
cardiac resynchronization therapy, 45–46
endocardial ICD leads, 35–36
pacemaker leads, 26
Stratos 338 200 LV-T CRT-P (Biotronik), 418, 418t
stress, and battery drain, 9–10
subcutaneous leads and arrays
Boston Scientific, 37
functional issues, ICD, 253–54, 253f
Medtronic, 37
Sudden Brady Response (Boston Scientific), 159
sudden cardiac death
defibrillation implant testing predicting, 386
ICDs and risk of, 309, 309f
morbidity and mortality, 229
superior vena cava (SVC) coils, 28
supraventricular tachycardia, 147, 327–29
Swing sensor (Sorin), 186
Symphony ICD (Sorin), 188, 195
syncope
atrioventricular block and, 80
low first-shock strength and, 382
neurocardiogenic, 158–60, 190
slow ventricular tachycardia and, 357
vasovagal, 153, 191, 193

Tachyarrhythmia Chronic System Study (TCSS), 43
tachycardias
atrial, 147, 152–53 (*See also* antitachycardia pacing (ATP))
detection algorithms, 317–27, 318t
endless loop, 85, 90, 91f, 93f
pacemaker mediated, 157–58
supraventricular, 147, 327–29
SVT/VT discriminators, 327–29
ventricular (*See* ventricular tachycardia (VT))
Talent ICD (Sorin), 188, 195
TARP (total atrial refractory period), 72–73, 73f
Telectronics devices. *See also* St. Jude Medical devices
Accufix lead recalls, 26–27
electrode pullback specifications, 61t
Encor leads, 26, 27, 236f
telemetry, 5, 6
Teligen CRT-D (Boston Scientific), 267t
Tendril lead (St. Jude Medical), 25f
Tensi-Lock (Medtronic), 255
test shocks, 374
thoracotomy, 27–28, 239
threshold measuring algorithms. *See* automatic threshold measuring algorithms
thromboembolism, 389
timing cycles. *See also* dual chamber pacing
algorithm abnormalities vs. pacemaker malfunction, 65

atrial-based, 71–72
biventricular pacing, 405–13
dual chamber pacing, 66–76
magnet response, 76–78
single chamber pacing, 65–66, 66f, 67t
torque, as MRI effect, 433–34
total atrial refractory period (TARP), 72–73, 73f
transtelephonic monitoring (TTM), 5–6
Transvene lead (Medtronic), 33, 41, 249f, 257–58
Treppe effect, 189
T waves
high amplitude, 272
oversensing
after paced beats, 273, 274f–275f, 276–79
after sensed beats, 271–73, 271f, 272f
operative intervention, 279
pacemakers vs. ICDs, 270–71
Twiddler's syndrome, 256

undersensing
amplifier saturation and, 137, 137f
atrial, 124–25, 126f
defined, 124
functional, 128–29, 128f, 129f
ventricular, 125, 126f, 127f
unipolar pacing systems, 20–21, 20f
lead conductors, 23
oversensing and, 129
upper limit of vulnerability
as clinical tool
conditions for efficacy, 377–79, 377f, 378f
vulnerability safety margin testing, 379–81, 380b, 381b
critical points, 375–76, 376f, 377
in defibrillation efficacy assessment, 375–77
defibrillation hypothesis, 376–77
discrepancies from defibrillation threshold, 378–79
as ICD implant criterion, 370
in ICD shock therapy, 310–11, 310f, 311f
vulnerable zone, 375–76, 376f, 377–78, 377f, 378f
upper rate limit
in dual chamber pacing, 72, 73f
PVARP and, in biventricular pacing, 406–8, 407f, 408f
in sensor-driven pacing, 197–98

Valsalva maneuver, 282f, 283
vasovagal syncope, 153, 191, 193
VDD pacing mode, 405
Ventak ICDs (Boston Scientific/Guidant), 337f, 343, 2335–336
ventricular acceleration, 354, 354f–355f, 356
Ventricular Autothreshold (ELA Medical), 169, 176
ventricular contraction
left, synchronized, 399, 400
premature (*See* premature ventricular contraction (PVC))
ventricular fibrillation (VF)
causes of, 309
defibrillation threshold testing risk and, 388–89
ICD shock therapy for, 309–14, 386–86
ICD vs. pacemaker sensing, 266, 267
refractory, 389
ventricular inhibited pacing (VVI), 8, 66
Ventricular Intrinsic Preference (VIP), PAVI extensions (St. Jude Medical), 84, 85t
ventricular pacing, right. *See* right ventricular pacing
Ventricular Post-Paced Start (St. Jude Medical), 277
ventricular proarrhythmia
from long PAVIs, 92, 94, 94f
minimal ventricular pacing and risk of, 107–9, 107f, 108f
ventricular refractory period (VRP), 66, 362–63
Ventricular Sense Response (Medtronic), 411
ventricular sensitivity, 267t
ventricular tachycardia (VT)
competitive pacing prevention during, 80
cycle length and ATP success, 299
detection interval in single chamber pacing, 361–62
long PAVIs and detection failure, 89–90, 89f. 90f
Ventritex leads (St. Jude Medical), 33, 61t, 249
verapamil, 384
verification, initial, 168, 169t
VF. *See* ventricular fibrillation (VF)
virtual electrode depolarization, 311–12, 312f
Virtuoso (Medtronic), 267, 270
Vitality ICDs (St. Jude Medical), 185–86, 341, 343
Vitatron devices
pacemaker generator recalls, 15t
Refined Ventricular Pacing (RVP), PAVI extensions, 84–85
voltage doubler, 11

VRP (ventricular refractory period), 66, 362–63
VT. *See* ventricular tachycardia (VT)
VT Therapy Timeout (St. Jude Medical), 304, 330–33, 331f, 332f
vulnerability, upper limit. *See* upper limit of vulnerability
vulnerable zone, 375–76, 376f
VV interval
  in biventricular pacing, 419–30
  definition, 419
  in dual chamber pacing, 323
  optimization of delay
    clinical trials, 421–22
    introduction to, 419–20
    techniques, 419b, 422–30
  rhythm identification and, 350, 352
VVIR pacing mode, 405

waveform, shock, 383
wavelet dynamic discrimination criterion, 318
wire, drawn brazed strand, 31, 31f, 245, 245f

Zephyr XL (St. Jude Medical), 12
zinc mercuric oxide batteries, 6